Y0-BZA-420

Lysosomal
Disorders of the Brain

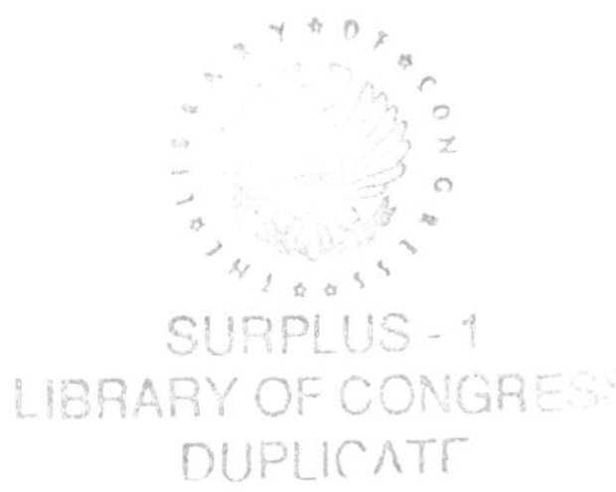

Lysosomal Disorders of the Brain

Recent Advances in Molecular and Cellular Pathogenesis and Treatment

Frances M. Platt
Department of Biochemistry, University of Oxford, Oxford, UK

and

Steven U. Walkley
Department of Neuroscience, Albert Einstein College of Medicine, New York, USA

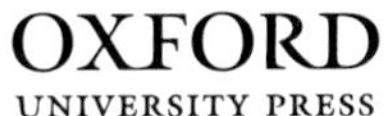

OXFORD
UNIVERSITY PRESS

Great Clarendon Street, Oxford OX2 6DP

Oxford University Press is a department of the University of Oxford.
It furthers the University's objective of excellence in research, scholarship,
and education by publishing worldwide in

Oxford New York
Auckland Bangkok Buenos Aires Cape Town Chennai
Dar es Salaam Delhi Hong Kong Istanbul Karachi Kolkata
Kuala Lumpur Madrid Melbourne Mexico City Mumbai Nairobi
São Paulo Shanghai Taipei Tokyo Toronto

Oxford is a registered trade mark of Oxford University Press
in the UK and in certain other countries

Published in the United States
by Oxford University Press Inc., New York

First published 2004

British Library Cataloguing in Publication Data

Data available

ISBN 0-19-850878-6

10 9 8 7 6 5 4 3 2 1

Typeset by Integra Software Services Pvt Ltd., Pondicherry, India
Printed in Great Britain
on acid-free paper by Biddles, King's Lynn, UK

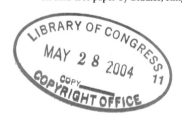

Preface

Nearly 50 years have passed since Christian de Duve discovered the presence, in cells, of enzymes with acidic pH optima and predicted the existence of a specialized organelle, the lysosome, to contain them. Shortly thereafter, H.G. Hers (see Foreword) made the seminal discovery that genetic deficiencies in such enzymes could underlie a group of enigmatic disorders known as 'storage diseases'. These diseases, numbering less than two dozen at the time, had emerged as clinical entities beginning in the late nineteenth and early twentieth centuries. Careful investigations by clinicians and scientists like Bernard Sachs, Frederick Batten, Max Bielschowsky, Károly Schaffer, Gordon Holmes, and others over the years led to the creation of a detailed classification system based on eponyms and the identity of storage materials within cells. While the inherited nature of these diseases became apparent early on, an explanation as to why materials were accumulating in cells had to await the modern advances in biochemistry and cell biology that culminated in Hers' discovery. Perhaps no group of inherited diseases better reflects the progress of twentieth-century medicine than the storage disorders: from enigmatic clinical conditions to inborn errors of metabolism in the truest Garrodian sense, to disorders exquisitely defined by gene, protein, and clinical condition. Now, with the optimism of twenty-first-century medicine, the biomedical research community even sees hope for correction of these otherwise primarily fatal neurological conditions through a variety of novel therapies. And, while the ultimate strategy here may be the direct replacement of defective genes in all affected cells, some of what we have learned about these conditions teaches us that this may not always be necessary, particularly in those diseases where gene products are shared between cells. Furthermore, with greater knowledge of affected metabolic pathways, it may be possible to circumvent storage or the effects of storage through other means, even pharmacological ones. While the challenge of therapy remains enormous, it is quite clear that advances here are closely linked to a need for significantly greater understanding as to how the original protein defect leads to widespread cell and organ dysfunction. No longer is it adequate to know simply the gene and protein defect and what clinical outcome it generates. As is revealed time and time again by the chapters herein, our concept of lysosomes and storage diseases has now expanded well beyond the simple scenario of enzyme defect causing storage, in turn causing fatal disease. The array of proteins linked to storage diseases has multiplied, with some not being enzymes at all and/or not residing within lysosomes, and with this expansion has come the potential for far greater insight into the ultimate housekeeping tasks confronting all cells, particularly long-lived neurones. Thus, it is evident that lysosomal diseases, like other rare inborn errors of metabolism, have enormous potential as tools for learning about the biology of normal cell systems, with this knowledge in turn catalysing advances in therapeutic strategies.

In approaching the organization of this book, we have chosen not to emphasize the established system of classification of lysosomal diseases based on the identity of stored materials but rather to use one centred on molecular defects. This is not because we feel that the time-honoured way of speaking about and knowing these diseases should be replaced, but rather because we believe that the value of these diseases as tools of discovery is far more readily apparent through a system of nomenclature which emphasizes the function of defective proteins. Our goal here too, we will unabashedly confess, is to draw in our cell biology and neuroscience colleagues who perhaps have not considered the richness of storage diseases as a focus for research. If this book serves no other purpose but this, it will have been well worth the enormous time and effort it has involved.

No topic of the magnitude of lysosomal disorders could easily be covered by a single author, or indeed by a pair of authors, and we are extremely grateful to the many contributors to this book who have lent their time and effort to this project. We all realize the enormous debt owed to others in the field who have in many cases worked on lysosomes and lysosomal diseases throughout their careers and have established the very foundations on which this book rests. While not authors in this particular book, they have nonetheless inspired and encouraged us all. So, we particularly thank Roscoe Brady, Robert Desnick, Christian de Duve, Hans Galjaard, Roy Gravel, Stuart Kornfeld, Arnold Reuser, William Sly, and David Wenger, each of whom has contributed so enormously over the last many decades to advance the field of lysosomal diseases. In addition to these individuals, the editors would like to make special mention of others who have made important contributions to our own personal development and interest in storage diseases, including Tim Cox, Rick Proia, Konrad Sandhoff, and Bryan Winchester (FMP), and also Henry Baker, Robert Jolly, Hugo Moser, Dominick Purpura, Isabelle Rapin, Kinuko and Kunihiko Suzuki, and Robert Terry (SUW). We thank Robert McGlynn and Gloria Stephney for the images used on the cover. We are indebted to Mylvaganam Jeyakumar for compiling the tables central to Chapter 2. We also thank Hugh Perry for suggesting that this book be written, in part to raise awareness of this group of rare diseases within the larger community of scientists and clinicians interested in neurodegenerative diseases.

Finally, we dedicate this volume to the countless victims of lysosomal diseases and to their families. It is our hope that through further research we can learn more, and ultimately, we can *do* more in terms of crafting successful therapies for all of these devastating and tragic diseases.

F.M. Platt
Oxford

S.U. Walkley
New York

Foreword

An Historical Perspective

The concept of inborn lysosomal disease is the logical deduction of a series of observations I made in type II glycogenosis in 1963 that I will briefly recall (see also: Hers 1983).

Type II glycogenosis as an inborn lysosomal disease

In 1932, Pompe described the case of a 7-month-old girl who died suddenly of idiopathic hypertrophy of the heart. Histochemical investigation revealed a large excess of glycogen in nearly all tissues. The disease became known as Pompe disease, or generalized glycogenosis, and was classified by Gerty Cori (1954) as type II glycogenosis because it was the second type amongst the four known at that time, in which the structure of glycogen was normal. Remarkably, all the enzymes known to participate in glycogen degradation displayed normal activity. Furthermore, the patients were not hypoglycaemic and their ability to break down glycogen was attested by a rise in blood sugar after epinephrine injection.

My discovery of acid maltase deficiency in this disease (Hers 1963) was pure serendipity. It had been indeed shown by Walker and Wheland (1960) that the debranching of glycogen, catalysed by amylo-1,6-glucosidase, occurs in two steps, one of them being the (α-1,4→α-1,4) transfer of either an oligoglycan or a single glucosyl unit. It was with the aim of discovering a subgroup of type III glycogenosis (deficiency in amylo-1,6-glucosidase) that I developed an assay for a hypothetical glucosyltransferase. This assay was based on the measurement of radioactivity in glycogen after incubation in the presence of [^{14}C]maltose and gave a positive result with extracts of normal human livers or muscles. I also tested a series of pathological tissues originating from patients with various types of glycogenosis. To my surprise, all type III samples catalysed the reaction normally, but all type II samples were inactive.

It then appeared that my assay was measuring the transferase activity of a maltase (also called α-glucosidase, since it is not specific for maltose but is also active on other α-glucosides, including glycogen and synthetic substrates such as *p*-nitrophenyl-α-D-glucoside) and had nothing to do with amylo-1, 6-glucosidase, which actually operates as an oligoglucan transferase. Routine investigation revealed that this glucosidase was most active at pH 4 and that it was sedimentable in a fresh liver homogenate but was recovered in the supernatant when the homogenate had been previously frozen and thawed. Working in the laboratory of Christian de Duve, I knew that these properties were those of a lysosomal enzyme. The lysosomal appurtenance of this acid maltase was then firmly established by its property of structure-linked latency and of sedimentability (Lejeune *et al.* 1963).

The pathogeny of type II glycogenosis

The role of a lysosomal α-glucosidase in glycogen metabolism was far from clear at that time. The concept of lysosomes had been defined by de Duve and co-workers in 1955, and in the early speculations over the role of these 'lytic bodies', it was postulated that some kind of injury to the lysosomal membrane was a prerequisite to the action of the hydrolases on cytosolic structures. At the same time when the deficiency of α-glucosidase was discovered, this 'suicide-bag' hypothesis was progressively replaced by the concept of cellular autophagy. Whereas lysosomes had been identified by Essner and Novikoff (1960) with the pericanalicular dense bodies, Ashford and Porter (1962) extended the concept to the digestive vacuoles in which mitochondria, at various stages of breakdown, could be recognized. In this 'autophagic' concept, a small area of cytoplasm containing various cellular constituents, including glycogen, becomes walled off from the rest of the cytoplasm by a membrane. An autophagic vacuole is thus formed and fuses with lysosomes, and all of the cytoplasmic constituents are then digested by the lysosomal hydrolases. This was believed to be a normal process which continuously occurred in living cells and ensures the catabolic part of cellular turnover. The role of the α-glucosidase was obviously to destroy the glycogen segregated within the vacuoles.

This view was illuminating in various respects. Indeed, it indicated that there are two pathways of glycogenolysis in cells. One of them, as described in all textbooks of biochemistry, is phosphorolytic and hormonally controlled. It is normal in type II glycogenosis, and its operation explains why the patients are not hypoglycaemic and respond normally to the hyperglycaemic stimulation of epinephrine and glucagon. The second mechanism, previously unsuspected, is hydrolytic and lysosomal. Its role is not to supply glucose to the cell but to destroy the glycogen that has been engulfed in the autophagic vacuoles. This glycogen is indeed not accessible to phosphorylase, from which it is separated by the lysosomal membrane. In the absence of acid maltase, it accumulates in the vacuoles and corresponds to the polysaccharide present in excess in type II glycogenosis.

If the above interpretation was correct, the glycogen-loaded vacuoles would be visible with the electron microscope. As first shown by Baudhuin *et al.* (1964), both the liver parenchymal cells and Kupffer cells of patients contain large vacuoles (up to 8 μm in diameter) delineated by a single membrane and filled with easily recognizable particulate glycogen. Except for the absence of pericanalicular dense bodies (the normal lysosome structure), the rest of the cytoplasm was normal and contained a normal amount of glycogen. A similar postmortem analysis revealed that this cytoplasmic glycogen had completely disappeared (most likely by phosphorolytic degradation induced by anoxia), whereas the vacuolar glycogen remained untouched.

The concept of inborn lysosomal disease (Hers 1965)

At the time when the above observations were made, a dozen acid hydrolases were known to be present in lysosomes. Their role was believed to most likely involve the digestion of cellular constituents normally present in the cell and engulfed in autophagic vacuoles, as well as of various macromolecules that could have entered cells by endocytosis. My previous experience with the several sub-types of glycogen storage disease had taught me that practically any enzyme can be found inactive due to a mutation of the corresponding gene. It was therefore almost certain that the accident that had happened to acid α-glucosidase also happened to at least some of the other lysosomal hydrolases and that this was responsible for a definite storage disease characterized by the same morphological hallmark: hypertrophy and overloading of lysosomes. This finding thus offered a unitarian explanation for a series of well-known lipidoses or mucopolysaccharidoses such as Gaucher, Niemann–Pick, or Hurler diseases. The latter, also known as gargoylism, was of particular interest because of the simultaneous storage of both glycolipids and mucopolysaccharides, which I had indeed considered as a possibility in a lysosomal disease. My assumption was that, similar to α-glucosidase (see above), other lysosomal hydrolases were not specific for one substrate molecule but for one linkage, which might be present in both a glycolipid and a mucopolysaccharide. The deficiency of a single hydrolase may therefore be responsible for the accumulation of very different complex macromolecules. Because of their lack of specificity, these enzymes can be assayed on a low-molecular weight substrate obtained by chemical synthesis. The heterogeneity of the depot can be seen under the electron microscope, with glycolipids appearing often as zebra bodies in the nervous tissues, whereas mucopolysaccharides accumulate in apparently empty vacuoles in the liver. The vacuolar aspect of the liver provided the first indication that Hurler disease was actually a lysosomal disease (Van Hoof and Hers 1964). Nevertheless, it took nearly 10 years to get this view accepted because the theory current at the time was that Hurler disease was caused by an excess production of acid mucopolysaccharides (Matalon and Dorfman 1966). It was only after Friedman and Weissmann (1972) succeeded in synthesizing *p*-nitrophenyl-α-L-iduronide that the deficiency of L-iduronidase was easily demonstrated in several patients (Bach *et al.* 1972; Matalon and Dorfman 1972) and that the concept of inborn lysosomal disease as described above became progressively accepted. Similarly, fucosidosis was recognized (Van Hoof and Hers 1968) as early as 1968, thanks to the commercial availability of *p*-nitrophenyl-α-L-fucoside.

In 1973, together with François Van Hoof, I edited a multi-author book entitled *Lysosomes and Storage Diseases*, in which more than 20 storage disorders were classified as lysosomal in origin. Now, 30 years latter, this number exceeds 40 (see Chapter 2). Whereas the general mechanism described above remains valid, the situation has become more complex and the field has greatly expanded, as revealed by the descriptions of several other disease mechanisms leading to storage in Chapters 4–10 of this book. Furthermore, numerous therapeutic attempts using enzyme replacement, gene therapy, bone marrow transplantation and substrate reduction have been made and the mechanism by which the overloading of lysosomes affects cell functioning has been extensively studied. Considering the quality of the authors that have been selected by the editors, there is no doubt that this book will make a valuable contribution, not only to lysosomal diseases of brain, but also to the whole field of cell biology.

H.G. Hers

References

Ashford, T. P. and Porter, K. R. (1962). Cytoplasmic components in hepatic cell lysosomes. *J Cell Biol*, **12**, 198–202.

Bach, G., Friedman, R., Weissmann B., and Neufeld E. F. (1972). The defect in the Hurler and Scheie syndromes: Deficiency of L-iduronidase. *Pro Natl Acad Sci USA*, **69**, 2048–51.

Baudhuin, P., Hers, H. G., and Loeb, H. (1964). An electron microscopic and biochemical study of Type II glycogenosis. *Lab Invest*, **13**, 1139–52.

Cori, G. T. (1954). Glycogen structure and enzyme deficiencies in glycogen storage disease. *Harvey Lect*, **48**, 145–71.

de Duve, C., Pressman B. C., Gianetto R., Wattiaux, R., and Appelmans, F. (1955). Tissue fractionation studies: Intracellular distribution patterns of enzymes in rat-liver tisssue. *Biochem J*, **64**, 604–17.

Essner, E. and Novikoff A. B. (1960). Human hepatocellular pigments and lysosomes. *J Ultrastruct Res*, **3**, 374–91.

Friedman and Weissmann (1972). The phenyl – and -L-idopyranosiduronic acids and some other aryl glycopyranosiduronic acids. *Carbohydrate Res*, **24**, 123–31.

Hers, H. G. (1963). α-Glucosidase deficiency in generalised glycogen storage disease (Pompes disease). *Biochem J*, **86**, 11–16.

Hers, H. G. (1965). Inborn lysosomal diseases. *Gastroenterology (Editorial)*, **48**, 625–33.

Hers, H. G. (1983). From fructose to fructose-2,6-bisphosphate with a detour through lysosomes and glycogen. In *Selected Topics in the History of Biochemistry* (ed. by G. Semenza), pp. 71–101. Elsevier Biomedical Press.

Hers, H. G. and Van Hoof, F. (ed.) (1973). *Lysosomes and Storage Diseases.* pp. 666. Academic Press, New York.

Lejeune, N., Thines-Sempoux D., and Hers, H. G. (1963). Intracellular distribution and properties of α-glucosidases in rat liver. *Biochem J*, **86**, 16–21.

Matalon, R. and Dorfman, A. (1966). Hurlers syndrome: Biosynthesis of acid mucopolysaccharides in tissue culture. *Proc Natl Acad Sci USA*, **56**, 1310–16.

Matalon, R. and Dorfman, A. (1972). Hurlers syndrome, an α-L-iduronidase deficiency. *Biochem Biophys Res Commun*, **47**, 959–64.

Pompe, J. C. (1932). Over idiopatische hypertrophie van het hart. *Ned Tijdschr Geneeskd*, **76**, 304–11.

Van Hoof, F. and Hers, H. G. (1964). L'ultrastructure des cellules hépatiques dans la maladie de Hürler (Gargoylisme). *Compte-Rendus de l'académie des Sciences*, **259**, 1281–3.

Van Hoof, F. and Hers, H. G. (1968). Mucopolysaccharidosis by absence of α-fucosidase. *Lancet*, **i**, 1198.

Walker, G. J. and Wheland, W. J. (1960). Stucture of the muscle-phosphorylase limit dextrin of glycogen and amylopectin. *Biochem J*, **76**, 254–68.

Contents

List of contributors

d'Azzo, Alessandra
Department of Genetics
St Jude Children's Research Hospital
332 North Lauderdale Street
Memphis, TN 38105
USA

Borissenko, Ljudmila V.
Georg-August-Universität Göttingen
Abt. Biochemie II
Heinrich-Düker-Weg 12
37073 Göttingen, Germany

Butters, Terry D.
Glycobiology Institute
Department of Biochemistry
University of Oxford
South Parks Road
Oxford OX1 3QU, UK

Crawley, Allison C.
Lysosomal Diseases Research Unit
Department of Chemical Pathology
Women's and Children's Hospital
North Adelaide SA 5006, Australia

Dierks, Thomas
Georg-August-Universität Göttingen
Abt. Biochemie II
Heinrich-Düker-Weg 12
37073 Göttingen, Germany

Dobrenis, Kostantin
Department of Neuroscience,
Rose F. Kennedy Centre for Research in Mental Retardation and Human Development, Albert Einstein College of Medicine
1410 Pelham Parkway South
Bronx, NY 10461
USA

Fey, Jens
Georg-August-Universität Göttingen
Abt. Biochemie II
Heinrich-Düker-Weg 12
37073 Göttingen, Germany

von Figura, Kurt
Georg-August-Universität Göttingen
Abt. Biochemie II
Heinrich-Düker-Weg 12
37073 Göttingen, Germany

Hasilik, Andrej
Institute of Physiological Chemistry
Philipps-University
Karl-von-Frisch-Str. 1
35033 Marburg, Germany

Hers, Henry-Gery
Laboratoire de Chimie Physiologique
Christian de Dure Institute of Cellular Pathology, and Université Catholique de Louvain
B-1200 Brussels
Belgium

Hopwood, John J.
Lysosomal Diseases Research Unit
Department of Chemical Pathology
Women's and Children's Hospital
North Adelaide, SA 5006,
Australia

Ioannou, Yiannis A.
Departments of Human Genetics, Gene Therapy and Molecular Medicine
Box 1498
The Mount Sinai School of Medicine
One Gustave L. Levy Place
New York, NY 10029
USA

Kolter, Thomas
Kekulé-Institut für Organische Chemie und Biochemie, Gerhard-Domagk-Str 1,
D-53121 Bonn,
Germany

Lemansky, Peter
Institute of Physiological Chemistry
Philipps-University
Karl-von-Frisch-Str. 1
35033 Marburg, Germany

Macheleidt, Oliver
Kekulé-Institut für Organische Chemie und Biochemie, Gerhard-Domagk-Str 1,
D-53121 Bonn,
Germany

Malm, Dag
Institute of Clinical Medicine
University Hospital of Northern-Norway
N-9038 Tromsø
Norway

Maxfield, Frederick R.
Department of Biochemistry
Weill Medical College of Cornell University
1300 York Avenue
New York, NY 10021
USA

Mukherjee, Sushmita
Department of Biochemistry
Weill Medical College of Cornell University
1300 York Avenue
New York, NY 10021
USA

Neufeld, Elizabeth F.
Department of Biological Chemistry
The David Geffen School of Medicine
University of California Los Angeles
CHS 33–257
650 Charles Young Drive South
Los Angeles, CA 90095–1737
USA

Pearce, David A.
Center for Aging and Developmental Biology
Department of Biochemistry and Biophysics
University of Rochester School of Medicine and Dentistry
Rochester, NY 14642
USA

Peng, Jianhe
Georg-August-Universität Göttingen
Abt. Biochemie II
Heinrich-Düker-Weg 12
37073 Göttingen, Germany

Platt, Frances M.
Department of Biochemistry
University of Oxford
South Parks Road
Oxford OX1 3QU, UK

Sandhoff, Konrad
Kekulé-Institut für Organische Chemie und Biochemie, Gerhard-Domagk-Str 1,
D-53121 Bonn,
Germany

Sands, Mark S.
Washington University School of Medicine
Departments of Internal Medicine and Genetics
P. O. Box 8007
660 South Euclid Avenue
St Louis, MO 63110
USA

Schmidt, Bernhard
Georg-August-Universität Göttingen
Abt. Biochemie II
Heinrich-Düker-Weg 12
37073 Göttingen, Germany

Taylor, Rosanne M.
Faculty of Veterinary Science
University of Sydney, B19
NSW 2006
Australia

Walkley, Steven U.
Department of Neuroscience
Rose F. Kennedy Center for Research in Mental Retardation and Human Development
Albert Einstein College of Medicine
1410 Pelham Parkway South Bronx, NY 10461,
USA

Winchester, Bryan G.
Biochemistry, Endocrinology & Metabolism Unit
Institute of Child Health
30 Guildford Street
London WCIN IEH, UK

Wraith, J. Edmond
Willink Biochemical Genetics Unit
Royal Manchester Children's Hospital
Manchester M27 4HA, UK

Prologue

The doctor as parent

The doubt

The year is 1983. In the dim light of the nursing room of the birth clinic there was nothing specifically wrong to be seen, but I felt uneasy watching my newborn daughter Silje, my first child. The other infants in the room in one way or the other seemed different. Then I felt guilty. How could I think like this? Being my first child I supposed that a father's feelings were commonly poorly developed shortly after birth. After all, whereas my wife had experienced motherhood over the last 9 months, I had only been a father for the last 15 minutes. However, both in the first and in the following health checks I was reassured that everything was all right, and subsequently I felt relieved.

In the fourth month of pregnancy, there had been problems with premature labour. These were successfully treated with medicines, although this not being the standard procedure. As a recently educated medical doctor, I wondered what caused this complication. We had been in China, Thailand, and Malaysia. Could my wife have been infected with some microbes? We had consumed clams and fish that might have been caught in the polluted harbour of Hong Kong and eaten at restaurants where the plates were washed in cold water before being dried on the naked pavement.

In her first year of life, Silje had abdominal pain that seemed to last forever and never-ending colds that hindered her breathing at night. We sometimes used a midwife's suction device to alleviate this problem. Once she had pneumonia. Was it common that small children were so often sick? Periods of diarrhoea made us suspect coeliac disease. We changed her diet but without effect.

Months went by, Silje was dressed up and my wife sewed her bonnets to protect her eyes from the sun. But the bonnets became too small all the time, and new ones had to be sewn. It made us uneasy, but our first child was so perfect that nothing could possibly be wrong! On the health check at 8 months, there was an increase in head circumference from 50th to the 99th percentile, but the paediatrician again reassured us that there surely was nothing wrong.

Nevertheless, I worried and referred her for ultrasound of the head. I remember making a joke about her head looking a bit like the helmets of the Italian cycling team (the Olympic games were held in Los Angeles in the summer of 1984). The examination showed that increased pressure of the cerebrospinal fluid had compressed her brain so that her cerebral ventricles were dilated. The X-ray of the skull visualized her cerebral windings imprinted on the inside of the skull. Computerized tomography was performed with me at the operator's desk. Picture by picture, I could see how the ventricles were cruelly enlarged.

The only treatment for Silje's condition of hydrocephalus was surgical, relieving the cerebrospinal pressure with an artificial duct. The neurosurgical department of the national hospital was situated in one of the older buildings, presenting with high roofs and long, cold corridors as gloomy as our own state of mind. I accompanied Silje to her first operation. It was not going to be her last. The anaesthetist was an old friend from a former workplace, and

I thought back to good long evenings together when life was unbearably easy, and the future looked bright and happy. Life is so changeable.

The operation was uncomplicated, and as Silje returned, we sat on her bed. She was lying on her back with an infusion in her hand. Her head was shaven, which made her look even more grotesque. How could I have been so blind? The forehead was very prominent. Would the hydrocephaly return? How would her mental capacity develop? We found some comfort in stories about other children with normal development after similar operations but did not really believe in it. On the walls—pictures of children previously operated on. How were they doing? I remembered child patients from my days as a medical student with their big heads and staring eyes. I did not reflect upon the tragedy for the families then, but now we found ourselves in the very same situation.

The next day, one of the elder doctors visited us. He was the neurosurgeon who had introduced this operation method in Norway. He sat next to Silje and watched her carefully without uttering a word. It was a strange look that I could not interpret. He said nothing, but a few days later she was transferred to the paediatric department. After extensive investigations nothing wrong was found except something undefinable in the urine.

The autumn that year was beautiful with ripe apples, pears, and cherries on the trees in the garden. Winter turned into spring, but Silje, now 2 years old, still could not walk. We explained this with her enlarged head. At last, in early summer, she managed to cross the floor with her big head waving from side to side. We were proud. But one night, my wife awakened me in bed, crying. 'We are going to lose her', she said. The uneasiness had moved into our mind for good.

I was then offered a position as a researcher and teacher at the University of Tromsø, my hometown. It is situated at 71° North, near the top of Norway, thus north of Siberia. Winter came. Silje was now 3 years old and walked around unsteadily. We could not understand why she constantly kept falling to the ground. Once she fell from the chair and got a deep cut in the forehead. There was a lot of snow that winter, and in the garden there was a 4-m-high pile of snow. It was perfect for sledging. I had to support and drag Silje up to let her slide down. The other children made it themselves without any problems. Why was she so weak and they not?

The confirmation

My wife became pregnant again, and we looked forward to the birth of the new child and to give Silje a sibling in April the following year.

In autumn that year, as Silje was to complete 4 years, she was suddenly sick and bedridden again. A new computerized tomographic scan confirmed the return of the hydrocephalus. She had to be operated on again, and as my wife arrived at the national hospital she met with the same doctor that had seen Silje previously. When he realized that Silje had no specific diagnosis after the first round of investigations, and that my wife was pregnant in the fourth month, he could not conceal his worry. He revealed that he suspected a serious metabolic disease and consequently ordered that she be re-examined. Much to our relief, also this time the tests came out negative.

The following spring, Emilie was born. She looked much stronger and healthier than Silje but had shortened Achilles tendons that needed an operation. A few weeks later, my wife noticed a-year-old girl in the neighborhood who in many ways resembled Silje. She was now 5 years old but had no language in spite of extensive training. Testing showed a mild mental retardation, but she also had an excellent memory, such as to remember exactly where the guests were seated in her birthday party years earlier.

In a new attempt to make a diagnosis, a young doctor at the local hospital decided to check a fibroblast culture from Silje for a metabolic disease since he had found vacuoles in the lymphocytes. Weeks later, he told me that the disease was probably α-mannosidosis. He had also previously diagnosed our neighbourhood girl with the same disease. I immediately went to the library where I found the first description from 1967 by Ockerman in Lund. A 4-year-old boy who had the same characteristics as Silje: large head, prominent forehead, bent spine, hearing deficiency, and frequent infections. The post-mortem showed accumulation of sugars in all tissues. My blood froze as my eyes hit the words 'The boy died'. What kind of horrid disease was this? The world seemed unreal. What were we awaiting?

The article informed me that the disease was caused by an inborn error of metabolism and immediately the suspicion came to my mind. Could Emilie have the same disease? Although she seemed so strong and healthy compared to her sister, we were alarmed. Later, the test showed that she, too, had the disease. We felt it to be devastating and unfair. With a recessive mode of inheritance, there should only be a 25% risk that the first child should be affected and only a 6.25% chance of two children in a row being affected. We had two children with α-mannosidosis. There was no justice.

The search

I systematically searched 'Current Contents' for research on mannosidosis. Being a researcher myself, I was used to thinking that everything can be elucidated and that all problems can be solved. However, this problem seemed so huge and intimate that the idea of myself doing research was uncomfortable. But the enzyme was not isolated and characterized, the gene was not cloned, and the disease-causing mutations were unknown. Month after month, I found no new publications on mannosidosis. It was almost insulting. How could such a serious disease be so uninteresting?

In one *in vitro* study, zinc had been found to increase residual α-mannosidosis activity, but results from single trials on calves and a boy with the disease were discouraging. Exchange of bone marrow with chimeric calves showed reduced accumulation of material in the body but not in the brain. In 1987, Will *et al.* treated a child with mannosidosis with bone marrow transplantation (BMT). The boy died after 18 weeks due to procedure-related complications. At the postmortem examination, peripheral tissues were largely free of deposit material, but in the brain very little enzyme activity was found, and histology showed extensive vacuolization. In 1994, Walkley performed BMT in kittens with α-mannosidosis. Here, the cats developed perfectly normally and the otherwise specific pathology in brain tissue could not be seen. This discrepancy in the findings of Walkley and Will could be explained by: (1) species differences; (2) that the timing of BMT is paramount and that the Will boy was transplanted too late; (3) that the heavy immunosuppressive treatment given to the Will boy before he died might have influenced enzyme production; (4) there could have been insufficient time following BMT to restore changes in the brain; or (5) since his mother was the donor, she would have been a carrier and inadequate enzyme production (25–50%) might be suspected.

But again, in 1998, Wall successfully performed BMT on a 22-month-old infant with α-mannosidosis. At the evaluation 15 months later, they reported that the BMT had resulted in the correction of bone disease and sinopulmonary disease and a stabilization of neurocognitive function. With one unsuccessful and one successful case published, it was premature to conclude anything about the benefits of BMT, and I was still uncertain.

At that time I participated in a transplant meeting. After seeing horrid pictures of children having graft-versus-host reactions and learning that mortality using HLA-identical non-familial donor was 25%, I found out that BMT did not seem the way to go. . . .

We wanted at least one healthy child and took the chance of another pregnancy for the third time in late 1989. Now having the specific diagnosis, we were able to undertake prenatal diagnostics. The result showed a foetus without α-mannosidosis, and Clara was later born healthy. This was at last joyful news after much bad news. A reflection was that if Silje's diagnosis had been clear before Emilie was conceived, Emilie would probably have been aborted and the life-long problem of the family been half as large. With a lovely 4-year-old Emilie stumbling around, the thought seemed absurd.

In 1991, I went to the Department of Medical Genetics holding the 100 more or less relevant articles on the topic with the request of initiating research. A group was established with university teachers and students from the fields of molecular biology, biochemistry, and clinical medicine. The University even salaried a research fellow at my request. The 'Tromsø/Mannosidosis Group' was born. Eight years later, the group had finished the first leg, and were the first to publish the correct gene sequence, the organization of the gene, and isolate, sequence, and characterize the enzyme from a number of species. In parallel, DNA samples and clinical data were collected from patients worldwide, enabling us to find and describe the first 40 mutations and the genotype–phenotype correlation.

In one long-term study on some patients it was claimed that the development of α-mannosidosis tends to stabilize after puberty. The affected families embraced this concept, of course. After searching for comfort myself in this 'Hypothesis of Stabilization' for some years, I experienced doubt, mainly because of personal communications from colleagues telling me about their patients. Through my work I had made contact with numerous colleagues from Europe, the US, and Australia, but also Russia. In 1998, we had a poster in Vienna, where we presented the disease-causing mutation in two patients of Italian origin. They had been bedridden for 20 years due to metabolic myopathy, arthropathy, and/or cerebellar atrophy. I reviewed the literature and had to realize that mannosidosis is an insidiously progressive disease with complications occurring at any age.

The possibility

At the same time, colleagues started forwarding the requests of their α-mannosidosis patients to me. Many questions were about my personal and professional attitude to BMT. My responses were general 'Pro et Contra' answers without a firm recommendation, not to interfere with the families' relationship with their doctor, who in the end was the responsible doctor in charge. In spite of acknowledging the progressive nature of the disease, the risks made me reluctant. A couple in the US who in spite of my advice decided to do BMT confused me. The relativity of a decision: There are humans willing to take risks and others who are not. Furthermore, there are societies where mental and physical retardation is a bigger disaster than in other societies.

Silje and Emilie reacted very differently to their situations. Silje easily accepted her condition being different, but Emilie never did. Whereas Silje plainly acknowledged that things were difficult and that her body was weak, Emilie focused on her faults: 'I am bad', 'I am stupid', 'I am ugly', or 'I want to cut my tongue out'. She was shy and by her reactions to the environment we could read that she had low self-esteem. We should not give her a long hug because she was not worth it, but at the same time she could cry if Clara got a longer good-night hug than her. We had a 9-year-old child with a reactive depression!

From the sixties, a number of metabolic diseases had been experimentally treated with BMT. The rationale was that blood is a mighty organ whose cells could deliver the enzyme that was missing. As previously mentioned, the first BMT was performed in 1987 on an 8-year-old boy with α-mannosidosis. There were obviously no good donors at hand since the mother donated parts of her own bone marrow (the mother is seldom HLA identical). At that time, there was a 30–50% risk of the patient dying due to procedure-related complications. Not unexpectedly, the patient developed a graft versus host reaction and died from pneumonia that could not be controlled.

Even though this complication could be expected, the outcome was so depressing that no other BMTs were performed as a treatment for α-mannosidosis over the next 8 years. It is strange how the scientific community, which should maintain a cool head, instead reacted almost emotionally by not doing further trials over a number of years. Thus, scientists seem to have a warm heart also. If there had been a related HLA-identical donor available, the chance of avoiding procedure-related death would have been 90–95%, in which case the first experiment could have been followed by many more trials, answering the question whether BMT is beneficial or not. What bad luck that the first experiment had such an unhappy ending!

At that time, I established a primitive home page on the university server to provide a supportive network to families worldwide. It also offered advice and the exchange of experiences by mail. From the fall of 1996, I received a number of requests from families in the US, Australia, New Zealand, Germany, Canada, Czechoslovakia, and Finland searching for advice regarding BMT. Here my double role became evident: as an MD and affected family member. The MD role would not complicate communication between patient and physician. But especially in the requests from the US, it seemed to be common to request second opinions. The affected family member role urged me to give as good advice as possible. I tried to circumvent the problem by giving 'personal' rather than 'professional' advice. But what is the difference? Once a doctor, always a doctor, 'He was born as a man, died as a doctor'.

Most of the early publications on α-mannosidosis were single case reports presented by colleagues satisfied with making a rare diagnosis. Their observations were presented and then put aside. But the essential question remained: What is the natural course of the disease in the long run? Through my Internet contacts I was able to find a number of patients with serious complications after puberty, and through contact with colleagues I found just as many. I then contacted one of the senior authorities on BMT as a therapy for inborn errors of metabolism. His recommendation was more straightforward than I ever had heard before. I also communicated with Steven Walkley, whom I had met some years earlier. He had performed BMT in kittens with α-mannosidosis and had observed that they developed normally. More importantly, there were no signs of the microscopic changes in brain, typical of this disease. At last, I contacted the leading scientists working on gene therapy that confirmed this as not being an alternative of the near future.

So I had to realize that: (1) mannosidosis is an insidiously progressive disease with complications occurring at any age, (2) BMT would probably remedy extracerebral complications and had been shown to prevent the neurodegenerative process in cats, and (3) gene therapy was not at hand.

The ethics

Thinking through these options, we HLA-typed the children: Clara (who had none of the mutations causing the disease in our family) turned out to be the perfect donor for Emilie but unfortunately not for Silje. So the logic led us to the choice between the 10% chance of death versus the 90% chance of a 'rebirth'. As an MD, I was used to thinking about risk, but this was personal. What is 10% risk of death when you as parents choose to do BMT? Lining up your 10 children and shooting one! How could our luck turn out, having 25% risk of the first child being affected and 6.25% chance of both the first-born children being affected? We had a lousy relationship with probability statistics.

So this led to several ethical considerations: Have parents the right to expose a child to a 10% risk of dying? On the other hand: Is it right not to give the child the 90% chance to get well? Are parents competent to judge this? Or are they the only ones who could possibly know?

Many parents would, in the case of prenatal diagnosed α-mannosidosis, opt for a late abortion: Could a fatal BMT be seen as an 'Ultra-late abortion', because the parents are unhappy with their product—the child? How should one apply the principle of informed consent in this case? Should we accept a death risk of 10% in Emile but not a risk of 20% in Silje? Where is the limit, and who defines it?

The benefit of BMT had been shown in a feline model, and worldwide only four patients (whom I had heard of by personal communication) had been treated with BMT. The first died, whereas the others were subjectively healthy after an observation time of 2 years. Where is the distinction between experimental and established treatment?

So, there were three alternatives regarding Emile and BMT:

1. A BMT is performed and is uneventful, and everything is all right.
2. A BMT is performed and she dies of procedure-related complications, leaving us with grief and guilt.
3. A BMT is not performed and the complications will disable her gradually, leaving us with a bad conscience.

In essence, we had the opportunity to do something beneficial for the child. How could we refrain from it? We felt we had no choice. It was like sitting on a runaway train.

Luckily, the haematologists at the BMT specialist centre accepted the indications, with the comment 'When a doctor is willing to do BMT on his own child, then there can be no doubt about the conviction'. The BMT was performed in the summer of 1997 with Clara as a happy donor. The procedure had the ordinary, but no extraordinary, complications, and at day 20 Emile could have a walk and enjoy a Coke™ in the 'Park of Vigeland' in Oslo. Later tests showed a close to 100 engraftment. Clara's comment: 'Now that my blood is her blood, she is half me'!

After the BMT, her muscular pain vanished, her muscular strength improved, and she even could play tennis and squash. Neuropsychological test, however, indicated a progressive impairment.

The problems

In 1995, a German colleague in Mainz told me that he wished there was a patient support group for these patients who rightly felt very alone in the world. At that time, I joined a university course in the use of the Internet. When searching for the word 'α-mannosidosis' on

Altavista, I received only one response from Paul Murphy in Atlanta. It turned out that he and his wife Debbie had a daughter with this disease. The daughter Taryn was the same age as Silje, and we exchanged experiences. We decided to start an international organization, mainly to provide information to affected families (and their doctors), but also with the aim to help and enhance research in the field of mannosidosis.

This led to several home pages, the most important being http://www.mannosidosis.org and http://www.fm.uit.no/~dagm/index.htm. Through the Internet, I have received mail daily from parents (mainly mothers) in search of information. Through this media, I have come to know numerous admirable people fighting for their children's quality of life. Some of the affected children were functioning well, but others were confined to a wheelchair or even bedridden. Other families reported complications such as infections, arthritis, muscular pain, and psychosis. The latter condition seemed to affect the families most, both emotionally and practically.

I came across situations I would call a social catastrophe. A father in the US who had changed jobs shortly before the diagnosis of the child got no cover from his health insurance, claiming the condition was pre-existing! In many cases, the consequences of having a child with mannosidosis led to one of the parents being unable to work. Other survival strategies were to plan life's movements in detail.

A family in Louisiana with 8- and 9-year-old daughters with α-mannosidosis impressed me the most. One of the children had never walked. The other was very weak and could only walk short distances. The children were operated for reflux disease and had a catheter through her skin to be given food directly into the stomach with syringe. The mother had a full-time job feeding the daughters. Thus, a family with a handicapped child is truly a handicapped family.

As for our family, the impact of the disease has been huge. It can be everyday problems. When going shopping every move has to be thoroughly planned because of short walking distances. A car must be spacious and practical. The house must be planned for wheel-chairs. For a number of years, my wife worked at night to be at home for the children during daytime, and I chose the liberal working conditions at the university for the same reasons. And there were luxury problems: We had to skip all dreams of deep-water sailing, since we could not risk hydrocephalus in the open sea. We could not have holidays in Africa, where the return flights are scarce. Once on a holiday in Thailand, Silje got a psychosis and the travel back through the airports of Bangkok and Copenhagen, with a 17-year-old with staring eyes pointing her tongue at fellow passengers was a special experience.

However, the benefits of our destiny have been many. On a personal level, I have learnt and been intrigued by the beauty of molecular medicine. It has induced research, which is important to me. This year, the Tromø Mannosidosis Group received US$ 1.67 million from the European Union together with nine other partners in Europe. As parents, we have learned to endure problems even in despair, and Clara has learned to handle her affected older sisters. To meet other scientists seriously and affectionately engaged in the understanding of lysosomal storage diseases has been an experience I would not be without. However, most rewarding has been the meeting with other parents all around the world, and I truly admire their affection, their engagement, and their determination to make the lives of their children meaningful. I have discovered how unique life is. Now, having seen so many aspects of life, I see clearer than before, making every day richer for myself.

D. Malm

Section I

Overview of lysosomes and storage diseases

Chapter 1

The endosomal–lysosomal system

Frederick R. Maxfield and Sushmita Mukherjee

Introduction

Mammalian cells are often highly differentiated and functionally specialized, and they exhibit complex patterns of communication with their neighbouring cells. This is achieved in part by the materials (such as nutrients, hormones, neurotransmitters, ligands modulating signal transduction systems, etc.) internalized by the cells from the extracellular milieu. The internalized molecules may be secreted by neighbouring cells or transported from elsewhere. Most specialized cells, including neurones and glia, preferentially internalize specific sets of molecules. This is achieved by the expression of specific cell-surface receptors that bind their ligands with high affinity. The receptor–ligand complex is subsequently internalized into the cell, often via the well-characterized clathrin-mediated endocytic pathway. Once inside the cell, the receptor–ligand complex enters a series of acidic endosomal compartments. In many, although not all, cases, the low pH of endosomes causes a dissociation of the ligand from its receptor. The precise subset of endosomes that receptors and/or ligands are transported to plays a major role in determining the eventual functioning of these molecules.

Although the receptor-mediated endocytosis is the most common and the best-studied example of endocytosis, it is by no means the only mechanism by which materials are internalized into cells. Several other forms of endocytosis have been well documented in the literature—including phagocytosis (the mechanism for internalizing large molecules such as bacteria into cells), pinocytosis and macropinocytosis (mechanisms for internalizing large volumes of extracellular fluid), and caveolar endocytosis (endocytosis of a specialized subset of molecules that localize in the 60 nm flask-shaped cell-surface structures called caveolae). In some cases, molecules that are internalized by different cell-surface processes enter common endosomal structures. For the purposes of this chapter, we primarily concentrate on receptor-mediated endocytosis.

The endosomal–lysosomal system: the 'early' and 'late' endocytic compartments

Definitions and ambiguities in definitions

In order to appreciate the complexities of the endocytic process, it is necessary to have a description of the organelles that participate in this process. However, in spite of extensive efforts, the identity of different classes of endosomes can often be quite ambiguous. One difficulty is the extensive and rapid traffic of molecules among different endocytic organelles. Consequently, at any given time, many so-called 'markers' of a given organelle can be found in several types of endocytic organelles, and this can make the interpretation of the routes taken by tracers difficult. Furthermore, the sorting is not 100% efficient at each step. For example, most transferrin (Tf) returns to the cell surface without passing through the Golgi apparatus, but a small percentage of internalized Tf does get into the Golgi apparatus (Stoorvogel *et al.* 1988).

In spite of the uncertainties in the definitions of different compartments, there is a general consensus regarding the basic configuration of the endocytic organelles and relationships among them. In Fig. 1.1, we present a schematic representation of the endocytic pathways in a non-specialized, non-polarized cell. The steps in the pathway that are more uncertain have been indicated with question marks.

By several criteria, the endocytic organelles can be broadly divided into 'early' and 'late' compartments (Mukherjee *et al.* 1997). Early endosomes include all the intracellular organelles that are on the major receptor recycling pathway. Internalized molecules must pass through portions of the early endosome system to reach the late endosomes. Late endosomes are compartments that are involved in the breakdown of internalized cargo or delivery to the *trans*-Golgi network (TGN). They lack significant levels of Tf and recycling receptors but contain low-density lipoprotein (LDL), α_2-macroglobulin (α_2-M), and other ligands that are degraded by cells after internalization. Lysosomes come after the late endosomes on the degradative pathway, and they are involved in the final breakdown of internalized cargo as well as in the storage of indigestible material.

The early endosome system can be divided into at least two separate compartments. Sorting endosomes contain recycling molecules such as Tf as well as ligands that will be degraded such as LDL. There is a physically separate portion of the early endosome system, called the endocytic recycling compartment (ERC), that contains recycling molecules but lacks molecules that will be degraded (Yamashiro *et al.* 1984). Some protein markers of these compartments, such as specific rab proteins, as well as the early endosomal antigen 1 (EEA1), are shown in Table 1.1.

The cation-independent mannose-6-phosphate receptor (CI-MPR) is frequently used as a marker of the late endocytic compartments. This receptor, which transports lysosomal hydrolases from the TGN to late endosomes, has a relatively complex itinerary (Kornfeld and Mellman 1989; Kornfeld 1992). Late endosomes are often defined as organelles lacking Tf and other recycling components but containing CI-MPRs. The CI-MPR does not enter lysosomes, and this can be used as a criterion to distinguish between late endosomes and lysosomes. Lysosomes contain endocytosed indigestible fluid-phase markers such as dextrans, but they lack the CI-MPR. It should be noted that this definition of lysosomes as CI-MPR-negative compartments (Kornfeld and Mellman 1989; Kornfeld 1992) is very useful in differentiating between types of organelles, but it represents a change from an earlier, widely used definition of lysosomes as hydrolase-rich, acidic organelles that carried out the catabolism of internalized material. Much of the hydrolysis of internalized molecules probably occurs in the compartments that are now classified as late endosomes. Late endosomes and lysosomes are enriched in a family of heavily glycosylated proteins known as LAMPs (lysosome-associated membrane proteins) or lgps (lysosomal membrane glycoproteins) (Kornfeld and Mellman 1989; Kornfeld 1992). Since CI-MPRs are in late endosomes but not lysosomes, an experimentally useful way to characterize lysosomes is as the lgp-positive, CI-MPR-negative organelles (Kornfeld and Mellman 1989).

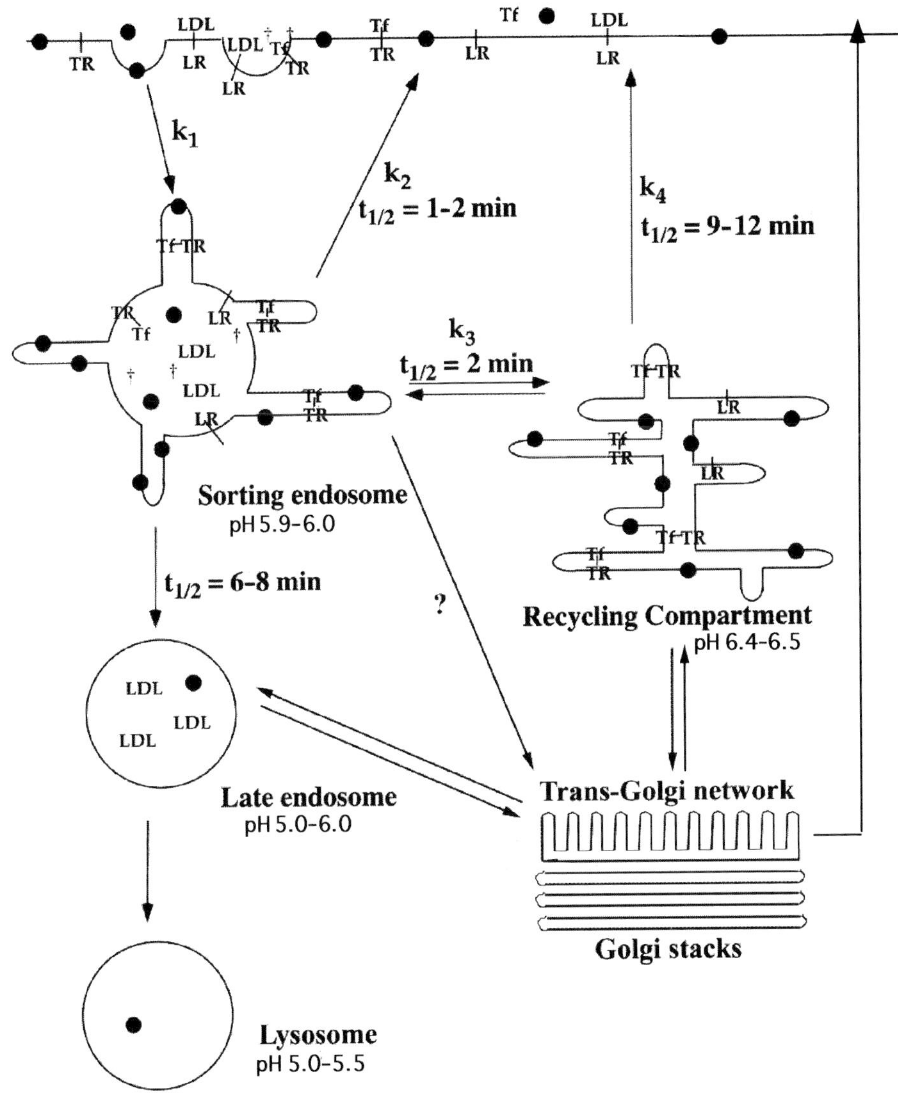

Fig. 1.1 Schematic representation of the itineraries followed by several prototypical endocytic markers in CHO cells. The lumenal pH of each of these organelles is also shown. Various ligand–receptor complexes are internalized from the plasma membrane *via* coated pits. These include the transferrin receptor (TR) bound to iron-loaded transferrin (Tf), low-density lipoprotein (LDL) bound to its receptor (LR), and lipids (•). Once in the sorting endosomes (pH 5.9–6.0), LDL and the iron bound to Tf (†) get released into the lumen of these organelles. Subsequently, a majority of the membrane-bound components (LR and apo-transferrin bound to TR after the release of Fe from Tf) enter the recycling compartment and eventually recycle back to the cell surface. The sorting endosome, in time, gives rise to the late endosome (pH 5.0–6.0). The lumen of this compartment thus contains ligands such as LDL that were earlier released into the lumen of sorting endosomes. The late endosomes eventually give rise to the lysosomes (pH 5.0–5.5) that contain all the released ligands. The lysosomal enzymes are optimally active in the low pH environment of the late endosomes/lysosomes, leading to the eventual degradation of released ligands and the storage of indigestible material in the lysosomes.

Table 1.1 Properties of Various Endosomal Compartments

	Compartment				
	Early endocytic compartments		Late endocytic compartments		
Properties	**Sorting endosomes**	**Recycling compartment**	**ECV-MVB**	**Late endosomes**	**Lysosomes**
Distribution	Peripheral	Variable: dispersed throughout cytoplasm or juxtanuclear	Throughout cytoplasm	Mainly perinuclear	Mainly perinuclear
Morphology	Tubulovesicular, cisternal (internal membranes)	Tubular with varicosities	Spherical with internal membranes	Complex structure with internal membranes (often onion-like)	Variable: tubular or similar to late endosomes
pH	5.9–6.0	6.4–6.5	<6.0	5.0–6.0	5.0–5.5
Receptors and membrane proteins	Recycling receptors (e.g. transferrin receptor and LDL receptor) and ligands destined for lysosome (e.g. LDL)	Recycling receptors (e.g. transferrin receptors) do not have lysosomally destined molecules (e.g. LDL)		M6P receptor, lgps, and LAMPs	lgps and LAMPs
GTP-binding proteins	Rab4, Rab5, and Rab11			Rab7 and Rab9	
Other proteins	EEA1	Rme-1			

Morphology

Sorting endosomes

Sorting endosomes have a tubulovesicular morphology with a vesicular portion that is typically 250–400 nm in diameter. Tubules radiating from these vesicular bodies are 50–60 nm in diameter and up to 4 μm long (Geuze *et al.* 1983; Gruenberg *et al.* 1989). A consequence of this geometry is that the bulk of the volume (60–70%) is in the vesicular portion, while most of the surface area (50–80%) is in the tubules (Marsh *et al.* 1986; Griffiths *et al.* 1989). By itself, this distribution provides a simple basis for partially sorting membrane components from soluble contents of the endosome (see later).

The endocytic recycling compartment

The ERC is composed of a collection of tubules with diameters of approximately 50–70 nm (Yamashiro *et al.* 1984; Ghosh *et al.* 1994). The diameter of these tubules is similar to that of the tubules emanating from the sorting endosomes, suggesting that the tubules bud off from the sorting endosome and deliver membrane-associated components to the recycling compartment. The tubules of the recycling compartment may be interconnected, and this network is often the most prominently labelled part of the early endosomal system. The tubules of the early endosome system have varicosities (Hopkins *et al.* 1990; Tooze and Hollinshead 1991) and coats (Tooze and Hollinshead 1991; Stoorvogel *et al.* 1996) associated with them. The recycling compartment is physically distinct from sorting endosomes, as judged by optical microscopy and electron microscopy (Yamashiro *et al.* 1984; Ghosh *et al.* 1994), and the two compartments maintain different pH values (Presley *et al.* 1993).

In many cells (e.g. CHO), the recycling compartment is densely concentrated in the pericentriolar region, and it appears as a bright peri-nuclear spot when viewed by 'widefield' fluorescence microscopy. This distribution is somewhat similar to that of TGN, which is also largely composed of tubular elements (Pagano *et al.* 1989; Ladinsky *et al.* 1994). However, the ERC is distinct from the TGN. Even in CHO cells where the two are adjacent to each other, the separation between the TGN and the recycling compartment is large enough to be resolved by confocal microscopy (Ghosh *et al.* 1998). In other cells (e.g. Hep2), the recycling compartment has a more widely dispersed tubular distribution (Ghosh *et al.* 1994), and the distribution of the ERC seems to be dependent upon the distribution of a subset of stable microtubules in various cell types (Lin *et al.* 2002). In non-polarized cells, the function of the ERC and the kinetics of passage of molecules through it appear to be unrelated to its morphological distribution in the cell. This is most evident from studies of a temperature-sensitive mutant CHO cell line in which the ERC is dispersed at elevated temperature, but the kinetics of recycling are unaltered. The ERC tubules often appear aligned along microtubules, and if the microtubules are disrupted following nocodazole treatment, the recycling compartment becomes fragmented (McGraw *et al.* 1988). Nevertheless, this disruption of localization does not have a large effect on the kinetics or efficiency of endocytic recycling (McGraw *et al.* 1988).

Late endosomes

Late endosomes are similar in size to sorting endosomes, but in thin-section electron microscopy, they appear to have more internal vesicular profiles and have also been named multivesicular bodies (MVBs). In fact, these 'vesicle' profiles are often inward invaginations of the membrane and not detached vesicles (van Deurs *et al.* 1993). Certain receptors, including the epidermal growth factor (EGF) receptor and lipids like lyso-bis-phosphatidic acid (LBPA), have been localized to these internal vesicle profiles (Kobayashi *et al.* 1998), and it has been proposed that this retention plays an important role in the catabolism of lipids and proteins. Late endosomes undergo extensive vesicular traffic with the TGN in order to acquire newly synthesized lysosomal enzymes and to return the MPRs back to the TGN (Kornfeld and Mellman 1989). In addition, there is extensive mixing of contents among late endosomes (Desjardins 1995). In general, late endosomes are nearer to the centre of the cell than sorting endosomes, and the late endosomes have the microtubule minus-end-directed motor, dynein, associated with them (Aniento *et al.* 1993; Oda *et al.* 1995).

Lysosomes

Lysosomes are heterogeneous in their morphology and are thus harder to categorize by appearance (Holtzman 1989; Kornfeld and Mellman 1989). Typically, a lysosome, when viewed by electron microscopy, appears as an electron-dense organelle (the so-called 'dense body'), delimited by a single membrane (Holtzman 1989). However, these structures are often similar in size to other intracellular compartments such as late endosomes (Holtzman 1989; Kornfeld and Mellman 1989). In addition, lysosomes may have forms other than dense bodies (Holtzman 1989). Among the variety of lysosomal shapes are the multilamellar structures seen in type II alveolar cells (Holtzman 1989) and the long tubular lysosomes seen in macrophages (Swanson *et al.* 1987). Some of the electron-dense lysosomes show a clear region ('halo') just inside the organelle membrane when viewed by electron microscopy (Holtzman 1989). This region is rich in carbohydrates and is believed to protect the lysosomal membrane proteins from degradation by the acidic hydrolases (Holtzman 1989).

Acidification

Various endosomes have characteristic pH values that are essential for their proper functioning. Extensive characterization of the pH of endocytic compartments has been carried out in CHO cells (Yamashiro and Maxfield 1987; Presley *et al.* 1993) and in other fibroblasts (Tycko and Maxfield 1982; Sipe and Murphy 1987). In CHO cells, sorting endosomes have a pH of 5.9–6.0, and the recycling compartment has a pH of 6.4–6.5. The late endosomes containing lysosomally directed markers such as fluorescent dextrans and α_2-M have a pH below 6.0, and the pH of lysosomes in these cells is between 5.0 and 5.5. The pH values for endosomes in CHO cells are shown in a schematic diagram (Fig. 1.1) and are also presented in Table 1.1. Endosomes in rat hippocampal neurones also exhibit acidic pH (5.0–6.5), although passage through these highly acidic compartments does not appear to be mandatory for the endocytic phase of synaptic vesicle cycling (Augenbraun *et al.* 1993).

One of the major functions of endosomes is to dissociate ligands from their receptors, after which many receptors are recycled to the cell surface, while the ligands are degraded. This is achieved, in a large part, by the low pH in the compartment. Several ligands, including insulin, EGF, LDL, and α_2M, dissociate from their receptors in the sorting endosomes (Mukherjee *et al.* 1997). Also, at the acidic pH of sorting endosomes, iron is released from Tf, while apo-transferrin remains bound to its receptor in the acidic endosomes (Dautry-Varsat *et al.* 1983; Mukherjee *et al.* 1997). Some ligands require a pH lower than that found in sorting endosomes to be released from their receptors. For example, mannose-6-phosphate (M6P) ligands are released from the CI-MPR at about pH 5.8 and lower, i.e. predominantly in the late endosomes.

Endosomal acidity is achieved by an ATP-dependent proton pump (vacuolar H^+-ATPase) which is a member of a family of multi-subunit proton pumps (al Awqati 1986; Gluck 1993) (Chapter 9). Early endosomes, but not late endosomes, contain the Na^+/K^+-ATPase (Cain *et al.* 1989; van Weert *et al.* 1995). The Na^+/K^+-ATPase would generate an inside positive membrane potential which would make it more difficult for the electrogenic vacuolar H^+-ATPase to pump protons into the endosome. Its presence in early sorting endosomes is thought to be required for their relatively low acidification (Sato and Toyama 1994). Other ion transporters such as chloride channels may also affect and regulate the pH of endosomes (al Awqati 1986). A suggested mechanism by which changes in membrane potential can affect the steady-state pH of an endosome involves changes in the coupling between proton translocation and ATP hydrolysis by the vacuolar proton pump as the proton concentration and/or positive charge in the compartment builds up (Gluck 1993).

The endocytic process

Plasma membrane distribution of molecules as determinants of internalization

It should be noted that although receptor–ligand complexes that localize at the clathrin-coated pits are rapidly internalized, these are not the only molecules that are endocytosed into a cell. In fact, almost all plasma membrane-bound molecules are internalized into cells, albeit at varying rates. It appears that many of these molecules just enter forming pits by default and are neither enriched nor depleted from these regions. There are, however, molecules that are internalized more slowly than would be expected from random incorporation into forming vesicles. For example, the influenza haemagglutinin (HA) molecule has been shown to be internalized at a rate significantly slower than the bulk membrane internalization (Lazarovits and Roth 1988).

Receptor-mediated endocytosis of molecules that concentrate in the coated pits leads to their very efficient clearance from the cell surface. Clathrin-coated pits are approximately 150 nm invaginated structures on the plasma membrane that occupy approximately 2% of the plasma membrane surface on human fibroblasts and on rat hepatocytes. Some receptors are constitutively concentrated in coated pits (e.g. the LDL receptor), but others become concentrated upon ligand binding (e.g. the EGF receptor or the Fc receptor type II) (Mukherjee *et al.* 1997). Interestingly, a study using time lapse imaging of GFP-clathrin showed that pits pinch off roughly about one per minute and tend to form repeatedly at definite sites on the plasma membrane while excluding other regions (Gaidarov *et al.* 1999).

Peptide internalization motifs

Specific targeting of most receptors to coated pits occurs as a result of interactions between recognition (internalization) motifs in their cytoplasmic domains with intracellular proteins that form part of the clathrin coat (Kirchhausen 2000; Wakeham *et al.* 2000).

Two types of conserved sequences of amino acids in the cytoplasmic tails of transmembrane proteins have been shown to facilitate localization into and internalization by clathrin-coated pits associated with the plasma membrane. The best characterized of these are tetrapeptide sequence NPXY for the LDL receptor or YXRF for the Tf receptor

(Trowbridge *et al.* 1993), often with an additional bulky hydrophobic group (that need not be aromatic) more towards the N-terminus (or in a more membrane proximal position). The structural basis for interaction of internalization motifs with adaptins has been elucidated by X-ray crystallography (Marks *et al.* 1997; Pearse *et al.* 2000).

A second type of signal for clathrin-mediated uptake includes the leucine- (Letourneur and Klausner 1992) and lysine- (Itin *et al.* 1995) based cytoplasmic sequences. Several proteins (e.g. the CD4 antigen or the human $FcIIB_2$ receptor) that participate in receptor-mediated endocytosis, but lack a tyrosine-based internalization motif, contain di-leucine internalization motifs in their cytoplasmic domains (Miettinen *et al.* 1992). It is interesting to note that while the di-leucine motif promotes the internalization of CD3γ chain of the T-cell antigen receptor (Letourneur and Klausner 1992), it seems to be ineffective in the internalization of CI-MPR (Lobel *et al.* 1989). Very recently, it has been shown that for CI-MPR as well as its cation-dependent counterpart (CD-MPR), the di-leucine motif in fact plays a role in Golgi to late endosome sorting, by binding to a novel class of adaptor-like proteins, called Golgi-localized, gamma-ear-containing, ARF-binding proteins (GGAs) (Puertollano *et al.* 2001; Zhu *et al.* 2001).

Other internalization mechanisms

Lipid domains and lipid-linked proteins

All endocytic processes necessarily involve the uptake of lipid components of the membrane. In many cases, these lipids and lipid-linked proteins enter membrane invaginations non-selectively and are passively incorporated in the forming endocytic compartment. By such mechanisms, lipid components would be in newly formed endocytic compartments at the same relative concentrations found in the plasma membrane, and this non-selective uptake would result in the clearance of lipids at a rate similar to the overall rate of membrane surface clearance. However, in several cases, it is clear that lipids and lipid-linked proteins do not randomly incorporate into coated pits or other endocytic structures. They may be selectively included or excluded. For example, a glycosphingolipid, GM1, has been shown to be predominantly localized in caveolae by ultrastructural studies (Parton 1994).

The Shiga toxin produced by *Shigella dysenteriae 1* provides an interesting example of receptor-mediated endocytosis via a glycosphingolipid receptor on the plasma membrane. The binding of the toxin causes aggregation of its glycosphingolipid receptors in clathrin-coated pits, and the toxin-bound receptor aggregate is then endocytosed (Sandvig *et al.* 1989). It is possible that this internalization involves the interaction of the glycosphingolipid receptor with a transmembrane protein that contains an internalization motif. Alternatively, self-association of these glycosphingolipids may give rise to aggregates that have a preference for coated pit localization. There is evidence for a similar localization in the coated pits of the complex between urokinase and its type-1 inhibitor, bound to the glycosylphosphatidylinositol (GPI)-linked urokinase receptor (uPAR), due to an interaction of uPAR with the α-2-macroglobulin receptor and glycoprotein 330 (Kjoller *et al.* 1995). It was suggested recently that in some cell types, a GFP–GPI construct as well as a proportion of cholera and Shiga toxins (subunit B of both) is endocytosed independent of the clathrin machinery and then delivered to the Golgi complex (Nichols *et al.* 2001). Both clathrin-dependent and clathrin-independent internalization pathways have also been shown for sphingolipid analogues (Chen *et al.* 1997; Puri *et al.* 2001).

It is possible that specific partitioning of some membrane proteins into specialized membrane domains is a mechanism for reducing the rate of their uptake by clathrin-mediated endocytosis (Ghosh and Webb 1994; Simson *et al.* 1995). For example, alternatively spliced FcRγII-B1 differs from FcRγII-B2 in having an in-frame insertion of 47 amino acids in the cytoplasmic domain. When both isoforms are separately transfected into receptor-negative fibroblasts, FcRγII-B2 is efficiently endocytosed through coated pits, while FcRγII-B1 is actively excluded from these pits. A tail-minus FcRII mutant is neither enriched nor specifically depleted from the coated pits, whereas transplanting the insert to the carboxy terminus of the FcRγII-B2 tail results in an almost complete inhibition of coated pit localization (Miettinen *et al.* 1992). Similarly, chimeras of the influenza HA (which is normally internalized very slowly into cells) containing foreign transmembrane domains, either alone or in addition to foreign cytoplasmic domains, were endocytosed at nearly the rate for the bulk membrane, whereas a single tyrosine mutation in its cytoplasmic domain increased its rate of endocytosis to approach those obtained for efficiently endocytosed receptors (Lazarovits and Roth 1988). Interestingly, FcRγII-B1 (Miettinen *et al.* 1992), influenza HA (Lin *et al.* 1998), as well as several crosslinked GPI-anchored proteins (Harder *et al.* 1998; Ilangumaran and Hoessli 1998; Schroeder *et al.* 1998) are all localized in the cold triton-insoluble raft-like domains, and this localization may interfere with their efficient internalization via the clathrin-mediated pathway.

Another example of non-random internalization of lipids was shown using concentration-dependent excimer (excited state dimer) formation which shifts the fluorescence emission of a short-chain BODIPY-sphingomyelin analogue (Chen *et al.* 1997). The plasma membrane was labelled at a concentration low enough so that it had no excimers, but within 7 s of endocytosis, a fraction of the endosomes contained BODIPY excimers, indicating that the BODIPY-lipid had become concentrated in these endosomes. The lipid analogues may have segregated into enriched domains just prior to endocytosis, or a subset of the endosomes may have segregated these analogues into domains, giving rise to excimers. In either case, the lipid became concentrated into some type of domains within seconds of endocytosis.

The inclusion into forming phagosomes of two fluorescent lipid analogues with identical head groups, $DiIC_{16}(3)$ and *FAST*DiI, was compared (Pierini *et al.* 1996). $DiIC_{16}(3)$ has long and saturated tails that prefer to reside in more ordered lipid domains, whereas *FAST*DiI has unsaturated tails that preferentially partition into disordered regions. During the phagocytosis of 6 micrometre beads, rat basophilic leukaemia cells specifically excluded $DiIC_{16}(3)$, but not *FAST*DiI, from the forming phagosomes. Thus, there are several examples of preferential partitioning of certain lipids into vesicles forming at the plasma membrane. In the comparison between the DiI analogues, partitioning between the coexisting domains of varying fluidities appears to be one determinant of this sorting.

Ubiquitination

Protein ubiquitination occurs via an amide linkage of the carboxyterminal of a 76-residue protein, ubiquitin, to the ϵ-amino groups of lysyl residues of target proteins. Often, several ubiquitin molecules form a chain, and poly-ubiquitinated proteins are specifically targeted for degradation by the 26S protease complex, whose catalytic core comprises a 20S protease complex termed the proteasome (Ciechanover 1994). A distinct process, involving transfer of a single ubiquitin, can lead to regulated endocytosis of cell-surface proteins and delivery to the lysosomes or vacuoles in both yeast (Hicke and Riezman 1996; Soetens *et al.* 2001) and mammalian cells (Wiley and Burke 2001). In fact, such ubiquitin-mediated internalization possibly modulates signalling by various tyrosine kinase receptors in mammalian cells. Specifically, signalling upon internalization is enhanced for TrkA and NGF and diminished for the insulin receptor, whereas certain specific signals are enhanced while others are diminished for the EGF receptor (Wiley and Burke 2001). It is interesting to note that ubiquitin shares a specific structural motif with other proteins implicated in clathrin-mediated endocytosis, including Eps15 and Epsin (Hofmann and Falquet 2001), as well as a di-leucine internalization motif (Nakatsu *et al.* 2000).

Internalization, vesiculation, and uncoating of the internalized vesicles

The mechanism by which the ends of the coated pit membranes fuse and eventually pinch off as coated vesicles remains unclear. It is ATP-dependent, since in ATP-depleted cells, the coated pits invaginate and sequester receptors efficiently, but vesicle budding is blocked (Schmid and Carter 1990). Dynamin is a GTPase whose role in vesicle budding during endocytosis and the possible mechanisms of achieving this fission have been investigated (Sever *et al.* 2000). This protein can self-assemble into a helical structure that wraps around lipids, and this may help pinch the necks of forming vesicles (Koenig and Ikeda 1989). A role has been proposed for the actin cytoskeleton as a downstream target of dynamin action, possibly via interaction with profilin and other binding partners of dynamin (Qualmann *et al.* 2000). Several accessory factors have been implicated in the dynamin-mediated scission of the invaginated coated pit. Primary among them are: synpatojanin, a polyphosphoinositide phosphatase that regulates the pool of phosphoinositides important for endocytosis (McPherson *et al.* 1996); amphiphysin and endophilin, multifunctional adaptors that facilitate the recruitment of coat proteins to the lipid bilayer as well as the recruitment of dynamin and synaptojanin to the coat (Wiggle and Mcmahon 1998; Schmidt *et al.* 1999); intersectin, a large, multidomain scaffold protein (Hussain *et al.* 1999); syndapin or pacsin, which helps link the endocytic machinery with the actin cytoskeleton (Qualmann and Kelly 2000); epsin and eps15, which bind each other as well as other coat components (Sengar *et al.* 1999). It has been proposed that the collapse of the membrane neck of a budding vesicle is driven by an interplay between the dynamin collar and the bending elastic energy of the neck membrane (Kozlov 2001). In fact, a change in the curvature of the membrane may be achieved, at least in part, by the transfer of an arachidonate to lysophosphatidic acid by the lysophosphatidic acid acyl transferase activity of endophilin 1 (Schmidt *et al.* 1999).

After receptors and their ligands are brought into the cell via clathrin-coated pits, the vesicles are uncoated by a 70 kDa ATP-dependent heat shock protein cognate (Braell *et al.* 1984; Schmid 1997). Another uncharacterized factor is needed to dissociate the adaptors from the membrane (Hannan *et al.* 1998).

Itineraries of endocytosed molecules

Entry and exit from sorting endosomes

Molecules that enter cells via clathrin-coated pits can be found in sorting endosomes within 1 min after the vesicles pinch off from the surface (Dunn *et al.* 1989). Sorting endosomes are short-lived organelles with a half-life of roughly 8 min (Dunn and Maxfield 1992). The kinetics of accumulation of various molecules in sorting endosomes indicates that there are many fusions that continue to deliver newly endocytosed molecules during this time. Also, during this time, material destined for recycling continues to leave the SE for the ERC or the plasma membrane.

Rapid recycling to the plasma membrane

Although the rate of recycling of an internalized membrane protein or lipid after delivery to the ERC has been estimated to be 10–12 min (Mayor *et al.* 1993) or slower, several studies have indicated that at least a fraction of the internalized molecules may recycle much faster. For example, more than 25% of a fluorescent lipid analogue, C_6-NBD-SM, was found to be returned to the cell surface with a half-time of about 2 min after being internalized by CHO cells (Presley *et al.* 1993). Similarly, about 50% of internalized sucrose is released from fibroblasts back into the medium with a half-time of 6–8 min (Besterman *et al.* 1981). A more precise recent study using several lipid analogues and a series of cell types showed that after a brief internalization pulse, 42–62% of an internalized lipid analogue recycled with a $t_{1/2}$ of 1–2 min (Hao and Maxfield 2000). Furthermore, it was shown that this rapid recycling pathway involves passage through the sorting endosomes. It is possible that the rapid component of recycling was not detected in earlier experimental protocols, since they were not specifically designed to examine the kinetics of rapid processes. In some cells, the rapid recycling is essential for biological functions. For instance, in rabbit reticulocytes, the high rate of iron uptake is sustained by recycling Tf receptors with a half-time of about 90 s, with efficient stripping of the iron from Tf in acidified endosomes (Iacopetta and Morgan 1983). Endocytic membrane recycling in renal proximal tubule was found to occur with a $t_{1/2}$ of 1.5 min (Birn *et al.* 1993). This process appears to help recover small molecules such as vitamins from the urine.

The sorting decision

Understanding the mechanisms for high-fidelity sorting of internalized ligands and receptors to their correct destinations has been a major goal of cell biologists. As discussed below, sorting depends on molecular recognition between receptors and other proteins, on the physical properties (e.g. shape or pH) of the endocytic organelles, on the regulation of fusion and vesicle formation by endosomes, and on the molecular properties of the ligands and receptors. In general, the recycling mechanisms are more efficient than lysosomal targeting. For example, each LDL receptor recycles about 150 times (Goldstein *et al.* 1985), each asialoglycoprotein receptor close to 250 times (Schwartz and Rup 1983), and each Tf receptor up to 300 times (Omary and Trowbridge 1981). On the other hand, between 25 and 50% of internalized asialoglycoprotein escapes degradation in the lysosomes and is returned intact to the cell surface in HepG2 cells (Simmons and Schwartz 1984). Also, approximately 20% of internalized α_2M is returned undegraded during each endocytic passage in CHO cells (Yamashiro *et al.* 1984), and approximately 40% of internalized insulin is recycled and released (Levy and Olefsky 1987).

Physical sorting

Physical sorting is based on properties such as the geometry and pH of the organelle, association of molecules with the membrane or the lumenal fluid, size of particles, solubility, etc. The accumulation of LDL in the sorting endosome is an example of physical sorting. Once they enter the acidified endosomes, LDL molecules (and many other ligands) are released from their receptors, and there is no evidence that binding to other proteins plays any role in their ultimate delivery to late endosomes and lysosomes. Indeed, soluble markers such as fluorescein isothiocyanate–dextran accumulate in sorting endosomes and are delivered to lysosomes by the same mechanism as LDL. The accumulation of LDL in sorting endosomes can be accounted for by the retention of most of the fluid volume in the vacuolar portion of the tubulovesicular sorting endosomes. If recycling components bud off as narrow diameter tubules from the sorting endosomes, very little volume will be carried off towards the recycling pathway. Furthermore, the diameter of LDL molecules (approximately 22 nm) (Brown and Goldstein 1986; Chapman 1986) is nearly half the internal diameter of the tubules associated with sorting endosomes, and the excluded volume for such a large particle may aid in the sorting process.

If retention of soluble molecules in sorting endosomes is based on physical sorting, what about the rapid and efficient export of membrane components? It appears that physical sorting is also a major determinant of this process. No specific peptide sequences have been identified that are required for rapid, efficient removal from sorting endosomes. Many mutant receptors with very short cytoplasmic domains (as little as four amino acids) (Jing *et al.* 1990) as well as lipid analogues (Mukherjee and Maxfield 2000) and GPI-anchored proteins (Mayor *et al.* 1998) have been shown to be internalized slowly but recycled efficiently by cells. This has led to the hypothesis that recycling constitutes the default pathway for the bulk of the internalized plasma membrane, and active sorting would be necessary to target membrane components to alternate locations, such as late endosomes/lysosomes or the TGN. It is not known whether there is sorting to determine which molecules return to the cell surface directly after exiting the sorting endosome and which are delivered to the ERC. The lipid probes examined so far follow both routes.

Physical characteristics may play a partial role in the retention of certain membrane components in sorting endosomes. For example, EGF receptor is found on the inward invaginations of MVBs (Haigler *et al.* 1979). This removes the receptor from the main outer membrane lining the lumen of the endosome, and thus it is not available for removal via tubule budding.

Membrane domains/rafts in endocytosis

A different sort of physical basis for the retention of membrane molecules in the sorting endosome would be the existence of specialized microenvironments or domains in the membrane (Mukherjee and Maxfield 2000; Gruenberg 2001). It is known that crosslinking a recycling receptor with antibodies will redirect it towards the lysosome (Mellman and Plunter 1984). This implies that aggregation and oligomerization of proteins can play a role in sorting endosome retention. An aggregated complex in a membrane is a specialized membrane sub-domain that is excluded from the default recycling pathway. A simple explanation would be that this domain is too large and/or rigid to be included in the sorting endosome's tubules. The size of a crosslinked aggregate can affect its sorting. Oligomerized Tf (10-mers) were directed to the recycling compartment, but very large Tf multimers were directed out of the recycling pathway and degraded, similar to the effects of receptor crosslinking by antibodies (Marsh *et al.* 1995). The redirection of crosslinked Tf receptors was not dependent on the cytoplasmic domain.

Lipid acyl chain properties and the resultant partitioning preferences also regulate the sorting and trafficking of lipid analogues in sorting endosomes (Mukherjee *et al.* 1999).

Disordered domain preferring lipid analogues includes $DiIC_{12}(3)$ and *FAST*DiI, which have short and unsaturated tails, respectively. Both of these lipid analogues exited the sorting endosomes rapidly and efficiently. Conversely, $DiIC_{16}(3)$ with long and saturated tails was retained in the sorting endosomes and then trafficked to the late endosomes/lysosomes. These results are consistent with other observations. While the short-chain phosphatidylcholine and sphingomyelin analogues (C_6-NBD-PC and C_6-NBD-SM) have been shown to recycle (Koval and Pagano 1989), rhodamine-labelled phosphatidylethanolamine (Kok *et al.* 1990) and several naturally occurring glycosphingolipids (van Echten and Sandhoff 1993) that contain long, saturated acyl chains are delivered to the late endosomal pathway.

Differential fluidity and curvature-based domains can be used to understand the mechanisms of lipid sorting in the sorting endosomes (Mukherjee *et al.* 1999). The sorting endosomes have a tubulovesicular morphology, with a vesicular region (often containing inner involutions), from which long, narrow-diameter tubules emanate (Mukherjee *et al.* 1997). It has been previously demonstrated that while the tubules of the sorting endosomes repeatedly pinch off to deliver material to the ERC, the vesicular region, in time, gives rise to the late endosomes (Mukherjee *et al.* 1997). Thus, the differential trafficking of the lipid analogues would correspond to a situation in which the long-chain lipids are retained in the vesicular part of the sorting endosomes and are prevented from entering into the tubules that carry material towards the recycling pathway.

Preferential retention of certain lipids has been demonstrated in the forming late endosomes. These organelles have an extensive system of internal vesicles and membrane whorls, and the internal *versus* the limiting membranes of these organelles have been shown to sort proteins and lipids differently (Mukherjee *et al.* 1997). Several long-chain, saturated glycosphingolipids are enriched in these inner involutions (Wilkening *et al.* 1998). Furthermore, a negatively charged lipid, LBPA, has been recently shown to be concentrated in the internal membranes (Kobayashi *et al.* 1998). Interestingly, these LBPA-enriched internal membranes, and not the limiting membranes of late endosomes, were shown to be critical to the correct sorting of other transmembrane proteins such as MPR from the late endosomes to the TGN (Kobayashi *et al.* 1998). Such retention is severely altered in lysosomal storage disorders such as Neimann Pick C (NPC), where a mutation in a transmembrane protein, NPC1, causes an overaccumulation of cholesterol and other lipids and proteins, resulting in a log-jam of late endocytic trafficking (Mukherjee and Maxfield 1999; Lusa *et al.* 2001) (See Chapter 9). Similar mechanisms appear to operate for a large number of sphingolipid storage disorders (Puri *et al.* 1999).

Cholesterol-mediated modulation of trafficking has also been reported for the GPI-anchored proteins in the ERC (Mayor *et al.* 1998), as well as for the delivery to the TGN either from the SE/ERC or from the LE (Kobayashi *et al.* 1999; Grimmer *et al.* 2000). Recently, cholesterol was reported to play a major role in the transport of cholera toxin from endosomes to the Golgi apparatus in hippocampal neurones (Shogomori and Futerman 2001).

Iterative fractionation: a mechanism for high-efficiency physical sorting

The tubulovesicular geometry of the sorting endosome provides a partial explanation for the efficient sorting of membrane components. Up to 80% of the sorting endosome's membrane area is in its tubules (Marsh *et al.* 1986; Griffiths *et al.* 1989). This means that the majority of the lipid in the sorting endosome membrane should be in the tubules. If there is no impediment to mobility for the sorting endosome's membrane proteins, they should be distributed uniformly throughout its surface, and the majority of these receptors should be in the tubules. Budding off of these tubules will carry off a high fraction of the diffusible membrane components and relatively little volume.

The geometrical mechanism is not sufficient to account for the high efficiency of recycling in a single sorting operation. However, if tubule budding is repeated many times during the lifetime of the sorting endosome, highly efficient recycling can be achieved by this simple physical mechanism (Rome 1985; Dunn *et al.* 1989). In fact, the kinetic measurements of ligand accumulation into and exit from sorting endosomes provide direct evidence for exactly this type of iterative fractionation process (Dunn *et al.* 1989; Mayor *et al.* 1993; Ghosh *et al.* 1994). For several minutes, vesicles carrying newly endocytosed molecules are delivered to sorting endosomes. At the same time, tubules continue to bud from them. With each tubule budding from the sorting endosome, more of the recycling receptors are removed, and the sorting endosome becomes more enriched in the released ligand. Thus, while the recycling receptors are removed from the sorting endosome, the released ligands accumulate in it.

Signal-mediated sorting

Although most membrane components efficiently recycle back to the cell surface, some of them are preferentially targeted to the late endosome/lysosome pathway. If recycling of membrane components is largely a default phenomenon, signals would be required for the retention of these components in the sorting endosomes until they are delivered to the late endosomes. Although less is known about the nature of signals required for sorting endosome retention, sequences on the retained proteins have been proposed to play a role in trafficking to late endosomes. For example, chimeras consisting of the LDL receptor's cytoplasmic domain and the CI-MPR's transmembrane and extracellular domain colocalized with unaltered CI-MPRs in the cell (Dintzis *et al.* 1994). This suggested that the CI-MPR has a retention signal in its extracellular or transmembrane domain. In addition, a cytoplasmic region containing a di-leucine sequence has been suggested to play a role in the trafficking of the CI-MPR to late endosomes (Johnson and Kornfeld 1992). Sequences in the EGF receptor have also been suggested to play a role in targeting the receptor to late endosomes and lysosomes (Honegger *et al.* 1987). In a study designed to understand the structural requirements for the internalization and lysosomal targeting of the major histocompatibility complex class II invariant chain, it was found that specific di-leucine sequences on the cytoplasmic tail as well as sequences in the transmembrane region differentially affected internalization and lysosomal targeting (Kang *et al.* 1998). While one of the two di-leucine motifs was necessary and sufficient for internalization, either were sufficient for lysosomal targeting. The transmembrane sequences, on the other hand, were only responsible for lysosomal localization and not internalization. Similarly, in a study on the cytoplasmic domain sequence requirements for internalization and TGN localization of the endoprotease, furin, it was shown that while both a classical tyrosine-based motif and an acidic cluster sequence (SDSEEDE) were responsible for internalization, the acidic cluster alone was responsible for the retrieval of furin from the endosomes to the TGN (Simmen *et al.* 1999).

Delivery from sorting endosomes to late endosomes

The passage of material from early sorting endosomes to late endosomes has been an area of active research. Two general models were proposed (Gruenberg and Maxfield 1995). In one model (vesicle shuttle model), the early endosomes would be stable organelles from which transport vesicles would pinch off to deliver endosome contents to late endosomes. This would be similar to vesicle traffic mechanisms that operate between the endoplasmic reticulum and the Golgi apparatus. In the second model (maturation model), the entire contents of the early sorting endosomes would be transformed into late endosomes. Although there are some uncertainties about the detailed mechanisms (Gruenberg and Maxfield 1995), essentially all the volume contents of an early sorting endosome move as a unit as they are delivered to late endosomes. There is vesicular budding from the early sorting endosomes, but this is mainly to deliver recycling components to the ERC. Thus, the behaviour of the endosome contents is consistent with the predictions of a maturation model. Although no contents can be detected as a remnant after a sorting endosome has matured, it is not known whether the sorting endosome truly forms *de novo* or whether there is a nucleating site for the formation of new sorting endosomes such as a remnant from an earlier sorting endosome. Microtubules are required for the delivery of molecules from early endosomes to late endosomes (Gruenberg *et al.* 1989). Endosome carrier vesicles (ECVs), a vesicle population with the properties of the transition intermediate between early endosomes and late endosomes, can be isolated from cells that have been treated with microtubule-disrupting agents (Gruenberg *et al.* 1989).

It is interesting to note that changes in fusion compatibility of endosomes change at approximately the same time that the pH drops by about 0.5 pH units. Both of these are indicative of a change in membrane protein composition, but it is unclear what the relationship is between these two changes in properties. Bafilomycin A_1, a vacuolar H^+-ATPase inhibitor, slows the progression from sorting endosomes to late endosomes to lysosomes (van Weert *et al.* 1995; Aniento *et al.* 1996), suggesting that changes in pH may be required for some of these transformations. On the other hand, the pH of the organelles will be determined by their composition of transmembrane ion transporters, channels, and pumps, so some changes in membrane composition presumably precede the changes in pH.

The kinetics of maturation of sorting endosomes are consistent with a stochastic process that happens relatively abruptly (i.e. there is no slow diminution in fusion accessibility with newly endocytosed material) (Dunn and Maxfield 1992). One possibility is that the sorting endosomes attach to microtubules and are moved away from a site in the cell periphery where they are most available for fusion with newly internalized vesicles coming from the plasma membrane. If tubule budding continued after the sorting endosome moved, this would change the overall membrane composition of the organelle. Among the molecules removed and not replenished by new endocytosis would be the Na^+/K^+-ATPase which helps block full acidification of the endosomes (Cain *et al.* 1989; Fuchs *et al.* 1989). In turn, changes in organelle pH could lead to changes in protein conformation, some of which could affect the cytoplasmic domains of transmembrane proteins, leading to altered interactions with proteins that control vesicle docking and fusion. Although association with microtubules, changes in pH, and changes in membrane composition are all known to be important for transformation to late endosomes, the order of these changes and their detailed roles are not known.

Trafficking through the endocytic recycling compartment

The recycling compartment was detected over a decade ago (Hopkins 1983; Yamashiro *et al.* 1984) and was thought to be a way station on the route back to the plasma membrane for recycling receptors. However, recent results show that this organelle plays a more complex role in membrane trafficking, and it has sorting capabilities of its own.

Recycling to the plasma membrane

After leaving the sorting endosomes, most membrane proteins and lipids are found in the tubules of the ERC (Stoorvogel *et al.* 1988; Dunn *et al.* 1989; Mayor *et al.* 1993; Ghosh *et al.* 1994). In CHO cells, recycling Tf receptors exit from the recycling compartment with a half-time of about 10 min (Mayor *et al.* 1993), which closely matches the overall half-time for the exit of Tf from cells after steady-state labelling (McGraw and Maxfield 1990). Exit from the recycling compartment is the slowest step on the major recycling itinerary, and consequently the ERC is the major intracellular localization of internalized Tf receptors (Dunn *et al.* 1989; Mayor *et al.* 1993). In some cells, the ERC is highly concentrated in the peri-centriolar region (Yamashiro *et al.* 1984; Hopkins *et al.* 1994), but in other cell types, the ERC is widely dispersed throughout the cell. The distribution of the ERC depends, in part, on the distribution of a stable pool of microtubules (Lin *et al.* 2001), but the kinetics of export from the ERC to the plasma membrane do not seem to be related to the physical distribution of the organelle. For example, in Hep2 human carcinoma cells, the ERC is observed as small tubules throughout the cell, but the overall kinetics of Tf exit from sorting endosomes, delivery to the ERC, and exit from the ERC to the plasma membrane are very similar to the kinetics observed in CHO cells (Ghosh *et al.* 1994).

In non-polarized cells such as fibroblasts, exit from the recycling compartment and entry to the plasma membrane do not depend on specific positive signals. Recycling rates have been measured for several mutated Tf receptors, including some with only three amino acids in the cytoplasmic domain, and no differences in the rates of return to the plasma membrane could be detected (Jing *et al.* 1990; McGraw and Maxfield 1990). Furthermore, some fluorescent lipid analogues such as C_6-NBD-SM exit the recycling compartment and return to the plasma membrane with kinetics that are indistinguishable from those of the recycling Tf receptors (Mayor *et al.* 1993). A rab protein, rab11 (Ullrich *et al.* 1996), as well as RME-1, an Eps 15 homology (EH)-domain protein (Lin *et al.* 2001), have been shown to regulate recycling out of the ERC.

The recycling compartment not only returns material to the plasma membrane, but it can also send membrane components back to sorting endosomes in a retrograde manner (Ghosh and Maxfield 1995). Retrograde traffic is observed elsewhere in the cell (e.g. Golgi to endoplasmic reticulum) and is used to retrieve errantly trafficked proteins and maintain the distinct protein compositions of various organelles. Retrograde traffic within the early endosomal system may play a similar role in maintaining the distinct protein compositions of various endosomal compartments.

Sorting and regulation of recycling

Studies using covalently linked oligomers of transferrin (Tf_{10}), which bound approximately six Tf receptors at a time, revealed important aspects of sorting in the recycling compartment (Marsh *et al.* 1995). Tf_{10} was endocytosed and delivered to the recycling compartment where it was retained for a long time (exit $t_{1/2}$ of about 1 h). This retention was not dependent on the Tf receptor's cytoplasmic tail, since a mutant receptor lacking the tail was still retained when bound to Tf_{10}. Newly internalized Tf could enter and leave the tubules containing the Tf_{10} with normal kinetics while Tf_{10} was retained. This implies that the recycling compartment can sort Tf from Tf_{10} and retain the latter. The long retention of Tf_{10} demonstrated that the recycling compartment is long lived.

The retention of Tf receptor oligomers in the recycling compartment may be based on the formation of microdomains. Consistent with a role for such domains, it has been found that GPI-anchored proteins have slowed exit from the ERC (Mayor *et al.* 1998). The exit kinetics of the GPI-anchored folate receptor and another GPI-anchored protein, decay-accelerating factor (DAF), were examined in transfected CHO cell lines. Although their clearance from the surface was slow ($t_{1/2}$ approximately 30 min), both of these proteins entered the ERC. Their exit from the cell back to the cell surface was about 2.5-fold slower than the Tf receptor or C_6-NBD-SM in the same cells. When cellular cholesterol levels were reduced by about 40% by growing the cells in lipid-depleted serum with cholesterol synthesis inhibitors, the rate of recycling of the GPI-anchored proteins was increased to the same rate as Tf receptors and C_6-NBD-SM. The cholesterol lowering by this method had no effect on the internalization or externalization kinetics of Tf. These data suggest that cholesterol-rich microdomains may form in the recycling compartment, as has been proposed for the TGN (Mukherjee and Maxfield 2000), and these domains may play a role in the sorting of GPI-anchored proteins in both compartments. Studies with dehydroergosterol, a naturally occurring fluorescent cholesterol analogue, indicate that the ERC is a sterol-rich organelle (Mukherjee *et al.* 1998).

Intracellular retention of certain receptors may serve important physiological functions. For example, the ERC is one place where the insulin-responsive GLUT4 glucose transporter and the insulin-regulated aminopeptidase (IRAP) are retained (Lampson *et al.* 2000). Insulin regulation of GLUT4 trafficking underlies the role that adipose tissue and muscle play in the maintenance of whole-body glucose homoeostasis. A di-leucine sequence as well as a cluster of acidic amino acids have been shown to be required for this dynamic retention of IRAP in the ERC of fibroblasts (Johnson *et al.* 2001).

Passage through late endosomes and delivery to lysosomes

Sorting and trafficking through late endosomes are less well understood than in the early endosomal system. It is known that there is extensive mixing of the contents among late endosomes (Desjardins 1995). Mannose-6-phosphate receptors are concentrated in the TGN and delivered to late endosomes. In the acidic late endosomes, the enzymes dissociate from the MPRs, and the unoccupied receptors are recycled back to the TGN (Kornfeld 1992).

The CD-MPR has several sequences in its cytoplasmic tail mediating its intracellular traffic. It contains a di-leucine motif responsible for recruitment into TGN clathrin pits and two signals, one, a tetra-peptide motif with tyrosine, necessary for rapid internalization from the cell surface (Rohrer *et al.* 1995), and the other, a five-amino acid sequence, that is reported to be necessary for the prevention of its delivery to lysosomes. This motif contains two cysteines that are sites of palmitoylation (Schweizer *et al.* 1996), and modifications that prevent palmitoylation cause delivery to lysosomes. The transmembrane domain may also play a role in preventing delivery to lysosomes (Rohrer *et al.* 1995). Thus, this receptor may have specific positive signals that are required to prevent trafficking to lysosomes, implying that lysosomal delivery might otherwise be a default pathway. However, it is also possible that the deletions and mutations may have altered the receptors to unintentionally create a positive signal (e.g. aggregation or binding to another protein) that causes retention in the late endosomes. Further experiments will be required to test these possibilities. AP2-containing coats have been reported to assemble on mature lysosomes, and these coats have been proposed to regulate retrograde membrane traffic out of the lysosomal compartment (Traub *et al.* 1996).

Digestion and delivery to lysosomes

The delivery of late endosomal content to lysosomes is thought to occur by the fusion of late endosomes with pre-existing lysosomes. In addition, evidence for bi-directional traffic of soluble material between lysosomes and late endosomes has been reported (Jahraus *et al.* 1994). Transient fusions of lysosomes with late endosomes have been shown to account for this exchange of material between these two compartments. Overall, the precise mode of delivery of material from the late endosome to the lysosome is not well understood. Transport from late endosomes to lysosomes depends on the vacuolar proton pump, and neutralization of pH by bafilomycin A_1 prevents this transport (van Weert *et al.* 1995). Delivery of internalized molecules to MPR-negative lysosomes is relatively slow in many cell types. For example, in NRK cells, it required chase periods of a few hours to deliver most α_2-M-colloidal gold to lysosomes (Griffiths *et al.* 1988). By comparison, degradation of α_2-M by NRK cells occurs with a half-time of about 15 min (Maxfield *et al.* 1981), indicating that the degradation must occur in MPR-positive late endosomes.

One of the best known functions of endocytic pathways is the delivery of nutrients necessary for cell sustenance and growth. Macromolecules endocytosed by either the receptor-mediated or the phagocytic pathways are ultimately digested in the late endosomes or lysosomes to small molecules (typically <1 kDa). As a result of the digestion process, the lumenal concentration of nutrients such as amino acids and sugars rises well above the cytoplasmic concentrations. This concentration gradient across the vacuolar membrane then drives diffusion of the nutrients into the cytoplasm through specific channels or carriers (Tietze *et al.* 1989; Mancini *et al.* 1991).

Traffic to the *trans*-Golgi network

Although most membrane-bound proteins and lipids are delivered to the recycling pathway via the ERC, certain proteins such as furin (Molloy *et al.* 1994) and TGN38 (Banting and Ponnambalam 1997) are instead destined to enter the TGN. Interestingly, however, these two proteins appear to take two different pathways to the TGN. While TGN38 traffics to the ERC at a rate similar to other membrane markers before trafficking to the TGN from the ERC (Ghosh *et al.* 1998), furin instead remains with the sorting endosomes as they begin to mature into late endosomes and is then delivered to the TGN, entirely bypassing the ERC (Mallet and Maxfield 1999). This latter pathway is similar to the one that has been reported for the CI-MPR, which also appears to traffic from the plasma membrane to the late endosomes and on to the TGN before being recycled out (Duncan and Kornfeld 1988). On the other hand, Shiga toxin appears to follow a trafficking itinerary very similar to TGN38, completely bypassing the late endosomes and entering the ERC exclusively on its way to the TGN (Mallard *et al.* 1998). This pathway is rab11 dependent (Wilcke *et al.* 2000) and may involve association with detergent-resistant membrane domains (Falguieres *et al.* 2001). This is in agreement with the observation that the fatty acyl chain length of Gb3, the glycolipid receptor for Shiga toxin, is important for trafficking in A431 cells (Sandvig *et al.* 1996).

It appears that certain proteins may enter the TGN via a non-clathrin-mediated pathway. The endosome to Golgi transport pathway of the plant toxin ricin has recently been reported to be independent of clathrin and of rab9 and rab11 ATPases (Iversen *et al.* 2001) and to be modulated by cellular cholesterol levels (Grimmer *et al.* 2000).

It has been widely accepted that trafficking between the TGN and the LE occurs by recruitment into coated pits at the TGN and that these coats contain clathrin and AP1. This hypothesis appeared to be well founded, given the binding of both CD- and CI-MPRs to AP1 (Glickman *et al.* 1989). However, two recent studies (Puertollano *et al.* 2001; Zhu *et al.* 2001) show that AP1 may not play a major role in this step of trafficking of the receptors, but rather, they are recruited for transport from the TGN to late endosomes by binding to a novel class of adaptor proteins, the so-called GGAs. It has been proposed that the role of AP1 may be in binding these receptors in an endosomal compartment, which would then recycle them to the TGN (Tooze 2001).

Specialized aspects of endocytosis in neurones

Neurones as polarized cells

The axonal and somatodendritic membranes contain a rather distinct protein profile, which need to be sorted and targeted correctly. Endocytic recycling pathways have been shown to play a significant role in this process (Parton *et al.* 1992). In some ways the membrane trafficking in neurones resembles polarized epithelia (Simons *et al.* 1992). In many cases, proteins that are targeted to the apical surface of polarized epithelia such as MDCK are trafficked to the axonal surface (e.g. GPI-anchored proteins and GABA transporter), whereas those that are basolaterally localized are destined to the somatodendritic surface (e.g. Tf receptor and LDL receptor) (Bradke and Dotti 1998). This rule, however, does not hold in all cases. For example, (Na,K)-ATPase is basolateral in MDCK cells, whereas it is found in both axons and dendrites of hippocampal neurones (Bradke and Dotti 1998).

Axonal endocytosis

The distribution of the endosomal–lysosomal machinery in cultured sympathetic neurones has been studied in some detail (Overly *et al.* 1995; Overly and Hollenbeck 1996). Nearly all axonal endocytosis occurs at the growth cones or presynaptic sites. These areas exhibit unimodal pH distribution of mildly acidified recycling/sorting endosomes with a mean pH of 6.3 (Augenbraun *et al.* 1993; Overly and Hollenbeck 1996). However, a much stronger organelle acidification is observed between 50 and 150 μm from the growth cone, exhibiting a trimodal pH distribution, with the three endosomal populations centred around neutral range, a middle peak (pH 5.0–6.0) and a third that is strongly acidic (pH <5.0), which possibly represent the lysosomes (Overly and Hollenbeck 1996). Such trimodal frequency distribution suggests at least two distinct acidification steps assuring the progression of endocytic organelles along the endosomal–lysosomal pathway (see the discussion above on acidification of endosomes in non-neuronal cells). Furthermore, axonal branch points represent specialized domains with splayed microtubules (which are otherwise tightly bundled in the axonal shaft) and a collection of various organelles and mRNAs. The pH of the endosomes in these regions represents a broad unimodal distribution centred around 6.4. This is consistent with the branch points being specialized endocytic domains, perhaps functioning as a meeting point between retrograde transported endocytic organelles and antergograde moving Golgi-derived delivery vesicles.

The recycling of synaptic vesicles is a very clear example of specialized, rapid, local endocytic recycling (Slepnev and De Camilli 2000). In fact, it appears that the endocytosis is not random along the growth cone but is restricted to μm-sized regions termed 'hot spots' (Roos and Kelly 1999). This appears to be similar to the recent observations of clathrin-coated pit blinking (Gaidarov *et al.* 1999). When a nerve terminal is electrically stimulated, neurotransmitter-containing docked synaptic vesicles fuse with the presynaptic plasma membrane and release their contents into the synaptic cleft. Synaptic vesicle proteins are recovered from the plasma membrane by endocytosis, and the internalized vesicles acquire a new cargo of neurotransmitters. These new synaptic vesicles accumulate near the plasma membrane and are capable of undergoing additional rounds of docking and fusion. The recycling can be quite rapid, and internalized membrane can be returned to the cell surface within 2 min or less (Betz and Wu 1995; Sankaranarayanan and Ryan 2000).

Synaptic vesicles contain rab5, which is also found on early endosomes, and members of the rab3 family (rab3A and 3C), which are specific for synaptic vesicles and secretory granules (Slepnev and De Camilli, 2000). Rab3 in synaptic vesicles has GTP bound to it, while cytosolic rab3 is associated with GDI in the GDP-bound form. Rab3A and 3C dissociate from synaptic vesicles after stimulation of synaptic vesicle exocytosis, and an increase in the GDP : GTP ratio of rab3A, results. Exocytosis occurs normally in mice lacking rab3A, following normal stimulation, but repetitive stimulation causes synaptic depression. It is believed that rab3A is not needed for synaptic vesicle docking or fusion, but it is required to maintain a normal synaptic vesicle reserve during repetitive stimulation when synaptic vesicle recycling becomes rate limiting. Rabphilin-3A is a peripheral membrane synaptic vesicle protein that binds calcium and phospholipids and is associated with rab3A and 3C. Rabphilin-3A is thought to be an effector for rab3s, and a function of rab3A and 3C is to recruit rabphilin-3A to synaptic vesicles in a GTP-dependent manner.

In summary, the growth cone is involved in rapid endocytosis of trophic signals and other environmental signals, local recycling of the plasma membrane components, and the addition and proper localization of newly arriving biosynthetic material. Most of the endosomes here are mildly acidic and are part of the early endosome system. A small fraction of endosomes exit the growth cone in what is possibly a critical sorting step and are delivered retrogradely towards the cell body. This population becomes increasingly acidified as they approach the proximal parts of the axon. Some of the acidification occurs in the axonal shaft itself (50–150 μm from the growth cone). Axonal branch points represent the second probable site for further endosome acidification.

Thus, unlike the general assumption that late endosomes/lysosomes in neurones are limited to the somatodendritic regions, the above studies by Hollenbeck and colleagues show that lysosomes do exist within the axonal shaft (as suggested by previous electron microscopic investigations). Furthermore, changes in axonal lysosomal populations during development and after injury or hyperosmotic stress have been reported (see discussion in Overly and Hollenbeck, 1996). In fact, in the case of α-motor axons, the node–paranode regions have been reported to be the local degradative centres, participating in the lysosome-mediated degradation of material being transported from the axon to the cell body (Gatzinsky 1996).

Endocytosis plays an important role in the agonist-dependent internalization and desensitization of GPCRs (Laporte *et al.* 2000; Oakley *et al.* 2001; von Zastrow, 2001). This process can be mediated by a class of cytosolic adaptor proteins called β-arrestins. These proteins bind phosphorylated GPCRs as well as clathrin and AP2, thereby recruiting these phosphorylated GPCRs to coated pits so that they are efficiently internalized. While β-arrestin dissociates from certain receptors at the plasma membrane (such as β-2-adrenergic receptors), it remains bound to other GPCRs in the endosomes. Such a persistent complex of the GPCR/β-arrestin prevents receptor resensitization. Two types of GPCR desensitization have been reported, one which involves a rapid sequence of desensitization, sequestration in intracellular endosomal vesicles, and resensitization via recycling, whereas the other is long-term downregulation involving receptor proteolysis, at least a part of which appears to occur at the lysosomes. These different pathways and the degrees of cross-talk between them have been extensively discussed in a recent review (Tsao *et al.* 2001). In fact, it has been shown that the target-derived neurotrophic factor, NGF, signals through TrkA from the so-called 'signalling endosomes', as they are delivered from the axon terminal to the cell body (Howe *et al.* 2001). This signalling is essential for survival, differentiation, and maintenance of neurones.

Axonal endocytosis has provided valuable information about the molecular regulation of endocytosis in general. For example, the *shibire* mutation in *Drosophila*, which is a temperature-sensitive defect in the re-uptake of synaptic membranes, was found to be due to a mutation in dynamin (Chen *et al.* 1991; Sever *et al.* 2000). In both neurones and fibroblasts with the mutant dynamin, long invaginations with coats at the end could be seen, suggesting that dynamin is involved in the final sealing of a coated pit. Dynamin binds to amphiphysin, another protein found in growth cones of neurones. Interestingly, amphiphysin binds to the AP2 complex of coated vesicles, and this may provide the link between dynamin and coated pits. Many of the accessory proteins crucial to synaptic vesicle docking and fusion have also been found to be similar to those used in other aspects of membrane traffic (Sever *et al.* 2000; Slepnev and De Camilli 2000).

Dendritic endocytosis

As discussed above, dendritic endocytosis has often been reported to be akin to the basolateral endocytosis in MDCK cells. In fact, a specific somatodendritic targeting signal has been found in the cytoplasmic domain of the Tf receptor (West *et al.* 1997). This somatodendritic region contains ample early endosomes and lysosomes, constituting extensive tubular networks of early endosomes and MVB-like structures (Parton *et al.* 1992). Lysosomal protease inhibition has been reported to generate meganeurites and tangle-like structures reminiscent of Alzheimer disease and, in general, of ageing brain (Bednarski *et al.* 1997). In this regard, it is noteworthy that cultured microglial cells, which can internalize amyloid-like fibrillar Aβ, degrade the Aβ very poorly (Paresce *et al.* 1997; Chung *et al.* 1999). However, this degradation can be enhanced in some cases, since it appears that microglia are responsible for degrading amyloid deposits after immunization of mice against Aβ (Schenk *et al.* 1999).

Summary

Many endocytic processes in neurones and glia share similarities with analogous processes in other cells. Thus, much that has been learned from studies in cell types such as fibroblasts or polarized epithelia can be used as a starting point for understanding similar processes in the brain. Even endocytic processes that are highly specialized (e.g. synaptic vesicle uptake and recycling) share the use of common elements such as clathrin-coated pits and dynamin for pinching off vesicles and rab and SNARE proteins for regulating vesicle docking and fusion. The geometry and function of neurones does place special requirements on the endocytic system, such as the need to recycle and refill synaptic vesicles very rapidly.

Furthermore, the length of some neurones can require vesicles to travel very long distances to reach the somatodendritic region from the axons. The long life of neurones and the special requirements for vesicle transport and recycling may make these cells especially vulnerable to defects in the endosomal/lysosomal systems.

Acknowledgements

We are grateful for support from the Ara Parseghian Medical Research Foundation and from NIH grants NS 34761 and DK27083.

References

Aniento, F., Emans, N., Griffiths, G. and Gruenberg, J. (1993). Cytoplasmic dynein-dependent vesicular transport from early to late endosomes. *J. Cell Biol.* **123**(6 Pt 1): 1373–87.

Aniento, F., Gu, F., Parton, R. G. and Gruenberg, J. (1996). An endosomal beta COP is involved in the pH dependent formation of transport vesicles destined for late endosomes. *J. Cell Biol.* **133**(1): 29–41.

Augenbraun, E., Maxfield, F. R., St. Jules, R., Setlik, W., et al. (1993). Properties of acidified compartments in hippocampal neurons. *Eur. J. Cell Biol.* **61**(1): 34–43.

al Awqati, Q. (1986). Proton translocating ATPases. *Annu. Rev. Cell Biol.* **2**: 179–99.

Banting, G. and Ponnambalam, S. (1997). TGN38 and its orthologues: roles in post-TGN vesicle formation and maintenance of TGN morphology. *Biochim. Biophys. Acta* **1355**: 209–17.

Bednarski, E., Ribak, C. and Lynch, G. (1997). Suppression of cathepsins B and L causes a proliferation of lysosomes and the formation of meganeurites in hippocampus. *J. Neurosci.* **17**(11): p4006–21.

Besterman, J. M., Airhart, J. A., Woodworth, R. C. and Low, R. B. (1981). Exocytosis of pinocytosed fluid in cultured cells: kinetic evidence for rapid turnover and compartmentation. *J. Cell Biol.* **91**: 716–27.

Betz, W. J. and Wu, L. G. (1995). Synaptic transmission. Kinetics of synaptic-vesicle recycling. *Curr. Biol.* **5**(10): 1098–101.

Birn, H., Christensen, E. I. and Nielsen, S. (1993). Kinetics of endocytosis in renal proximal tubule studied with ruthenium red as membrane marker. *Am. J. Physiol.* **264**: F239–50.

Bradke, F. and Dotti, C. (1998). Membrane traffic in polarized neurons. *Biochim. Biophys. Acta* **1404**(1–2): p245–58.

Braell, W. A., Schlossman, D. M., Schmid, S. L. and Rothman, J. E. (1984). Dissociation of clathrin coats coupled to the hydrolysis of ATP: role of an uncoating ATPase. *J. Cell Biol.* **99**(2): 734–41.

Brown, M. S. and Goldstein, J. L. (1986). A receptor-mediated pathway for cholesterol homeostasis. *Science* **232**: 34–47.

Cain, C. C., Sipe, D. M. and Murphy, R. F. (1989). Regulation of endocytic pH by the Na^+,K^+-ATPase in living cells. *Proc. Natl. Acad. Sci. U.S.A.* **86**: 544–8.

Chapman, M. J. (1986). Comparative analysis of mamalian plasma lipoproteins. *Meth. Enzymol.* **128**: 70–143.

Chen, M., Obar, R., Schroeder, C., Austin, T., et al. (1991). Multiple forms of dynamin are encoded by shibire, a Drosophila gene involved in endocytosis. *Nature* **351**(6327): p583–6.

Chen, C. S., Martin, O. C. and Pagano, R. E. (1997). Changes in the spectral properties of a plasma membrane lipid analog during the first seconds of endocytosis in living cells. *Biophys. J.* **72**: 37–50.

Chung, H., Brazil, M., Soe, T. and Maxfield, F. (1999). Uptake, degradation, and release of fibrillar and soluble forms of Alzheimer's amyloid beta-peptide by microglial cells. *J Biol Chem* **274**(45): p32301–8.

Ciechanover, A. (1994). The ubiquitin-proteasome proteolytic pathway. *Cell* **79**(1): 13–21.

Dautry-Varsat, A., Ciechanover, A. and Lodish, H. F. (1983). pH and the recycling of transferrin during receptor-mediated endocytosis. *Proc. Natl. Acad. Sci. U.S.A.* **80**(8): 2258–62.

Desjardins, M. (1995). Biogenesis of phagolysosomes: the 'kiss and run' hypothesis. *Trends Cell Biol.* **5**: 183–6.

van Deurs, B., Holm, P. K., Kayser, L., Sandvig, K., et al. (1993). Multivesicular bodies in HEp-2 cells are maturing endosomes. *Eur. J. Cell Biol.* **61**(2): 208–24.

Dintzis, S. M., Velculescu, V. E. and Pfeffer, S. R. (1994). Receptor extracellular domains may contain trafficking information – studies of the 300-kDa mannose 6-phosphate receptor. *J. Biol. Chem.* **269**: 12159–66.

Duncan, J. R. and Kornfeld, S. (1988). Intracellular movement of two mannose 6-phosphate receptors: return to the Golgi apparatus. *J. Cell Biol.* **106**(3): 617–28.

Dunn, K. W., McGraw, T. E. and Maxfield, F. R. (1989). Iterative fractionation of recycling receptors from lysosomally destined ligands in an early sorting endosome. *J. Cell Biol.* **109**(6 Pt. 2): 3303–14.

Dunn, K. W. and Maxfield, F. R. (1992). Delivery of ligands from sorting endosomes to late endosomes occurs by maturation of sorting endosomes. *J. Cell Biol.* **117**(2): 301–10.

van Echten, G. and Sandhoff, K. (1993). Ganglioside metabolism. Enzymology, Topology, and regulation. *J. Biol. Chem.* **268**(8): 5341–4.

Falguieres, T., Mallard, F., Baron, C., Hanau, D., et al. (2001). Targeting of shiga toxin b-subunit to retrograde transport route in association with detergent-resistant membranes. *Mol. Biol. Cell* **12**(8): 2453–68.

Fuchs, R., Schmid, S. and Mellman, I. (1989). A possible role for Na^+, K^+-ATPase in regulating ATP-dependent endosome acidification. *Proc. Natl. Acad. Sci. U.S.A.* **86**: 539–43.

Gaidarov, I., Santini, F., Warren, R. A. and Keen, J. H. (1999). Spatial control of coated-pit dynamics in living cells. *Nature Cell Biol.* **1–7**.

Gatzinsky, K. (1996). Node-paranode regions as local degradative centres in alpha-motor axons. *Microsc Res Tech* **34**(6): p492–506.

Geuze, H. J., Slot, J. W., Strous, G. J. A. M., Lodish, H. F., et al. (1983). Intracellular site of asialoglycoprotein receptor-ligand uncoupling: double immunoelectron microscopy during receptor-mediated endocytosis. *Cell* **32**: 277–87.

Ghosh, R. N. and Webb, W. W. (1994). Automated detection and tracking of individual and clustered cell surface low density lipoprotein receptor molecules. *Biophys. J.* **66**: 1301–18.

Ghosh, R. N. and Maxfield, F. R. (1995). Evidence for nonvectorial, retrograde transferrin trafficking in the early endosomes of HEp2 cells. *J. Cell Biol.* **128**(4): 549–61.

Ghosh, R. N., Gelman, D. L. and Maxfield, F. R. (1994). Quantification of low density lipoprotein and transferrin endocytic sorting HEp2 cells using confocal microscopy. *J. Cell Sci.* **107**(Pt. 8): 2177–89.

Ghosh, R. N., Mallet, W. G., Soe, T. T., McGraw, T. E., et al. (1998). An endocytosed TGN38 chimeric protein is delivered to the TGN after trafficking through the endocytic recycling compartment in CHO cells. *J. Cell Biol.* **142**: 923–36.

Glickman, J. N., Conibear, E. and Pearse, B. M. F. (1989). Specificity of binding of clathrin adaptors to signals on the mannose-6-phosphate/insulin-like growth factor II receptor. *EMBO J.* **8**: 1041–7.

Gluck, S. L. (1993). The vacuolar H^+-ATPases: versatile proton pumps participating in constitutive and specialized functions of eucaryotic cells. *Int. Rev. Cytol.* **137C**: 105–37.

Goldstein, J. L., Brown, M. S., Anderson, R. G. W., Russell, D. W., et al. (1985). Receptor-mediated endocytosis: concepts emerging from the LDL receptor system. *Annu. Rev. Cell Biol.* **1**(1): 1–39.

Griffiths, G., Hoflack, B., Simons, K., Mellman, I., et al. (1988). The mannose 6-phosphate receptor and the biogenesis of lysosomes. *Cell* **52**(3): 329–41.

Griffiths, G., Back, R. and Marsh, M. (1989). A quantitative analysis of the endocytic pathway in baby hamster kidney cells. *J. Cell Biol.* **109**: 2703–20.

Grimmer, S., Iversen, T., van, D. B. and Sandvig, K. (2000). Endosome to Golgi transport of ricin is regulated by cholesterol. *Mol Biol Cell* **11**(12): p4205–16.

Gruenberg, J. (2001). The endocytic pathway: a mosaic of domains. *Nat Rev Mol Cell Biol* **2**(10): p721–30.

Gruenberg, J. and Maxfield, F. R. (1995). Membrane transport in the endocytic pathway *Curr. Opin. Cell Biol.* **7**(4): 552–63.

Gruenberg, J., Griffiths, G. and Howell, K. E. (1989). Characterization of the early endosome and putative endocytic carrier vesicles *in vivo* and with an assay of vesicle fusion *in vitro*. *J. Cell Biol.* **108**: 1301–16.

Haigler, H. T., McKanna, J. A. and Cohen, S. (1979). Direct visualization of the binding and internalization of a ferritin conjugate of epidermal growth factor in human carcinoma cells A-431. *J. Cell Biol.* **81**(2): 382–95.

Hannan, L. A., Newmyer, S. L. and Schmid, S. L. (1998). ATP- and cytosol-dependent release of adaptor proteins from clathrin-coated vesicles: a dual role for Hsc70. *Mol. Biol. Cell* **9**: 2217–29.

Hao, M. and Maxfield, F. R. (2000). Characterization of rapid membrane internalization and recycling. *J. Biol. Chem.* **275**(20): 15279–86.

Harder, T., Scheiffele, P., Verkade, P. and Simons, K. (1998). Lipid domain structure of the plasma membrane revealed by patching of membrane components. *J Cell Biol* **141**(4): 929–42.

Hicke, L. and Riezman, H. (1996). Ubiquitination of a yeast plasma membrane receptor signals its ligand-stimulated endocytosis. *Cell* **84**(2): 277–87.

Holtzman, E. (1989). *Lysosomes*. New York, Plenum Press.

Hofmann, K. and Falquet, L. (2001). A ubiquitin-interacting motif conserved in components of the proteasomal and lysosomal protein degradation systems. *Trends Biochem. Sci.* **26**(6): 347–50.

Honegger, A. M., Dull, T. J., Felder, S., Van Obberghen, E., et al. (1987). Point mutation at the ATP binding site of EGF receptor abolishes protein-tyrosine kinase activity and alters cellular routing. *Cell* **51**(2): 199–209.

Hopkins, C. R. (1983). Intracellular routing of transferrin and transferrin receptors in epidermoid carcinoma A431 cells. *Cell* **35**(1): 321–30.

Hopkins, C. R., Gibson, A., Shipman, M. and Miller, K. (1990). Movement of internalized ligand-receptor complexes along a continuous endosomal reticulum. *Nature* **346**: 335–39.

Hopkins, C. R., Gibson, A., Shipman, M., Strickland, D. K., et al. (1994). In migrating fibroblasts, recycling receptors are concentrated in narrow tubules in the pericentriolar area, and then routed to the plasma membrane of the leading lamella. *J. Cell Biol.* **125**(6): 1265–74.

Howe, C., Valletta, J., Rusnak, A. and Mobley, W. (2001). NGF signaling from clathrin-coated vesicles: evidence that signaling endosomes serve as a platform for the Ras-MAPK pathway. *Neuron* **32**(5): p801–14.

Hussain, N. K., Yamabhai, M., Ramjaun, A. R., Guy, A. M., et al. (1999). Splice variants of intersectin are components of the endocytic machinery in neurons and nonneuronal cells. *J. Biol. Chem.* **274**(22): 15671–7.

Iacopetta, B. J. and Morgan, E. H. (1983). The kinetics of transferrin endocytosis and iron uptake from transferrin in rabbit reticulocytes. *J. Biol. Chem.* **258**(15): 9108–15.

Ilangumaran, S. and Hoessli, D. C. (1998). Effects of cholesterol depletion by cyclodextrin on the sphingolipid microdomains of the plasma membrane. *Biochem. J.* **335**(Pt 2): 433–40.

Itin, C., Kappeler, F., Linstedt, A. D. and Hauri, H. P. (1995). A novel endocytosis signal related to the KKXX ER-retrieval signal. *EMBO J.* **14**(10): 2250–6.

Iversen, T. G., Skretting, G., Llorente, A., Nicoziani, P., et al. (2001). Endosome to golgi transport of ricin is independent of clathrin and of the rab9- and rab11-gtpases. *Mol. Biol. Cell* **12**(7): 2099–107.

Jahraus, A., Storrie, B., Griffiths, G. and Desjardins, M. (1994). Evidence for retrograde traffic between terminal lysosomes and the prelysosomal/late endosome compartment. *J. Cell Sci.* **107**(Pt 1): 145–57.

Jing, S. Q., Spencer, T., Miller, K., Hopkins, C., et al. (1990). Role of the human transferrin receptor cytoplasmic domain in endocytosis: localization of a specific signal sequence for internalization. *J. Cell Biol.* **110**(2): 283–94.

Johnson, K. F. and Kornfeld, S. (1992). A His-Leu-Leu sequence near the carboxyl terminus of the cytoplasmic domain of the cation-dependent mannose 6-phosphate receptor is necessary for the lysosomal enzyme sorting function. *J. Biol. Chem.* **267**(24): 17110–5.

Johnson, A. O., Lampson, M. A. and McGraw, T. E. (2001). A di-leucine sequence and a cluster of acidic amino acids are required for dynamic retention in the endosomal recycling compartment of fibroblasts. *Mol. Biol. Cell* **12**(2): 367–81.

Kang, S., Liang, L., Parker, C. D. and Collawn, J. F. (1998). Structural requirements for major histocompatibility complex class II invariant chain endocytosis and lysosomal targeting. *J. Biol. Chem.* **273**(32): 20644–52.

Kirchhausen, T. (2000). Clathrin. *Annu. Rev. Biochem.* **69**: 699–727.

Kjoller, L., Simonsen, A. C., Ellgaard, L. and Andreasen, P. A. (1995). Differential regulation of urokinase-type-1 inhibitor complex endocytosis by phorbol esters in different cell lines is associated with differential regulation of α_2-macroglobulin receptor and urokinase receptor expression. *Mol. Cell. Endocrinol.* **109**: 209–17.

Kobayashi, T., Stang, E., Fang, K. S., de Moerloose, P., et al. (1998). A lipid associated with antiphospholipid syndrome regulates endosome structure and function. *Nature* **392**: 193–7.

Kobayashi, T., Beuchat, M., Lindsay, M., Frias, S., et al. (1999). Late endosomal membranes rich in lysobisphosphatidic acid regulate cholesterol transport. *Nat Cell Biol* **1**(2): p113–8.

Koenig, J. H. and Ikeda, K. (1989). Disappearance and reformation of synaptic vesicle membrane upon transmitter release observed under reversible blockage of membrane retrieval. *J. Neurosci.* **9**(11): 3844–60.

Kok, J. W., ter Beest, M., Scherphof, G. and Hoekstra, D. (1990). A non-exchangeable fluorescent phospholipid analog as a membrane traffic marker of the endocytic pathway. *Eur. J. Cell Biol.* **53**: 173–184.

Kornfeld, S. (1992). Structure and function of the mannose 6-phosphate/insulin like growth factor II receptors *Annu. Rev. Biochem.* **61**(307): 307–30.

Kornfeld, S. and Mellman, I. (1989). The biogenesis of lysosomes. *Annu. Rev. Cell Biol.* **5**(483): 483–525.

Koval, M. and Pagano, R. E. (1989). Lipid recycling between the plasma membrane and intracellular compartments: transport and metabolism of fluorescent sphingomyelin analogues in cultured fibroblasts. *J. Cell Biol.* **108**(6): 2169–81.

Kozlov, M. M. (2001). Fission of biological membranes: interplay between dynamin and lipids. *Traffic* **2**(1): 51–65.

Ladinsky, M. S., Kramer, J. R., Furcinitti, P. S., McIntosh, J. R., et al. (1994). HVEM tomography of the trans-Golgi network: structural insights and identification of a lace-like vesicle coat. *J. Cell Biol.* **127**: 29–38.

Lampson, M. A., Racz, A., Cushman, S. W. and McGraw, T. E. (2000). Demonstration of insulin-responsive trafficking of GLUT4 and vpTR in fibroblasts. *J. Cell Sci.* **113**(22): 4065–76.

Laporte, S. A., Oakley, R. H., Holt, J. A., Barak, L. S., et al. (2000). The interaction of beta-arrestin with the AP-2 adaptor is required for the clustering of beta 2-adrenergic receptor into clathrin-coated pits. *J. Biol. Chem.* **275**(30): 23120–6.

Lazarovits, J. and Roth, M. (1988). A single amino acid change in the cytoplasmic domain allows the influenza virus hemagglutinin to be endocytosed through coated pits. *Cell* **53**(5): 743–52.

Letourneur, F. and Klausner, R. D. (1992). A novel di-leucine motif and a tyrosine-based motif independently mediate lysosomal targeting and endocytosis of CD3 chains. *Cell* **69**(7): 1143–57.

Levy, J. R. and Olefsky, J. M. (1987). The trafficking and processing of insulin and insulin receptors in cultured hepatocytes. *Endocrinology* **121**(6): 2075–86.

Lin, S., Gundersen, G. and Maxfield, F. (2002). Export from pericentriolar endocytic recycling compartment to cell surface depends on stable, detyrosinated (glu) microtubules and Kinesin [In Process Citation]. *Mol Biol Cell* **13**(1): p96–109.

Lin, S., Naim, H. Y., Rodriguez, A. C. and Roth, M. G. (1998). Mutations in the middle of the transmembrane domain reverse the polarity of transport of the influenza virus hemagglutinin in MDCK epithelial cells. *J Cell Biol* **142**(1): 51–7.

Lin, S. X., Grant, B., Hirsh, D. and Maxfield, F. R. (2001). RME-1 regulates the distribution and function of the endocytic recycling compartment in mammalian cells. *Nat. Cell Biol.* **3**: 567–72.

Lobel, P., Fujimoto, K., Ye, R. D., Griffiths, G., et al. (1989). Mutations in the cytoplasmic domain of the 275 kd mannose 6-phosphate receptor differentially alter lysosomal enzyme sorting and endocytosis. *Cell* **57**(5): 787–96.

Lusa, S., Blom, T., Eskelinen, E., Kuismanen, E., et al. (2001). Depletion of rafts in late endocytic membranes is controlled by NPC1-dependent recycling of cholesterol to the plasma membrane. *J Cell Sci* **114**(Pt 10): p1893–900.

Mallard, F., Antony, C., Tenza, D., Salamero, J., et al. (1998). Direct pathway from early/recycling endosomes to the Golgi apparatus revealed through the study of shiga toxin B-fragment transport. *J. Cell Biol.* **143**(4): 973–90.

Mallet, W. G. and Maxfield, F. R. (1999). Chimeric forms of furin and TGN38 are transported with the plasma membrane in the trans-Golgi network via distinct endosomal pathways. *J Cell Biol* **146**(2): 345–59.

Mancini, G. M., Beerens, C. E., Aula, P. P. and Verheijen, F. W. (1991). Sialic acid storage diseases. A multiple lysosomal transport defect for acidic monosaccharides. *J. Clin. Invest.* **87**(4): 1329–35.

Marks, M. S., Ohno, H., Kirchhausen, T. and Bonifacino, J. S. (1997). Protein sorting by tyrosine-based signals: adapting to the Ys and wherefores. *Trends Cell Biol.* **7**: 124–8.

Marsh, M., Griffiths, G., Dean, G. E., Mellman, I., et al. (1986). Three-dimensional structure of endosomes in BHK-21 cells. *Proc. Natl. Acad. Sci. U.S.A.* **83**: 2899–903.

Marsh, E. W., Leopold, P. L., Jones, N. L. and Maxfield, F. R. (1995). Oligomerized transferrin receptors are selectively retained by a lumenal sorting signal in a long-lived endocytic recycling compartment. *J. Cell Biol.* **129**(6): 1509–22.

Maxfield, F. R., Willingham, M. C., Haigler, H. T., Dragsten, P., et al. (1981). Binding, surface mobility, internalization, and degradation of rhodamine-labeled α_2-macroglobulin. *Biochemistry* **20**(18): 5353–8.

Mayor, S., Presley, J. F. and Maxfield, F. R. (1993). Sorting of membrane components from endosomes and subsequent recycling to the cell surface occurs by a bulk flow process. *J. Cell Biol.* **121**(6): 1257–69.

Mayor, S., Sabharanjak, S. and Maxfield, F. R. (1998). Cholesterol-dependent retention of GPI-anchored proteins in endosomes. *EMBO J.* **17**: 4626–38.

McGraw, T. E., Dunn, K. W. and Maxfield, F. R. (1988). Phorbol ester treatment increases the exocytic rate of the transferrin receptor recycling pathway independent of serine-24 phosphorylation. *J. Cell Biol.* **106**(4): 1061–6.

McGraw, T. E. and Maxfield, F. R. (1990). Human transferrin receptor internalization is partially dependent upon an aromatic amino acid on the cytoplasmic domain. *Cell Regul.* **1**(4): 369–77.

McPherson, P. S., Garcia, E. P., Slepnev, V. I., David, C., et al. (1996). A presynaptic inositol-5-phosphatase. *Nature* **379**(6563): 353–7.

Mellman, I. and Plunter, H. (1984). Internalization and degradation of macrophage Fc receptors bound to polyvalent immune complex. *J. Cell Biol.* **98**: 1170–7.

Miettinen, H. M., Matter, K., Hunziker, W., Rose, J. K., et al. (1992). Fc receptor endocytosis is controlled by a cytoplasmic domain determinant that actively prevents coated pit localization. *J. Cell Biol.* **116**(4): 875–88.

Molloy, S. S., Thomas, L., VanSlyke, J. K., Stenberg, P. E., et al. (1994). Intracellular trafficking and activation of the furin proprotein convertase: localization to the TGN and recycling from the cell surface. *EMBO J.* **13**: 18–33.

Mukherjee, S. and Maxfield, F. R. (1999). Cholesterol: stuck in traffic [news] [In Process Citation]. *Nat Cell Biol* **1**(2): E37–8.

Mukherjee, S. and Maxfield, F. R. (2000). Role of membrane organization and membrane domains in endocytic lipid trafficking. *Traffic* **1**: 203–11.

Mukherjee, S., Ghosh, R. N. and Maxfield, F. R. (1997). Endocytosis. *Physiol. Rev.* **77**: 759–803.

Mukherjee, S., Zha, X., tabas, I. and Maxfield, F. R. (1998). Cholesterol distribution in living cells: fluorescence imaging using dehydroergosterol as a fluorescent cholesterol analog. *Biophys. J.* **75**: 1915–25.

Mukherjee, S., Soe, T. T. and Maxfield, F. R. (1999). Endocytic sorting of lipid analogues differing solely in the chemistry of their hydrophobic tails. *J Cell Biol* **144**(6): 1271–84.

Nakatsu, F., Sakuma, M., Matsuo, Y., Arase, H., et al. (2000). A Di-leucine signal in the ubiquitin moiety. Possible involvement in ubiquitination-mediated endocytosis. *J. Biol. Chem.* **275**(34): 26213–9.

Nichols, B. J., Kenworthy, A. K., Polishchuk, R. S., Lodge, R., et al. (2001). Rapid cycling of lipid raft markers between the cell surface and Golgi complex. *J. Cell Biol.* **153**(3): 529–41.

Oakley, R. H., Laporte, S. A., Holt, J. A., Barak, L. S., et al. (2001). Molecular determinants underlying the formation of stable intracellular GPCR/{beta} arrestin complexes following receptor endocytosis. *J. Biol. Chem.*

Oda, H., Stockert, R. J., Collins, C., Wang, H., et al. (1995). Interaction of the microtubule cytoskeleton with endocytic vesicles and cytoplasmic dynein in cultured rat hepatocytes. *J. Biol. Chem.* **270**(25): 15242–9.

Omary, M. B. and Trowbridge, I. S. (1981). Biosynthesis of the human transferrin receptor in cultured cells. *J. Biol. Chem.* **256**(24): 12888–92.

Overly, C. and Hollenbeck, P. (1996). Dynamic organization of endocytic pathways in axons of cultured sympathetic neurons. *J. Neurosci.* **16**(19): p6056–64.

Overly, C., Lee, K., Berthiaume, E. and Hollenbeck, P. (1995). Quantitative measurement of intraorganelle pH in the endosomal-lysosomal pathway in neurons by using ratiometric imaging with pyranine. *Proc Natl Acad Sci U S A* **92**(8): p3156–60.

Pagano, R. E., Sepanski, M. A. and Martin, O. C. (1989). Molecular trapping of a fluorescent ceramide analogue at the Golgi apparatus of fixed cells: Interaction with endogenous lipids provides a trans-Golgi marker for both light and electron microscopy. *J. Cell Biol.* **109**: 2067–9.

Paresce, D., Chung, H. and Maxfield, F. (1997). Slow degradation of aggregates of the Alzheimer's disease amyloid beta-protein by microglial cells. *J Biol Chem* **272**(46): p29390–7.

Parton, R. G. (1994). Ultrastructural localization of gangliosides; GM_1 is concentrated in caveolae. *J. Histochem. Cytochem.* **42**(2): 155–66.

Parton, R., Simons, K. and Dotti, C. (1992). Axonal and dendritic endocytic pathways in cultured neurons. *J Cell Biol* **119**(1): p123–37.

Pearse, B. M., Smith, C. J. and Owen, D. J. (2000). Clathrin coat construction in endocytosis. *Curr. Opin. Struct. Biol.* **10**(2): 220–8.

Pierini, L., Holowka, D. and Baird, B. (1996). FcεRI-mediated association of 6-μm beads with RBL-2H3 mast cells results in exclusion of signaling proteins from the forming phagosome and abrogation of nomal downstream signaling. *J. Cell Biol.* **134**: 1427–39.

Presley, J. F., Mayor, S., Dunn, K. W., Johnson, L. S., et al. (1993). The End2 mutation in CHO cells slows the exit of transferrin receptors from the recycling compartment but bulk membrane recycling is unaffected. *J. Cell Biol.* **122**(6): 1231–41.

Puertollano, R., Aguilar, R. C., Gorshkova, I., Crouch, R. J., et al. (2001). Sorting of mannose 6-phosphate receptors mediated by the GGAs. *Science* **292**: 1712–6.

Puri, V., Watanabe, R., Dominguez, M., Sun, X., et al. (1999). Cholesterol modulates membrane traffic along the endocytic pathway in sphingolipid-storage diseases. *Nat Cell Biol* **1**(6): p386–8.

Puri, V., Watanabe, R., Singh, R. D., Dominguez, M., et al. (2001). Clathrin-dependent and -independent internalization of plasma membrane sphingolipids initiates two Golgi targeting pathways. *J. Cell Biol.* **154**(3): 535–47.

Qualmann, B. and Kelly, R. B. (2000). Syndapin isoforms participate in receptor-mediated endocytosis and actin organization. *J. Cell Biol.* **148**: 1047–62.

Qualmann, B., Kessels, M. M. and Kelly, R. B. (2000). Molecular links between endocytosis and the actin cytoskeleton. *J. Cell Biol.* **150**(5): F111–6.

Rohrer, J., Schweizer, A., Johnson, K. F. and Kornfeld, S. (1995). A determinant in the cytoplasmic tail of the cation-dependent mannose 6-phosphate receptor prevents trafficking to lysosomes. *J. Cell Biol.* **130**(6): 1297–306.

Rome, L. H. (1985). Curling receptors. *Trends Biochem. Sci.* **10**: 151.

Roos, J. and Kelly, R. (1999). The endocytic machinery in nerve terminals surrounds sites of exocytosis. *Curr. Biol.* **9**(23): p1411–4.

Sandvig, K., Olsnes, S., Brown, J. E., Petersen, O. W., et al. (1989). Endocytosis from coated pits of Shiga toxin: a glycolipid-binding protein from Shigella dysenteriae 1. *J. Cell Biol.* **108**(4): 1331–43.

Sandvig, K., Garred, O., van Helvoort, A., van Meer, G., et al. (1996). Importance of glycolipid synthesis for butyric acid-induced sensitization to shiga toxin and intracellular sorting of toxin in A431 cells. *Mol Biol Cell* **7**(9): 1391–404.

Sankaranarayanan, S. and Ryan, T. A. (2000). Real-time measurements of vesicle-SNARE recycling in synapses of the central nervous system. *Nature Cell Biol.* **2**(4): 197–204.

Sato, S. B. and Toyama, S. (1994). Interference with the endosomal acidification by a monoclonal antibody directed toward the 116 (100)-kD subunit of the vacuolar type proton pump. *J. Cell Biol.* **127**(1): 39–53.

Schenk, D., Barbour, R., Dunn, W., Gordon, G., et al. (1999). Immunization with amyloid-beta attenuates Alzheimer-disease-like pathology in the PDAPP mouse. *Nature* **400**(6740): p173–7.

Schmid, S. S. (1997). Clathrin-coated vesicle formation and protein sorting: an integrated process. *Annu. Rev. Biochem.* **66**: 511–48.

Schmid, S. L. and Carter, L. L. (1990). ATP is required for receptor-mediated endocytosis in intact cells. *J. Cell Biol.* **111**(6 Pt. 1): 2307–18.

Schmidt, A., Wolde, M., Thiele, C., Fest, W., et al. (1999). Endophilin I mediates synaptic vesicle formation by transfer of arachidonate to lysophosphatidic acid. *Nature* **401**(133–41).

Schroeder, R. J., Ahmed, S. N., Zhu, Y., London, E., et al. (1998). Cholesterol and sphingolipid enhance the Triton X-100 insolubility of glycosylphosphatidylinositol-anchored proteins by promoting the formation of detergent-insoluble ordered membrane domains. *J Biol Chem* **273**(2): 1150–7.

Schwartz, A. L. and Rup, D. (1983). Biosynthesis of the human asialoglycoprotein receptor. *J. Biol. Chem.* **258**(18): 11249–55.

Schweizer, A., Kornfeld, S. and Rohrer, J. (1996). Cysteine-34 of the cytoplasmic tail of the cation-dependent mannose 6-phosphate receptor is reversibly palmitoylated and required for normal trafficking and lysosomal sorting. *J. Cell Biol.* **132**: 577–584.

Sengar, A. S., Wang, W., Bishay, J., Cohen, S., et al. (1999). The EH and SH3 domain Ese proteins regulate endocytosis by linking to dynamin and Eps15. *EMBO J.* **18**: 1159–71.

Sever, S., Damke, H. and Schmid, S. L. (2000). Garrotes, springs, ratchets, and whips: putting dynamin models to the test. *Traffic* **1**(5): 385–92.

Shogomori, H. and Futerman, A. (2001). Cholesterol depletion by methyl-beta-cyclodextrin blocks cholera toxin transport from endosomes to the Golgi apparatus in hippocampal neurons. *J Neurochem* **78**(5): p991–9.

Simmen, T., Nobile, M., Bonifacino, J. S. and Hunziker, W. (1999). Basolateral sorting of furin in MDCK cells requires a phenylalanine-isoleucine motif together with an acidic amino acid cluster. *Mol. Cell Biol.* **19**(4): 3136–44.

Simmons, C. F. J. and Schwartz, A. L. (1984). Cellular pathways of galactose-terminal ligand movement in a cloned human hepatoma cell line. *Mol. Pharmacol.* **26**(3): 509–19.

Simons, K., Dupree, P., Fiedler, K., Huber, L. A., et al. (1992). Biogenesis of cell-surface polarity in epithelial cells and neurons. *Cold Spring Harb. Symp. Quant. Biol.* **57**: 611–619.

Simson, R., Sheets, E. D. and Jacobson, K. (1995). Detection of temporary lateral confinement of membrane proteins using single-particle tracking analysis. *Biophys. J.* **69**: 989–93.

Sipe, D. M. and Murphy, R. F. (1987). High resolution kinetics of transferrin acidification in Balb/c 3T3 cells: exposure to pH 6 followed by temperature sensitive alkalinization during recycling. *Proc. Natl. Acad. Sci. U.S.A.* **84**: 7119–23.

Slepnev, V. I. and De Camilli, P. (2000). Accessory factors in clathrin-dependent synaptic vesicle endocytosis. *Nature Rev. Neurosci.* **1**: 161–72.

Soetens, O., De Craene, J. O. and Andre, B. (2001). Ubiquitin is required for sorting to the vacuole of the yeast Gap1 permease. *J. Biol. Chem.* **276,** 43949–57.

Stoorvogel, W., Geuze, H. J., Griffith, J. M. and Strous, G. J. (1988). The pathways of endocytosed transferrin and secretory protein are connected in the trans-golgi reticulum. *J. Cell Biol.* **106**: 1821–29.

Stoorvogel, W., Oorschot, V. and Geuze, H. J. (1996). A novel class of clathrin-coated vesicles budding from endosomes. *J. Cell Biol.* **132**: 21–33.

Swanson, J., Bushnell, A. and Silverstein, S. C. (1987). Tubular lysosome morphology and distribution within macrophages depend on the integrity of cytoplasmic microtubules. *Proc. Natl. Acad. Sci. U.S.A.* **84**: 1921–5.

Tietze, F., Kohn, L. D., Kohn, A. D., Bernardini, I., et al. (1989). Carrier-mediated transport of monoiodotyrosine out of thyroid cell lysosomes. *J. Biol. Chem.* **264**(9): 4762–5.

Tooze, S. A. (2001). GGAs tie up the loose ends. *Science* **292**(5522): 1663–5.

Tooze, J. and Hollinshead, M. (1991). Tubular early endosomal networks in AtT20 and other cells. *J. Cell Biol.* **115**: 635–53.

Traub, L. M., Bannykh, S. I., Rodel, J. E., Aridor, M., et al. (1996). AP-2-containing clathrin coats assemble on mature lysosomes. *J. Cell Biol.* **135**: 1801–14.

Trowbridge, I. S., Collawn, J. F. and Hopkins, C. R. (1993). Signal-dependent membrane protein trafficking in the endocytic pathway *Annu. Rev. Cell Biol.* **9**(129): 129–61.

Tsao, P., Cao, T. and von Zastrow, M. (2001). Role of endocytosis in mediating downregulation of G-protein-coupled receptors. *Trends Pharmacol. Sci.* **22**(2): 91–6.

Tycko, B. and Maxfield, F. R. (1982). Rapid acidification of endocytic vesicles containing α_2-macroglobulin. *Cell* **28**(3): 643–51.

Ullrich, O., Reinsch, S., Urbe, S., Zerial, M., et al. (1996). Rab11 regulates recycling through the pericentriolar recycling endosome. *J. Cell Biol.* **135**: 913–24.

Wakeham, D. E., Ybe, J. A., Brodsky, F. M. and Hwang, P. K. (2000). Molecular structures of proteins involved in vesicle coat formation. *Traffic* **1**(5): 393–8.

van Weert, A. V. M., Dunn, K. W., Geuze, H. J., Maxfield, F. R., et al. (1995). Transport from late endosomes to lysosomes, but not sorting of integral membrane proteins in endosomes, depends on the vacuolar proton pump. *J. Cell Biol.* **130**: 821–34.

West, A., Neve, R. and Buckley, K. (1997). Identification of a somatodendritic targeting signal in the cytoplasmic domain of the transferrin receptor. *J. Neurosci.* **17**(16): p6038–47.

Wiggle, P. and McMahon, H. T. (1998). The amphiphysin family of proteins and their role in endocytosis at the synapse. *Trends Neurosci.* **21**: 339–44.

Wilcke, M., Johannes, L., Galli, T., Mayau, V., et al. (2000). Rab11 regulates the compartmentalization of early endosomes required for efficient transport from early endosomes to the trans-golgi network. *J. Cell Biol.* **151**(6): 1207–20.

Wiley, H. S. and Burke, P. M. (2001). Regulation of receptor tyrosine kinase signaling by endocytic trafficking. *Traffic* **2**(1): 12–18.

Wilkening, G., Linke, T. and Sandhoff, K. (1998). Lysosomal degradation on vesicular membrane surfaces. Enhanced glucosylceramide degradation by lysosomal anionic lipids and activators. *J Biol Chem* **273**(46): 30271–8.

Yamashiro, D. J. and Maxfield, F. R. (1987). Acidification of morphologically distinct endosomes in mutant and wild-type Chinese hamster ovary cells. *J. Cell Biol.* **105**(6 Pt. 1): 2723–33.

Yamashiro, D. J., Tycko, B., Fluss, S. R. and Maxfield, F. R. (1984). Segregation of transferrin to a mildly acidic (pH 6.5) para-Golgi compartment in the recycling pathway. *Cell* **37**(3): 789–800.

von Zastrow, M. (2001). Role of endocytosis in signalling and regulation of G-protein-coupled receptors. *Biochem. Soc. Trans.* **29**(Pt 4): p500–4.

Zhu, Y., Doray, B., Poussu, A., Lehto, V.-P., et al. (2001). Binding of GGA2 to the lysosomal enzyme sorting motif of the mannose 6-phosphate receptor. *Science* **292**: 1716–8.

Chapter 2

Lysosomal defects and storage

Frances M. Platt and Steven U. Walkley

Introduction

The first published reports on what are today recognized as lysosomal diseases appeared as early as the 1820s (Stengel 1826), but it was not until the latter part of the nineteenth and early twentieth centuries that sufficient clinical and pathological data accumulated to suggest that individual groups of diseases could be recognized. Gaucher, Niemann–Pick, and Tay–Sachs diseases were three such disease groupings that emerged during this time. Tay–Sachs mirrors these developments particularly well, having been originally seen clinically as a condition exhibiting blindness and accompanied by a characteristic ophthalmological finding, the cherry red spot (Tay 1881). This was followed by a series of remarkable studies by Sachs and his colleagues in which the clinical and pathological features were described in considerable detail, based initially on a single case (Sachs 1887) and later expanded to include others (Sachs 1903; Sachs and Strauss 1910). These findings led to the designation *familial amaurotic idiocy* to denote this condition's three most obvious characteristics: increased incidence in certain families, blindness, and mental retardation. Considerable debate ensued as to its aetiology and the reason for its familial characteristic, with one theory including the possibility of a toxic factor, perhaps one derived from the mother's milk (Hirsch 1898). Very early suggestions of 'inherent biochemical abnormalities' by clinicians at the Hospital for Sick Children at Great Ormond Street in London in the early 1900s (Poynton *et al.* 1906) may be reflective of Archibold Garrod's influence at that institution (Garrod 1909). This pathogenic concept was later emphasized by Bielschowsky (1921), who went so far as to suggest that administration of enzyme-containing extracts of normal developing brain might be curative.

During the early twentieth century, many other conditions with similar features were described and inevitably compared to Tay–Sachs and Niemann–Pick diseases, with the goal of including the new disorder as a sub-type or providing evidence to distinguish it from these diseases. Several disorders now recognized in the Batten disease (neuronal ceroid lipofuscinosis) category, for example, were at one time considered sub-types of amaurotic idiocy. Gargoylism or Hurler–Pfaundler syndrome, later to be known as mucopolysaccharidosis (Brante 1952), also emerged during this period and was accurately noted to represent a new type of disorder. Key features recognized in almost all of these diseases were the familial trait, the apparent normalcy of early life (in many cases), and a particular change seen pathologically in various cells of brain and sometimes other organs. This latter characteristic was thought to represent some type of material accumulating within the cell cytoplasm, from which grew the concept of 'storage'. That the abnormal material in cells was often lipid in character was clearly recognized in a variety of biochemical and histochemical studies, and the term 'lipidosis' came to be used to refer to many of these diseases. However, the term also had a broader usage and was applied to non-storage disorders involving abnormal lipid metabolism, including hyperlipidaemias and xanthomatoses (Thannhauser 1940). That is, whether the cellular accumulation of lipids was cell endogenous or derived from the blood was simply not known (see Sperry 1942). By 1960, with the discovery of lysosomes by de Duve and colleagues (1955), the idea that an enzyme defect might be the cause of, for example ganglioside storage in Tay–Sachs disease, began to draw adherents. In 1963, a general explanation of a unifying cause of storage diseases was established, based on the unequivocal demonstration of a deficiency in acid maltase, a lysosomal enzyme, in a type of glycogen storage disease (Foreword; Hers 1963). Inherent in this view was the idea of a 'primary' storage material which accumulated in abundance due to the absence of its catabolic enzyme. Identifying this material for a given disease, and the enzyme normally responsible for its degradation, thus became the central goal in disease diagnosis and classification.

When considering a large family of diseases, such as the lysosomal disorders, it clearly is helpful to sub-classify them on the basis of shared features. This provides a framework within which strategies for diagnosis and therapy can be developed and also provides a basis for comparing mechanisms of pathogenesis. The clinical spectrum associated with lysosomal disorders affecting brain is complex, overlapping, and highly variable and is therefore not particularly helpful as a sole taxonomic guide (Chapter 3). Nonetheless, clinical presentation, coupled with pathologic studies, formed the basis for early classification systems that typically bore eponyms for identification (Gaucher, Tay–Sachs, Niemann–Pick, Hurler, and so forth). However, growth of knowledge about these diseases and the types of primary materials accumulating naturally led to a classification system based on the identity of the stored molecules (mucopolysaccharidoses (MPSs), gangliosidoses, and so forth). To a significant degree, the nature of the storage material, coupled with key clinical and pathological characteristics, provides the most common classification system used today. A second means to categorize lysosomal diseases is to examine the underlying *cause* of disease and classify on the basis of the molecular mechanisms leading to storage. These different approaches are not mutually exclusive and both have important roles to play, giving different insights into the diseases and their underlying molecular mechanisms. In fact, modern classification systems typically used in most texts are hybrid schemes that conform to a substrate-based system but with those that defy incorporation into such a scheme being categorized by common mechanism(s) leading to storage. In this chapter, we present the advantages and disadvantages of these two classification systems and discuss why we have elected to organize this book on the basis of the underlying molecular mechanisms.

Traditional classification of lysosomal storage diseases

Lysosomal diseases are a group of inherited metabolic diseases characterized by intralysosomal accumulation of non-metabolized macromolecules. They are all autosomal recessive disorders except for Fabry disease and MPS type II, which are X-linked. While storage diseases are individually rare, they have a collective frequency of approximately 1:8000 live births (Meikle *et al.* 1999). They represent a significant health problem worldwide (Chapter 3) and devastate the lives of affected individuals and their families (Prologue). To date, at least 41 disorders have been described (Meikle *et al.* 1999). The vast majority involve pathology in the brain, and the complete listing of organ involvement for each disease is provided as Table 3.1 in Chapter 3.

Major progress in understanding lysosomal diseases came from the biochemical identification of storage molecule(s) characteristic of each disorder (Table 2.1). This was typically the prelude to identifying the genetic lesion responsible for each disorder. The biochemical nature of the storage material thus provides a convenient framework to sub-classify these diseases. The categories into which the diseases can be organized include the lipidoses (glycosphingolipidoses, including gangliosidoses), MPSs, glycogenoses, mucolipidoses, oligosaccharidoses, and neuronal ceroid lipofuscinoses (NCLs) (Batten family diseases). Where this system of classification flounders, however, is in dealing with disorders that span multiple categories (I-cell disease, sialidosis, and multiple sulfatase deficiency) and in its tendency to lump diseases with radically different causes into the same category (e.g. Niemann–Pick diseases types A and B with type C).

Lipidoses

The lipidoses include all storage diseases in which the major accumulating material is some type of lipid. Owing to the biochemical diversity of lipids, it is useful to subdivide this group to more precisely reflect the biochemical class of lipid stored. The majority of the lipidoses involve the storage of sphingolipids (SLs). The two diseases characterized by the storage of non-sphingolipid species are Wolman disease (lysosomal acid lipase deficiency) and cholesteryl ester storage disease (acid lipase deficiency) (Assmann and Seedorf 2001) (Chapter 3). Wolman disease and cholesteryl ester storage disease represent different extremes of a clinical spectrum, with the former disease being an acute, lethal disease of early infancy and the latter a more benign disease of childhood/adulthood. They both result from mutations in the same gene (acid lipase) but differ in the severity of the mutations. Wolman disease is virtually devoid of residual enzyme activity, whereas measurable enzyme is present in cholesteryl ester storage disease. The main storage products are cholesteryl esters and frequently triglycerides (Assmann and Seedorf 2001).

Sphingolipidoses

The major sub-group of SLs stored are the glycosphingolipids (GSLs). However, non-glycosylated SLs are also stored. For instance, in Farber disease, acid ceramidase is deficient and ceramide accumulates (Moser *et al.* 2001) (Chapters 3 and 4). Niemann–Pick diseases A and B result from sphingomyelinase deficiency, with primary storage of sphingomyelin and secondary storage of gangliosides (Schuchman and Desnick 2001) (Chapters 3 and 4). Niemann–Pick disease type C, like types A and B, also exhibits storage of sphingomyelin and gangliosides (hence its classification in the Niemann–Pick group) but is particularly well known for increases in cholesterol (Pentchev *et al.* 1994). Unlike types A and B, however, in type C, the molecular defects involve non-enzyme proteins which appear to have no direct relationship with sphingomyelinase, and thus provides a good example of the failings of the traditional system of nomenclature for storage diseases. (See further discussion below.)

Glycosphingolipidoses

The GSL diseases represent a major sub-category of storage disorders comprising approximately half of all cases (Meikle *et al.* 1999). GSLs have a common lipid backbone, ceramide, to which one or more monosaccharide is linked. The GSLs can be sub-classified biochemically on the basis of whether the first sugar residue linked to ceramide is glucose (glucosylceramide, GlcCer) or galactose (galactosylceramide, GalCer). The GalCer-based GSLs are stored in two

Table 2.1

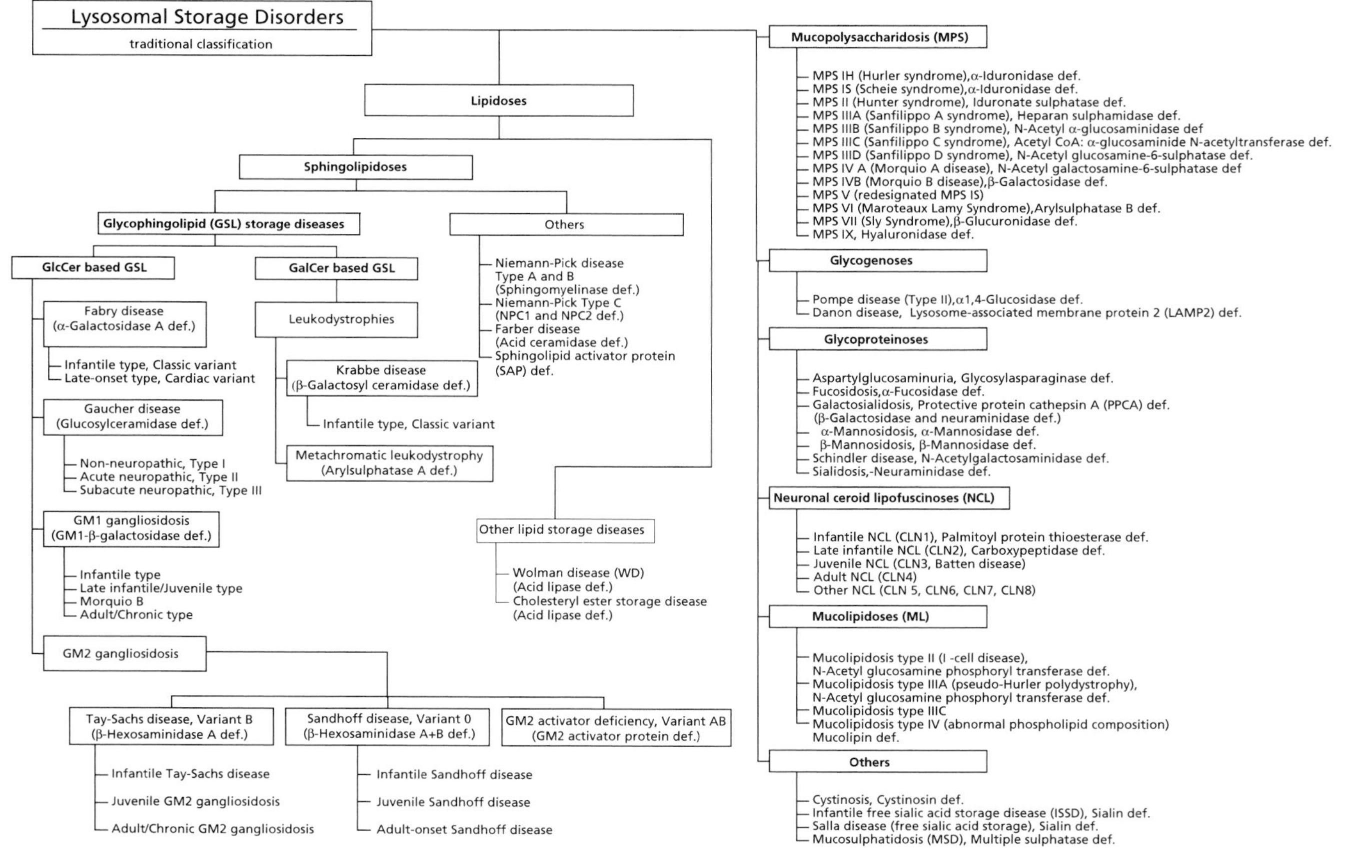

Lysosomal Storage Disorders
traditional classification
Lipidoses
Sphingolipidoses
Glycophingolipid (GSL) storage diseases
GlcCer based GSL
Fabry disease (α-Galactosidase A def.)
Infantile type, Classic variant
Late-onset type, Cardiac variant
Gaucher disease (Glucosylceramidase def.)
Non-neuropathic, Type I
Acute neuropathic, Type II
Subacute neuropathic, Type III
GM1 gangliosidosis (GM1-β-galactosidase def.)
Infantile type
Late infantile/Juvenile type
Morquio B
Adult/Chronic type
GM2 gangliosidosis
Tay-Sachs disease, Variant B (β-Hexosaminidase A def.)
Infantile Tay-Sachs disease
Juvenile GM2 gangliosidosis
Adult/Chronic GM2 gangliosidosis
Sandhoff disease, Variant 0 (β-Hexosaminidase A+B def.)
Infantile Sandhoff disease
Juvenile Sandhoff disease
Adult-onset Sandhoff disease
GM2 activator deficiency, Variant AB (GM2 activator protein def.)
GalCer based GSL
Leukodystrophies
Krabbe disease (β-Galactosyl ceramidase def.)
Infantile type, Classic variant
Metachromatic leukodystrophy (Arylsulphatase A def.)
Others
Niemann-Pick disease Type A and B (Sphingomyelinase def.)
Niemann-Pick Type C (NPC1 and NPC2 def.)
Farber disease (Acid ceramidase def.)
Sphingolipid activator protein (SAP) def.
Other lipid storage diseases
Wolman disease (WD) (Acid lipase def.)
Cholesteryl ester storage disease (Acid lipase def.)
Mucopolysaccharidosis (MPS)
MPS IH (Hurler syndrome),α-Iduronidase def.
MPS IS (Scheie syndrome),α-Iduronidase def.
MPS II (Hunter syndrome), Iduronate sulphatase def.
MPS IIIA (Sanfilippo A syndrome), Heparan sulphamidase def.
MPS IIIB (Sanfilippo B syndrome), N-Acetyl α-glucosaminidase def
MPS IIIC (Sanfilippo C syndrome), Acetyl CoA: α-glucosaminide N-acetyltransferase def.
MPS IIID (Sanfilippo D syndrome), N-Acetyl glucosamine-6-sulphatase def.
MPS IV A (Morquio A disease), N-Acetyl galactosamine-6-sulphatase def
MPS IVB (Morquio B disease),β-Galactosidase def.
MPS V (redesignated MPS IS)
MPS VI (Maroteaux Lamy Syndrome),Arylsulphatase B def.
MPS VII (Sly Syndrome),β-Glucuronidase def.
MPS IX, Hyaluronidase def.
Glycogenoses
Pompe disease (Type II),α1,4-Glucosidase def.
Danon disease, Lysosome-associated membrane protein 2 (LAMP2) def.
Glycoproteinoses
Aspartylglucosaminuria, Glycosylasparaginase def.
Fucosidosis,α-Fucosidase def.
Galactosialidosis, Protective protein cathepsin A (PPCA) def. (β-Galactosidase and neuraminidase def.)
α-Mannosidosis, α-Mannosidase def.
β-Mannosidosis, β-Mannosidase def.
Schindler disease, N-Acetylgalactosaminidase def.
Sialidosis,-Neuraminidase def.
Neuronal ceroid lipofuscinoses (NCL)
Infantile NCL (CLN1), Palmitoyl protein thioesterase def.
Late infantile NCL (CLN2), Carboxypeptidase def.
Juvenile NCL (CLN3, Batten disease)
Adult NCL (CLN4)
Other NCL (CLN 5, CLN6, CLN7, CLN8)
Mucolipidoses (ML)
Mucolipidosis type II (I -cell disease), N-Acetyl glucosamine phosphoryl transferase def.
Mucolipidosis type IIIA (pseudo-Hurler polydystrophy), N-Acetyl glucosamine phosphoryl transferase def.
Mucolipidosis type IIIC
Mucolipidosis type IV (abnormal phospholipid composition) Mucolipin def.
Others
Cystinosis, Cystinosin def.
Infantile free sialic acid storage disease (ISSD), Sialin def.
Salla disease (free sialic acid storage), Sialin def.
Mucosulphatidosis (MSD), Multiple sulphatase def.

diseases, Krabbe disease (globoid cell leukodystrophy) (Wenger *et al.* 2001) and metachromatic leukodystrophy (von Figura *et al.* 2001) (Chapters 3 and 4). The storage lipids are GalCer and its sulfated derivative sulfatide respectively. GalCer and sulfatide play important roles in the stability of myelin, and hence these diseases primarily involve demyelination of the central and peripheral nervous systems.

The other GSL storage diseases result from the storage of GlcCer-based GSLs (Fig. 8.1 in Chapter 8 and Table 15.1 in Chapter 15). This family of SLs can be further sub-classified on the basis of the glycan that is linked to ceramide. This can either involve neutral sugars linked to ceramide or they can be modified with one or more charged sialic acid residue and are termed gangliosides. GSLs are differentially expressed in different tissues. For instance, gangliosides are prominent components of the membranes of neurones and hence their storage primarily leads to neuropathology (Chapter 12). However, gangliosides are also expressed differentially by peripheral tissues and there is often visceral involvement in addition to the dominant neuropathology of the CNS (Chapter 3).

The storage diseases in which the GSL stored is a neutral species are Gaucher and Fabry diseases. Gaucher disease results from glucocerebrosidase deficiency and is classified into three sub-types (types 1, 2, and 3), although there is increasing evidence that the diseases represent different points in a clinical continuum. The storage lipid is GlcCer, the simplest member of this family of GSLs (Chapters 3 and 4) (Beutler and Grabowski 2001) and the first GSL to be synthesized in the GSL biosynthetic pathway. Fabry disease results from α-galactosidase A deficiency and causes the storage of ceramide trihexoside (Gb3) (Desnick *et al.* 2001) (Chapters 3 and 4).

The remaining GSL storage diseases all involve the storage of gangliosides and grouped collectively are termed the gangliosidoses. The asialo derivatives of these gangliosides can also be stored due to the action of lysosomal sialidases that can desialylate gangliosides. There are two main subdivisions of this group, that in which the storage GSL is GM1 ganglioside (GM1 gangliosidosis and Morquio B disease) and that in which GM2 is stored (the GM2 gangliosidoses) (Chapters 3 and 4). This latter group of diseases includes Tay–Sachs disease, Sandhoff disease, and GM2-activator protein deficiency. Unlike the previous disorders discussed, the defect in this latter disease is not in a hydrolase responsible for GSL catabolism. Hexosaminidase levels are normal in these individuals and instead the non-enzymatic co-factor (GM2-activator protein) essential for the function of this enzyme is deficient (Chapter 8 and below).

Mucopolysaccharidoses

This group of diseases lends itself well to the traditional classification scheme, as the substrates in question are related molecules and the enzymes form part of a common catabolic pathway. In addition, the causes of the diseases are primary defects in lysosomal enzymes (Chapter 4). The MPSs are a family of diseases resulting from defects in the genes encoding the enzymes involved in mucopolysaccharide catabolism (Neufeld and Muenzer 2001) (Chapters 3 and 4). Mucopolysaccharides (glycosaminoglycans) are complex glycoconjugates which include dermatan sulfate, heparan sulfate, keratan sulfate, chondroitin sulfate, and hyaluronan. Depending on the specific gene defect in question, the catabolism of one or more of these molecules is blocked, leading to the lysosomal storage of the deficient enzyme's substrate(s). There are 11 enzyme deficiencies characterized to date that lead to the numerous forms of MPS disease (types I–VII). While clinically diverse, even within single disorders, there are common features shared between all of the MPS disorders (Chapter 3).

Glycogenosis

There are many diseases of glycogen synthesis and catabolism (Chen 2001) affecting the quality or quantity of glycogen in the cytoplasm but only one that involves the storage of glycogen in the lysosome (Hirschborn and Reuser 2001). This disease fits into the substrate-based scheme of classification and is the prototypic lysosomal storage disease. It is variously termed glycogen storage disease type II (GSDII), Pompe disease, or acid maltase deficiency (Chapter 4). Glycogen (a branched glucose polymer) is the storage form of glucose in almost all cell types but is particularly abundant in liver and muscle. This disease is of historical significance, as it was the first lysosomal storage disease to be characterized (Hirschborn and Reuser 2001) (Foreword). The defective enzyme, acid α-glucosidase, is a lysosomal hydrolase that cleaves α-l,4 and α-1,6 glucosidic linkages and degrades glycogen that enters the lysosome from the cytosol as a result of a presumed autophagic process. The clinical picture is highly variable, but some degree of myopathy is present in all cases (Chapter 3). Another type of glycogen storage disorder that affects brain (Danon disease) has long been known to exhibit normal α-glucosidase activity (Hirschborn and Reuser 2001). Recently, this disorder was found to be secondary to a defect in the transmembrane lysosomal protein known as LAMP2, which possibly causes defects in autophagocytosis (discussed below).

Glycoproteinoses

Storage diseases generally grouped as glycoproteinoses, unlike many of the disorders discussed above, do not conveniently fit into a single category. Although frequently termed glycoprotein storage diseases, this is a misleading term, as frequently non-glycoprotein substrates are additionally stored, albeit at lower levels. Oligosaccharide storage disease is a slightly more accurate term but covers a multitude of different substrates. Also some of these diseases store monosaccharide-containing material rather than oligosaccharides. The essential problem with this disease category stems from the fact that multiple classes of glycoconjugates carry similar monosaccharides in similar glycosidic linkage to other sugar residues and are frequently catabolized by a common lysosomal enzyme. To add to the complexity, one member of this family of diseases (galactosialidosis) is not a primary hydrolase deficiency but rather is characterized by two hydrolase deficiencies arising from a defect in protective protein (Chapter 7).

It is worth reviewing a few points relating to these diseases to highlight how substrate-based classification schemes can be problematic. Aspartylglycosaminuria is a disease characterized by developmental delay (Chapter 3). The defective enzyme is aspartylglucosaminidase (glycosylasparaginase), which is ubiquitously expressed at low levels in all tissues (Chapter 4). Enzyme deficiency results in a failure to cleave the bond between the asparagine residue and *N*-acetylglucosamine, the final step in N-glycan catabolism. The storage molecule is a glycoprotein-derived monosaccharide linked to a single amino acid, a challenge to taxonomic categorization. The catabolic defect certainly affects an aspect of glycoprotein catabolism, but the term glycoprotein/oligosaccharide storage does not adequately describe the storage material itself, which must be the primary aim of systematizing the categories on the basis of substrate stored.

Fucosidosis is another member of this family of lysosomal disorders resulting from defects in the gene encoding α-fucosidase (Chapter 4). The disease involves psychomotor retardation and is often subdivided into a severe infantile type 1 and a milder disease phenotype (type II), although, in common with other lysosomal disorders, in reality there is probably a clinical continuum (Chapter 3). This enzyme contributes to the catabolism of multiple fucosylated glycoconjugates including glycoproteins, GSLs, and oligosaccharides. Its inclusion in a glycoprotein category only indicates part of the story. The mannosidoses (α- and β-mannosidosis) fit well within a glycoprotein storage family category, as mannose is restricted to glycoprotein substrates. In α-mannosidosis, all oligosaccharides isolated from urine have a single GlcNAc residue at the reducing terminus glycosidically-linked to multiple mannose residues. The major species found in patient urine is Manα1-3Manβ1-4GlcNAc. The major storage disaccharide found in β-mannosidosis patients is Manβ1-4GlcNAc. The storage molecule can become sialylated and constitutes approximately 10% of the total storage burden.

Sialidosis results from a primary defect in the lysosomal sialidase (neuraminidase), leading to the storage of multiple sialaylated glycoconjugates, including glycoproteins and gangliosides (Chapter 4). It is clinically and biochemically very similar (in terms of storage species) to galactosialidosis (Chapter 3), although the defect at the molecular level is quite different. As mentioned above, galactosialidosis has two enzyme deficiencies, β-galactosidase and neuraminidase. These deficiencies arise secondary to a defect in a different gene that encodes another lysosomal protein, protective protein/cathepsin A (PPCA) (Chapter 7, and below).

Schindler disease is a primary *N*-acetylgalactosaminidase deficiency that has been relatively recently recognized to be a lysosomal disorder (Chapters 3 and 4) (Desnick and Schindler 2001) and is another disease with complexity in terms of storage substrates, rendering classification difficult. While it is typically placed in the glycoprotein storage sub-family, all of the substrates have a characteristic and diagnostic terminal α-*N*-acetylgalacosamine residue and include O- and N-linked glycopeptides, GSLs (including forssman antigen), and keratan sulfate type II. The relative abundance of these different species in different tissues has not yet been fully elucidated (Desnick and Schindler 2001).

Mucolipidoses

The mucolipidosis (ML) category of lysosomal disease was designated for those disorders that exhibit similarities to both the MPSs and the sphingolipidoses (Spranger and Wiedemann 1970). ML type I was a classification originally assigned to a type of sialidosis (neuraminidase deficiency), but this designation is generally no longer used, as the number of types of sialidosis has expanded. Sialidosis is now more commonly categorized with oligosaccharide storage disorders (discussed above). ML types II and III, which are also known as I-cell disease and pseudo-Hurler polydystrophy, are unrelated to ML type I and in fact are caused by an unusual mechanism involving a defect in lysosomal enzyme targeting (Chapter 6, and discussed below). There is an additional disease, ML-IV, which bears clinical and biochemical similarity with the other ML disorders but is caused by an unusual metabolic defect in a transmembrane protein called mucolipin (Chapter 9, and discussed below). Thus, the ML group of disorders clearly demonstrates that categorization of lysosomal diseases using the clinical presentation coupled with the biochemical nature of the storage molecules can lead to odd collections of diseases with disparate aetiologies.

Neuronal ceroid lipofuscinoses

Perhaps the most enigmatic of the storage diseases, in terms of a group of disorders, have been those characterized by storage of so-called ceroid-lipofuscin. This term was coined in the early 1960s by Zemen and colleagues to describe the occurrence of autofluorescent lipopigment accumulation in neurones in several storage diseases (Zemen 1976). Also known as Batten disease (a term most commonly applied to the juvenile form of the disease group), the NCL disorders are now believed to encompass at least eight different genetic types (CLN1–CLN8). The nature of the primary storage material, oddly enough, still remains to be determined. Studies in recent years have shown that most forms of NCL disease are characterized by substantial accumulation of the c subunit of mitochondrial ATP synthase (see Chapter 12), but the reason for its elevation and relationship with the primary genetic defects and with disease pathogenesis remain poorly understood. The infantile forms of this disease (CLN1 defect) are also characterized by increased levels of saposins in tissues, although again without known cause. Accumulation of proteins within membrane-bounded organelles within neuronal perikarya, however, is consistent with these disorders being classed as lysosomal proteinoses (Palmer *et al.* 1986). This view is further reinforced by the finding that the defective proteins in CLN1 and CLN2 are both lysosomal enzymes (palmitoyl protein thioesterase and pepstatin-insentitive peptidase, respectively) (Hoffman and Peltonen 2001). Other defective proteins in this disease group (CLN3, CLN4, CLN5, and CLN6), however, are transmembrane proteins whose function has not been fully elucidated. CLN4 and CLN7 diseases remain undefined genetically.

Others

There are a number of lysosomal storage diseases that fail to fit conveniently into any of the above categories, once again reflecting the difficulty of a classification system based on the identity of the primary storage substrate, coupled with characteristic clinical and pathological findings. Examples of these diseases include multiple sulfatase deficiency (Chapter 5), which is caused by an abnormality in lysosomal enzyme processing secondary to a defect in a non-lysosomal enzyme, and cystinosis and free sialic acid storage diseases, which are caused by defects in transmembrane proteins. These disorders will be considered in greater detail below.

Classifying lysosomal diseases on the basis of molecular defect

Steady progress in recent years in understanding the molecular genetics of lysosomal storage disorders has revealed that many of the defective proteins responsible for storage are not lysosomal hydrolases (Fig. 2.1). Such discoveries not only have revealed that storage diseases with similar phenotypes can result from radically different molecular defects but also, with the advent of various therapeutic strategies, have raised awareness that utilization of such treatments must be tailored to these defects. For example, bone marrow transplantation theoretically might lead to improvement in Niemann–Pick disease type C if caused by a defect in NPC2 (a soluble lysosomal protein targeted via the mannose-6-phosphate receptor), whereas those cases due to NPC1 (a membrane-bound protein) would not. The discovery of non-lysosomal enzyme defects has also been remarkably revealing in terms of normal biology of cells, as is readily illustrated by the discovery that I-cell disease was caused by a phosphokinase, which in turn led to the discovery of the mannose-6-phosphate recognition system for lysosomal targeting (Natowicz *et al.* 1979). It is for these reasons that a classification system based on molecular defects, viewed in parallel with the traditional system, can be of value. Presently, six broad categories of molecular defects responsible for causing accumulation of materials within the endosomal–lysosomal system can be recognized and are the

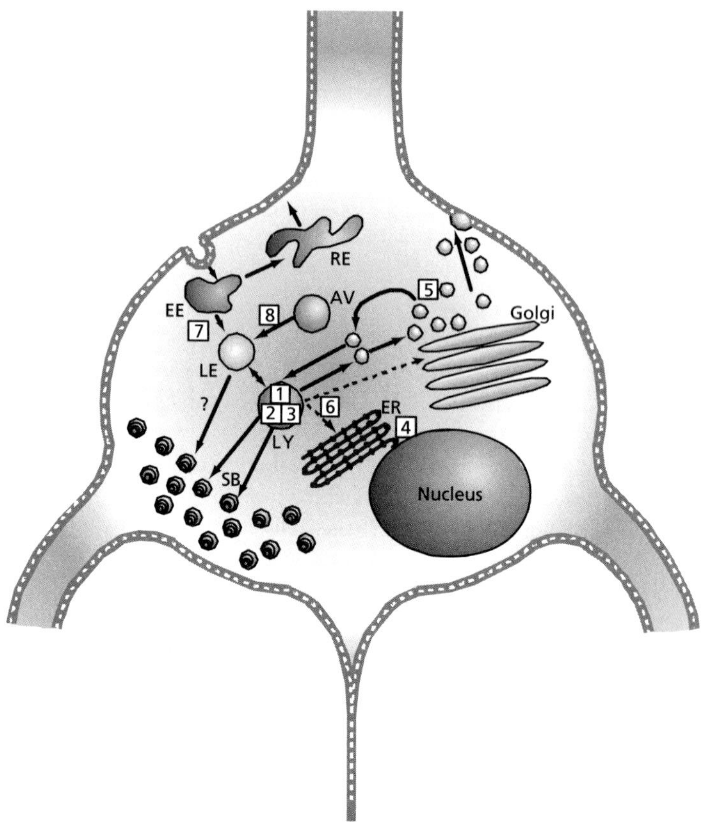

Fig. 2.1 Schematic illustration of a neurone and its endosomal–lysosomal system with known or putative sites of molecular defects leading to lysosomal storage disease. Storage bodies (SB) are generated by accumulation of materials within late endosomes (LE) and lysosomes (LY) (*double arrow* depicts functional continuity between these compartments). These vesicles are in close functional association with early endosomes (EE) and recycling endosomes (RE). Defects within the LE–LY compartment include those directly impacting lysosomal enzymes [1], protective protein [2], and activator proteins [3], as seen in Tay–Sachs, galactosialidosis, and GM2 gangliosidosis AB variant diseases, respectively. Lysosomal enzyme processing in the endoplasmic reticulum (ER) may be abnormal [4], as seen in multiple sulfatase deficiency. Lysosomal enzymes may be made and processed normally but fail to receive the mannose-6-phospate recognition marker during transit through the Golgi resulting in, for example, I-cell disease [5]. Abnormal movement of degraded materials (gangliosides and cholesterol) out of the LE–LY compartment secondary to defects in transmembrane proteins may lead to diseases like Niemann–Pick type C [6]. Other transmembrane proteins may facilitate earlier endocytic events [7] or autophagic processing and vesicle fusion [8] as seen in mucolipidoses IV and Danon disease, respectively (Modified from Walkley 2001). **See Plate 1.**

focus of Chapters 4–9. Included here are defects in genes encoding lysosomal enzymes, endoplasmic reticulum and Golgi-associated processing enzymes, protective proteins and other soluble lysosomal proteins, and transmembrane proteins related to substrate movement out of endosomes/lysosomes or involved with endosome fusion or related vesicular trafficking. Illustrated in Table 2.2 is an outline of storage diseases based on molecular defect. It is by no means a final categorization, for as we learn more about individual defects, particularly those affecting various transmembrane proteins, additional subdivisions or modifications will be

Table 2.2

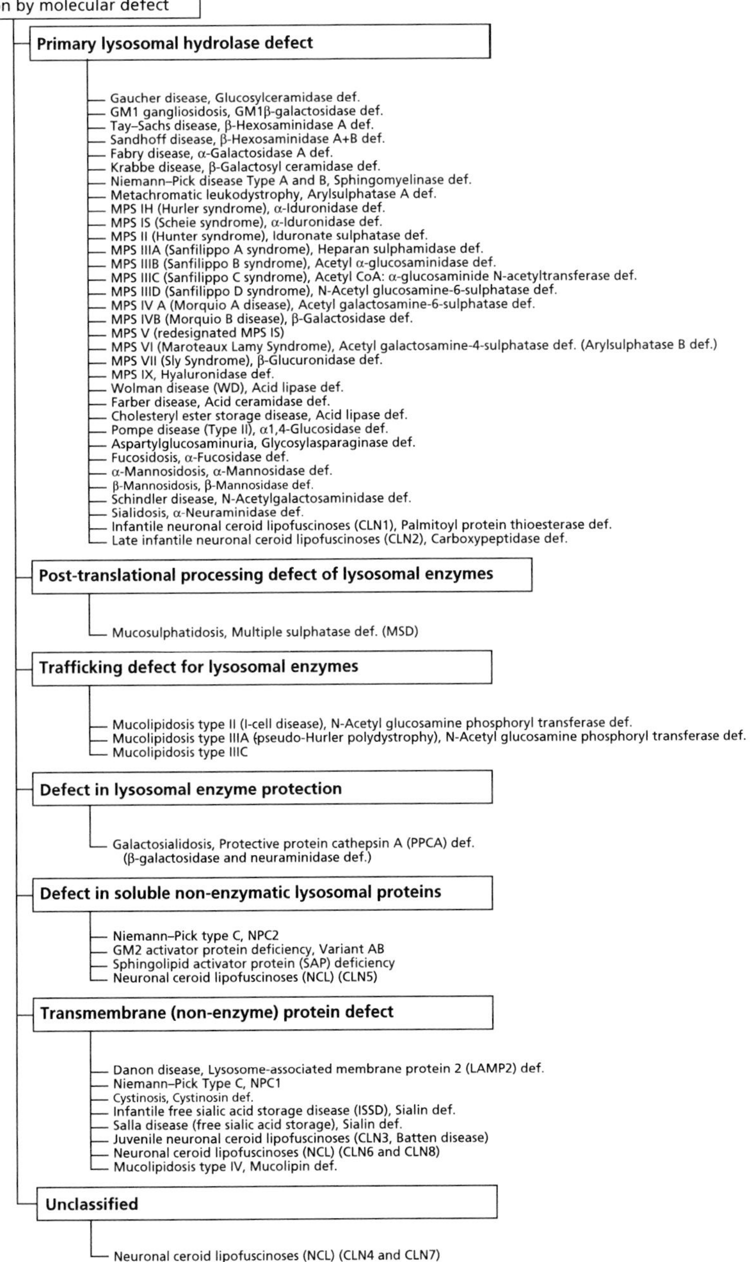

Lysosomal Storage Disorders
classification by molecular defect

- **Primary lysosomal hydrolase defect**
  - Gaucher disease, Glucosylceramidase def.
  - GM1 gangliosidosis, GM1β-galactosidase def.
  - Tay–Sachs disease, β-Hexosaminidase A def.
  - Sandhoff disease, β-Hexosaminidase A+B def.
  - Fabry disease, α-Galactosidase A def.
  - Krabbe disease, β-Galactosyl ceramidase def.
  - Niemann–Pick disease Type A and B, Sphingomyelinase def.
  - Metachromatic leukodystrophy, Arylsulphatase A def.
  - MPS IH (Hurler syndrome), α-Iduronidase def.
  - MPS IS (Scheie syndrome), α-Iduronidase def.
  - MPS II (Hunter syndrome), Iduronate sulphatase def.
  - MPS IIIA (Sanfilippo A syndrome), Heparan sulphamidase def.
  - MPS IIIB (Sanfilippo B syndrome), Acetyl α-glucosaminidase def.
  - MPS IIIC (Sanfilippo C syndrome), Acetyl CoA: α-glucosaminide N-acetyltransferase def.
  - MPS IIID (Sanfilippo D syndrome), N-Acetyl glucosamine-6-sulphatase def.
  - MPS IV A (Morquio A disease), Acetyl galactosamine-6-sulphatase def.
  - MPS IVB (Morquio B disease), β-Galactosidase def.
  - MPS V (redesignated MPS IS)
  - MPS VI (Maroteaux Lamy Syndrome), Acetyl galactosamine-4-sulphatase def. (Arylsulphatase B def.)
  - MPS VII (Sly Syndrome), β-Glucuronidase def.
  - MPS IX, Hyaluronidase def.
  - Wolman disease (WD), Acid lipase def.
  - Farber disease, Acid ceramidase def.
  - Cholesteryl ester storage disease, Acid lipase def.
  - Pompe disease (Type II), α1,4-Glucosidase def.
  - Aspartylglucosaminuria, Glycosylasparaginase def.
  - Fucosidosis, α-Fucosidase def.
  - α-Mannosidosis, α-Mannosidase def.
  - β-Mannosidosis, β-Mannosidase def.
  - Schindler disease, N-Acetylgalactosaminidase def.
  - Sialidosis, α-Neuraminidase def.
  - Infantile neuronal ceroid lipofuscinoses (CLN1), Palmitoyl protein thioesterase def.
  - Late infantile neuronal ceroid lipofuscinoses (CLN2), Carboxypeptidase def.
- **Post-translational processing defect of lysosomal enzymes**
  - Mucosulphatidosis, Multiple sulphatase def. (MSD)
- **Trafficking defect for lysosomal enzymes**
  - Mucolipidosis type II (I-cell disease), N-Acetyl glucosamine phosphoryl transferase def.
  - Mucolipidosis type IIIA (pseudo-Hurler polydystrophy), N-Acetyl glucosamine phosphoryl transferase def.
  - Mucolipidosis type IIIC
- **Defect in lysosomal enzyme protection**
  - Galactosialidosis, Protective protein cathepsin A (PPCA) def. (β-galactosidase and neuraminidase def.)
- **Defect in soluble non-enzymatic lysosomal proteins**
  - Niemann–Pick type C, NPC2
  - GM2 activator protein deficiency, Variant AB
  - Sphingolipid activator protein (SAP) deficiency
  - Neuronal ceroid lipofuscinoses (NCL) (CLN5)
- **Transmembrane (non-enzyme) protein defect**
  - Danon disease, Lysosome-associated membrane protein 2 (LAMP2) def.
  - Niemann–Pick Type C, NPC1
  - Cystinosis, Cystinosin def.
  - Infantile free sialic acid storage disease (ISSD), Sialin def.
  - Salla disease (free sialic acid storage), Sialin def.
  - Juvenile neuronal ceroid lipofuscinoses (CLN3, Batten disease)
  - Neuronal ceroid lipofuscinoses (NCL) (CLN6 and CLN8)
  - Mucolipidosis type IV, Mucolipin def.
- **Unclassified**
  - Neuronal ceroid lipofuscinoses (NCL) (CLN4 and CLN7)

in order. Indeed, for sake of discussion, we have further divided transmembrane defects into an additional three categories, for a total of eight classes of molecular defects (Fig. 2.2).

Primary lysosomal hydrolase defects

Most known forms of lysosomal storage diseases are caused by mutations in genes encoding individual catabolic enzymes (Chapter 4). Thus, included in this group are the classic conditions, Tay–Sachs and Gaucher diseases, infantile and late-infantile NCL disorders, and Niemann–Pick disease type A, as well as all of the MPSs. In all such cases, the endosomal–lysosomal system is deprived of a functional enzyme due to a mutation in the gene encoding that protein. Excluded from the group are numerous storage diseases including the Tay–Sachs-like condition known as GM2 gangliosidosis AB variant, Niemann–Pick disease type C, all types of the mucolipidoses, and most of the NCL disorders. Many individuals with defects in genes encoding hydrolases are actually compound heterozygotes and exhibit variable degrees of enzyme activity (Chapter 4) and thus variable phenotypic expression (Chapter 3). Individuals with single defective alleles (genetic carriers) for lysosomal hydrolases typically exhibit intermediate enzyme expression and are phenotypically normal. This may not always be the case such as female carriers of the X-linked Fabry disease and for non-enzyme proteins, e.g. NPC1, where partial deficiency may lead to at least rare cellular defects (Brown *et al.* 1996).

Post-translational processing defect of lysosomal enzymes

As mentioned above, several types of storage diseases have been discovered that essentially defy classification in the traditional scheme. One of these is multiple sulfatase deficiency, a disorder characterized by a striking reduction in catalytic activity of all 12 known sulfatases (Chapter 5) (Hopwood and Ballabio 2001). The substrates for these enzymes are diverse and include sulfated glycosaminoglycans, GSLs, glycopeptides, and hydroxysteroids. This disease arises due to a deficiency in a mechanism that modifies all of these enzymes to generate an α-formylglycine residue by oxidizing the thiol group in an active site cysteine. The cysteine is conserved in all mammalian sulfatases, hence the defect affects the catalytic activity of all sulfatases.

Trafficking defect of lysosomal enzymes

Functional deficiency of multiple lysosomal enzymes is also seen in the disorder known as I-cell disease (ML II) and in its related counterparts ML IIIA (pseudo-Hurler polydystrophy) and ML IIIC. These disorders are clinically similar to Hurler syndrome but do not exhibit mucopolysacchariduria (Chapters 3 and 6) (Kornfeld and Sly 2001). Pseudo-Hurler polydystrophy, ML IIIA, and its clinical variant ML IIIC are milder disorders than ML II with later onset of clinical signs. Both ML II and III diseases are the result of a defect in lysosomal enzyme transport within cells (including neurones) such that instead of being routed to the lysosome, the newly synthesized lysosomal enzymes are secreted from the cell. As a consequence, affected cells have prominent storage bodies, and elevated levels of lysosomal enzymes can be detected in the serum and body fluids. Failure to target the enzymes correctly results from an enzyme deficiency affecting the synthesis of the mannose-6-phosphate-recognition marker (Chapter 6). The recognition marker is synthesized in two steps in the Golgi, with the first step catalysed by UDP-*N*-acetylglucosamine: lysosomal enzyme *N*-acetylglucosaminyl-1-phosphotransferase. It is interesting that although the phosphotransferase is deficient in all cells, only some cell types are affected, implying that alternative transport pathways are also available (Kornfeld and Sly 2001). ML II and IIIA diseases have been shown to be allelic and are both characterized by defects in this Golgi-associated enzyme. ML IIIC, in contrast, exhibits normal activity of the phosphotransferase enzyme against artificial substrates. This enzyme has been found to be composed of three subunits ($\alpha_2\beta_2\gamma_2$) coded for by two different genes (α and β by one and γ by the other). Type II and IIIA diseases are known to be caused by defects in the α-β gene, and recently, ML IIIC has been reported to possess a defect specifically in the gene coding for the γ-subunit (Raas-Rothschild *et al.* 2000). This finding indicates that the γ-subunit of the enzyme is specifically responsible for lysosomal hydrolase recognition and provides the molecular mechanism for ML IIIC disease.

Defect in lysosomal enzyme protection

In one type of lysosomal storage disease, the catabolic enzymes are encoded, synthesized, and trafficked normally, but upon reaching the lysosome are themselves degraded. In this case, a protein, PPCA, associates with two enzymes (β-galactosidase and sialidase) during biosynthesis and the complex is routed to the lysosome where the enzymes are protected from intralysosomal proteolysis (Chapter 7). Patients with this disorder, which is known as galactosialidosis, accumulate a range of substrates including fully sialylated complex N-glycans and gangliosides. Galactosialidosis is dominated by the loss of sialidase activity since β-galactosidase largely acts downstream of the sialidase and therefore contributes little to the disease. For this reason, the disorder has clinical and pathological similarity to sialidosis, a disease caused by a primary sialidase deficiency (Chapters 3 and 4).

Defect in soluble non-enzymatic lysosomal proteins

In addition to lysosomal hydrolases and protective proteins described above, the lysosome also contains numerous soluble non-enzyme glycoproteins shown to be critical for lysosomal hydrolase function. These so-called activator proteins have been most commonly referred to as sphingolipid activator proteins (SAPs) or as saposins. The first of these proteins to be discovered was a co-factor for arylsulfatase A in the degradation of sulfatides (Fischer and Jatzkewitz 1978). Subsequent discoveries revealed four different types of SAP proteins (A–D), but with each produced through the proteolytic processing of a single precursor protein called prosaposin (Chapter 8). A fifth member of the group has also been described and is coded for on a separate gene. This protein, the GM2 activator, was found to be deficient in cases of GM2 gangliosidosis in which β-hexosaminidase appeared normal (Conzelmann and Sandhoff 1978). Like the other SAPs, the GM2 activator was believed to be essential in the degradation of GSLs with short oligosaccharide head groups through lifting this part of the molecule to allow enzymatic cleavage, hence its designation as a 'liftase' (Sandhoff and Kolter 1996). Several proteins with homology to SAPs (saposin-like or SAPIPs) have also been described recently, with all sharing similar lipid-(including phospholipid) and membrane-binding properties (Vaccaro *et al.* 1999). Some studies have also suggested that the GM2 activator protein may additionally function in lipid transport

(Mahuran 1998; Mundel *et al.* 1999), raising interesting questions about the overall role of these small glycoproteins in lysosomal function.

Yet another soluble lysosomal protein recently discovered is NPC2, an absence of which has been shown to be responsible for approximately 5% of cases of Niemann–Pick disease type C, a cholesterol-ganglioside lipidosis (Chapters 8, 9, and 12). NPC2 was previously identified in human epididymus and referred to as HE1 (Naureckiene *et al.* 2000). It is believed to be a cholesterol-binding protein, to be at least in part secreted from cells, and to be delivered to the lysosome by way of the mannose-6-phosphate pathway. While the function of NPC2 remains unknown, the similarity of the diseases caused by NPC1 and NPC2 deficiencies suggests that the two proteins may be acting in concert with retroendocytic substrate shuttling from the late endosomal system to the Golgi or other locations in the cell.

Transmembrane (non-enzyme) protein defects

The newest and most rapidly expanding group of molecular defects that have been documented as giving rise to storage in neurones and other cells involves transmembrane proteins. In most cases, the functions of these proteins remain poorly understood, but current evidence suggests that a variety of trafficking, vesicle fusion, and substrate shuttling mechanisms are probably involved (Fig. 2.1).

NPC1

The discovery that lysosomal sphingomyelinase was deficient in type A and type B Niemann–Pick diseases, but was normal in types C and D, left these latter forms of the Niemann–Pick disorders without any known cause. Furthermore, the discovery of a cholesterol homoeostatic defect in type C fibroblasts and the usefulness of a cholesterol challenge test for diagnosis led to an emphasis on cholesterol rather than GSLs as a primary storage material (Pentchev *et al.* 1985). The identity of the defective gene and protein responsible for the vast majority of type C and D cases were reported by Carstea and colleagues in 1997. The protein showed homology to patched and possessed a sterol-sensing domain, consistent with it playing a key role in retroendocytic shuttling of cholesterol. Its location in association with a transient late endosomal vesicle population further supported this role. However, while unesterified cholesterol has been found to be elevated in neurones lacking NPC1 (Zervas *et al.* 2001), storage of gangliosides is also known to be prominent. Recent studies (reviewed in Chapter 12) indicate that cholesterol storage in neurones of the murine NPC1 model is reduced when synthesis of GM2 and higher order gangliosides is prevented, a finding that raises significant questions about the primacy of cholesterol in this disease (Gondré-Lewis *et al.* 2003). One recent study (Davies *et al.* 2000) suggests that NPC1 is a eukaryotic version of a prokaryotic permease. Although the substrate moved in this way by the NPC1 protein was not determined, evidence did suggest that it was not cholesterol (Chapter 9).

Cystinosin

The lysosomal disease known as cystinosis arises due to a defect in the carrier-mediated transport of the amino acid cystine across the lysosomal membrane, resulting in intralysosomal crystalline cystine inclusions. The disease has a characteristic nephropathology with renal failure leading to premature death in affected individuals (Chapter 3). The gene of the lysosomal cystine carrier is located on chromosome 17p13 and encodes a protein called cystinosin that has seven transmembrane spanning domains (Chapter 9). This protein plays an essential role in cystine transport out of the lysosome. Chronic cystine-depleting therapy (using cysteamine) is effective, preserving renal function, provided therapy is initiated early (Gahl *et al.* 2001). One report has suggested that severe brain involvement can also occur in the absence of cystinosin (Jonas *et al.* 1987).

Sialin

The free sialic acid lysosomal storage diseases (Salla disease) and infantile free sialic acid storage disease (ISSD) result from the accumulation of free sialic acid in lysosomes (Aula and Gahl 2001) (Chapter 3) and are characterized clinically by psychomotor retardation (Chapter 3). Note the comparison with sialidosis, discussed above with the glycoproteinoses, which exhibits lysosomal storage of sialic acid-linked glycoconjugates. The free sialic acid storage diseases arise from impaired carrier-mediated transport of sialic acid (and to a lesser extent glucoronic acid and monocarboxylates such as lactate, pyruvate, and valproate) in the lysosomal membrane. The defective gene codes for sialin, an essential monosaccharide transporter protein that serves to remove from the lysosome monosaccharides and other ligands that arise as end products of glycoconjugate catabolism (Chapter 9).

Mucolipin

The genetic basis of a form of mucolipidoses (type IV), distinct from ML types I, IIIA, and IIIC discussed above, has also been recently elucidated (Sun *et al.* 2000) (Chapter 9). ML IV is characterized by early onset of growth and psychomotor retardation and severe visual impairments and, like the other MLs, exhibits features of both the sphingolipidoses and MPSs. Importantly, however, lysosomal enzymes required for the degradation of these compounds appear normal. Pagano and colleagues have examined ML IV fibroblasts in culture using fluorescent endocytic markers and have shown that lysosomal storage may be secondary to an abnormality in lipid efflux from these organelles (Chen *et al.* 1998). Interestingly, the defective gene in ML IV has been found to code for a protein (mucolipin) which has characteristics of members of the polycystin II sub-family of the *Drosophila* transient receptor potential (TRP) gene family (Clapham *et al.* 2001). Members of the TRP family exhibit a topology of six transmembrane segments and most have been implicated in a diverse array of cell functions including calcium entry following receptor activation, receptor-mediated excitation, and cell-cycle modulation. While these functions appear at odds with the presence of lipid storage in lysosomes, polycystin-2 in one report has been implicated in lipid transport towards basolateral membranes in primary kidney cell cultures (Charron *et al.* 2000). Furthermore, mutation of the *Caenorhabditis elegans* homologue of mucolipin (CUP-5) has recently been shown to cause enhanced uptake of fluid-phase markers, decreased degradation of endocytosed protein, and accumulation of large vacuoles (Fares and Greenwald 2001). Overexpression of CUP-5 caused an opposite phenotype consistent with this protein in some way regulating endocytosis.

LAMP2

Lysosomal membranes are known to contain a variety of highly N-glycosylated proteins, including LAMP1 and LAMP2. Recent studies have indicated that patients with an unusual form of glycogenosis known as Danon disease have defects in LAMP2 (Nishino *et al.* 2000) (Chapter 9). Interestingly, a recent report on a knockout of LAMP2 in mice has revealed a severe storage disease model characterized by abnormalities in the degradation of long-lived proteins in hepatocytes and other cells (Tanaka *et al.* 2000). Similarities between the mouse model and human Danon disease suggested that accumulation of autophagic material was central to the disease process, suggesting a link between LAMP2 function and the fusion of autophagocytic vacuoles with endosomes or lysosomes. In contrast, mice in which the gene for LAMP1 was knocked out showed no lysosomal pathology but did demonstrate a striking upregulation of LAMP2 protein (Andrejewski *et al.* 1999).

CLN proteins

Whereas the proteins found defective in and responsible for CLN1 and CLN2 diseases have been identified as a lysosomal thioesterase and peptidase, respectively (see above), all of the other forms of neuronal ceroid lipofuscinosis in which genes have been identified involve transmembrane proteins of unknown function. In most cases, the precise identity of membranes in which the proteins reside remains poorly understood. For example, although the CLN3 protein (battenin) has been identified in lysosomal membranes (Jarvela *et al.* 1998), other studies have suggested mitochondrial localization (Janes *et al.* 1996) (Chapter 9). Initial studies of the CLN5 protein suggested that it was a transmembrane protein, but more recent studies have challenged this view and suggested that it may be soluble lysosomal protein (Isosomppi *et al.* 2002). The recently discovered CLN6 protein (linclin) appears to be yet another type of membrane spanning protein of presently unknown location and function (Gao *et al.* 2002). The similarity of the clinical and pathological features of NCL disorders has suggested that many of these proteins may normally function together, possibly as protein complexes. Indeed, one recent study suggested that CLN5 polypeptides directly interact with both CLN2 and CLN3 proteins based on immunoprecipitation studies and *in vivo* binding assays (Vesa *et al.* 2002). CLN3 protein has also been implicated in the regulation of lysosomal pH (Pearce *et al.* 1999), yet another way that dysfunction of one of these proteins may interfere with the function of others, particularly given that CLN1 and CLN2 proteins are believed to be lysosomal enzymes.

Summary

Over the past decades, considerable progress has been made in understanding the underlying mechanisms leading to the storage of molecules in the lysosome. Although the majority of these diseases do arise through a direct lysosomal enzyme defect, as originally predicted, many others clearly do not. The latter have proved challenging to elucidate, and we still do not understand the cell biological basis for several of these diseases. Classification of related diseases can be very helpful in facilitating correct diagnosis, improving understanding, and designing appropriate therapies. The traditional classification systems based on the biochemical nature of the storage molecule(s) only provide partial insight into these disorders. For some disease categories it is helpful (e.g. MPSs), but for others, multiple substrates accumulate, and we still do not understand the pathobiology at the cellular level (e.g. NPC). In this chapter we have set out the pros and cons of both a substrate-based classification scheme and one that is based on molecular mechanism leading to storage. Both have different roles to play in aiding our understanding of these disorders and their biochemical and molecular relationships. However, it is certainly the case that a mechanism-based understanding is the only route to the rational development of therapies. It also gives a different perspective on the disease process, emphasizing the complexities of the underlying pathogenic cascades. In this book, we have therefore elected to organize topics on the basis of mechanisms leading to disease. By including summary diagrams of both traditional and mechanism-based classification schemes, we hope to provide a useful framework for the reader to understand the biochemical storage material characteristic of each disease but at the same time emphasize how this storage arises.

References

Andrejewski, N., Punnonen, E. L., Guhde, G. *et al.* (1999). Normal lysosomal morphology and function in LAMP-1-deficient mice. *J Biol Chem*, **274**, 12692–701.

Assmann, G. and Seedorf, U. (2001). Acid lipase deficiency: Wolman disease and cholesteryl ester storage disease. In *The metabolic and molecular bases of inherited disease* (Scriver, C. R., Beadet, A. L., Valle, D. and Sly, W. S., ed.), Vol. 3, pp. 3551–72. New York: McGraw-Hill.

Aula, P. and Gahl, W. A. (2001). Disorders of free sialic acid storage. In *The metabolic and molecular bases of inherited disease* (Scriver, C. R., Beadet, A. L., Valle, D. and Sly, W. S., ed.), Vol. 3, pp. 5109–20. New York: McGraw-Hill.

Beutler, E. and Grabowski, G. (2001). Gaucher disease. In *The metabolic and molecular bases of inherited disease* (Scriver, C. R., Beadet, A. L., Valle, D. and Sly, W. S., ed.), Vol. 3, pp. 3636–68. New York: McGraw-Hill.

Bielschowsky, M. (1921). Zur histopathologie und pathogenese der amaurotischen idiotie mit besonderer berücksichtigung der zerebellaren veränderungen. *J Psychol Neurol*, **26**, 123–99.

Brante, G. (1952). Gargoylism: a mucopolysaccharidosis. *Scand J Clin Lab Invest*, **4**, 43–8.

Brown, D., Thrall, M. A. and Walkley, S. U. (1996). Feline Niemann–Pick disease type C heterozygotes: Evidence of abnormal metabolic events in brain and viscera. *J Inherit Metabol Dis*, **19**, 319–30.

Carstea, E. D., Morris, J. A., Coleman, K. G. *et al.* (1997). Niemann–Pick C1 disease gene: Homology to mediators of cholesterol homeostasis. *Science*, **277**, 228–31.

Charron, A. J., Nakamura, S., Bacallao, R. and Wandinger-Ness, A. (2000). Compromised cytoarchitecture and polarized trafficking in autosomal dominant polycystic kidney disease cells. *J Cell Biol*, **149**, 111–24.

Chen, Y.-T. (2001). Glycogen storage diseases. In *The metabolic and molecular bases of inherited disease* (Scriver, C. R., Beadet, A. L., Valle, D. and Sly, W. S., ed.), Vol. 1, pp. 1521–51. New York: McGraw-Hill.

Chen, C. S., Bach, G. and Pagano, R. (1998). Abnormal transport along the lysosomal pathway in mucolipidosis type IV disease. *Proc Natl Acad Sci USA*, **95**, 6373–8.

Clapham, D. E., Runnels, L. W. and Strübing, C. (2001). The TRP ion channel family. *Nat Rev Neurosci*, **2**, 387–96.

Conzelmann, E. and Sandhoff, K. (1978). AB-variant of infantile GM2 gangliosidosis. Deficiency of a factor necessary for stimulation of hexosaminidase A-catalyzed degradation of ganglioside GM2 and glycolipid GA2. *Proc Natl Acad Sci USA*, **75**, 3979–83.

Davies, J. P., Chen, F. W. and Ioannou, Y. (2000). Transmembrane molecular pump activity of Niemann–Pick C1 protein. *Science*, **290**, 2295–8.

Desnick, R. J., Ioannou, Y. A. and Eng, C. M. (2001). Alpha-galctosidase A deficiency: Fabry disease. In *The metabolic and molecular bases of inherited disease* (Scriver, C. R., Beuadet, A. L., Valle, D. and Sly, W. S., ed.) , Vol. 3, pp. 3733–74. New York: McGraw-Hill.

Desnick, R. J. and Schindler, D. (2001). Alpha-*N*-acetylgalactosaminidase deficiency: Schindler disease. In *The metabolic and molecular bases of inherited disease* (Scriver, C. R., Beadet, A. L., Valle, D. and Sly, W. S., ed.), Vol. 3, pp. 3483–506. New York: McGraw-Hill.

de Duve, C., Pressman, B. C., Gianetto, R., Wattiaux, R. and Appelmans, F. (1955). Tissue fractionation studies: Intracellular distribution patterns of enzymes in rat-liver tissue. *Biochem J*, **64**, 604–17.

Fares, H. and Greenwald, I. (2001). Regulation of endocytosis by CUP-5, the *Caenorhabditis elegans* mucolipin-1 homolog. *Nat Genet*, **28**, 64–8.

von Figura, K., Gieselmann, V. and Jaeken, J. (2001). Metachromatic leukodystrophy. In *The metabolic and molecular bases of inherited disease* (Scriver, C. R., Beadet, A. L., Valle, D. and Sly, W. S., ed.), Vol. 3, pp. 3695–724. New York: McGraw-Hill.

Fischer, G. and Jatzkewitz, H. (1978). The activator of cerebroside sulfatase. A. Model of the activation. *Biochim Biophys Acta*, **528**, 69.

Gahl, W. A., Theone, J. G. and Schneider, J. A. (2001). Cystinosis: A disorder of lysosomal membrane transport. In *The metabolic and molecular bases of inherited disease* (Scriver, C. R., Beadet, A. L., Valle, D. and Sly, W. S., ed.), Vol. 3, pp. 5085–108. New York: McGraw-Hill.

Gao, H., Boustany, R. N., Espinola, J. A. *et al.* (2002). Mutations in a novel *CLN6*-encoded transmembrane protein cause variant neuronal ceroid lipofuscinosis in man and mouse. *Am J Hum Genet*, **70**, 324–35.

Garrod, A. (1909). *Inborn errors of metabolism*. Oxford: Oxford University Press.

Gondré-Lewis, M., McGlynn, R. and Walkley, S. U. (2003). Cholesterol accumulation in NPC1-deficient neurons is ganglioside-dependent. *Current Biology* **13**, 1324–9.

Hers, H. G. (1963). α-glucosidase deficiency in generalised glycogen storage disease (Pompe's disease). *Biochem J*, **86**, 11–16.

Hirsch, W. (1898). The pathological anatomy of a fatal disease of infancy with symmetrical changes in the region of the yellow spot. *J Nerv Ment Dis*, **25**, 529.

Hirschborn, R. and Reuser, A. J. J. (2001). Glycogen storage disease type II: acid alpha-glucosidase (acid maltase) deficiency. In *The metabolic and molecular bases of inherited disease* (Scriver, C. R., Beadet, A. L., Valle, D. and Sly, W. S., ed.), Vol. 3, pp. 3389–420. New York: McGraw-Hill.

Hoffman, S. and Peltonen, L. (2001). The neuronal ceroid lipofuscinoses. In *The metabolic and molecular bases of inherited disease*, (Scriver, C. R., Beaudet, A. L., Sly, W. S. and Valle, D., ed.), 8th edn., Vol. 3, pp. 3877–94. New York: McGraw-Hill.

Hopwood, J. J. and Ballabio, A. (2001). Multiple sulfatase deficiency and the nature of the sulfatase family. In *The metabolic and molecular bases of inherited disease* (Scriver, C. R., Beadet, A. L., Valle, D. and Sly, W. S., ed.), Vol. 3, pp. 3725–32. New York: McGraw-Hill.

Isosomppi, J., Vesa, J., Jalanko, A. and Peltonen, L. (2002). Lysosomal localization of the neuronal ceroid lipofuscinosis CLN5 protein. *Hum Mol Genet*, **11**, 885–91.

Janes, R. W., Munroe, P. B., Mitchison, H. M., Gardiner, R. M., Mole, S. E. and Wallace, B. A. (1996). A model for Batten disease protein CLN3: Functional implications from homology and mutations. *FEBS Lett*, **399**, 75–7.

Jarvela, I., Sainio, M., Rantamaki, T. *et al.* (1998). Biosynthesis and intracellular targeting of the CLN3 protein defective in Batten disease. *Hum Mol Genet*, **7**, 85–90.

Jonas, A. J., Conley, S. B., Marshall, R., Johnson, R. A., Marks, M. and Rosenberg, H. (1987). Nephropathic cystinosis with central nervous system involvement. *Am J Med*, **83**, 966.

Kornfeld, S. and Sly, W. S. (2001). I-Cell disease and pseudo-Hurler polydystrophy: disorders of lysosomal enzyme phosphorylation and localisation. In *The metabolic and molecular bases of inherited disease* (Scriver, C. R., Beadet, A. L., Valle, D. and Sly, W. S., ed.), Vol. 3, pp. 3469–82. New York: McGraw-Hill.

Mahuran, D. J. (1998). The GM2 activator protein, its role as a co-factor in GM2 hydrolysis and as a general glycolipid transport protein. *Biochim Biophys Acta*, **1393**, 1–18.

Meikle, P. J., Hopwood, J. J., Clague, A. E. and Carey, W. F. (1999). Prevalence of lysosomal storage disorders. *JAMA*, **281**, 249–54.

Moser, H., Linke, T., Fensom, A. H., Levade, T. and Sandhoff, K. (2001). Acid ceramidase deficiency: Farber lipogranulomatosis. In *The metabolic and molecular bases of inherited disease* (Scriver, C. R., Beadet, A. L., Valle, D. and Sly, W. S., ed.), Vol. 3, pp. 3573–88. New York: McGraw-Hill.

Mundel, T. M., Heid, H. W., Mahuran, D. J., Kriz, W. and Mundel, P. (1999). Ganglioside GM2-activator protein and vesicular transport in collecting duct intercalated cells. *J Am Soc Nephrol*, **10**, 435–43.

Natowicz, M. R., Chi, M. M.-Y., Lowry, O. H. and Sly, W. S. (1979). Enzymatic identification of mannose 6-phosphate on the recognition marker for receptor-mediated pinocytosis of β-glucuronidase by human fibroblasts. *Proc Natl Acad Sci USA*, **76**, 4322–7.

Naureckiene, S., Sleat, D. E., Lackland, H. *et al.* (2000). Identification of HE1 as the second gene of Niemann–Pick C disease. *Science*, **290**, 2298–301.

Neufeld, E. F. and Muenzer, J. (2001). The mucopolysaccharidoses. In *The metabolic and molecular bases of inherited disease* (Scriver, C. R., Beadet, A. L., Valle, D. and Sly, W. S., ed.), Vol. 3, pp. 3421–52. New York: McGraw-Hill.

Nishino, I., Fu, J., Tanji, K., Yamada, T. *et al.* (2000). Primary LAMP-2 deficiency causes X-linked vacuolar cardiomyopathy and myopathy (Danon's disease). *Nature*, **406**, 906–10.

Palmer, D. N., Barns, G., Husbands, D. R. and Jolly, R. D. (1986). Ceroid lipofuscinosis in sheep. II. The major component of the lipopigment in liver, kidney, pancreas, and brain is low molecular weight protein. *J Biol Chem*, **261**, 1773–7.

Pearce, D. A., Nosel, S. A. and Sherman, F. (1999). Studies of pH regulation by Btn1p, the yeast homolog of human Cln3p. *Mol Genet Metab*, **66**, 320–3.

Pentchev, P. G., Comly, M. E., Kruth, H. S. *et al.* (1985). A defect in cholesterol esterification in Niemann–Pick disease (type C) patients. *Proc Natl Acad Sci USA*, **82**, 8247–51.

Pentchev, P., Blanchette-Mackie, J. and Dawidowicz, E. A. (1994). The NP-C gene: a key to pathways of intracellular transport. *Trends Cell Biol*, **4**, 365–9.

Poynton, F. J., Parsons, J. H. and Holmes, G. (1906). A contribution to the study of amaurotic family idiocy. *Brain*, **29**, 180–208.

Raas-Rothschild, A., Cormier-Daire, V., Bao, M. *et al.* (2000). Molecular basis of variant pseudo-Hurler polydystrophy (mucolipidosis IIIC). *J Clin Invest*, **105**, 673–81.

Sachs, B. (1887). On arrested cerebral development, with special reference to its cortical pathology. *J Nervous Mental Dis*, **14**, 541–53.

Sachs, B. (1903). On amaurotic family idiocy. A disease chiefly of the gray matter of the central nervous system. *J Nervous Mental Dis*, **30**, 1–13.

Sachs, B. and Strauss, I. (1910). The cell changes in amaurotic family idiocy. *J Exp Med*, **12**, 685–95.

Sandhoff, K. and Kolter, T. (1996). Topology of glycosphingolipid degradation. *Trends Cell Biol*, **6**, 98–103.

Schuchman, E. H. and Desnick, R. J. (2001). Niemann–Pick disease types A and B: acid sphingomylinase deficiency. In *The metabolic and molecular bases of inherited disease* (Scriver, C. R., Beadet, A. L., Valle, D. and Sly, W. S., ed.), Vol. 3, pp. 3589–610. New York: McGraw-Hill.

Sperry, W. M. (1942). The biochemistry of the lipidoses. *J Mt Sinai Hosp*, **9**, 799–817.

Spranger, J. W. and Wiedemann, H. R. (1970). The genetic mucolipidoses. *Human-Genetik*, **9**, 113.

Stengel, C. (1826). Account of a singular illness among four siblings in the vicinity of Røraas, Etr Christiania, **1**, 47–352, reprinted In *Ceroid Lipofuscinosis (Batten disease)* (Armstrong, D., Koppang, N. and Rider, J. A., ed.). Elsevier Biomedical Press.

Sun, M., Goldin, E., Stahl, S., Falardeau, J. L. *et al.* (2000). Mucolipidosis type IV is caused by mutations in a gene encoding a novel transient receptor potential channel. *Hum Mol Genet*, **9**, 2471–8.

Tanaka, Y., Guhde, G., Suter, A., Eskelinen, E.-L. *et al.* (2000). Accumulation of autophagic vacuoles and cardiomyopathy in LAMP-2-deficient mice. *Nature*, **406**, 902–6.

Tay, W. (1881). Symmetrical changes in the region of the yellow spot in each eye of an infant. *Trans Ophthalmol Soc U.K.*, **1**, 155.

Thannhauser, S. J. (1940). *Lipidoses: diseases of the cellular lipid metabolism.* London: Oxford University Press.

Vaccaro, A. M., Salvioli, R., Tatti, M. and Ciaffoni, F. (1999). Saposins and their interaction with lipids. *Neurochem Res*, **24**, 307–14.

Vesa, J., Chin, M. H., Oelgeschlager, K., Isosomppi, J., DellAngelica, E. C., Jalanko, A., Peltonen, L. (2002). Neuronal ceroid lipofuscinoses are connected at molecular level: interaction of CLN5 protein with CLN2 and CLN3. *Mol Biol Cell*, **13**, 2410–20.

Walkley, S. U. (2001). Lysosomal storage diseases: New proteins from old diseases provide new insights in cell biology. *Curr Opin Neurol*, **14**, 805–10.

Wenger, D. A., Suzuki, K., Suzuki, Y. and Suzuki, K. (2001). Galactosylceramide lipidosis: globoid cell leukodystrophy (Krabbe disease). In *The metabolic and molecular bases of inherited disease* (Scriver, C. R., Beadet, A. L., Valle, D. and Sly, W. S., ed.), Vol. 3, pp. 3669–94. New York: McGraw-Hill.

Zemen, W. (1976). The neuronal ceroid-lipofuscinoses. *Prog Neuropath*, **3**, 203–23.

Zervas, M., Dobrenis, K. and Walkley, S. U. (2001). Neurons in Niemann–Pick disease type C accumulate gangliosides and cholesterol and undergo dendritic and axonal alterations. *J Neuropathol Exp Neurol*, **60**, 49–64.

Chapter 3

Clinical aspects and diagnosis

J. Edmond Wraith

Introduction

The lysosomal storage disorders, like many other metabolic and genetic diseases, show a remarkably variable clinical phenotype. In some patients, the presentation may be in the neonatal period with hydrops fetalis, whereas in others, even with the same enzyme deficiency (but probably a different genetic mutation), onset may be late into adult life. However, for most patients, the onset of symptoms is in the first months or years of life following an often unremarkable and apparently normal period of early development.

The first signs may be some slowing of development and other neurological signs; in other patients, some visceromegaly or a dysmorphic facial appearance may be noted. Recognition of these clinical signs can assist in the selection of appropriate diagnostic tests. A number of the initial tests performed will be screening tests, as there can be considerable clinical overlap between different enzyme deficiencies, e.g. Niemann–Pick type B and Gaucher disease. A very useful property of lysosomal enzymes is the fact that although they are highly specific towards the structure and linkage of the terminal moiety on a complex macromolecule, the overall structure may not be important. It is therefore possible to measure lysosomal enzyme activities using a variety of relatively simple water-soluble substrates incorporating coloured or fluorescent groups. Such assays are commonly used for diagnostic studies. Table 3.1 lists the different disorders as well as the screening test, diagnostic test, preferred method of prenatal diagnosis, and a brief clinical synopsis for each condition.

General clinical presentation

Whilst classification based on storage product helps decide which biochemical tests are appropriate with each diagnosis, it does not help with the clinical approach to diagnosis as there is considerable clinical overlap between different groups of lysosomal disorders (see also Chapter 2). In this review, I will describe the clinical signs and symptoms in general and then concentrate in some detail on a few selected disorders that illustrate more specific modes of presentation. The neonatal presentation of lysosomal disorders has recently been reviewed (Wraith 2002).

Hydrops fetalis

Hydrops fetalis is the pathological accumulation of serous fluid within the fetal body cavities, often associated with generalized fetal and placental oedema. It is the end result of a number of possible pathologies associated with fetal cardiac failure, anaemia, or hypoproteinaemia.

Table 3.1 Lysosomal storage disorders

Disease	Enzyme deficiency	Storage material	Chromosome location	Gene mutations	Screening test	Diagnostic test	Prenatal diagnosis	Main clinical features
MPS								
MPS I (Hurler, Scheie, Hurler/Scheie)	Iduronidase	DS, HS	4p16.3	W402X, Q70X plus many others	Urine GAGs	WBC enzyme assay	CVB*	HSM, CNS, SD, DYS, OPH, CAR
MPS II (Hunter)	Iduronate-2-sulfatase	DS, HS	Xq27–28	No common mutations	Urine GAGs	Plasma enzyme assay	CVB†	HSM, CNS, SD, DYS, OPH, CAR, SK
MPS III (Sanfilippo)								
IIIA	Heparan-*N*-sulfatase	HS	17q25.3	R245H,R74C and many others	Urine GAGs	WBC enzyme assay	CVB	CNS, SD (+/−), DYS (+/−)
IIIB	*N*-Acetyl-glucosaminidase	HS	17q21.1	No common mutations	Urine GAGs	Plasma enzyme assay	CVB	CNS, SD (+/−), DYS (+/−)
IIIC	Acetyl CoA glucosamine *N*-acetyl transferase	HS	Uncertain	Unknown	Urine GAGs	WBC enzyme assay	CVB	CNS, SD (+/−), DYS (+/−)
IIID	*N*-acetyl-glucosamine-6-sulfatase	HS	12q14	Very few patients studied	Urine GAGs	WBC enzyme assay	CVB	CNS, SD (+/−), DYS (+/−)
MPS IV (Morquio)								
IVA	N-acetyl-galacto-samine 6-sulfatase	KS	16q24	I113F (UK and Ireland)	Urine GAGs	WBC enzyme assay	CVB	SD, CAR, OPH (+/−)
IVB	β-galactosidase	KS	3p21-pter	No common mutations	Urine GAGs	WBC enzyme assay	CVB	SD, CAR

Table 3.1 *(continued)*

Disease	Enzyme deficiency	Storage material	Chromosome location	Gene mutations	Screening test	Diagnostic test	Prenatal diagnosis	Main clinical features
MPS VI (Maro–teaux Lamy)	*N*-acetyl-galactos-amine-4-sulfatase	DS	5q13-q14	No common mutations	Urine GAGs	WBC enzyme assay	CVB	HSM, SD, DYS, OPH, CAR
MPS VII (Sly)	β-glucuronidase	HS, DS	7q21.1-q22	Very few patients studied	Urine GAGs	WBC enzyme assay	CVB	HF, HSM, CNS, SD, DYS, OPH, CAR
MPS IX	Hyaluronidase	HA	3p21.3	Very few patients studied	None	Cultured cells	Unknown	U/K
Mucolipidoses								
ML I (Sialidosis I)	Neuraminidase	SA	10pter-q23	No common mutations	Urine sialic acid	Cultured cells	Cultured cells	CNS, CRS, SD (+/−)
ML II (I-cell)	Transferase[$]	Many	4q21-23	Unknown	Urine oligos	Plasma enzyme assays	Cultured cells AF	HSM, CNS, SD, DYS, OPH, CAR
ML III (pseudo-Hurler)								
IIIA	As ML II	Many	4q21-23	Unknown	Urine oligos	Plasma enzyme assays	Cultured cells or AF	HSM (+/−), CNS (+/−), SD, DYS (+/−), CAR
IIIC	Transferase-δ-subunit	Many	16p	Very few patients studied	Urine oligos	Plasma enzyme assays	Cultured cells or AF	As ML IIIA
ML IV	Mucolipin-I	Many	19p13.2-13.3	R750W (20%)	None	Histology of CVB	Histology CNS, OPH	

Sphingolipidoses

GM1 Ganglio-sidosis	β-Galactosidase	GM1, KS, oligos, glycolipids	3p21-3pter	No common mutations	Urine oligos	WBC enzyme assay	CVB	HF, CNS, SD (+/−), CRS
GM2 Gangliosidosis								
Tay–Sachs	β-Hexosam-inidase A	GM2 Globoside, oligos glycolipids	15q23-24	Two Common Ashkenazi mutations	None	WBC enzyme assay	CVB	CNS, CRS
Sandhoff	β-Hexosam-inidase A and B	GM2 oligos	5q13	Common maronite mutation	None	WBC enzyme assay	CVB	CNS, CRS
GM2 Ganglio-sidosis	GM2 Activator	GM2 glycolipids	5q32-33	Very few patients studied	None	Cultured cells and natural substrate	Unknown	CNS, CRS
Globoid cell leukodystrophy Krabbe	Galacto-cerebrosidase	Galactosyl-ceramides	14q31	502T/del (40%)	None	WBC enzyme assay	CVB	CNS
MLD	Arylsul-phatase A	Sulfatides	22q13-3	VS2+1G→A and P426L (50%)	None	WBC enzyme assay	CVB	CNS
MLD	Saposin B activator (sap B)	Sulfatides, GM1 glycolipids	10q21	Very few patients studied	None	Sulfatide loading of cultured cells	In theory sulfatide loading of cultured cells +/or DNA	CNS
Fabry disease	α-Galactosidase	Galacyosyl-sphingolipids oligos	Xq22	No common mutations	None	WBC enzyme assay	CVB	SKA, REN CAR

Table 3.1 *(continued)*

Disease	Enzyme deficiency	Storage material	Chromosome location	Gene mutations	Screening test	Diagnostic test	Prenatal diagnosis	Main clinical features
Gaucher disease	β-glucosidase	Gluco-ceramide	1q21	N370S, 84gg, L444P IVS2+1, D409H, R463C	None	WBC enzyme assay	CVB	HSM, BM—Type I HSM, BM, OPH, CNS—Types II/III
Gaucher disease	Saposin C-activator	As above	10q21	Very few patients studied	None	Unknown	Unknown	As II/III
Farber disease	Ceramidase	Ceramide	8p22-21.2	Very few patients studied	None	WBC enzyme assay	CVB	CNS, SK, HSM (+/−)
Niemann–Pick A and B	Sphingo-myelinase	Sphingo-myelin	11p15.1-15.4	L302P, R496L, fs330, ΔR608	None	WBC enzyme assay	CVB	A—HSM, CRS, CNS B—HSM,
Glycoproteinoses								
α-Mannosidosis	α-Mannosidase	α-Mannosides	19p13.2-q12	R750W (20%)	Urine oligos	WBC enzyme assay	CVB	HSM, SD, DYS, CAR, CNS (+/−)
β-Mannosidosis	β-Mannosidase	β-Mannosides	4p	Very few patients studied	Urine oligos	WBC enzyme assay	CVB	CNS, HSM (+/−)
Fucosidosis	Fucosidase	Fucosides glycolipids	1p24	No common mutations	Urine oligos	WBC enzyme assay	CVB	CNS, SKA
Aspartylglucos-aminuria	Aspartylglucos-aminidase	Aspartyl-glucosamine	4q32-33	C163S (90% of Finnish patients)	Urine oligos	WBC enzyme assay	CVB	CNS, DYS, SD (+/−)
Schindler disease	α-Galacto-sidase B	*N*-acetyl-galactosamide glycolipids	22q13.1-13.2	Very few patients studied	Urine oligos	WBC enzyme assay	CVB	CNS, SD, SKA

Glycogen								
Pompe disease	α-Glucosidase	Glycogen	17q23	No common mutations	ECG characteristic	Lymphocyte enzyme assay	CVB	CAR
LIPID								
Wolman disease and cholesterol ester storage disease (CESD)	Acid lipase	Cholesterol esters	10q23.2-23.3	c.894 G > A	None	WBC Enzyme assay	CVB	CNS, HSM
Niemann–Pick C	Unknown	Cholesterol sphingolipids	Two genes: NPC 1—18q NPC 2—14q24.3	11061T Very few patients	Filipin staining of cultured cells	Cholesterol esterification studies	Cultured cells (not always possible)	HSM, OPH, CNS,
Monosaccharide aminoacids and monomers								
ISSD (infantile sialic acid storage disease)	Sialic acid transporter	Sialic acid glucuronic	6q14-q15	R39C/other mutation	Urine oligo	Cultured cells	AF	HF, DYS, HSM, CNS, SD
Salla disease	As ISSD	As ISSD	As ISSD	R39C homo	As ISSD	As ISSD	As ISSD	CNS (+/−)
Cystine	Cystine transporter	Cystine	17p13	Common del.	Renal tubular disease	WBC cystine	Cultured cells	REN
Cobalamin F disease	Cobalamin transporter	Cobalamin	Unknown		MMA, Hcy	Cultured cells	Cultured cells	CNS
Danon disease	LAMP-2	Cytoplasmic debris and glycogen	Xq24	Very few patients studied	None	Unknown	Unknown	CAR

Table 3.1 *(continued)*

Disease	Enzyme deficiency	Storage material	Chromosome location	Gene mutations	Screening test	Diagnostic test	Prenatal diagnosis	Main clinical features
PEPTIDES								
Pycnodysostosis	Cathepsin K	Bone proteins	1q21	Very few patients studied	X-Ray	Poss. DNA	Poss. DNA	SD
S-Acylated proteins								
Neuronal Ceroid lipofusc-inosis (Batten disease)								
CLN 1 (infantile)	Palmitoyl protein thioesterase	Saposins	1p32	R122W (Finland)	Histology	Cutured cells and DNA	DNA	CNS, RET
CLN 2 (late infantile)	Pepstatin insensitive carboxy-peptidase	Sub-unit C mitochondrial ATP synthase	11p15.5	Two common mutations in exon 6 = 60%	Histology	Cultured cells and DNA	DNA	CNS, RET
CLN 3 (juvenile)	Membrane protein	As CLN 2	16p21	Common deletion (c462-677del)	Histology	DNA	DNA	CNS, RET
CLN 4 (adult, Kuf disease)	Unknown	As CLN 2	Unknown	Unknown	Histology	Histology	Unknown	RET, CNS (+/−)
CLN 5 (late infantile, Finnish variant)	Membrane protein	As CLN 2	13q22	Common deletion (c1175delAT)	Histology	DNA	DNA	CNS, RET
CLN 6 (late-infantile variant)	Membrane protein	As CLN 2	15q-q23	Very few patients studied	Histology	Histology	Unknown	CNS, RET

CLN 7 (late-infantile variant)	Unknown	Unknown	Unknown	Very few patients studied	Histology	Histology	Unknown	CNS, RET
CLN 8 (progreessive epilepsy with mental retardation, EPMR)	Membrane protein	As CLN 2	8p23	Very few patients studied	Histology	Histology	Unknown	CNS, RET
Multiple enzyme deficiencies								
Multiple sulfatase deficiency	C(α)-Formylglycine generating enzyme	Sulfatides, glycolipids, GAGs	Unknown	Unknown	Urine GAGs	WBC and plasma enzyme assays	CVB	CNS, ICTH, HSM (+/−), SD (+/−)
Galactosialidosis	Neuraminidase and β-galactosidase protective protein	Oligos, sialic acid	20q13.3	Very few patients studied	Urine oligs	Cultured cells	Cultured cells	HF, CNS, SD, HSM

*Low activity in CVB—caution recontamination with maternal decidua.

†Always do fetal sexing as some unaffected female fetuses will have very low enzyme results.

‡Difficult because of cross-reactivity from other sulfatases.

$UDP-*N*-acetylglucosamine: lysosomal enzyme *N*-acetylglucosaminyl-l-phosphotransferase.

AF, amniotic fluid; BM, bone marrow failure; CAR, cardiac disease; CNS, regression; CRS, cherry-red spot; CVB, chorion villus biopsy; DS, dermatan sulfate; HS, heparan sulfate; KS, keratan sulfate; HA, hyaluronic acid; SA, sialic acid; DYS, dysmorphic appearance; GAGs, glycosaminoglycans; HF, hydrops fetalis; HSM, hepatosplenomegaly; ICTH, icthyosis; Oligos, oligosaccharides; OPH, eye signs—corneal clouding or ophthalmoplegia; REN, renal disease; RET, primary retinopathy; SD, dysostosis multiplex; SK, dermatological signs; SKA, angiokeratoma; WBC, white blood cell; +/−, sign not always present or mild.

Non-immune hydrops fetalis can be caused by a wide variety of fetal, placental, and maternal disorders. Fetal mortality is high and it is important to diagnose lysosomal storage diseases presenting in this way so that the appropriate genetic advice can be offered to the family. Table 3.2 indicates the disorders that have been associated with this presentation, and the whole topic has been extensively reviewed (Machin 1989; Stone and Sidransky 1999).

A lysosomal storage disease is more likely if there is a history of recurrent episodes and if the parents are consanguineous. Detailed anatomical examination by ultrasound should attempt to diagnose underlying placental and fetal abnormalities. Fetal echocardiography should be performed to exclude congenital heart lesions, and a fetal karyotype should be carried out to exclude aneuploidy. Cell-free fluid should be analysed for metabolite excretion (oligosaccharides and glycosaminoglycans) and a culture established for subsequent enzyme assay. Fetal blood sampling has a very limited role in the diagnosis of a storage disease in this situation as the volume of blood that can be removed is so small. It may, however, be indicated to check for fetal anaemia, haemoglobin variants, or other causes of haemolytic disease (e.g. fetal RBC enzyme defects). The fetal and neonatal mortality rate for non-immune hydrops fetalis is very high (Norton 1994), and a detailed physical examination of the placenta, fetus, or neonate is essential to exclude a lysosomal storage disease. The placenta may appear pale and bulky on gross examination and histology should confirm lysosomal vacuolation (Nelson *et al.* 1993; Soma *et al.* 2000). In cases where no amniotic fluid has been obtained, a placental cell line from a piece of chorion should be established for subsequent enzyme analysis. Often, the presence of severe hydrops makes identification of specific dysmorphic features difficult to appreciate. In addition, the fetus may be macerated or aborted at a very early stage of the pregnancy, making physical examination very difficult. In those infants who survive until late in pregnancy or who are live-born, a careful physical and radiological examination is required.

Table 3.2 Disorders known to have presented with hydrops fetalis

Mucopolysaccharidosis type I
Mucopolysaccharidosis type IV
Mucopolysaccharidosis type VII (common)
Mucolipidosis I (sialidosis I)
Mucolipidosis II (I-cell disease)
GM1 Gangliosidosis (common)
Farber disease
Gaucher disease type II
Niemann–Pick A
Niemann–Pick C
Wolman disease
Infantile sialic acid storage disease (common)
Multiple sulfatase deficiency
Galactosialidosis (common)

Dysmorphism

Patients with a storage disorder often have a facial appearance which is characteristically labelled 'coarse', although most parents find the term objectionable. A combination of subcutaneous storage and involvement of the facial bones in the dyostosis produces the typical appearance seen in its most developed form in mucopolysaccharidosis type IH (Hurler syndrome, Fig. 3.1). Underdevelopment of the mid-facial skeleton and the firm puffiness associated with subcutaneous storage result in a retrusse nose and a 'blurring' of the facial features. The lips and tongue are thickened and the hair is often abundant and dull. The persistent nasal discharge detracts further from the child's general appearance. A dark synophyris is a characteristic finding and affected children are often hirsute.

In some disorders (e.g. mucolipidosis II, GM1 gangliosidosis, and infantile sialic acid storage disease, ISSD), facial dysmorphism (usually termed 'Hurler-like') can be identified at birth. In other conditions the abnormalities only become apparent slowly with time and there is a gradual evolution of the facial phenotype over the early years of life. It is important to remember that some disorders (e.g. metachromatic leukodystrophy, Krabbe, Tay–Sach and Sandhoff diseases) are associated with a normal facial appearance and general absence of dysmorphology.

Dysostosis multiplex

Dysostosis multiplex (Fig. 3.2) is the general term used to describe the bony changes seen in many of the lysosomal storage diseases. In a similar way to the dysmorphism the most exaggerated bony changes are seen in the mucopolysaccharide (MPS) disorders (especially MPS IH, Hurler syndrome), and an attenuated form of the skeletal dysplasia is seen in mucolipidoses and the glycoproteinoses. In some storage diseases, skeletal involvement results from a different mechanism. For instance, in Gaucher disease bone marrow involvement with marrow cavity expansion and vascular compromise producing abnormalities of remodelling, bone infraction, and pathological fracture (Pastores 2000). Dysostosis multiplex appears to be due to a defect in bone formation and turnover. The earliest changes are seen in the medial borders of the clavicle and then in the ribs that result in a characteristic 'oar' shape with a narrow vertebral end and an expanded sternal edge. The diaphyses of the long bones are expanded, and in the vertebrae a characteristic 'beaking' is seen, most classically at L1. Odontoid dysplasia is almost always seen in

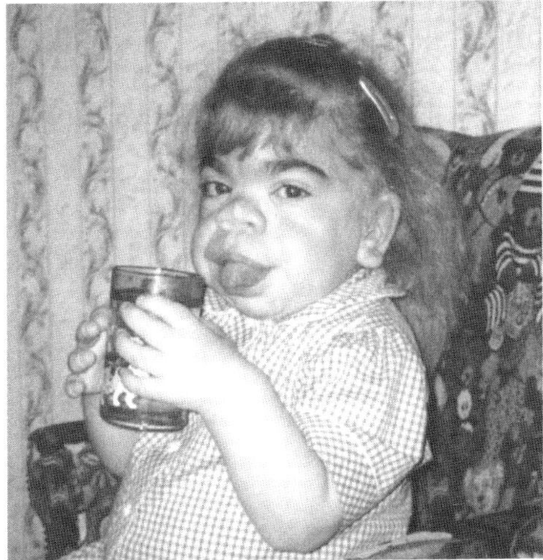

Fig 3.1 Typical facial appearence of 'storage' in a patient with MPS type IH (Hurler syndrome).

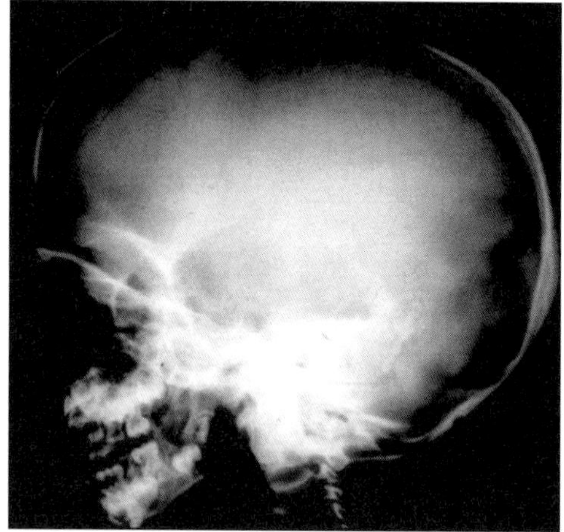

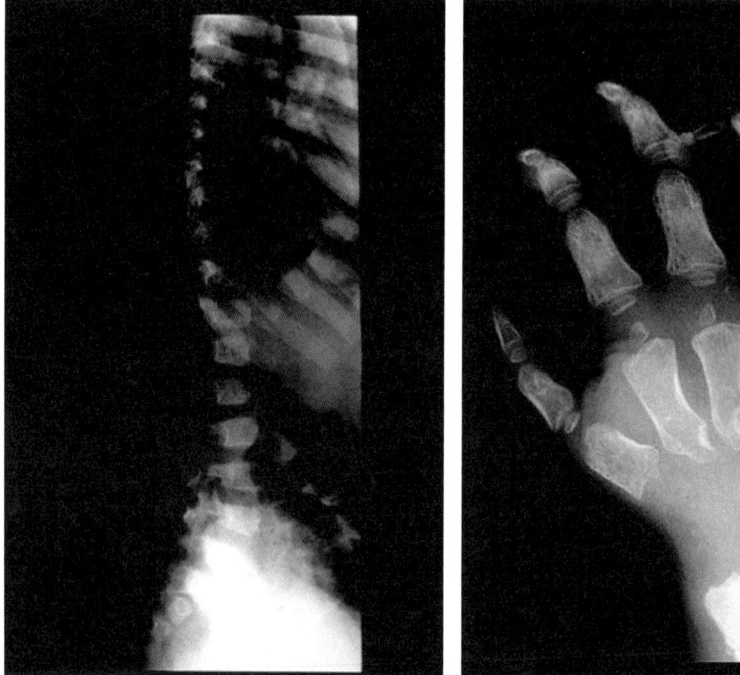

Fig. 3.2 Dysostosis multiplex. (a) Lateral skull X-ray–scaphiocephalic shape with expanded sella turcica; (b) lateral spine—note hypoplastic and beaked lumbar vertebrae; (c) hand and wrist—pointed proximal metacarpal bones.

fully developed dysostosis multiplex, and this is important to remember as it renders the cranio-cervical junction unstable in these patients. Other minor changes such as proximal tapering of the metacarpals are also common. In truth, almost no bone is spared in this generalized skeletal dysplasia.

Two lysosomal storage diseases deserve special comment as their skeletal dysplasia is more specific. In mucopolysaccharidosis type IV (MPS IV, Morquio syndrome), the skeletal dysplasia is spondyloepiphyseal in nature and results in a very severe form of short-trunk dwarfism. In severely affected patients, hip dislocation and long-bone involvement ensure that the affected individual rarely achieves a height in excess of 100 cm. The extreme vertebral flattening (platyspondyly) is also associated with a very hypoplastic odontoid process, making the patient vulnerable to atlanto-axial subluxation subsequent cervical myelopathy. In addition, as the patients' age, a restrictive respiratory defect secondary to the small thoracic volume is almost inevitable and is a common cause of death in this disorder.

Cathepsin K is a recently identified lysosomal cysteine proteinase, abundant in osteoclasts, where it is felt to play a vital role in the resorption and remodelling of bone (Saftig *et al.* 1998). A deficiency of this enzyme was shown to be associated with the skeletal dysplasia pycnodysostosis (Gelb *et al.* 1996), the disorder thought to be the cause of Toulouse–Lautrec's disability (Maroteaux and Lamy 1965). In addition to short stature (150–160 cm), affected individuals have a generalized increase in bone density, wormian bones of the skull with open fontanelles, partial absence of the distal phalanges, and bone fragility. In addition, both of these disorders are associated with specific dental abnormalities that are more severe than the dental anomalies seen in other lysosomal storage diseases. In MPS IV the enamel is thin, the cusps are pointed, and the incisors are spade shaped. The thin enamel is pitted on its buccal surface, and the affected teeth are prone to dental caries (Rolling *et al.* 1999). In pycnodysostosis, the dental findings usually include unerupted teeth and malocclusion (Ferguson *et al.* 1991).

Hepatosplenomegaly

In those disorders where somatic storage is usual (as opposed to primary storage within the central nervous system, CNS), hepatosplenomegaly is a common finding. In some conditions, e.g. Niemann–Pick diseases A, B, and C and Gaucher disease, enlargement of the liver and spleen will often be the major presenting clinical sign. In some patients, the organs are massively enlarged and almost fill the abdomen (Fig. 3.3). In mucopolysaccharidoses and

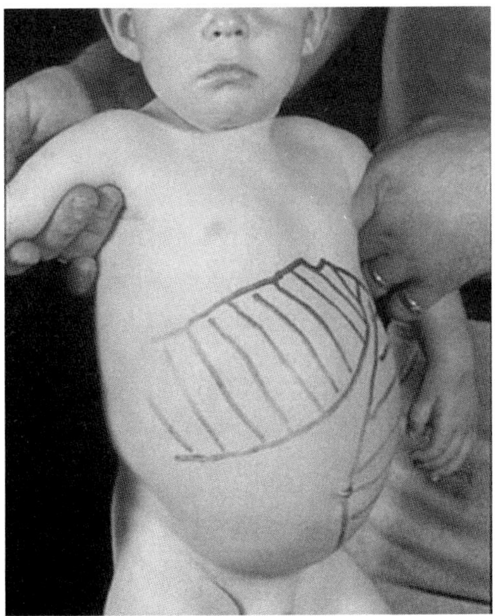

Fig. 3.3 Organomegaly in a patient with Gaucher disease.

glycoproteinoses, the function of the organs is not compromised despite significant enlargement. Niemann–Pick type B and Gaucher disease, however, can be associated with significant liver impairment. In Niemann–Pick diseases type C, a significant number of patients will present with liver failure, usually in the newborn period. If the infant survives, it can be many years before other symptoms of the disease become apparent (Jaeken *et al.* 1980).

In Niemann–Pick and Gaucher diseases, the enlarged abdominal organs can cause respiratory embarrassment by splinting the diaphragm. This is exacerbated by pulmonary infiltration, which is a common complication of these disorders. In other conditions, e.g. mucopolysaccharidoses, the enlargement of the liver and spleen raises intra-abdominal pressure to such a degree that herniae are common at points of weakness, such as at the umbilicus or in the inguinal region.

Central nervous system disease

Table 3.3 lists those disorders that primarily affect the CNS with little or no somatic abnormality such as organomegaly or dysostosis. The cause of the CNS dysfunction in lysosomal storage diseases is multifactorial and reviewed in detail in other chapters (see Chapter 12). The end result is a characteristic pattern of abnormalities that produce signs and symptoms helpful to the diagnostic process. A common thread across many disorders is the tempo of the illness. The majority of infants are normal at birth, and the neurological abnormalities evolve over a period of time following a variable period of normal progress. The developmental profile is characterized by regression, with the loss of previously acquired skills being the hallmark of this process. Most affected patients are macrocephalic (classically seen in Tay–Sachs disease) as a result of storage within the CNS. It should be noted, however, that patients with mucolipidosis II (I-cell disease) often have a small head circumference and premature sutural fusion. Indeed, sutural synostosis seems to occur more commonly in lysosomal storage diseases when compared to the normal population.

In addition to excessive storage, a number of disorders affect the cerebral white matter, leading to demyelination, often visible on MRI scanning as central white matter involvement and usually termed 'leukodystrophy' e.g. metachromatic leukodystrophy. In disorders affecting myelination in this way, presentation is usually with motor problems such as clumsiness and ataxia progressing to increasing spasticity with time and

Table 3.3 Lysosomal storage diseases associated with primary CNS dysfunction

• Metachromatic leukodystrophy
• Krabbe disease
• Tay–Sachs and Sandhoff disease
• Sialidosis I
• Mucolipidosis IV
• Schindler disease
• Neuronal ceroid lipofuscinoses
• Cobalamin F disease

ultimately associated with cognitive involvement as well. The age at the onset of symptoms and the speed of progression of the disease varies depending on the specific enzyme deficiency. Very acute-onset neurological abnormalities are seen for instance in Krabbe leukodystrophy where many patients in retrospect have abnormalities from the newborn period (Hagberg 1984).

In addition to the motor problems, the majority of patients will develop other evidence of CNS dysfunction. Episodes of hyperacusis (sensitivity to sound) are often followed by the development of frank seizures that may be generalized, tonic–clonic, myoclonic, or mixed. The incidence of seizures in the different enzyme deficiencies is variable but can be the dominant symptom in some disorders, e.g. the neuronal ceroid lipofuscinoses (NCLs). Sensory loss with blindness and deafness is common, and severe learning disability is the usual end result in those disorders with a major CNS component.

The extreme variability of the disorders leads to a different mode of presentation in attenuated, adult forms of the disease. In these patients a psychiatric presentation is more likely with very late or no cognitive decline (Rapola 1994).

Ophthalmological signs

A variety of eye abnormalities are seen in lysosomal storage diseases. Blindness from progressive retinal or central involvement is a late feature of many disorders (e.g. NCLs), but some are associated with more specific physical signs.

Corneal clouding due to abnormalities in glycosaminoglycan metabolism is seen in patients with mucopolysaccharidoses types I, IV, VI, and VII. In mucolipidosis type IV, corneal opacification is often the presenting feature. Many other disorders such as the oligosaccharidoses and glycoproteinoses will develop some corneal clouding, often at a later stage of the illness and sometimes only visible with a slit-lamp examination.

In Fabry disease, eye signs are common and can be helpful in delineating female carriers of this X-linked disorder. In the cornea, haziness followed by streak-like opacities occurs as the disease progresses and many patients develop a posterior cataract (Sher *et al.* 1979). In addition, in this disorder and in fucosidosis, the retinal vessels are often very tortuous.

The most quoted ocular abnormality associated with lysosomal storage diseases is the macular cherry-red spot (Fig. 3.4). This has been classically linked with Tay–Sachs disease but is seen in a number of others (Table 3.4). It is also important to note that as retinal ganglion cells are progressively lost later in the course of the disorders, the macular abnormality may become less apparent with time.

Other eye abnormalities include disorders of ocular mobility. In Gaucher disease type III and Niemann–Pick C, supranuclear ophthalmoplegia are classic physical signs leading to a defect in the initiation of either vertical or horizontal saccades. In both disorders, this may be the only neurological abnormality for many years.

Cardiovascular system

The classic LSD associated with cardiomyopathy is glycogen storage disease type II (Pompe disease). The infantile form of the disease has severe cardiac involvement with massive cardiomegaly, grossly abnormal electrocardiogram, and rapidly progressive cardiac failure leading to death in early infancy. The juvenile and adult forms of the disease have no overt cardiac involvement.

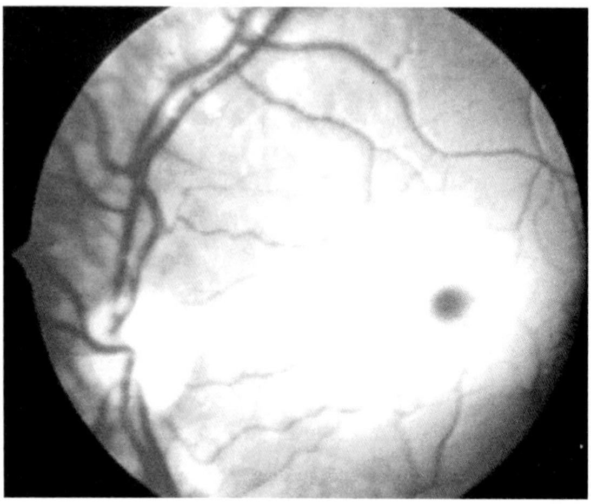

Fig. 3.4 Cherry red spot–Tay–Sachs disease. **See Plate 2.**

Table 3.4 Disorders associated with a macular cherry-redspot

Sialidosis I
Galactosialidosis
Tay–Sachs disease
Sandhoff disease
GM1 gangliosidosis
Niemann–Pick A (common) C (rare)
Metachromatic leukodystrophy (rare)
Krabbe disease (rare)
Farber disease (rare)

A cardiac variant of Fabry disease is also well documented. Affected patients have residual α-galactosidase activity and have little or no disease outside the heart. The patients present in middle age with a non-obstructive, hypertrophic, cardiomyopathy affecting mainly the left ventricle, leading to episodes of syncope and ischaemia (Yoshitama *et al.* 2001).

Cardiac storage occurs in other lysosomal storage diseases and cardiomyopathy can be the mode of presentation in some of the mucopolysaccharidoses (Fong *et al.* 1987). Heart valve lesions are also frequent findings especially in the mucopolysaccharidoses, oligosaccharidoses, and glycoproteinoses, and valve replacement surgery has been performed in some adults with these disorders (Fischer *et al.* 1999).

Renal disease

In affected males (and some females) with Fabry disease, progressive renal dysfunction is a major cause of early death. Initially, podocyte involvement leads to proteinuria and haematuria, often first detected in adolescence. As the disease progresses, the sphingolipid storage within the walls of the blood vessels leads to progressive glomerulosclerosis and end-stage renal failure. Dialysis and renal replacement therapy used to be the only treatment for affected patients, but the introduction of enzyme replacement therapy hopefully will prevent this complication. Severe renal failure may also occur in galactosialidosis, often after a period of proteinuria approaching the level seen in the nephrotic syndrome.

Cutaneous manifestations

A wide variety of cutaneous manifestations are seen on patients with lysosomal storage diseases. Some are very specific, e.g. the silvery papules seen on the trunk of boys with mucopolysaccharidosis type II (Hunter syndrome), whereas some are common and non-specific, e.g. angiokeratomas. The latter abnormality is due to storage within the vascular endothelium, and they are seen in their most florid form in males with Fabry disease. In affected patients, clusters of dark-red, flat, slightly verrucous lesions are seen most commonly on the trunk, perineum, and upper thighs (Fig. 3.5). With age, in many other disorders, angiokeratoma become more prominent. They are seen notably in fucosidosis, α- and β-mannosidosis, Schindler disease, GM1 gangliosidosis, sialidosis I and II, and galactosialidosis.

Specific clinical presentation and progression

This section should be read in conjunction with Table 3.1.

Mucopolysaccharidoses

All of the MPS disorders are chronic, progressive disorders (Wraith 1995) that usually present in one of three ways:

- as a dysmorphic syndrome—MPS I, II, VI, and VII
- as a severe neurological disorder with little somatic disease—MPS III
- as a skeletal dysplasia—MPS IV

The prototype for this group is MPS IH (α-iduronidase deficiency), a condition that exhibits most of the pathology associated with lysosomal storage diseases including extreme heterogeneity. Affected children are dysmorphic and have dysostosis and hepatosplenomegaly (see above). The early clinical course is dominated by upper airway obstruction with frequent

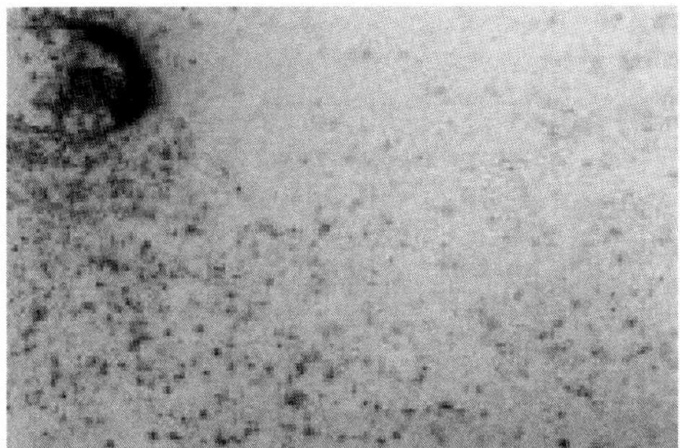

Fig. 3.5 Abdominal angiokeratomas in a patient with Fabry disease. **See Plate 3**.

ear, nose, and throat infections. Short stature, abdominal distension, and learning difficulties all contribute to a characteristic and well-known phenotype (shared by MPS VI—without the learning disability and MPS VII). Progressive cardiac and respiratory disease with neurodegeneration usually leads to death before the end of the first decade. Adults with the attenuated form of the disease (MPS IS, Scheie disease) are often of normal height and have no learning difficulties. Typical symptoms are joint stiffness, corneal clouding, carpal tunnel syndrome, and mild skeletal changes. Progressive mitral and aortic valve disease may also be present. Between these two extremes, there is a clinical continuum usually referred to as MPS I/S, Hurler/Scheie disease.

MPS II (Hunter's syndrome) is X-linked and produces a clinical syndrome similar to MPS I, but corneal clouding is absent. Attenuated forms of the disease are also common. A particular problem in these men appears to be the development of cervical compromise due to abnormalities at the cranio-cervical junction (Parsons *et al.* 1996).

MPS III (Sanfilippo disease types A, B, C, and D) is a very different disorder (Cleary and Wraith 1993). Somatic features are mild, diagnosis is often delayed, and insomnia and severe behavioural disturbance dominate the condition. Progressive loss of skills continues, and death occurs in a vegetative state around the end of the second decade of life.

MPS IV illustrates the third mode of presentation for patients with MPS. The condition is a primary skeletal dysplasia, and affected patients have more in common with patients with other primary bone disorders (e.g. achondroplasia) than they have with other MPS subtypes. Extreme short stature is usual with an adult height of around 100 cm. As mentioned, these patients are at particular risk from cervical myelopathy, and most survivors develop restrictive respiratory disease as adults.

Mucolipidoses

This group consists of at least three very different biochemical disorders:

- mucolipidosis I caused by neuraminidase deficiency
- mucolipidosis II and III due to a defect in lysosomal enzyme targeting
- mucolipidosis IV associated with an ill-defined transport defect in the late steps of endocytosis (Bassi *et al.* 2000).

Isolated neuraminidase deficiency (distinct from combined neuraminidase/β-galactosidase deficiency due to a defect in protective protein, galactosialidosis) is associated in the literature with two phenotypes, usually referred to as sialidoses I and II. It is unclear how many of the reported type II patients are isolated deficiencies rather than examples of the combined enzyme defect.

Sialidosis I due to isolated neuraminidase deficiency is also known as 'cherry-red spot myoclonus' syndrome that accurately describes this phenotype. Presentation is usually in childhood with failing vision. Drop attacks (myoclonic seizures) and ataxia are usually present by teenage years, and slow progression leads to severe disability in adult life. Cognitive abilities are not affected, and unlike the combined enzyme defect, somatic features are not present.

Mucolipidoses II and III share the same biochemical defect and represent two ends of the same spectrum. A failure of lysosomal targeting (discussed in detail in another chapter) results in a functional defect in several lysosomal hydrolases. In severely affected patients, this is a dramatic disorder with symptoms present from birth. There is dysmorphism, a specific skeletal dysplasia, and often a severe cardiomyopathy. The bone changes include osteopenia, periosteal cloaking, neonatal or *in utero* fractures, and dysharmonic epiphyseal ossification (Herman and McAlister 1996). Death occurs in infancy in severely affected patients. Mucolipidosis III tends to present in childhood with joint stiffness. Affected patients are unable to raise their arms above their heads. Fingers become clawed, and there is often associated carpal tunnel syndrome. Ball and socket joints seem to be most affected, and a severe hip dysplasia can cause considerable disability in affected adults. Life expectancy can be normal and intellectual involvement tends to be mild.

Mucolipidosis IV is a disorder found primarily in patients of Ashkenazi Jewish origin and presents with a combination of corneal clouding and learning disability in the absence of other somatic abnormalities. Patients usually survive well into adult life. The biochemical defect is not fully elucidated but seems to involve a protein (called mucolipin-I) that appears to have a role in the trafficking of late endosomes and lysosomes.

Sphingolipidoses

In this group of disorders there is a progressive accumulation of complex lipids that are often important, integral components of cell membranes, and as such, neurodegeneration is a common feature here.

GM1 gangliosidosis

Infantile-, juvenile-, and adult-onset forms of this disorder are recognized and all are caused by a deficiency of β-galactosidase. The severe form of the condition can present with hydrops fetalis and is associated with neonatal dysmorphism, severe hepatosplenomegaly, cherry-red spot, and skeletal dysplasia. Seizures and progressive learning difficulties lead to early death.

In the adult, there is usually no visceral involvement and the condition usually presents with dystonia and dysarthria. Myoclonic seizures and a slow intellectual decline have been reported in some patients (Yoshida *et al.* 1992). As expected, the juvenile form of the disease produces an intermediate phenotype, with death occurring in the first or second decade of life.

GM2 gangliosidosis

Three different genetic disorders (clinically identical) contribute to this group: Tay–Sachs (more prevalent in Ashkenazi Jews), Sandhoff diseases, and GM2 activator protein deficiency.

Wide clinical variation is again a feature of these disorders, although most clinicians will only be familiar with the classical infantile forms of the disease. These present in the first months of life with a combination of hypotonia and hyperacusis. Developmental delay is obvious by the end of the first year of life. More dramatic neurological dysfunction becomes apparent within the second year, with loss of visual attentiveness, increasing spasticity, and seizures. Infants are macrocephalic and have a cherry-red spot on fundal examination. Death usually occurs around the third year of life.

Late-onset forms of the disease are usually, but not invariably, associated with hexosaminidase A deficiency (adult Tay–Sachs disease). A variety of presentations have been described in this age group including psychosis, dystonia, and anterior horn cell disease (Harding *et al.* 1987). An adult variant of Sandhoff disease has been reported presenting with spinocerebellar degeneration (Oonk *et al.* 1979).

Globoid cell leukodystrophy (Krabbe disease)

Krabbe disease is caused by a deficiency of the enzyme galactocerebrosidase that results in the accumulation of a toxic intermediate psychoscine (Wenger 2000). The end result is a severe demyelination of both the CNS and the peripheral nervous system. In the infantile form or classic Krabbe disease the disorder is aggressive and relentless. It usually starts in the early weeks of life, although some patients have symptoms in the neonatal period. Hyperpyrexia, irritability, crying, dystonic spasms, and fixed opisthotonic posturing are typical. Death usually follows the onset of loss of bulbar function at around the age of 12–18 months. Nerve conduction velocities are delayed due to demyelination of the peripheral nervous system, and the protein content of cerebrospinal fluid (CSF) is always elevated.

In late-onset forms the clinical presentation can be very variable (Kolodny *et al.* 1991). Intellectual deterioration is not inevitable, and optic atrophy, slowly progressive spasticity, and tremor are more common.

Metachromatic leukodystrophy

The vast majority of patients have a primary defect in arylsulfatase A (ASA) activity. A small minority have a defect in the saposin B activator protein necessary for normal enzyme activity. Once again, a very wide clinical spectrum has been reported, but by far the commonest mode of presentation is the late-infantile form of the disease (von Figura *et al.* 2001). Affected patients present between the ages of 12 and 18 months with motor impairment secondary to a disturbance of both the CNS and the peripheral nervous systems. There is very little visceral involvement outside of the nervous system. The disease progresses rapidly with nystagmus, optic atrophy, dementia, seizures, and spastic quadriplegia. Most patients die well before the end of the first decade. Juvenile patients often present (between the ages of 5 and 15 years) with school failure or behavioural disturbance, often on a background of 'slow learning'. Seizures may occur and the rate of progression of the disease can be very variable, with some patients deteriorating rapidly (Haltia *et al.* 1980), whilst others survive 10–15 years after diagnosis.

Adult-onset metachromatic leukodystrophy usually presents with psychiatric manifestations. Patients develop personality change, depression, and occasionally frank psychosis (Hyde *et al.* 1992). In a psychiatric setting, subtle neurological abnormality such as mild ataxia or diminished tendon reflexes can easily be missed. A more obviously organic symptom such as a seizure may precipitate further investigation, and if this includes imaging, the typical white matter changes are found, leading to the diagnostic investigations.

Fabry disease

This X-linked disorder unlike the majority of other lysosomal storage diseases is primarily a disease of adults, although symptoms can be dated back to childhood in most affected patients. The primary pathology is in the endothelial cells, perithelium, and smooth muscle cells of blood vessels, cardiac myocytes, autonomic spinal ganglia, renal podocytes, glomerular epithelium, and tubules.

Although most of the severely affected patients are male, the disorder produces significant pathology in female heterozygotes, prompting the suggestion that the disease may be X-linked dominant (Beck 2001, personal communication). Typical presentation is in late childhood, with episodes of burning discomfort in the extremities (acroparasthesiae) which may be provoked by exertion. Unexplained pyrexias with associated hypohidrosis occur, and eventually the characteristic skin lesions (angiokeratoma corporis diffusum) lead to referral to the dermatology clinic where the majority of diagnoses are made. The angiokeratomas are clusters of dark red papules, often with a verrucous surface, present in the bathing trunk area, umbilicus, and upper thighs of affected men. Women also get angiokeratomas, but in females they tend to be more widespread but less abundant.

Serious organ involvement follows in most affected men, and by middle age, most have both significant renal impairment and cardiovascular disease. Ophthalmological abnormalities include both corneal and lenticular opacities (see above).

In some patients isolated cardiac involvement occurs ('cardiac variant'). In these patients hypertrophic cardiomyopathy is the only finding, with no angiokeratomas, renal involvement, or acroparasthesiae.

In severely affected females, cardiomyopathy and end-stage renal failure can occur.

Gaucher disease

Glucocerebrosidase deficiency produces a clinical spectrum that ranges from a perinatal lethal form of the disease to one that is asymptomatic (Pastores 2000). The undigested substrate, glucosylceramide (derived primarily from senescent RBCs and tissue debris in the periphery and membrane gangliosides in the brain), is stored primarily in cells of the monocyte/macrophage lineage.

Although three discrete phenotypes are described (types I, II, and III), it is important to remember that like all lysosomal storage diseases there is a clinical continuum in affected patients:

1. Type I (adult-onset, non-neuronopathic disease) is especially prevalent in Ashkenazi Jewish individuals where the carrier frequency is 1 : 15. The main pathology is seen in the skeleton, liver, spleen, bone marrow, and lungs. The bone disease is especially pernicious and progresses without treatment from osteopenia and sclerotic lesions to osteonecrosis and pathological fracture. The major weight-bearing joints of the lower limb are particularly vulnerable. The spleen is usually massively enlarged, and hypersplenism contributes to the haematological abnormalities. Splenic infarction can produce severe abdominal pain and mimic an abdominal emergency. Although liver enlargement is usual, cirrhosis and hepatic failure are very rare. Bone marrow infiltration leads to thrombocytopenia, and ultimately, anaemia and neutropenia result from a combination of bone marrow failure and hypersplenism. Frequent episodes of bleeding following minor trauma or excessive bruising are common. Pulmonary hypertension, interstitial lung disease, and lobar consolidation are less common complications of type I disease.
2. Types II and III (neuronopathic Gaucher disease) represent a spectrum of disease, both ends of which include some form of neurological involvement. Type II disease is severe and acute in onset and can be associated with a colloidian skin abnormality or hydrops fetalis (Stone *et al.* 2000). More commonly, bulbar involvement with a characteristic triad of strabismus, trismus, and opisthotonus is present from the early weeks or months of life. Myoclonic seizures may also occur in the context of a rapidly progressive disorder, often fatal in the first 2 or 3 years of life (Conradi *et al.* 1984). Type III disease is a chronic disorder, and oculomotor apraxia may be the only neurological abnormality (at least initially). Systemic symptoms are often severe in this form of the disease, and some patients will eventually show neurological progression (Erikson 1986).

3. Patients homozygous for the D409H mutation present with a cardiac variant of the disease. The disorder is characterized by the evolution of mitral and aortic valve calcification. Corneal opacities, ocular motor apraxia, and splenomegaly may also be present (Bohlega *et al.* 2000).

Farber disease

Ceramidase deficiency is a very rare disorder associated with intracellular storage of ceramide. The condition can present before birth with fetal hydrops, but most commonly presents in the early weeks of life with a combination of hoarseness, lymphadenopathy, hepatosplenomegaly, and characteristic nodules around joints and over bony prominences. A cherry-red spot may develop, and affected children have global learning difficulties. Death usually occurs in the first 18–24 months from pulmonary involvement. The disorder is heterogeneous with a number of described sub-types (Moser *et al.* 2001).

Sphingomyelinase deficiency–Niemann–Pick disease types A and B

Type A Niemann–Pick is a severe disorder presenting in the early weeks of life with marked neurological and visceral symptoms. Massive hepatomegaly, hypotonia, severe feeding problems, and seizures are often present. A cherry-red spot is present in most patients by the end of the first year. The clinical picture can be dominated by severe respiratory symptoms secondary to a severe pulmonary infiltration that on X-ray resembles an interstitial pneumonitis. Foam cells are usually found on bone marrow aspiration (Fig. 3.6) and death usually occurs in early infancy.

Type B disease follows a much more chronic course, and survival into adult life is usual. Affected patients may have massive splenomegaly and hypersplenism, and in addition cirrhosis of the liver can occur. Neurological involvement is very rare, and the clinical picture can be dominated by respiratory problems secondary to pulmonary infiltration.

Type B disease can be mistaken clinically for non-neuronpathic Gaucher disease.

Glycoproteinoses

α- and β-mannosidosis

α-Mannosidosis is a disorder with features in common with the mucopolysaccharidoses. Mild dysostosis multiplex, facial dysmorphism, middle ear disease, and mild-to-moderate learning difficulties are common in affected patients. An associated immune deficiency can also be present (Malm *et al.* 2000), but most patients survive into middle age.

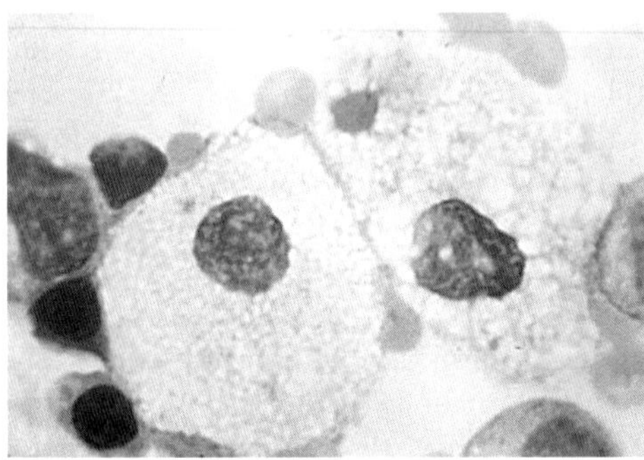

Fig. 3.6 Foam cells in the bone marrow of a patient with Niemann–Pick B disease. **See Plate 4.**

β-Mannosidosis has been diagnosed in very few patients, and there appears to be no consistent phenotype. Dysostosis multiplex and facial dysmorphism do not occur, but neurological involvement can be severe (Cooper *et al.* 1990).

Fucosidosis

A very wide clinical spectrum is seen in affected patients with fucosidosis (Willems *et al.* 1991). All patients have progressive neurodegeneration, and in severely affected patients this may be the only abnormal finding, with death occurring very early in infancy. Patients with more attenuated forms of the disease have more classic features of storage with dysmorphism, angiokeratoma, and visceromegaly. Skeletal abnormalities are generally mild, and corneal clouding is not a feature of this disease.

Aspartylglucosaminuria

This disorder is rare except in Finland where it has a prevalence approaching 1 : 18 000 (Arvio *et al.* 1993). Affected patients are rather like patients with mucopolysaccharidosis type III (Sanfilippo disease) and present with behavioural disturbance and aggression. A coarse facial appearance and intellectual decline is present by the end of the first decade of life, and as adults the vast majority of patients are in sheltered accommodation. Organomegaly and dysostosis multiplex are generally very mild, and most patients survive long into adult life.

α-*N*-Acetylgalactosaminidase deficiency (Schindler disease)

This is a very rare disorder, and the few reported patients have a very variable phenotype (Desnick and Schindler 2001). At the severe end of the spectrum is a disorder associated with severe neurodegeneration with no visceral involvement. In the few attenuated patients described, extensive angiokeratomas, other vascular lesions, and lymphoedema are prominent.

Glycogen

Acid glucosidase deficiency (Pompe disease)

The age of onset of this disorder divides it into three sub-types: infantile, juvenile, and adult-onset disease. As expected, the severity is related to the age of onset and the infantile form has a very poor prognosis because it is associated with cardiac muscle involvement. It tends to present with generalized hypotonia, feeding difficulties, macroglossia, and cardiac failure. The muscles have a firm, 'woody', feel. The electrocardiogram is characteristic with bizarre QRS complexes and deep septal Q waves. Death usually occurs from cardiac failure in the first year of life.

The juvenile and adult forms of the disease have no cardiac involvement and have variable skeletal muscle involvement. Death usually results from respiratory failure (often before adult age in the juvenile patient), but some patients live into old age with increasing motor disability.

Lipid

Acid lipase deficiency

Accumulation of cholesterol esters and triglycerides secondary to acid lipase deficiency leads to the allelic disorders, Wolman disease and cholesterol ester storage disease. The severe variant is associated with hepatosplenomegaly, malabsorption, and severe failure to thrive (Assmann and Seedorf 2001). Calcification of the adrenal glands is usually seen on radiological study and death occurs in the first 6 months. Cholesterol eater storage disease is a more slowly progressive disorder that presents in adult life with liver dysfunction and the effects of severe atherosclerosis.

Niemann–Pick disease type C (NPC)

NPC is a complex disorder(s) associated with abnormalities in cholesterol and sphingolipid trafficking within the cell (Chapter 9). At least two different genes (*NPC1* and *NPC2*) are involved, although most patients (95%) have mutations in *NPC1* (see also Chapter 9). Extreme heterogeneity is seen in this disorder that can present with hydrops fetalis or liver failure in the newborn period or remain asymptomatic throughout life (Fensom *et al.* 1999). The most classic clinical presentation is in mid-childhood with an insidious onset of supranuclear gaze palsy, ataxia, and seizures. Dementia follows, and the associated dystonia and dysphagia are major management problems. A very mixed pattern of epilepsy may occur, but episodes of cataplexy and gelastic seizure are absolutely characteristic and, if present in a child with a progressive disorder, are virtually diagnostic of NPC. The *NPC2* gene has recently been shown to be the *HE1* gene, a ubiquitously expressed soluble lysosomal protein identified previously as a cholesterol-binding protein (Naureckiene *et al.* 2000) (Chapter 8).

Monosaccharide, aminoacids, and monomers

This group contains a number of different disorders including some conditions, e.g. cystinosis, usually not considered with other metabolic disorders.

Infantile sialic acid storage disease (ISSD) and Salla disease

Only these two allelic disorders will be considered in this chapter. The defective gene (*SLC17A5*) encodes the lysosomal free sialic acid transporter (Aula *et al.* 2000) and results in an accumulation of free sialic acid within the lysosomes. The severe neonatal form of the disease (ISSD) is often associated with fetal hydrops fetalis, and survivors have dysmorphism, organomegaly, and severe learning difficulties. Dysostosis multiplex is rare, and corneal clouding is not a feature of the disease. In Finland, the disorder most often presents with an attenuated form of the disease known as Salla disease. A founder mutation in the gene (*R39C*) leads to learning difficulty, ataxia, mild hepatosplenomegaly, and facial dysmorphism. Most patients live a normal lifespan.

Peptides

Pycnodysostosis

This disorder has been described in some detail earlier. It is a primary skeletal dysplasia due to a defect in cathepsin K, characterized by short stature and osteosclerosis. The diagnosis is suggested by the radiological findings.

S-Acylated proteins

Neuronal ceroid lipofuscinoses

This group of disorders, collectively, constitutes the most common group of progressive brain diseases in children (Tyynela and Sreopanki 2000). All of the disorders are progressive and can present at all ages. Atypical forms of the disease are common, and a high index of suspicion is necessary to establish a prompt diagnosis (Nardocci *et al.* 2000). Dementia, motor problems, epilepsy, and blindness are prominent features in affected patients. Experienced pathologists can help in diagnosis by characterizing the ultra-structural appearance of the storage material. At a clinical level, seizures in affected patients may be extremely resistant to treatment.

Multiple enzyme deficiencies

Multiple sulfatase deficiency

In multiple sulfatase deficiency, there is reduced activity of all sulfatases to their natural substrates due to defective modification of their active site (see Chapter 5). A complex disorder can result from this multiple enzyme deficiency state, but the most common phenotype resembles that of late-infantile metachromatic leukodystrophy. In a few patients, the dysmorphism associated with MPS disease has been noted along with a mild dysostosis multiplex (Burk *et al.* 1984). The disorder is steadily progressive and usually leads to death in early infancy.

Galactosialidosis

In galactosialidosis, there is functional deficiency of both neuraminidase and β-galactosidase due to defect in protective protein/cathepsin A. Sialic acid-rich oligosaccharides accumulate within the lysosomes and give rise to a variable clinical phenotype which may include hydrops fetalis (early infantile). Late-infantile and juvenile/adult forms are more attenuated with variable dysostosis and dysmorphism, cherry-red spots, myoclonus, and ataxia. Angiokeratoma can be abundant, and all patients have progressive learning difficulties. In the adult form of the disease the patient may survive well into adult life.

Establishing the diagnosis

In general terms, there is no simple diagnostic screening test which will detect all these disorders. The tests chosen will be guided by the clinical picture, and in many patients a battery of screening tests on both blood and urine will be necessary to establish the exact biochemical diagnosis. Many different algorithms have been produced to aid the diagnostic process, but in clinical practice these are of little value because of the considerable heterogeneity seen with this group of disorders. If a clinician strongly suspects the presence of an lysosomal storage disease, but initial biochemical studies are normal, a tissue biopsy should be studied by electron microscopy to confirm the presence of lysosomal distension. If present, further investigation is necessary and disorders not readily detected by blood or urine testing, e.g. activator protein or saposin deficiency, should be considered. Skin fibroblast culture is mandatory in this situation for diagnosis.

Although Table 3.1 gives information about the screening and diagnostic tests needed for each disorder, a few general points need to be made.

Initial diagnosis of an MPS disorder should be based on urine glycosaminoglycan excretion analysed by an electrophoretic method. Spot urine tests are inaccurate and may miss cases of MPS III and IV. If glycosaminoglycans are normal but MPS-like features are present, a disorder of glycoprotein metabolism or a mucolipidosis needs to be excluded. For these disorders thin-layer chromatography of urine oligosaccharide excretion may suggest a possible diagnosis, but specific enzyme analysis using plasma, leukocytes, or skin fibroblasts will also be necessary. For the other lysosomal storage disorders, specific enzyme assays should be performed and these are often offered as a screen of several enzymes performed on the same blood sample. More specialized tests on fibroblasts will be needed for the transport and activator protein defects.

Mutation analysis

Molecular analysis cannot be used as the primary method of diagnosis because of the number of potential mutations within each gene (Chapter 4). However, it is important to try and clearly define the molecular pathology, as this allows for genotype/phenotype correlation and accurate carrier testing.

For some disorders (see Table 3.1) there are common mutations within certain population groups, but for the majority of patients extensive sequencing efforts will be needed to establish genotype.

Carrier testing

If prenatal diagnosis is to be offered in future pregnancies based on enzyme assay, it is important to measure activity in the parents who are presumed obligate heterozygotes. The usual presumption is that if the enzyme level in the parents is easily distinguished from the proband, this will also be true for other carriers within the family and prenatal diagnosis would not lead to the situation where a carrier fetus could mistakenly be assumed to be affected. In other situations, carrier testing for recessive disorders is usually not indicated or possible. The overlap between normal and carrier is so great that carrier testing based on enzyme activity is too inaccurate except in certain circumstances, e.g. Tay–Sachs disease.

For X-linked disorders (e.g. Fabry and MPS II), carrier detection in females within the family is essential, but this should be based on mutation analysis. For recessive disorders, carrier testing could also be done by mutation analysis, but the value of this approach is limited by the few disorders that are associated with common mutations. In genetic isolates or in consanguineous families, carrier detection by mutation analysis may help reproductive choice by identifying possible unions within the family or group which would be at higher risk of an affected child.

Summary

Disorders associated with abnormal lysosomal storage are present from conception and as a result produce a clinical phenotype that evolves with time. The clinical diagnosis becomes easier with the passage of time but the introduction of potential therapies has made early diagnosis a priority. Clues to the presence of a lysosomal disorder can be found in the tempo of the illness especially if the central nervous system is involved. Loss of a previously acquired developmental milestone (regression) is very characteristic of this group of conditions. Clinical clues can include a dysmorphic appearance or the presence of characteristic skeletal involvement (dysostosis multiplex), but in some disorders e.g. Pompe disease or Krabbe disease these do not occur.

The approach to diagnosis has to involve 'screening' as there can be considerable clinical overlap between conditions and it is not always possible to make a clear clinical distinction. Both urine and blood testing are necessary and the majority of diagnoses can now be confirmed at a molecular level. Prenatal diagnosis is possible for all.

References

Arvio, Autio, S. and Louhiala, P. (1993). Early clinical symptoms and incidence of aspartylglucosaminuria in Finland. *Acta Paediatr*, **82**, 469–71.

Assmann, G. and Seedorf, U. (2001). Acid lipase deficiency: Wolman disease and cholesteryl ester storage disease. In *The metabolic and molecular bases of inherited disease* eds. (Scriver, C. R., Beaudet, A. L., Sly, W. S ., Valle, D, ed.), pp. 3551–73. New York: McGraw-Hill.

Aula, N., Salomaki, P., Timonen, R., Verheijen, F., Mancini, G., Mansson, J. *et al.* (2000). The spectrum of SLC1tA5-gene mutations resulting in free sialic acid-storage diseases indicates some genotype-phenotype correlation. *Am J Hum Genet*, **67**, 832–40.

Bassi, M. T., Manzoni, M., Monti, E., Pizzo, M. T., Ballabio, A. and Borsani, G. (2000). Cloning of the gene encoding a novel integral membrane protein mucolipidin – and identification of the two major founder mutations causing mucolipidosis type IV. *Am J Hum Genet*, **67**, 1110–20.

Bohlega, S., Kambouris, M., Shahid, M., Al Homsi, M. and Al Sous, W. (2000). Gaucher disease with oculomotor apraxia and cardiovascular calcification. (Gaucher Type III C) *Neurology*, **54**, 261–3.

Burk, R. D., Valle, D., Thomas, G. H., Miller, C., Moser, A., Moser, H. *et al.* (1984). Early manifestations of multiple sulfatase deficiency. *J Pediatr*, **104**, 574–61.

Cleary, M. A. and Wraith, J. E. (1993). Management of mucopolysaccharidosis type. III. *Arch Dis Childh*, **67**, 403–6.

Conradi, N. G., Sourander, P., Nilsson, O., Svennerholm, L. and Erikson, A. (1984). Neuropathology of the Norrbotnian type of Gaucher disease. Morphological and biochemical studies. *Acta Neuropathol*, **65**, 99–109.

Cooper, A., Hatton, C. E., Thornley, M. and Sardharwalla, I. B. (1990). Alpha- and beta-mannosidoses. *J Inherit Metab Dis*, **13**, 538–48.

Desnick, R. J. and Schindler, D. (2001). α-N-acetylgalactosaminidase deficiency: Schindler disease. In *The metabolic and molecular bases of inherited disease* (Scriver, C. R., Beaudetm A. L., Sly, W. S., Valle, D, ed.), pp. 3483–507. New York: McGraw-Hill.

Erikson, A. (1986). Gaucher disease – Norrrbottnian type (III). *Acta Paediatr Scand*, **326**, 1–43.

Fensom, A. H., Grant, A. R., Steinberg, S. J., Ward, C. P., Lake, B. D., Logan, E. *et al.* (1999). An adult with a non-neuronpathic form of Niemann–Pick C disease. *J Inherit Metab Dis*, **22**, 84–6.

Ferguson, J. W., Brown, R. H. and Cheong, L. Y. (1991). Pycnodysostosis associated with delayed and ectopic eruption of permanent teeth. *Int J Pediatr Dent*, **1**, 35–41.

Fischer, T. A., Lehr, H. A., Nixdorf, U. and Meyer, J. (1999). Combined aortic and mitral stenosis in mucopolysaccharidosis type I-S (Ullrich–Scheie Syndrome), **81**, 97–9.

Fong, L. V., Menahem, S., Wraith, J. E. and Chow, C. W. (1987). Endocardial fibroelastosis in mucopolysaccharidosis type VI, 362–4.

Gelb, B. D., Shi, G. P., Chapman, H. A. and Desnick, R. J. (1996). Pycnodysostosis, a lysosomal disease caused by cathepsin K deficiency. *Science*, **273**, 1236–8.

Hagberg, B. (1984). Krabbe's disease: clinical presentation of neurological variants. *Neuropediatrics*, **15**, 11–5.

Haltia, T., Palo, J., Haltia, M. and Icen, A. (1980). Juvenile metachromatic leukodystrophy. Clinical, biochemical, and neuropathologic studies in nine cases. *Arch Neurol*, **37**, 42–6.

Harding, A. E., Young, E. P. and Schon, F. (1987). Adult onset supra-nuclear ophthalmoplegia, cerebellar ataxia and neurogenic proximal muscular weakness in a brother and sister: another hexosaminidase A deficiency syndrome. *J Neurol Neurosurg Psychiatr*, **50**, 687.

Herman, T. E. and McAlister, W. H. (1996). Neonatal mucolipidosis II (I-cell disease) with disharmonic epiphyseal ossification and butterfly vertebral body. *J Perinatol*, **16**, 400–2.

Hyde, T. M., Ziegler, J. C. and Weinberger, D. R. (1992). Psychiatric disturbances in metachromatic leucodystrophy. *Arch Neurol*, **49**, 401–6.

Jaeken, J., Proesmans, W., Eggermont, E., Van Hoof, F., Den Tandt, W., Standaert, L. *et al.* (1980). Niemann–Pick type C disease and early cholestasis in three brothers. *Acta Paediatr Belg*, **33**, 43–6.

Kolodny, E. H., Raghavan, S. and Krivit, W. (1991). Late-onset Krabbe disease (globoid cell leukodystrophy): clinical and biochemical features of 15 cases. *Dev Neurosci*, **13**, 232–9.

Machin, G. A. (1989). Hydrops revisited: Literature review of 1,414 cases published in the 1980s. *Am J Med Genet*, **34**, 366–90.

Malm, D., Halvorsen, D. S., Tranebjaerg, L. and Sjursen, H. (2000). Immunodeficiency in alpha-mannosidosis: a matched case-control study on immunoglobulins, complement factors, rece density, phagocytosis and intracellularkilling in leucocytes. *Eur J Pediatr*, **159**, 699–703.

Maroteaux, P. and Lamy, M. (1965). The malady of Toulouse–Lautrec. *JAMA*, **191**, 715.

Moser, H. W., Linke, T., Fensom, A. H., Levade, T. and Sandhoff, K. (2001). Acid ceramidase deficiency: Farber lipogranulomatosis. In *The metabolic and molecular bases of inherited disease* (Scriver, C. R., Beaudet, A. L., Sly, W. S., Valle, D, ed.), pp. 3573–89. New York.: McGraw-Hill.

Nardocci, N., Morbin, M., Bugiani, M., Lamantea, E. and Bugiani, O. (2000). Neuronal ceroid lipofuscinoses: detection of atypical forms. *Neurol Sci*, **21**, (Suppl. 3): S57–61.

Naureckiene, S., Sleat, D. E., Lackland, H., Fensom, A., Vanier, M. T., Watti, R. *et al.* (2000). Identification of HE 1 as the second gene of Niemann–Pick C disease. *Science*, **290**, 2298–301.

Nelson, J., Kenny, B., O'Hara, D., Harper, A. and Broadhead, D. (1993). Foamy changes of placental cells in probable beta glucuronidase deficiency associated with hydrops fetalis. *J Clin Pathol*, **46**, 370–1.

Norton, M. E. (1994). Nonimmune hydrops fetalis. *Semin Perinatol*, **18**, 321–32.

Oonk, J. G., van der Helm, H. J. and Martin, J. J. (1979). Spinocerebellar degeneration: hexosaminidase A and B deficiency in two adult sisters. *Neurology*, **29**, 380–4.

Parsons, V. J., Hughes, D. G. and Wraith, J. E. (1996). Magnetic resonance imaging of the brain, neck and cervical spine in mild Hunter's syndrome (mucopolysaccharidosis type II). *Clin Radiol*, **51**, 719–23.

Pastores, G. M. (2000). Gaucher Disease. In *Gene clinics* (http:/ /geneclinics.org/profiles/-gaucher/details.htm).

Pastores, G. M., Patel, M. J. and Firooznia, H. (2000). Bone and joint complications related to Gaucher disease. *Curr Rheumatol Rep*, **2**, 175–80.

Rapola, J. (1994). Lysosomal storage diseases in adults. *Pathol Res Pract*, **190**, 759–66.

Rolling, I., Clausen, N., Nyvad, B. and Sindet-Pedersen, S. (1999). Dental findings in three siblings with Morquio's syndrome. *Int J Paediatr Dent*, **9**, 219–24.

Saftig, P., Hunziker, E., Wehmeyer, O., Jones, S., Boyde, A., Rommerskirch, W. *et al.* (1998). Impaired osteoclastic bone resorption leads to osteoporosis in cathepsin-K-deficient mice. *Proc Natl Acad Sci USA*, **95**, 13453–8.

Sher, N. A., Letson, R. D. and Desnick, R. J. (1979). The ocular manifestations in Fabry's disease. *Arch Ophthalmol*, **97**, 671–6.

Soma, H., Yamada, K., Osawa, H., Hata, T., Oguro, T. and Kudo, M. (2000). Identification of Gaucher cells in the chorionic villi associated with recurrent hydrops fetalis. *Placenta*, **21**, 412–6.

Stone, D. L. and Sidransky, E. (1999). Hydrops fetalis: lysosomal storage disorders. In *Extremis. Adv Pediatr*, **46**, 409–40.

Stone, D. L., Carey, W. F., Christodoulou, J., Sillence, D., Nelson, P., Callahan, J. *et al.* (2000). Type 2 Gaucher disease: the collodion baby phenotype revisited. *Arch Dis Childh*, **82**, F163–6.

Tyynela, J. and Suopanki, J. (2000). Biochemical aspects of neuronal ceroid lipofuscinoses. *Neurol Sci*, **21**, S21–5.

von Figura, K., Gieselmann, V. and Jaeken, J. (2001). Metachromatic leucodystrophy. In *The metabolic and molecular bases of inherited disease* (Scriver, C. R., Beaudet, A. L., Sly, W. S., Valle, D, ed.). New York.: McGraw-Hill.

Wenger, D. A. (2000). Krabbe disease. *Gene Clin* (http:/ /www.geneclinics.org/profiles/krabbe/details.html).

Willems, P. J., Gatti, R., Darby, J. K., Romeo, G., Durand, P., Dumon, J. E. *et al.* (1991). Fucosidosis revisited: a review of 77 patients. *Am J Med Genet*, **38**, 111–31.

Wraith, J. E. (1995). The mucopolysaccharidoses: a clinical review and guide to management. *Arch Dis Childh*, **72**, 263–7.

Wraith, J. E. (2002). Lysosmal disorders. *Semin Neonatol*, **1**, 75–83.

Yoshida, K., Oshima, A., Sakuraba, H., Nakano, T., Yangagisawa, N., Inui, K. *et al.* (1992). GM1 gangliosidosis in adults: clinical and molecular analysis in 16 Japanese patients. **31**, 328–32.

Yoshitama, T., Nakao, S., Takenaka, T., Teraguchi, H., Sasaki, T., Kodama *et al.* (2001). Molecular genetic, biochemical, and clinical studies in three families with cardiac Fabry's disease. *Am J Cardiol*, **87**, 71–5.

Section II

Molecular mechanisms of storage

Chapter 4

Primary defects in lysosomal enzymes

Bryan G. Winchester

Introduction

Approximately 45 genetically distinct lysosomal storage diseases have been described (Meikle *et al.* 1999). Over two thirds of these diseases are due directly to defects in genes encoding lysosomal enzymes, which are predominantly hydrolases with acidic pH-optima. Deficiencies of lysosomal enzymic activities can also arise indirectly through genetic defects in enzymes involved in the post-translational processing (Chapter 5), intracellular transport (Chapter 6), or protection (Chapter 7) of the lysosomal enzymes. Deficiencies in the activities of the hydrolases acting on insoluble substrates such as membrane-associated sphingolipids can also arise because of defects in sphingolipid activator proteins (Chapter 8), which are encoded by distinct genes. [Lysosomal storage diseases can also result from defects in lysosomal membrane components (Chapter 9).] The activity of lysosomal enzymes is closely linked to cellular function. Although some cells may have specialised lysosomes with a different complement of enzymes, e.g. osteoclasts, most lysosomal enzymes are ubiquitously expressed in cells, albeit at different levels, to reflect the function of the cell type. When there is a defect in a lysosomal enzyme, the rate of intralysosomal accumulation of the substrates of that enzyme will depend upon the normal load of those substrates presented to the lysosomes of each cell type and upon the amount of residual enzymic activity. If the cell is the main site of catabolism of a particular substrate, e.g. gangliosides in neurones, then tissues containing these cells will be the prime site of storage and development of the pathology. The amount of residual activity required to prevent storage from occurring will depend on the load and the solubility of the substrate. Very little activity may be required, and there is a very sensitive relationship between the residual activity and the threshold of storage (Conzelmann and Sandhoff 1983). Some non-pathogenic mutations decrease the activity markedly without initiating storage, the so-called pseudodeficiencies (Zlotogora and Bach 1985; Thomas 1994). Lysosomal enzymes have strict specificities towards natural substrates, but the structural features that constitute that specificity may be present in more than one naturally occurring lysosomal substrate. Lysosomal β-galactosidase acts on β1→3 and β1→4 galactosidic linkages in a range of glycoconjugates, albeit with different aglycone moieties. In consequence, the storage products of a particular enzymic deficiency are often heterogeneous. Representatives of most classes of macromolecules are turned over in the lysosomes of one type of brain cell or another. Therefore, even if the prime site of lysosomal storage due to a specific enzymic defect is outside the brain, e.g. glycogen in glycogen storage disease type II, there is probably a slow but insidious build up of storage material in some brain cells. This may only manifest itself clinically late in the disease process, or if the primary lesions have been decreased by treatment. Thus, all lysosomal enzyme defects, with perhaps a few exceptions such as pycnodysostosis in which the defective enzyme, cathepsin K, is not expressed appreciably in brain cells, should be considered as causing brain disease to a lesser or greater extent.

The lysosomal hydrolases undergo specific and essential post-translational modification en route from their site of synthesis on ribosomes associated with the rough endoplasmic reticulum (ER) to their site of action, the lumen of the lysosome. This includes the removal of an N-terminal signal peptide, and asparagine-linked glycosylation in the ER, processing of the N-linked glycans, and acquisition of the mannose-6-phosphate lysosomal recognition marker in the Golgi apparatus and partial proteolysis to form the active conformation. Mutations in the structural gene for an enzyme may affect any of these steps in the maturation of the enzyme. This has to be taken into account when interpreting the effects of mutations on the function of an enzyme.

Molecular genetics of lysosomal enzyme deficiencies

A deficiency of a lysosomal enzyme has been shown to be the primary defect in the majority of neuronal storage disorders (see Table in Chapter 2). All of these disorders are inherited in an autosomal recessive manner except Danon, Fabry and Hunter diseases, which are X-linked. The genes encoding the lysosomal enzymes that are deficient in neuronal storage disorders have all been cloned and characterized (Gieselmann 1995), except acetyl coenzyme A(CoA): α-glucosamine-*N*-acetyltransferase (Sanfilippo disease type C). The genes are widely distributed over the chromosomes, and there is no evidence of polycistronic genes for the enzymes in a particular lysosomal catabolic pathway. Enzymes may, however, aggregate to form functional multienzyme complexes. Pseudogenes for several lysosomal enzymes have been found. Most of them are gene fragments, which have probably arisen by unequal crossover or unequal sister chromatid exchanges. Recombinant mutant alleles produced by crossover events between the functional and pseudogenes have been detected in Gaucher and Hunter diseases. The functional significance of transcription of some pseudogenes in lysosomal storage diseases is not known. Other loci can affect the level of expression of a lysosomal enzyme, e.g. *FUCA2* and α-*L*-fucosidase (Eiberg *et al.* 1984).

The cloning of the lysosomal enzyme genes has allowed the determination of the mutations in individual cases and families. The genotype can be useful in predicting the course of some diseases and as an aid in diagnosis. Carrier detection for genetic counselling is much more reliable by DNA analysis than enzymology or metabolite measurement. An increasingly important use of genotyping is selection of patients for the new forms of therapy becoming available.

Lysosomal storage diseases are clinically very heterogeneous, and the variety and nature of the mutations in the gene encoding the deficient enzyme are the major causes of this heterogeneity. Many types of mutations and causative genetic mechanisms have been found in lysosomal enzyme deficiencies, including single-base substitutions producing missense, nonsense, or splice-site mutations, deletions, insertions, complex mutations, and chromosomal rearrangements. Triplet repeat expansion, although found in several neurological disorders, has not been observed for any lysosomal neuronal disorder. The severity and rate of accumulation of storage material will inversely depend on the amount of residual enzymic activity in the lysosomes. In general, large insertions, deletions, and rearrangements of the gene, mutations, that produce frameshifts and nonsense mutations, will produce null alleles. Mutations in splice-site consensus sequences will usually lead to a null allele because of the absence or decrease of normally spliced mRNA or exon skipping. Sometimes, however, partial use of the mutated consensus sequence or the use of an alternative splice site generates some activity. It is important to study the mRNA for mutations that affect transcription.

It is difficult to predict the effects of missense mutations even with knowledge of the structure of the enzyme (Terp *et al.* 2002). However, substitution of an amino acid involved in the catalytic mechanism or necessary for interaction with another protein will generally decrease or abolish the activity. Alteration of an amino acid, which is highly conserved in the enzyme from different species, or a drastic change in the chemical nature of the side chain, will probably lead to loss of function. Expression of a missense mutation *in vitro* can indicate whether the mutation abolishes activity. Conversely, if a mutation does not abolish activity *in vitro*, the intracellular transport, processing, or aggregation of the mutant enzyme must be checked before concluding that a mutation is non-pathogenic. A sequence change or polymorphism that does not cause the disease itself may enhance (Islam *et al.* 1996) or lessen the effect of another sequence change.

The clinical phenotype can also give information about mutations. If a severely affected patient is homozygous for a mutation, then that mutation almost certainly produces a null allele. If that mutation is found as a compound heterozygote in a less severely affected patient, then the second mutation probably gives rise to some residual activity. Similarly, homozygosity for a mutation in a patient with milder phenotype indicates a mutation producing residual activity.

Although other genetic and physiological factors can clearly modify the phenotype in an individual, even within a family (intrafamilial variation), the severity of an autosomal recessive disease will largely be determined by the combination of alleles by the principle of gene dosage. In X-linked disorders, the clinical phenotype of males will predominantly depend on the nature of the single mutation. In female carriers of Fabry disease, random lyonization of the X-chromosomes in different cells can give rise to clinical symptoms. In contrast, female Hunter heterozygotes do not manifest any symptoms unless there is non-random inactivation or an abnormality of the X-chromosome. In all lysosomal storage diseases, there is a continuum of clinical severity, which is a reflection of the wide range of mutations found in each disorder.

Relating mutations to the structure and function of lysosomal enzymes

The ultimate purpose of determining the mutations in individual patients is to understand how they affect the structure, intracellular transport, and activity of the affected enzyme. This information will increase our understanding of the molecular basis of the disease in that individual and perhaps point to approaches to therapy. A full understanding of the relationship between mutations in a gene and their effects on an enzymic protein will only be possible when the three-dimensional structure of the enzyme–substrate/inhibitor complex has been established and the functional significance of the structural domains established. Such information is becoming available for human lysosomal enzymes (Table 4.1). However, if the three-dimensional structure of an enzyme is not available, it may be possible to predict some of its structural features from sequence data and comparison with structures of

Table 4.1 3-D structures of human lysosomal enzymes

Enzyme	EC. number	Lysosomal Disease	Comments	Reference
Cathepsin A	EC.3.4.16.5	Galactosialidosis	Precursor and mature forms, 2.2 Å	Rudenko *et al.* 1995,1998
Cathepsin B	EC.3.4.22.1	–	2.15 Å	Musil *et al.* 1991
Cathepsin D	EC.3.4.23.5	Neuronal ceroid lipofuscinosis in Swedish landrace sheep and mice	2.5 Å, complex with inhibitor	Baldwin *et al.* 1993
Cathepsin F		–	1.7 Å	Somoza *et al.* 2002
Cathepsin G	EC.3.4.21.20	–	1.8 Å	Hof *et al.* 1996
Cathepsin K	–	Pycnodysostosis	Proenzyme, 3.2 Å Mature enzyme, complex with inhibitor	Sivaraman *et al.* 1999 McGrath *et al.* 1997; Zhao *et al.* 1997
Cathepsin L	EC.3.4.22.15	–	Proenzyme, 2.2 Å Mature enzyme at 2.5 Å	Coulombe *et al.* 1996 Fujishima *et al.* 1997
Cathepsin S	–	–	2.5 Å	McGrath *et al.* 1998
Cathepsin V	–	–	1.6 Å	Somoza *et al.* 2000
Cathepsin X	–	–	2.67 Å	Guncar *et al.* 2000
Palmitoyl protein thioesterase 1	–	Infantile ceroid lipofuscinosis	2.25 Å Bovine	Bellizzi *et al.* 2000
Palmitoyl protein thioesterase 2	–	–	2.7 Å	Calero *et al.* 2003
Aspartylglucosaminidase	EC.3.2.2.11	Aspartylglucosaminuria	2.0 Å	Oinonen *et al.* 1995 Tikkanen *et al.* 1996
α Chain of β-hexosaminidase	EC.3.2.1.52	GM2 gangliosidosis Tay–Sachs variant	Modelled on β-chain	Mark *et al.* 2003

β Chain of β-hexosaminidase		GM2 gangliosidosis Sandhoff disease	Homology modelling	Sakuraba *et al.* 2002
β-Hexosaminidase B	EC.3.2.1.52	GM2 gangliosidosis Sandhoff disease	2.3 Å 2.4 Å	Maier *et al.* 2003 Mark *et al.* 2003
GM2 activator protein	–	Variant AB GM2 gangliosidosis	2.0Å	Wright *et al.* 2000
Acid lipase	EC.3.1.1.13	Wolman	Modelled on human gastric lipase	Roussel *et al.* 1999
Neuraminidase	EC.3.2.1.18	Sialidosis	Modelled on bacterial sialidases	Bonten *et al.* 2000 Lukong *et al.* 2000 Naganawa *et al.* 2000
Arylsulfatase A	EC.3.1.6.8	Metachromatic leucodystrophy	2.1 Å	Lukatela *et al.* 1998; von Bulow *et al.* 2001
Saposin B	–	Variant of metachromatic leucodystrophy	2.2 Å	Ahn *et al.* 2003
Arylsulfatase B	EC.3.1.6.1	MPS VI	2.5 Å	Bond *et al.* 1997
β-glucocerebrosidase (acid β-glucosidase)	EC.3.2.1.45	Gaucher	2.0 Å	Dvir *et al.* 2003
α-*N*-acetyl-galactosaminidase	EC.3.2.1.49	Schindler	1.9 Å Chicken α-*N*-acetyl-galactosaminidase	Garman *et al.* 2002a
α-Galactosidase	EC.3.2.1.22	Fabry	Modelled on chicken α-*N*-acetylgalactosaminidase	Garman *et al.* 2002a,b
α-Mannosidase	EC.3.2.1.24	α-Mannosidosis	2.7 Å, bovine	Heikinheimo *et al.* 2003
N-acetylgalactosamine-6-sulfatase	EC.3.1.6.4	MPS IVA	Modelled on ASA A and B	Sukegawa *et al.* 2000
β-Glucuronidase	EC.3.2.1.31	MPS VII	2.6 Å	Jain *et al.* 1996

related enzymes by molecular modelling techniques (Durand *et al.* 2000). Only 25% sequence identity between two molecules of approximately the same size is required to build a useful three-dimensional model of the protein of unknown structure by homology modelling techniques. This approach has been used to predict the three-dimensional structures of some lysosomal enzymes (Table 4.1). Even if the three-dimensional structure of an homologous protein is not available, it may still be possible to predict some structural features of a protein by using two-dimensional hydrophobic cluster analysis to probe the sequence data of a family of closely related proteins (Callebaut *et al.* 1997). Hydrophobic cluster analysis has been used to model the catalytic domains of a group of five lysosomal glycosidases (β-galactosidase, β-glucocerebrosidase, β-glucuronidase, α-*L*-iduronidase, and β-mannosidase), which are all members of the clan GH-A of glycoside hydrolases on the basis of protein sequence and mechanistic similarities (Durand *et al.* 1997). Although the levels of sequence identity amongst the five enzymes are low, below the threshold limit of usefulness of linear searches such as BLAST of 25–30%, they are all predicted to have a similar catalytic domain. Furthermore, many known disease-causing mutations in the diseases associated with deficiencies of the five enzymes have been shown to affect key residues in the active site. This approach can also be used to refine three-dimensional structural information to gain further understanding of the effect of mutations on enzymic function in, for example, β-glucuronidase.

Six and possibly eight lysosomal sulfatases belong to the sulfatase family of enzymes (Parenti *et al.* 1997; Hopwood and Ballabio 2001), which share many structural features, including the specific post-translational modification of an active-site cysteine to Cα-formylglycine (see Chapter 5). The sequence homology amongst the sulfatases ranges from 20 to 60%, with the active site and the N-terminal region being especially conserved. Arylsulfatases A and B have nearly one third amino acid sequence identity, with many other amino acids being conservative changes, and their three-dimensional structures, as determined by X-ray diffraction (Bond *et al.* 1997; Lukatela *et al.* 1998), are very similar. Many mutations have been identified in the conserved active-site residues of different lysosomal sulfatases, providing evidence for their pathogenicity, but the molecular basis of the exquisite substrate specificity of the lysosomal sulfatases remains to be elucidated.

The other major group of lysosomal hydrolases for which three-dimensional structural information is available is the cathepsins, which are subdivided according to the critical amino acid in their active sites into cysteine proteases (B, C, F, H, K, L, O, S, V, W, and X), aspartic proteases (D and E), and serine proteases (A and G). Although many of the cathepsins are ubiquitously distributed, others have very specific tissue expression patterns, e.g. cathepsin S in lymphatic tissues, where it plays an important role in processing major histocompatibility complex-II (MHC-II) complexes in antigen presentation. The three-dimensional structures of ten cathepsins have been established (Table 4.1). Six of these belong to the cysteine protease family, but only two human lysosomal storage diseases have been attributed definitely to a deficiency of a cysteine protease, cathepsin K in pycnodysostosis (Gelb *et al.* 1996) and cathepsin C in Papillon–Lefèvre syndrome (Toomes *et al.* 1999). The overall folding of cathepsins B and K is similar, but cathepsin B has a 10-amino acid loop covering its active site, which may be related to its specificity as a dipeptidyl carboxypeptidase (McGrath *et al.* 1997; Zhao *et al.* 1997; Sivaraman *et al.* 1999). The structure of cathepsin D, an aspartic acid protease, has provided insight into the structural features recognized by the phosphotransferase in the formation of the lysosomal recognition marker, mannose-6-phosphate (Baldwin *et al.* 1993), and the substrate specificity (Majer *et al.* 1997). The crystal structure (Rudenko *et al*, 1995, 1998) and molecular pathology of the precursor of the multifunctional serine protease, cathepsin A, or the human protective protein are discussed in Chapter 7.

Genotype/phenotype correlation in groups of neuronal storage disorders

It is instructive to review the genotype/phenotype relationship for individual enzymic defects by disease group rather than by enzyme specificity, because this focuses on common clinical features associated with different lysosomal catabolic pathways.

Lipidoses

The lipidoses account for about half of the lysosomal storage diseases. Most of these disorders involve the central nervous system (CNS) because of the importance of glycolipids in neuronal function. In a few lipidoses, the predominant clinical features are not neurological and death results from other aspects of lipid storage. For example, although there is deposition of lipid in some neural cells in the severe form of acid lipase deficiency (Wolman disease), it is the accumulation of triglycerides and cholesteryl esters in liver, spleen, and adrenals leading to abdominal distension, steatorrhoea and other gastrointestinal problems that causes death by 1 year. There is no deposition of lipid in the CNS in the less severe phenotype (cholesteryl ester storage disease). In most typical cases of the rare disorder, Farber disease, which is due to a deficiency of lysosomal acid ceramidase, the characteristic symptoms and an early death result from granulomatosis, but there is also progressive impairment of psychomotor development. A sub-group of patients is characterized by progressive neurological deterioration and seizures, without excessive storage in the viscera. The pathways for the lysosomal catabolism of the glycosphingolipids and other lipids are well documented (Winchester 1996; Kolter and Sandhoff 1999) (Fig. 4.1).

GM2 gangliosidoses

The GM2 gangliosidoses are characterized by the massive accumulation of GM2 gangliosides (GM2) and related lipids in lysosomes, predominantly in neurones. Three gene products are involved in the lysosomal catabolism of GM2 gangliosides, the α- and β-subunits of β-*N*-acetyl-*D*-hexosaminidase (*HEXA* and *HEXB*), and the GM2 activator protein (*GM2A*) (Mahuran 1999; Gravel *et al.* 2001; Sandhoff 2001). The monomeric subunits of β-*N*-acetyl-*D*-hexosaminidase have inactive catalytic sites but combine to form active dimers, known as hexosaminidase A (αβ), hexosaminidase B (ββ), and hexosaminidase S (αα). All these forms of hexosaminidase are specific for the hydrolysis of terminal, non-reducing β-glycosidically linked *N*-acetylglucosamine or *N*-acetylgalactosamine. However, they have different substrate specificities because of differences in the specificities of the catalytic sites on the α- and β-subunits (Sandhoff 2001) (Fig. 4.2). The α-subunit catalytic site can act on neutral or negatively charged glycolipids, oligosaccharides, glycosaminoglycans (GAGs), and synthetic substrates. In contrast, the β-subunit acts preferentially on neutral, water-soluble natural and synthetic substrates. To be degraded *in vivo*, lipophilic GM2 gangliosides must combine with the GM2 activator protein to form a complex. Only hexosaminidase A (αβ) can act on the GM2 ganglioside/GM2 activator protein complex.

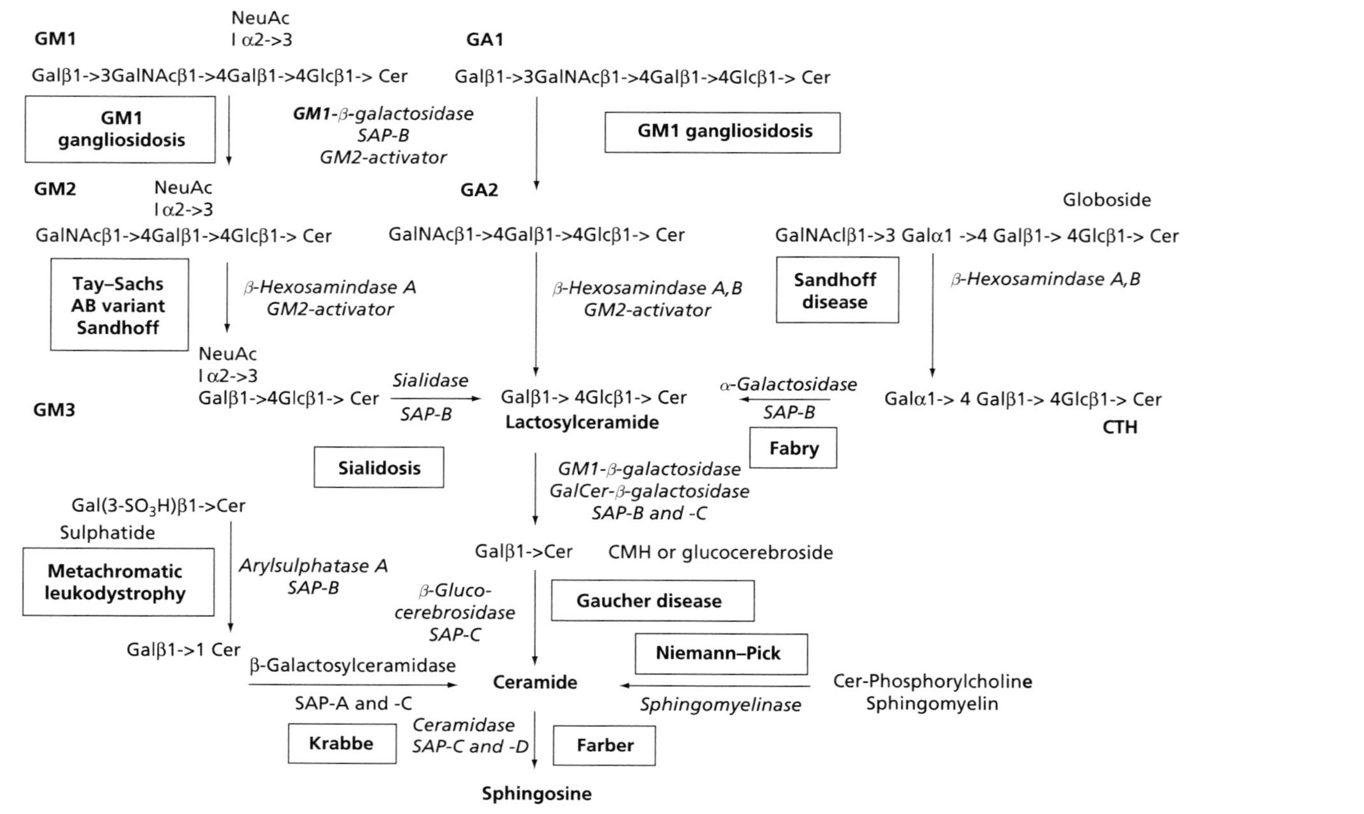

Fig. 4.1 Lysosomal catabolism of some glycosphingolipids.

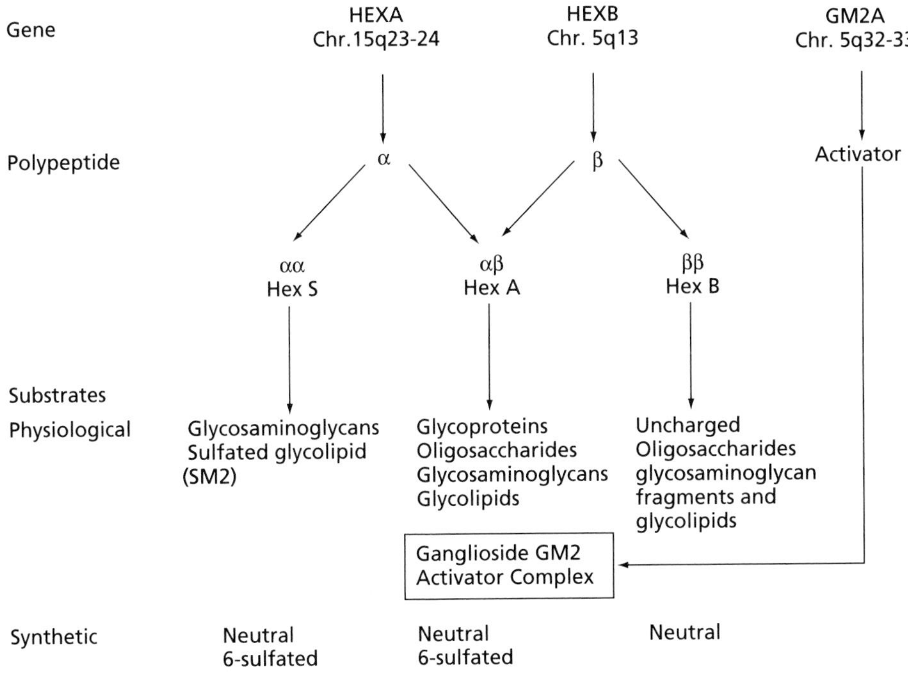

Fig. 4.2 β-Hexosaminidase system. SOURCE: Modified from Sandhoff, 2001.

Mutations in the HEXA gene lead to Tay–Sachs disease, variant B, in which there is a deficiency of hexosaminidase A (αβ) and hexosaminidase S (αα) but normal hexosaminidase B (ββ). In Sandhoff's disease, mutations in *HEXB* lead to deficiencies of both hexosaminidase A and hexosaminidase B (variant O) but not of hexosamindase S. Mice with the double knockout of *HEXA* and *HEXB* accumulate mucopolysaccharides as well as GM2 gangliosides, suggesting that β-hexosaminidase also has a role in the degradation of GAGs (Sango *et al.* 1996). Human recombinant hexosaminidase S is active *in vitro* towards sulfated oligosaccharides, the synthetic sulfated substrate (MUGS), the sulfated glycolipid SM2, and neutral substrates, consistent with the presence of two α-subunit active sites (Hepbildikler *et al.* 2002). This suggests that hexosaminidase S catalyses the hydrolysis of an important group of substrates *in vivo*. Human patients with deficiencies of both the α-subunit and the β-subunit of hexosaminidase have not been reported. A deficiency of the GM2 activator protein due to mutations in *GM2A* (variant AB) prevents the formation of the GM2 ganglioside/GM2 activator protein complex. Therefore, the accumulation of GM2 can arise from a defect in any of the three genes, *HEXA*, *HEXB*, or *GM2A*. In addition to GM2, a range of other glycolipids and oligosaccharides accumulate in the GM2 gangliosidoses, depending on which gene is mutated. The different forms of GM2 gangliosidosis are very similar clinically but all present in a wide range of severity and age of onset.

Mutations in the *HEXA* gene

Over 100 different mutations have been reported in the *HEXA* gene (database, http://data.mch.mcgill.ca). All of the nonsense mutations and the deletions and insertions that produce frameshifts give rise to the severe infantile form of GM2 gangliosidosis or classic infantile Tay–Sachs disease either in the homozygous state or in combination. They are all null alleles producing no CRM + material. Most splice-site mutations also fall into this category. A 7.6 kb deletion at the 5′-end of the gene, which extends into exon 1, was the first mutation to be discovered. It occurs in French Canadians and probably arose as a result of recombination between two Alu sequences. Two mutations account for the majority of mutant alleles in cases of infantile Tay–Sachs disease in Ashkenazi Jews, in whom the incidence has been estimated to be 1 in 4100 live births (Gravel *et al.* 2001). A 4 bp insertion in exon 11 is more common (75–80% of alleles) and causes a frameshift and premature stop codon. Although mRNA is transcribed normally, it is unstable, despite the mutation being near the 3′-end of the gene (Boles and Proia 1995). The second common mutation (15% of alleles) is a donor splice-site mutation, IVS12 + 1G→C, which leads to abnormal splicing and trace amounts of mRNA with or without exon 12 (Ohno and Suzuki 1988*a*). Common mutations due to founder effects have been found in several other isolated ethnic groups in addition to Ashkenazi Jews and French Canadians (Gravel *et al.* 2001). Many other combinations of null alleles cause infantile Tay–Sachs disease in individual families. If the family is consanguineous, the patients are generally homozygous for a rare mutation; if not, they are usually compound heterozygotes for a recurrent mutation and a rare mutation. These null alleles of the α-subunit cause loss of hexosaminidase A activity in a wide variety of ways. They include aberrant splicing of the RNA (IVS9 + 1G→A; Akli *et al.* 1990), defective intracellular transport or processing of the α-subunit (E482K; Nakano *et al.* 1988), failure of the α- and β-subunits to associate (R504C; Paw *et al.* 1990), and substitution of a functional group in the active site (S210F; Akli *et al.* 1991).

Other mutations either in the homozygous state or in combination with a null allele give rise to the less severe variants of Tay–Sachs disease, because they result in some residual hexosaminidase A activity. Splice-site mutations in which some normal mRNA is produced have been shown to lead to the late infantile (570G→A; Akli *et al.* 1990) or chronic (IVS7–7G→A; Fernandes *et al.* 1997) forms of the disease. Amino acid substitutions producing residual activity result in juvenile onset in patients homozygous for G250D (Trop *et al.* 1992) or compound heterozygotes for R499H or R504H with the null allele 1278insTATC (Paw *et al.* 1990). Patients homozygous for G269S have a relatively mild, late onset form of the disease (D'Azzo *et al.* 1984), whereas patients homozygous for another mutation in the same codon, G269D, have the severe infantile form (Akerman *et al.* 1997), illustrating the subtle effects of amino acid changes.

The mutation R178H inactivates the α-subunit but does not affect the association of the α- and β-subunits or the activity of the β-subunit (Ohno and Suzuki 1988*b*). As a result, the mutant dimeric hexosaminidase A behaves like hexosaminidase B and hydrolyses uncharged substrates predominantly. Homozygotes for this so-called B1 variant have the juvenile disease, but compound heterozygotes for the B1 mutation and a null allele have a more severe phenotype with late infantile onset. Two other mutations have been found in the same codon: R178 C produces a similar B1 phenotype, whereas R178L leads to the severe infantile form. Arginine 178 is close to the substrate-binding site in the proposed model for the ternary complex of hexosaminidase A, GM2 activator protein or GM2 ganglioside (see below, Mark *et al.* 2003). These mutations again illustrate the subtle consequences of changes in the amino acid side chain. An homologous arginine is present in the β-subunit, but its mutation has not been reported. Mutation of another residue in the α-subunit, aspartic acid 258 (D258H), also results in the B1 variant phenotype (Bayleran *et al.* 1987).

Two close and similar mutations, R247W and R249W (Cao *et al.* 1997), lead to a pseudo-deficiency of hexosaminidase A (Vidgoff *et al.* 1973), in which the α-subunit has lost activity towards synthetic substrates but retains activity towards GM2 ganglioside and is not, therefore, disease-causing. Surprisingly, the loss of activity towards the synthetic substrates is due to a decrease in stability rather than to a change in substrate recognition. Most mutations in both the *HEXA* gene and the *HEXB* gene affect the stability or processing of the subunits rather than their function (Mahuran 1999).

Mutations in the *HEXB* gene

Mutations in the β-subunit lead to a combined deficiency of β-hexosaminidases A and B or Sandhoff disease. Most of the 25 known mutations are associated with the severe infantile form of the disease, which is clinically similar to classic infantile Tay–Sachs disease. The most common mutation, accounting for approximately 30% of Sandhoff alleles, is a deletion of 16 kb at the 5′ end of the gene that removes the *HEXB* promoter, exons 1–5, and part of intron 5 (Neote *et al.* 1990). It is probably generated by recombination between two *Alu* repeat sequences. Homozygotes for this mutation have the severe, infantile-onset disease. Other combinations of null alleles including small deletions, several splice-site mutations and amino acid substitutions have been reported in severe, infantile-onset cases (Gravel *et al.* 2001).

Mutations resulting in residual enzymic activity are found in patients with later onset or less severe forms of the disease, either in the homozygous state or as compound heterozygotes with a known null allele or another mutation. One mutation, P417L, is found in a homozygous state in a juvenile case of Sandhoff disease (Wakamatsu *et al.* 1992) but as a compound heterozygote with a null allele in a family in which the presentation varied from very mild to asymptomatic (McInnes *et al.* 1992). A possible explanation for this anomalous gene dosage effect is that, although the mutation is exonic, it actually affects splicing by the variable use of a cryptic splice site and exon skipping. In consequence, the proportions of the different transcripts are highly variable, between tissues and patients even within a family (Wakamatsu *et al.* 1992). Furthermore, P417L occurs in a complex allele cis with S225R, and in homozygous state, this gives rise to the severe infantile disease (Fujimaru *et al.* 1998). Presumably, the second sequence change further decreases the amount of normal mRNA. The different phenotypes associated with this mutation emphasize the importance of detailed investigations of the genetic mechanisms of mutations before clinical use of the information. Several mutations clustered near the C-terminal, e.g. R505Q (Bolhuis *et al.* 1993), lead to a thermolabile β-subunit, which in association with a null allele results in the chronic disease or even asymptomatic individuals.

Mutations in the *GM2A* gene

The five mutations that have been discovered in the *GM2A* gene all occur in the homozygous state and lead to a severe infantile form of GM2 gangliosidosis, due to the absence of hexosaminidase A activity towards GM2 ganglioside (Mahuran 1999). The crystal structure of the GM2 activator protein has been published (Wright *et al.* 2000). For details of the molecular explanation of the effects of these mutations see Chapter 8.

Structure/function; hexosaminidase

The X-ray crystal structures of β-hexosaminidase B alone (Mark *et al.* 2003) and in complexes with inhibitors (Mark *et al.* 2003; Maier *et al.* 2003) have been published recently. The two β-subunits in the dimer are related at their interface by a two-fold axis of symmetry. Each subunit consists of a two-domain, kidney-shaped protein containing three disulfide-linked polypeptides. Domain 1 contains a six-stranded anti-parallel β-sheet and two α-helices buried against domain 2, which consists predominantly of a $(\alpha/\beta)_8$ barrel with the active site located in loops on the C-terminal side of the barrel. The architecture of the active site is consistent with the previously predicted double-displacement retention mechanism for the hydrolysis of glycosides with E355 acting as a general acid-base catalyst. Most known missense mutations occur in the region of contact between the subunits or disturb the dimer interface indirectly, indicating the importance of dimer formation for activity. For example the C534Y mutation, which is associated with an acute infantile form of Sandhoff disease destroys a disulfide bridge (C534-551C) that maintains the conformation of the C-terminus and a large section of the dimer interface (Sakuraba *et al.*, 2002). In contrast the P417L mutation occurs in a β-loop in domain 2 and leads to a milder form of the disease.

As the α- and β-subunits of β-hexosaminidase have 60% identity and the catalytic and interface (20/25) residues are highly conserved, the structure of the β-subunit is a good basis for modelling the α-subunit and the αβ dimer (β-hexosaminidase A) (Mark *et al.* 2003; Maier *et al.* 2003). The shape of the model of the αβ heterodimer is very similar to that of the ββ-homodimer but it also has a large groove into which the GM2 activator protein could dock. A loop on the α-subunit, which is predicted to be involved in the docking, is not present on the β-subunit because it is removed post-translationally. Its absence probably contributes to the more restricted substrate specificity of the β-subunit. The postulated quaternary complex of α- and β-subunits, GM2 activator protein and GM2 ganglioside positions the terminal GalNAc residue on GM2 ganglioside within the α-subunit active site. The sialic acid on the GM2 ganglioside can form an ionic bond with an arginine side chain (R424) in the β-subunit. R424 is replaced by L453 in the β-subunit and two other amino acid changes, βD426 -> αE394 and βD452 -> αN423 also probably contribute to the altered specificity.

Thus the X-ray crystal structures of β-hexosaminidase B and the GM2 activator protein, have provided great insight into the molecular understanding of the lysosomal catabolism of GM2 ganglioside and related substrates and GM2 gangliosidosis.

GM1 gangliosidosis/MPS IVB (gene *BGAL*; Chr. 3p21.3; enzyme: β-D-galactosidase; EC 3.2.1.23)

A deficiency of lysosomal β-galactosidase is present in patients with GM1 gangliosidosis and Morquio disease type B (MPS IVB), which represent the two extremes in a spectrum of clinical phenotype resulting from mutations in the β-galactosidase gene (Callahan 1999; Suzuki *et al.* 2001). β-Galactosidase has a relatively wide specificity and acts on β1→4 galactosidic linkages in N-glycans and keratan sulfate and on β1→3 and β1→4 galactosidic linkages in glycolipids. Therefore, a deficiency of the enzyme leads to a mixture of storage products, which depend upon the substrate specificity of the mutated enzyme. A secondary deficiency of β-galactosidase can arise from defects in the protective protein cathepsin A (galactosialidosis) (see Chapter 7). The hydrolysis of GM1 and lactosyl ceramide are stimulated *in vitro* by saposin B and saposins B and C, respectively (Kolter and Sandhoff 1999), but mutations in saposin B do not give rise to GM1 gangliosidosis. A second, genetically distinct lysosomal β-galactosidase, galactocerebrosidase (EC 3.2.1.46), which acts on galactosylceramide and galactosylsphingosine and is deficient in globoid cell leukodystrophy, can substitute.

Historically, GM1 gangliosidosis has been classified into three forms: infantile type I, late infantile/juvenile type 2, and adult/chronic type 3, with the majority of patients having type 1. GM1 and its asialo derivative GA1 accumulate in the brain in all three types, and galactose-terminated oligosaccharides are excreted in the urine of types 1 and 2. Some GAG derived from keratan sulfate is excreted in the urine of type 1 patients, who have severe skeletal dysplasia, but it is not believed to contribute to the pathology. The amount of residual enzymic activity and the level of storage material correlate with the severity and rate of neurological deterioration. In contrast, keratan sulfate is the major storage product in Morquio B patients, but it is different from that excreted by GM1 type I patients. Morquio B patients have extensive skeletal dysplasia but normal intelligence. There is no CNS involvement, consistent with lack of storage of GM1 ganglioside. However, the biochemical and clinical distinction between the GM1 gangliosidosis and Morquio B diseases is disappearing, as more cases are investigated in depth. The *BGAL* gene encodes a protein of 677 amino acids, which is processed to a mature form of 64 kDa, which aggregates to a homomultimer of approximately 700 kDa with the help of the protective protein (Oshima *et al.* 1987*a*; Morreau *et al.* 1991). An alternative transcript encodes a β-galactosidase-like protein (called S-Gal), which is inactive towards synthetic β-galactosidase substrates and is not transported to lysosomes (Callahan 1999). It appears to be a component of the elastin-binding receptor, which has a lactose-binding site. Over 40 different mutations have been found in the *BGAL* gene, including nonsense, frameshift, and splice-site mutations, duplications, insertions, and a predominance of missense mutations. GM1 gangliosidosis is extremely heterogeneous, and there is no obvious relationship between the type and position of the mutation and the phenotype. Most mutations give rise to no activity in expression studies because of defects in the biosynthesis, transport, or aggregation of the mutant protein. Combinations of these mutations give rise to the severe infantile disease. Mutations with measurable residual activity are associated with the juvenile (R201C), adult (I51T, T82M), and Morquio B (W273L) variants either in homozygotes or in compound heterozygotes. The second allele can modify the rate of progression of the disease in adult GM1, and individuals homozygous for the mild mutations may be asymptomatic (Chakraborty *et al.* 1994).

There is a high correlation between mutation W273L and Morquio B disease (Paschke *et al.* 2001). Interestingly, in one Morquio B case, W273L is found in conjunction with R482H, which gives rise to the severe infantile form homoallelically. Trp273 is a highly conserved residue close to the putative active-site catalytic nucleophile, Glu286. It has been postulated that Trp273 plays an important role in the binding of keratan sulfate by promoting stacking between the indole ring and pyranose backbone of the substrate (McCarter *et al.* 1997). This could explain the phenotypic differences, as mutations in Trp273 would not affect the catalytic mechanism or interaction with saposin B and would not cause accumulation of GM1. Conversely, mutations that affect the binding of saposin B would not affect the strong binding of keratan sulfate. Many missense mutations do affect folding and hence perhaps interaction with saposin B and aggregation. However, some mutant enzymes, e.g. R148S, retain some residual activity. In such situations, keratan sulfate might be bound and hydrolysed preferentially because of its intact binding site. W273L has not been found in cases where the predominant storage product is GM1 ganglioside.

Thus genetic analysis and molecular modelling of the active-site domain are beginning to provide a molecular basis for the different phenotypes.

Gaucher disease (gene: GBA; Chr. 1q21; enzyme: acid β-glucosidase or β-glucocerebrosidase; EC 3.2.1.45)

Lysosomal or acidic β-glucosidase catalyses the hydrolysis of the β-glucosidic linkage in glucosylceramide and its deacylated derivative, glucosyl sphingosine, in the presence of saposin C. The deficiency of β-glucosidase in Gaucher disease leads to the accumulation of these glycolipids in cells of the monocyte/macrophage system (Beutler and Grabowski 2001). There is marked elevation in the liver, spleen, and brain of the major storage product, glucosylceramide, which is widely distributed normally at low levels as an intermediate in the biosynthesis and catabolism of glycosphingolipids. High concentrations of glucosylsphingosine, which is not normally present in detectable amounts, are found in the liver and spleen of all Gaucher patients but in the brains of patients only with the neuronopathic forms of the diseases (Orvisky *et al.* 2000; Beutler and Grabowski 2001). The structures of the storage products reflect their tissue of origin, with only the brain storage products in the neuronopathic forms of the disease being of neural origin. The enzyme kinetics, substrate specificty, and physicochemical properties of acidic β-glucosidase have been extensively studied (Grabowski and Horowitz 1997; Beutler and Grabowski, 2001; Qi and Grabowski, 2001). The enzyme has 497 amino acids and its 3-D structure has been determined at 2.0 Å resolution by X-ray crystallography (Dvir *et al.* 2003). Saposin C binds to the enzyme in the presence of negatively charged phospolipids to induce the active conformation. A genetic defect in saposin C leads to a deficiency of acidic β-glucosidase *in vivo* (Christomanou *et al.* 1986). Unlike most other lysosomal hydrolases, acidic β-glucosidase is strongly associated with the lysosomal membrane, but it does not posses a transmembrane domain and is a perpiheral membrane protein (Imai 1985). It also differs from other lysosomal hydrolases in not undergoing further proteolytic processing after removal of the signal peptide and in not being transported to the lysosomes via the mannose-6-phosphate pathway (Erickson *et al.* 1985; Aerts *et al.* 1988). The lysosome-associated membrane proteins, LAMP-1 and LAMP-2, may be involved in the transport of acidic β-glucosidase (Zimmer *et al.* 1999). Four of five of the potential N-glycosylation sites are occupied by a mixture of complex and high-mannose glycans (Berg-Fussman *et al.* 1993), which give rise to multiple forms of the enzyme. Glycosylation is essential for the formation of the active conformation and stabilization of the enzyme.

Three clinical phenotypes of Gaucher disease are recognized on the basis of the absence (type 1) or presence and rate of progression of neurological involvement (acute type 2 and chronic type 3) (Beutler and Grabowski 2001; Elstein *et al.* 2001). Gaucher disease is panethnic and is the most common lysososmal storage disease in most populations, with a frequency of 1 in 50–100 000. Type I is the most common and is particularly prevalent in Ashkenazi Jews, in whom the predicted prevalence is 1 in ~850 (Elstein *et al.* 2001). Genotyping is providing some insight into the molecular basis of the different phenotypes (Koprivica *et al.* 2000; Beutler and Grabowski 2001; Elstein *et al.* 2001). The gene for acidic β-glucosidase, *GBA*, has been fully characterized (Sorge *et al.* 1985; Tsuji *et al.* 1986), and over 200 mutations, including point, frameshift, and splice-site mutations, deletions, insertions, and recombinant alleles, have been reported (Koprivica *et al.* 2000; Elstein *et al.* 2001; Qi and Grabowski 2001). A pseudogene with a high degree of homology is located about 16 kb downstream of the functional gene (Horowitz *et al.* 1989). It is transcribed but does not form a protein product because it lacks an open-reading frame. Its close homology to the functional gene leads to recombination events and causes problems in the detection of pathogenic mutations in the functional gene (Grabowski and Horowitz 1997; Cormand *et al.* 2000). Recombinant alleles are found in approximately 20% of patients (Koprivica *et al.* 2000).

Four common mutations, N370S, c.84–85insG, IVS2 + 1G→A and L444P, account for over 93% of the mutations in type I Jewish patients but only 49% in non-Jewish type I patients (Koprivica *et al.* 2000). The mutations, c.84–85insG and IVS2 + 1G→A, produce null alleles and are never found homoallelically and are only found rarely in non-Jewish type I patients. *In vitro* expression of the N370S mutation leads to a stable enzyme with residual activity. Possession of one N370S allele protects against neurological disease, and individuals homozygous for N370S may even be asymptomatic (Cox and Schofield 1997). Other mutations found in combination with null alleles in type I patients are deduced or have been shown to produce residual activity.

The mutation L444P produces an unstable enzyme with negligible activity. Homozygosity for the L444P mutation is generally associated with type 3, but it has been found in all three phenotypes. It is common in the Norrbottnian genetic isolate due to a founder effect. It is often found as part of a complex allele with recombination between the functional and pseudogenes. Patients apparently homozygous for L444P should always be checked for complex alleles. Mutation R463C, which produces a stable enzyme with a little residual activity on *in vitro* expression (Hong *et al.* 1990), is also common in type 3 patients (Koprivica *et al.* 2000). L444P, R463C, and other mutations that are found in combination with null alleles in type 3 patients must produce insufficient activity to prevent the accumulation of glucosylceramide of neural origin in neurones.

The severe fatal type 2 Gaucher disease results from a combination of two very severe alleles. Most recombinant alleles are null alleles, and homozygosity for a recombinant allele results in early lethality (Stone *et al.* 2000). Homozygosity for several missense mutations and combinations of L444P with one of these mutations or a known null allele also result in type 2. Type 2 patients who are homozgous for L444P have been reported, but it is not known whether one of their alleles is in fact a recombinant allele. Homozygosity for D409H is associated with an unusual phenotype reminiscent of the mucopolysaccharidosis, MPS IH (Abrahamov *et al.* 1995).

Knowledge of the 3-D structure of β-glucocerebrosidase is beginning to provide a molecular basis for the relationship between mutations and clinical phenotype (Dvir *et al.* 2003). The enzyme has three domains. The active site is in domain III, which consists of a $(\beta/\alpha)_8$ TIM barrel and is homologous to other enzymes in the glucosidase hydrolase A clan. The two putative catalytic groups, the carboxyl side chains of E235 and E340, are about 5 Å apart, which is consistent with retention of configuration in the catalytic mechanism The common mutation N370S is located on one of the α-helices in the catalytic domain at the interface with domain II. It is too far away from the active site for direct involvement. Several other mutations are found on this helix, all pointing into the barrel. Mutations occur in residues near the active site e.g. H311, A341 and C342. One side of the active site is lined with aromatic side chains, which may be involved in substrate recognition. Mutations in residues close to this lining, such as V394L, may disrupt the active conformation. Two mutations associated with a milder form of the disease, R463C and R496H, are situated in domain II, which resembles an immunoglobulin fold with two β-pleated sheets. The severe mutation, L444P, is also located in domain II but in the hydrophobic core of the IgG-like domain and probably disrupts the conformation leading to an unstable protein. This non-catalytic domain may regulate the interaction of β-glucocerebrosidase with substrate or saposin C. Domain I, which contains the N-terminus and three β-pleated sheets has relatively few known mutations but seven mutations, including the common severe mutation, D409H, occur in a C-terminal strand in this domain.

There is great variation in phenotype in Gaucher disease, even amongst patients with the same genotype. The expression of the ancillary gene, saposin C, disruption of contiguous genes in the gene-rich region on chromosome 1 (Tayebi *et al.* 2000) and environmental factors (Cox and Schofield 1997) may all contribute to the phenotype.

Globoid cell leukodystrophy (Krabbe disease) (gene: *GALC*; Chr. 14q243-32.1; enzyme: galactocerebrosidase or galactosyl ceramidase/galactocerebroside β-galactosidase; EC 3.2.1.46)

Galactocerebrosidase catalyses the hydrolysis of the β-galactosidic linkages in various galactolipids, galactosylceramide, galactosylsphingosine, monogalactosyldiglyceride, and possibly lactosylceramide. As galactosylceramide and its sulfated derivative, sulfatide, are found almost exclusively in myelin, which is synthesized in oligodendrocytes, a deficiency of galactocerebrosidase essentially leads to a disorder of the white matter of the CNS and peripheral nervous systems (Wenger *et al.* 2000, 2001). However, the total concentration of galactosylceramide in the brain does not increase. It has been suggested that the accumulation of the toxic galactosylsphingosine (psychosine) leads to the early destruction of the oligodendroglia (Suzuki 1998; Im *et al.* 2001). The majority of patients (approximately 90%) have a severe infantile disease, but patients with a later onset, even in adulthood, have been described. The age of onset and progress of the disease are highly variable even in patients with the same genotype.

Galactocerebrosidase is a very hydrophobic protein, and its activity towards galactosylceramide is stimulated *in vitro* by phosphatidyl serine and saposins A and C. The human brain enzyme is synthesized as an 80 kDa precursor, which is processed to two subunits of 50–53 and 30 kDa, both of which are required for activity. The cDNA encodes a predicted protein of 669 amino acids, including a signal peptide of 26 amino acids (Chen *et al.* 1993), which suggests that most of the potential glycosylation sites are occupied in the mature enzyme. Over 60 mutations have been found in the *GALC* gene (Wenger *et al.* 2000, 2001). The majority of patients are compound heterozygotes, but several missense mutations have been found in homozygous form, permitting their designation as null or mild alleles with the caveat of marked variability of phenotype. A 30 kb deletion, which removes all of the coding region for the 30 kDa subunit and part of the 50 kDa subunit, accounts for 40–50% of the alleles in infantile patients of European ancestry and 35% in infantile Mexican patients (Rafi *et al.* 1995). Some mutations, which presumably produce enzyme with residual activity, are homoallelic in juvenile/adult (G270D) or adult patients (I66M, L629R). Patients, who are compound heterozygotes for G270D, and the large deletion have a juvenile or adult phenotype but with tremendous variation in severity.

The *GALC* gene is highly polymorphic, and about 80% of disease-causing mutations occur on alleles with at least one polymorphism. These polymorphisms affect the activity in normal and mutant alleles. The most common polymorphism, I546T, which has a frequency of 40–50% in the general population, decreases activity by up to 70%. The common deletion is always found in association with 502T. A genotype of one deleted and one polymorphic allele can lead to late-onset disease with normal activity towards galactosylsphingosine (Harzer *et al.* 2002). These polymorphisms are responsible for the wide reference ranges of activities in carriers and normal individuals and for some, but certainly not all, of the variation within a disease genotype.

Metachromatic leukodystrophy (gene: *ASA*; Chr. 22q13; enzyme: arylsulfatase A or cerebroside-3-sulfatase; EC 3.1.6.8)

Metachromatic leukodystrophy (MLD) results from a deficiency of arylsulfatase A (ASA), which catalyses the hydrolytic removal of sulfate from 3-*O*-sulfated galactose–containing glycolipids in the presence of saposin B (von Figura *et al.* 2001). The loss of ASA activity usually results from mutations in the structural gene for the enzyme (*ASA*) but can occur rarely from defects in saposin B (Shapiro *et al.* 1979). Arylsulfatase A activity is also affected in multiple sulfatase deficiency disorder. The sulfatides (galactosylceramide-3-sulfates), which are predominantly found in the myelin sheath in the CNS and peripheral nervous system and in the kidney, are the major sphingosine-containing storage products. The lysosomal catabolism of lactosyl ceramide-3-sulfate, galactosylpsychosine sulfate, and 3-*O*-sulfated galactosyl-glycerolipids (seminolipid), which occurs in the testes and spermatozoa, is also blocked. There is great variation in the age of onset and severity of MLD, with infantile, juvenile, and adult forms of the disease being recognized clinically. Biochemical studies suggest that the severity of MLD depends upon the amount of residual enzymic activity. Arylsulfatase A is synthesized as a 507-amino acid precursor, which loses a signal peptide and is glycosylated in the ER, before acquiring the lysosomal recognition marker in the Golgi and being transported to the lysosomes via the mannose-6-phosphate receptor pathway. Like other eukaryotic sulfatases, ASA undergoes the characteristic modification of an active-site cysteine to C^{α}-formylglycine. However, it does not undergo further proteolytic processing. Arylsulfatase A forms a homo-octamer of four dimers at acidic pH. The *ASA* gene is well characterized (Kreysing *et al.* 1990) and over 60 mutations have been reported (von Figura *et al.* 2001). The majority (>80%) are missense mutations, but several deletions and splice-site mutations have been found. Most of the mutations have only been found in a single family, but three mutations occur with a higher frequency in patients of European descent (Berger *et al.* 1997). The donor splice-site mutation, IV2 + 1 (formerly called I mutation), is a null allele, and patients homozygous for this mutation have the most severe infantile form of MLD. In contrast, the missense mutation, P426L, results in an enzyme that is synthesized and transported to the lysosomes normally but has low residual activity and is unstable intralysosomally due to defective oligomerization (von Bulow *et al.* 2002). Homozygosity for this mutation results in the adult or juvenile forms of MLD, and patients who are compound heterozygotes for P426L and a null allele have juvenile MLD (Polten *et al.* 1991). However, patients heterozygous for P426L have presented in infancy (Barth *et al.* 1993), indicating that other genetic and environmental factors can influence the course of the disease. These two mutations account for about 50% of the mutations and the third mutation, I179S, for about 12%. Other mutations are prevalent in different ethnic groups, and the common European mutations are not found in Japanese patients, in whom the severe mutation, G99D, is present in 30% of the alleles (Eto *et al.* 1993).

The three-dimensional structure of the enzyme has been established by X-ray crystallography (Lukatela *et al.* 1998). The core of the enzyme consists of two β-pleated sheets that are sandwiched between helices. The enzyme has strong structural homology to alkaline phosphatase. The modified active-site cysteine is hydrogen-bonded to several residues conserved between ASA and arylsulfatase B. A divalent metal ion is located at the bottom of a substrate-binding pocket, which also contains residues conserved in the sequences of other sulfatases. Arylsulfatase A has a unique cysteine-rich C-terminal region that is free of mutations but does contain a polymorphism, R496H (Ricketts *et al.* 1998). No mutations have been found in the catalytic residues and about 60% occur in the non-structured loop regions. Proline 426 is located in the minor central β-pleated sheet. Mutations in Asp335 and Arg370, which form an intramolecular salt bridge in the crystal structure, lead to a variety of clinical phenotypes. Expression of D335V showed that the mutant enzyme is retained in the ER with complete loss of activity (Hess *et al.* 1996). Conversion of Arg370 to tryptophan (R370W) or to glutamine (R370Q) leads to severe or mild forms of the disease, respectively (von Figura *et al.* 2001). The crystal structures of complexes of two inactive active-site mutants of ASA with an artificial substrate have provided further insight into the molecular mechanism of action (Von Bulow *et al.* 2001). However, despite the three-dimensional structure, it remains difficult to predict the effect of missense mutations.

X-ray crystallography of saposin B suggests that a homodimer with a large hydrophobic cavity can extract lipids to form a soluble lipid-protein substrate for arylsulfatase A (Ahn *et al.* 2003).

A marked decrease of ASA activity, 5–15% residual activity, which does not cause any clinical or biochemical signs of MLD, is found in 1–2% of Europeans (Dubois *et al.* 1975). This so-called pseudodeficiency of ASA was initially shown to be due to a complex allele containing two polymorphisms, N350S and 1524 + 95G→A (Gieselmann *et al.* 1989). N350S abolishes a glycosylation site and results in a smaller but active enzyme, whereas 1524 + 95G→A disrupts the polyadenylation signal 95 bp downstream from the termination codon and decreases the concentration of the major 2.1 kb mRNA by approximately 90%. Thus, the polyadenylation polymorphism is responsible for the marked decrease in ASA synthesis. In fact, it was subsequently shown that both polymorphisms occur independently and that their distribution varies widely in different populations (Zlotogora *et al.* 1994; Ricketts *et al.* 1996; Ott *et al.* 1997). The existence of the pseudodeficiency complicates enzymic diagnosis of MLD, especially if a disease-causing mutation occurs on an allele carrying the polyadenylation polymorphism. A functional sulfatide-loading test may be needed to resolve the problem (Leistner *et al.* 1995). Expression studies *in vitro* suggest that polymorphisms on the same allele can contribute to the decrease in enzymic activity and to the severity of the disease, but it is not known whether this occurs *in vivo* (Regis *et al.* 2002).

Fabry disease (gene: *GLA*; Chr. Xq21.3-Xq22; enzyme: α-galactosidase A; EC 3.2.1.22)

Fabry disease is an X-linked disorder resulting from a deficiency of α-galactosidase A (Desnick *et al.* 2001). In consequence, there is progressive accumulation within lysosomes of glycosphingolipids with terminal α-galactosyl residues, globotriaosylceramide, and to a lesser extent galabiosylceramide and blood group B substances. This predominantly occurs in the endothelial, perithelial, and smooth muscle cells of blood vessels, but there is deposition in many other cell types. Male hemizygotes with typical clinical presentation have negligible residual α-galactosidase activity and mostly no detectable α-galactosidase protein (Desnick *et al.* 2001). However, clinical variants, who may be asymptomatic, mildly affected, or mainly show cardiac manifestations, do generally have residual activity. Paradoxically, several male Fabry patients with classic clinical symptoms have been reported with normal activity *in vitro*. The α-galactosidase in female heterozygotes ranges from near zero to normal due to random inactivation of the X-chromosome, and heterozygotes can only be detected reliably by molecular genetic techniques (Whybra *et al.* 2001). Some female heterozygotes are asymptomatic, but others are as severely affected as typical hemizygotes, and symptoms may be confined to a single organ because of the random nature of the X-inactivation. The extreme of this mosaicism is seen in two identical female twin carriers who showed very different phenotypes due to uneven X-inactivation (Redonnet-Vernhet *et al.* 1996). There is no correlation between activity measured in plasma or white blood cells, genotype, and severity in heterozygotes. α-Galactosidase A is synthesized as a precursor of 50 kDa, which undergoes processing to a mature lysosomal form of 46 kDa and is transported to the lysosomes via the mannose-6-phosphate pathway (Lemansky *et al.* 1987). The active enzyme is a homodimer of about 110 kDa and requires saposin B to act on its natural substrates *in vivo*. A second lysosomal enzyme, α-galactosaminidase or α-galactosidase B, also acts on synthetic substrates for α-galactosidase *in vitro*. The two enzymes are structurally related (46.9% amino acid sequence identity) but are encoded by different but evolutionary related genes (Wang and Desnick 1991). A model of human α-galactosidase has been constructed based on the crystal structure of chicken α-galactosaminidase (Garman *et al.* 2002 *a, b*). The *GLA* gene has been fully characterized (Bishop *et al.* 1986; Kornreich *et al.* 1989), and over 200 different mutations have been reported. They include missense and nonsense mutations, RNA processing defects, gene rearrangements (approximately 5%), small insertions and deletions, and four complex mutations, in which more than one mutational event appears to have occurred. Most are private mutations, but some are recurrent, a few of which have been shown by haplotyping to occur in distantly related members of the same family. The majority of the recurrent mutations occur in CpG dinucleotides. All except a few missense mutations give rise to null alleles and the classic phenotype in hemizygotes. A group of atypical patients, who lack the typical early symptoms, present with a late-onset cardiomyopathy or cardiomegaly. These 'cardiac variants' have missense mutations that give rise to residual α-galactosidase A activity: A20P, G66Q, N215S, M269V, M269I, S279E, and R301Q, (Sakuraba *et al.* 1990; Ishii *et al.* 1992). The mutations, Q279E and R301Q, do not alter the kinetic properties of α-galactosidase A but decrease the amount reaching the lysosomes, presumably because of retention in the ER (Kase *et al.* 2000). Female heterozygotes with 'cardiac' mutations do not all have decreased α-galactosidase activity (Yoshitama *et al.* 2001). Other atypical patients with missense mutations, e.g. M72V, have been described with a slower course of the disease or limited range of symptoms (Okumiya *et al.* 1998), suggesting that there is a spectrum of phenotypes depending on the amount and distribution of the residual α-galactosidase A activity. Some of the mutations found in the variants, e.g. R112H, R301Q, and G328R (Ashton-Prolla *et al.* 2000), are also found in patients with the classic phenotype, suggesting that other factors affect the phenotype. Two mutations E66Q and R112C, which separately give rise to residual activity, constitute a null allele in combination (Beier *et al.* 1999). Intrafamilial variation is found with some null alleles, e.g. W226X (Knol *et al.* 1999). Manifesting female heterozygotes with decreased α-galactosidase A activity but no mutations in the *GLA* gene are also known (Handa *et al.* 2000). A mutation in the 5′-untranslated region of the *GLA* gene, – 30G→A, which is found in 0.5% of normal individuals gives rise to elevated plasma α-galactosidase A (Fitzmaurice *et al.* 1997). Although disease-causing mutations are distributed over the whole model of α-galactosidase A, they fall into two classes, those that disrupt the active site of the enzyme and those that affect the stability of the folded protein. Mutations associated with the classic phenotype tend to affect residues in the centre of the molecule, whereas those associated with less severe phenotypes tend to not to disrupt the hydrophobic core (Garman *et al.* 2000 *b*).

Niemann–Pick disease types A and B (gene: *ASM*; Chr. 11p15.1-p15.4; enzyme: acid sphingomyelinase; EC 3.1.4.12)

Niemann–Pick disease types A and B (NP-A and -B) result from a primary deficiency of acid sphingomyelinase (ASM) activity, which results in the accumulation of sphingomyelin in a variety of cells but in particular in cells of the monocyte–macrophage lineage (Kolodny 2000; Schuchman and Desnick 2001). In contrast, in Niemann–Pick type C (NPC), there is a defect in the intracellular processing of low-density lipoprotein-derived cholesterol, which gives rise to similar clinical features. There is a marked deficiency of ASM (1–3% residual activity) in NPD type A, which is a progressive neurodegenerative disorder with infantile onset and death at 2–3 years. The residual activity is higher in NPB, giving rise to a less severe form of the disease with neurological involvement generally limited to cherry-red macula. The phenotype is more variable in NPB, and there is probably a continuum of age of onset and severity, reflecting the amount and distribution of residual ASM activity. Assays that measure the hydrolysis of accumulated lysosomal sphingomyelin *in situ* can distinguish between NPA and typical NPB patients (Rodriguez-Lafasse and Vanier 1999). The accumulation of sphingomyelin (up to 50 times normal) in the viscera (hepatosplenomegaly) and reticuloendothelial system is similar in NPA and -B, but it only accumulates in the brain of NPA and not NPB patients (Strasberg and Callahan 1998; Rodriguez-Lafasse and Vanier 1999). The lyso form of sphingomyelin, sphingosylphophorylcholine, is also markedly increased in the liver and spleen of both types but again is only found in NPA brain (Rodriguez-Lafasse and Vanier 1999). It is tempting to suggest that this lysosphingolipid is the cause of the neurodegeneration in NPA, as has been suggested for the psychosines in Krabbe and neuronopathic Gaucher disease (Berger *et al.* 1995). However, an enzymic pathway for the deacylation of sphingomyelin has not been described in human tissues.

Acid sphingomyelinase is a zinc-dependent glycoprotein of 629 amino acids, which has a signal peptide of 46 amino acids and is processed and transported to the lysosomes via the mannose-6-phosphate pathway (Schuchman and Desnick 2001). There is a SAP-like domain in the N-terminal region (C89-C165), which is linked to the rest of the protein by a proline-rich sequence. This probably acts as an endogenous detergent *in vivo*, obviating a requirement for a saposin. Many cells can secrete ASM, and it has been suggested that the deficiency of the extracellular ASM may contribute to the pathology of NPD (Schissel *et al.* 1996). The *ASM* gene has been cloned and fully characterized (Schuchman *et al.* 1991, 1992), and over 50 different mutations have been found in NPD patients. Most of these are private mutations, but recurrent mutations have been reported in both NPA and NPB patients. Three common mutations (L302P, R496L, and fsP330) constitute 92% of the alleles in Ashkenazi Jews, who account for about two thirds of NPA patients and in whom the carrier frequency is about 1 in 80 (Schuchman and Desnick 2001). Expression studies show that all three are null alleles, explaining the severe type of disease in these patients. Combinations of other proven or putative null alleles have been found in non-Jewish type A patients. R496L has been found in combination with DR608 in a Jewish type B patient. Expression of DR608 produced activity, and this mutation has been found in other Jewish type B patients and is predominant in North African type B patients (Vanier *et al.* 1993). Several other mutations give rise to activity on expression (e.g. G242R) or have been found in homoallelic form

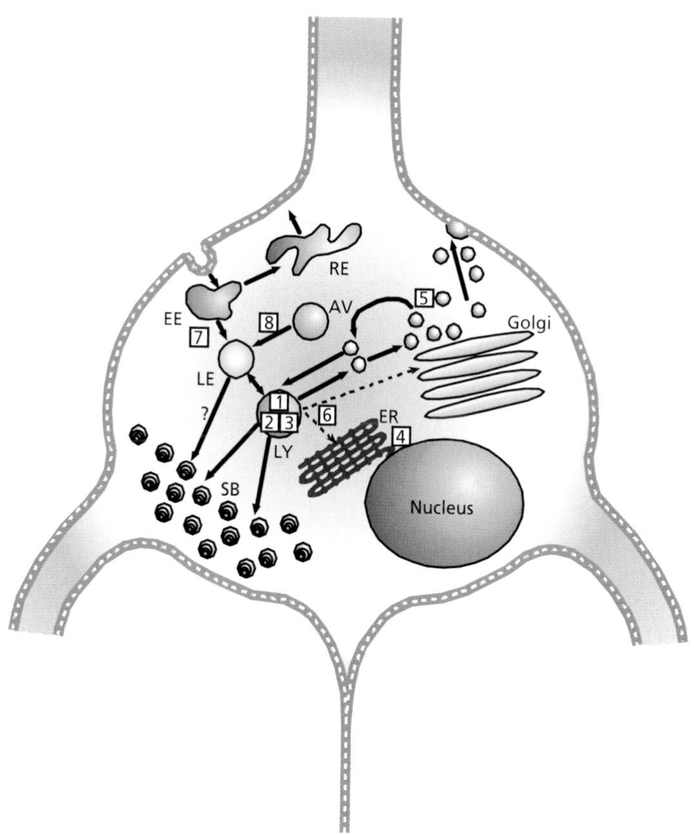

Plate 1 Schematic illustration of a neurone and its endosomal–lysosomal system with known or putative sites of molecular defects leading to lysosomal storage disease. Storage bodies (SB) are generated by accumulation of materials within late endosomes (LE) and lysosomes (LY) (*double arrow* depicts functional continuity between these compartments). These vesicles are in close functional association with early endosomes (EE) and recycling endosomes (RE). Defects within the LE–LY compartment include those directly impacting lysosomal enzymes [1], protective protein [2], and activator proteins [3], as seen in Tay–Sachs, galactosialidosis, and GM2 gangliosidosis AB variant diseases, respectively. Lysosomal enzyme processing in the endoplasmic reticulum (ER) may be abnormal [4], as seen in multiple sulfatase deficiency. Lysosomal enzymes may be made and processed normally but fail to receive the mannose-6-phospate recognition marker during transit through the Golgi resulting in, for example, I-cell disease [5]. Abnormal movement of degraded materials (gangliosides and cholesterol) out of the LE–LY compartment secondary to defects in transmembrane proteins may lead to diseases like Niemann–Pick type C [6]. Other transmembrane proteins may facilitate earlier endocytic events [7] or autophagic processing and vesicle fusion [8] as seen in mucolipidoses IV and Danon disease, respectively (Modified from Walkley 2001.).

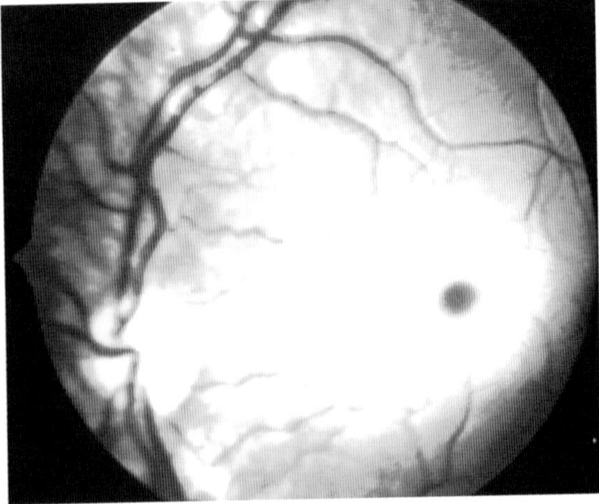

Plate 2 Cherry red spot–Tay–Sachs disease.

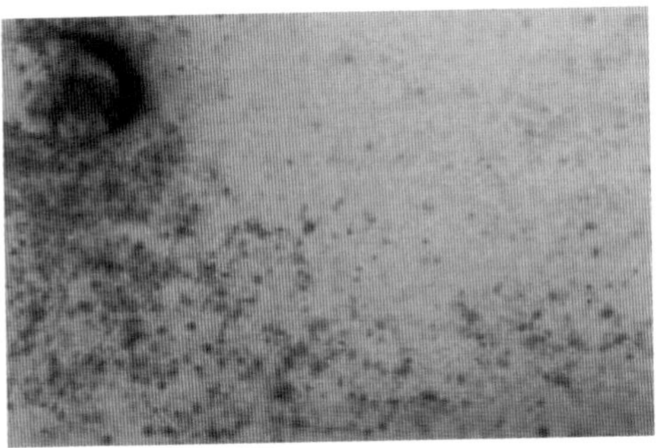

Plate 3 Abdominal angiokeratomas in a patient with Fabry disease.

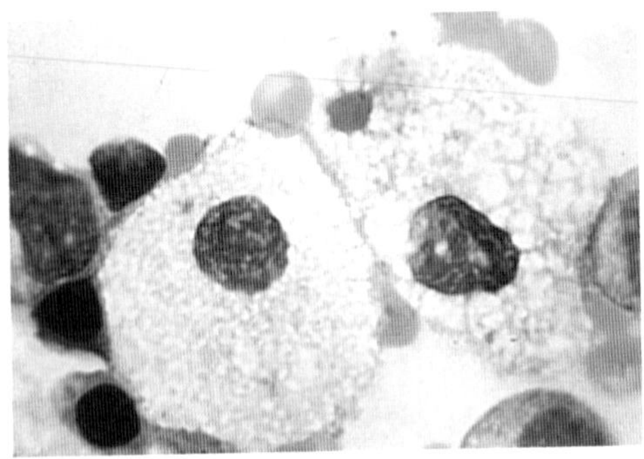

Plate 4 Foam cells in the bone marrow of a patient with Niemann–Pick B disease.

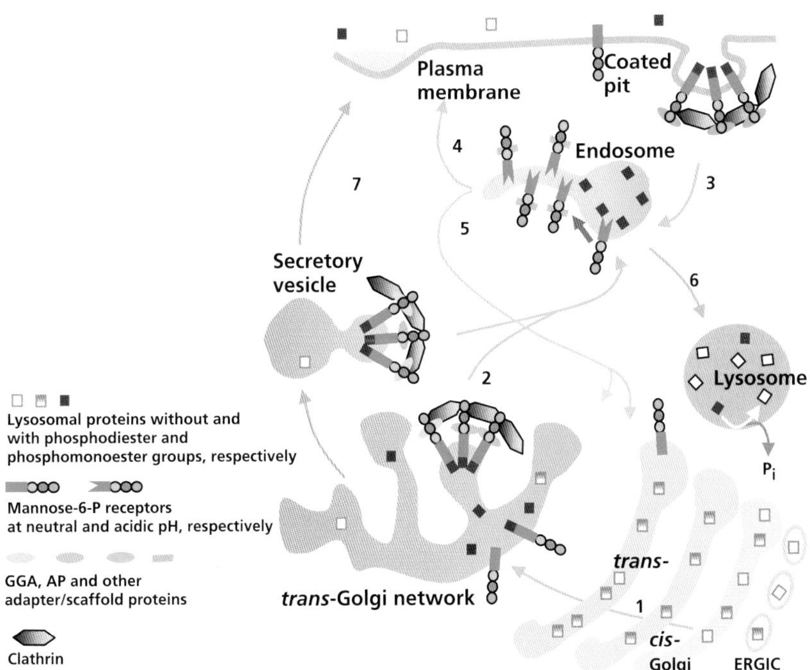

Plate 5 Modification and transport of soluble lysosomal proteins into lysosomes. **1**: After synthesis, glycosylation and folding in the RER proteins are transported into and through the ERGIC and Golgi cisternae; most of the soluble lysosomal enzymes that bear a recognition signal for N-acetyl-glucosaminyl phosphotransferase become phosphorylated. **2**: The phosphorylated glycoproteins leaving the *trans*-Golgi cisternae bear covered mannose 6-phosphate residues. In the *trans*-Golgi network (TGN) uncovering takes place and the uncovered M6P-residues mediate binding to M6P-receptors. In the TGN and possibly the secretory vesicles phosphatidyl inositol-bisphosphate and Arf-1 initiate the formation of a protein scaffold, in which the cytosolic domains of the receptors, Rab, GGA, AP-1 and coat (clathrin) proteins promote budding of vesicles. A vesicle detachment is assisted by dynamin and followed by uncoating and fusion with early and/or late endosomes. **3**: Phosphorylated lysosomal enzymes that escape sorting and become secreted may be captured by the original or a remote cell bearing the CI-MPR at the plasma membrane. The formation of coated pits and endocytic vesicles involves besides CI-MPR, Arf-6, AP-1, clathrin also dynamin that facilitates the detachment. Following uncoating, these vesicles fuse with early endosomes. In the acidic interior of endosomes phosphorylated lysosomal enzymes dissociate from their receptors and their proteolytic processing is initiated. **4** and **5**: In early and late endosomes cargo-free receptors interact with a retrieval machinery that mediates their return to the plasma membrane and *trans*-Golgi. For the sake of brevity the scheme does not differentiate between the recycling, early and late endosomes that have their characteristic sets of proteins facilitating the recycling. **6**: The contents of the late endosomes are delivered to lysosomes, where a dephosphorylation and even a partial deglycosylation of lysosomal enzymes may proceed and the proteolytic maturation is completed. **7**: Default secretion of lysosomal proteins that have escaped segregation into the lysosomal pathway.

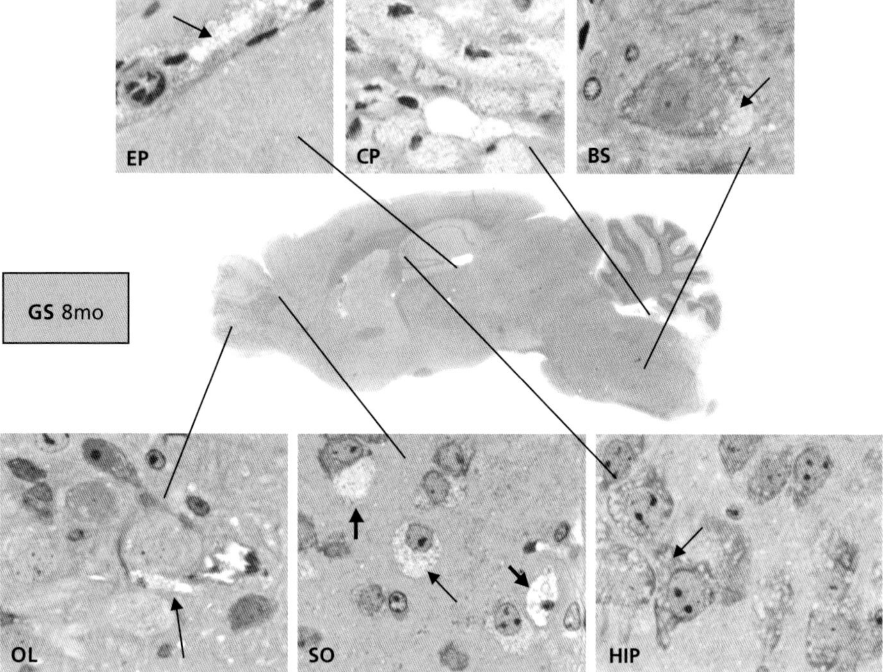

Plate 6 The brain of a galactosialidosis (GS) mouse aged 8 months was fixed in 10% neutral-buffered formalin and embedded in glycol methacrylate. Sections of 1 μm thickness were stained with toluidine blue. The different regions of the brain that were photographed are indicated in the parasagittal section in the middle panel. *Top row*: ependyma (EP), choroid plexus (CP), and brainstem (BS). *Bottom row*: anterior olfactory (OL), subolfactory (SO), and hippocampus.

(e.g. S436R) in type B patients. Possession of one of these milder alleles appears to be sufficient to prevent the neuronopathy associated with NPA. Other mutations produce less residual activity than the typical type B mutations and lead to an intermediate phenotype with a protracted neuropathic disease. One such mutation, W391G, produces an enzyme which is synthesized and transported to the lysosomes normally but is unstable (Ferlinz *et al.* 1995). Thus, mutation analysis is beginning to provide a genotype/phenotype correlation for NPA and -B, but other factors can affect the severity, particularly neurological involvement, as is shown by intrafamilial variation in patients with an intermediate phenotype (Pavlu and Elleder 1997; Obenberger *et al.* 1999).

Glycoproteinoses or oligosaccharide storage diseases

The lysosomal degradation of glycoproteins containing *N*-linked glycans occurs in two stages (Winchester 1996; Michalski and Klein 1999; Thomas 2001). Firstly, the polypeptide is degraded by lysosomal proteases or cathepsins to produce a mixture of amino acids, dipeptides, and glycoasparagines. The glycoasparagines are then degraded in a highly ordered, bi-directional series of enzymic steps, as shown for a representative *N*-linked complex glycan in Fig. 4.3. α-1-6-Linked fucose is removed from the core *N*-acetylgucosamine before the oligosaccharide is released from the asparagine by aspartylglucosaminidase. The chitobiose linkage is then hydrolysed by endo-β-*N*-acetylglucosaminidase (chitobiase) to complete the digestion of the linkage region. Subsequently, monosaccharides are removed sequentially from the non-reducing end by exoglycosidases. High-mannose and hybrid glycans are degraded by similar pathways. Storage disorders are known for deficiencies of each enzyme except endo-β-*N*-acetylglucosaminidase (chitobiase). The chitobiosidic linkage can also be cleaved at a later stage in the pathway by the exoglycosidase, β-hexosaminidases A or B, thereby compensating for a deficiency of the endoglycosidase. It is interesting that only humans and rodents express the chitobiase and other mammals use the alternative pathway normally. The lysosomal catabolism of O-linked glycans has not been investigated so thoroughly, and it is not known whether exhaustive proteolysis occurs before the breakdown of the oligosaccharide. As many of the glycosidic linkages in O-linked glycans are the same as in glycolipids, e.g. β-galactoside or β-*N*-acetylgalactosaminide, or in *N*-linked glycans, it is assumed that the same enzymes are involved in their hydrolysis. The linking bond, GalNAc (1→O) ser/thr, is hydrolysed by α-*N*-acetylgalactosaminidase, which also hydrolyses the same linkage in keratan sulfate type II and GalNAcα (1→3) Gal bonds in glycoproteins and glycosphingolipids. Therefore, oligosaccharides will accumulate in other lysosomal storage diseases in which the predominant clinical features relate to the storage of other compounds, e.g. GM1 and GM2 gangliosidoses. In contrast, α-mannosidosis and aspartylglucosaminuria are probably pure glycoproteinoses because the bonds hydrolysed by the deficient enzymes do not occur appreciably in other structures. All of the enzymes involved in the lysosomal catabolism of glycoproteins have been cloned, but the crystal structure is only known for aspartylglucosaminidase, α-mannosidase and α-*N*-acetylgalactosaminidase (Table 4.1).

Fucosidosis (gene: *FUCA1*; Chr. 1p34; enzyme: α-L-fucosidase; EC 3.2.1.51)

Fucosidosis results from a deficiency of α-L-fucosidase, which acts on α1→2, α1→3, α1→4 and α1→6 fucosidic linkages predominantly to galactose or *N*-acetylglucosamine in

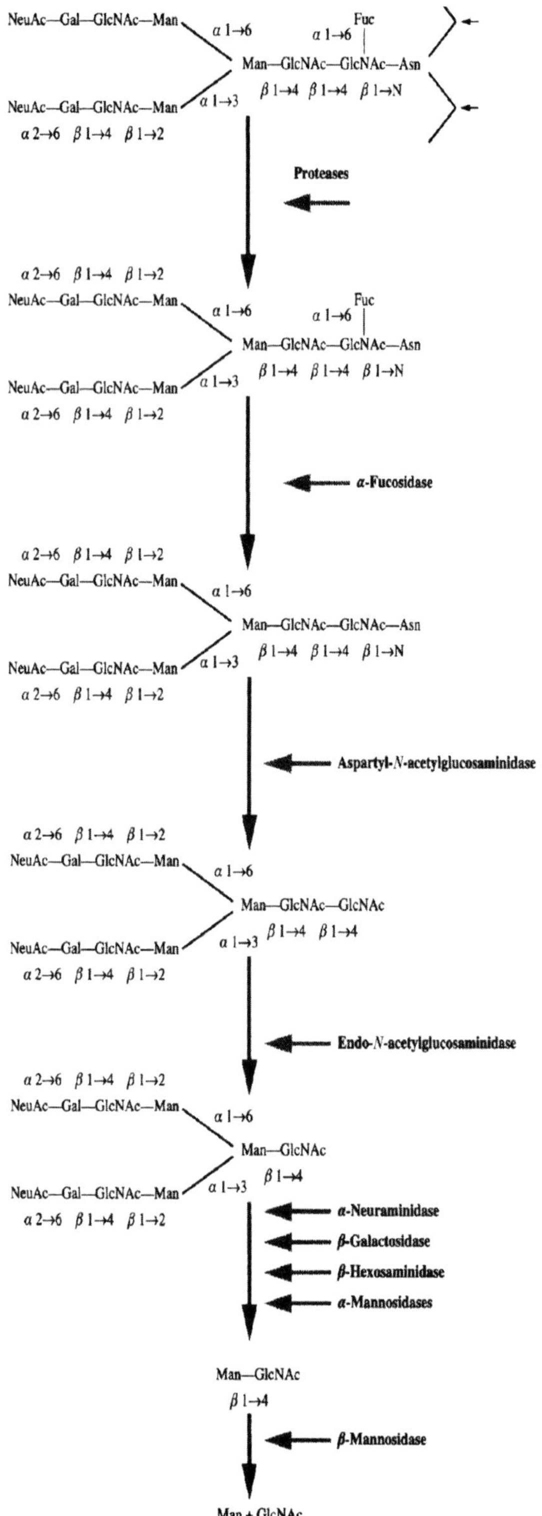

Fig. 4.3 Lysosomal degradation of a typical complex N-linked glycan of glycoproteins.

glycosphingolipids and oligosaccharides. Although it is a typical lysosomal hydrolase and is transported to the lysosomes by the mannose-6-phosphate pathway, it has a relatively wide activity-pH range. It aggregates readily to give active dimers, trimers, and tetramers, with one active site per monomer of approximately 50 kDa (White *et al.* 1987). A carboxy group with a pK_a value of 3.7–3.8, which could stabilize a fucosyl oxocarbonium ion transition state, has been implicated in the catalytic mechanism (White *et al.* 1987; Winchester *et al.* 1990). Since isolation of the *FUCA1* gene (Kretz *et al.* 1992), over 20 different mutations have been identified (Willems *et al.* 1999; Thomas 2001). Most of the patients are homozygous for private mutations, with over 40% resulting from consainguineous marriages, consistent with fucosidosis being a rare autosomal recessive disorder. One mutation, Q422X, has been found in eight families and is the basis for the relatively high incidence in families originating from the Calabria region of Italy. Four patients are homozygous for missense mutations in conserved amino acids. Three were severely affected, but the fourth, who has the mutation, L450R, is a 46-year-old patient with a less severe phenotype (Fleming *et al.* 1998). Another patient with the chronic, infantile form of fucosidosis is a compound heterozygote for a stop codon and a large deletion of all the exons but has a relatively mild clinical course despite the absence of mRNA (Akagi *et al.* 1999). Originally, fucosidosis was classified as type I or II on the basis of age of onset and clinical severity. However, patients with the same genotype, including siblings, have been reported with the two clinical phenotypes (Willeems *et al.* 1991). As most of the mutations lead to negligible α-L-fucosidase activity and protein, other factors must determine the variation in phenotype. A pseudogene (*FUCA1P*) on chromosome 2 is 80% colinear with *FUCA1* (Carrit and Welch 1987; Kretz *et al.* 1992) and a locus on chromosome 6 (*FUCA2*) regulates the level of α-L-fucosidase in fibroblasts and plasma but not leucocytes (Eiberg *et al.* 1984). There is no structural similarity between *FUCA1* and *FUCA2*.

Aspartylglucosaminuria (gene: *AGA*; Chr. 4q32–33; enzyme: *N*-(β-*N*-acetylglucosaminyl)-1-asparaginase or aspartylglucosaminidase; EC 3.5.1.26)

Aspartylglucosaminuria results from a deficiency of aspartylglucosaminidase (glycosylasparaginase), which hydrolyses the amide bond between the innermost core *N*-acetylglucosamine residue in N-linked glycans and the side chain of asparagine (Aronson 1999; Aula *et al.* 2001). The enzyme does not appear to act on intact glycoproteins and only releases glycans from glycosylasparagines. It requires the prior removal of any α-1–6-linked fucose on the core *N*-acetylglucosamine residue by α-L-fucosidase before it will cleave the amide bond (Barker *et al.* 1988; Noronkoski and Mononen 1997). The biosynthesis (Ikonen *et al.* 1993) and the three-dimensional structure of aspartylglucosaminidase (Oinonen *et al.* 1995) have been investigated thoroughly, allowing a good understanding of the consequences of specific mutations on the enzymic activity (Saarela *et al.* 2001). It is synthesized as a single precursor polypeptide, which loses a signal peptide and undergoes preliminary folding and dimerization in the ER. The dimeric precursor is activated by autodigestion of the peptide bond between aspartic acid 205 and threonine 206 to form a tetramer consisting of two α- and two β-subunits of 27 and 17 kDa, respectively. The enzyme is glycosylated and acquires the mannose-6-phosphate marker in the Golgi and is delivered to the lysosome where final maturation of both subunits takes place. The three-dimensional structure of aspartylglucosaminidase (AGA) shows that it is a member of the N-terminal nucleophile protein family with a central four-layer sandwich of α-helices and β-sheets. The α-amino group of the exposed threonine 206 at the N-terminal of the β-subunit acts as a base to enhance the nucleophilicity of the OH-group in the catalytic mechanism. Aspartylglucosaminuria is particularly common in Finland, where a common mutation (C163S) found in conjunction with a polymorphism R161Q accounts for 98% of the mutant alleles. This is due to a founder effect, and there is a carrier frequency of 1 in 40. This mutation prevents the formation of a disulfide bridge and dimerization, leading to the loss of the enzymic activity. Over 25 different mutations have been reported worldwide (Saarela *et al.* 2001). Two thirds of them are missense mutations, which cause the introduction of bulkier side chains. They have been predicted by a combination of expression studies, immunolocalization, and modelling to disrupt dimerization, to destabilize the enzyme, to prevent disulfide formation, or to affect active-site functional residues. The effects of small deletions and insertions and nonsense codons have also been investigated. The mutations have been classified as having a mild, moderate, or severe effect on the basis of these studies, and there is good agreement between the predicted and observed effects in patients.

Sialidosis (mucolipidosis I) (gene:NEU1; Chr. 6p21.3; enzyme: neuraminidase (sialidase); EC 3.2.1.18)

At least three different human neuraminidases, with different sub-cellular locations (cytosol, plasma membrane, and lysosomes), pH-optima, and substrate specificities, exist (Achyuthan and Achyuthan 2001). The lysosomal neuraminidase is very labile and normally exists as a functional complex with the protective protein, β-galactosidase and perhaps *N*-acetylgalactosamine-6-sulfatase (see Chapter 7). Therefore, a deficiency of lysosomal neuraminidase activity can arise from mutations in the structural genes for neuraminidase or the protective protein. A deficiency of lysosomal neuraminidase is responsible for both the less severe sialidosis type I (cherry-red spot myoclonus syndrome) and the severe sialidosis type II (Lowden and O'Brien 1979; Thomas 2001). The enzyme releases α-2→3- and 2→6-linked neuraminic acids from both oligosaccharides and gangliosides (Ulrich-Bott *et al.* 1987). The *NEU1* gene has been cloned (Bonten *et al.* 1996; Pshezhetsky *et al.* 1997) and mutations in patients have been analysed (Bonten *et al.* 2000; Naganawa *et al.* 2000; Lukong *et al.* 2001; Penzel *et al.* 2001). A model of human lysosmal neuraminidase, which has been constructed using homology modelling, based on bacterial and influenza virus sialidases (Lukong *et al.* 2000), has been used to predict the structural changes caused by the mutations. Using this information in conjunction with expression studies and characterization of any residual activity in patient cells, it has been possible to explain the variation in clinical phenotype in sialidosis in cellular and molecular terms (Pshezhetsky and Ashmarina 2001; Itoh *et al.* 2002). There is a good correlation between severity and residual enzymic activity. Mutation of the putative active-site tyrosine, Y370C, completely abolishes activity, and patients homozygous for this mutation have the severe sialidosis type II. Several other missense mutations lead to complete loss of activity either in homozygosity or in combination with a null allele. Biochemical data and modelling suggest that they disrupt folding and destabilize the enzyme, thereby preventing its transport to lysosomes (L363P) or interaction with the protective protein (L270F). Other missense mutations, e.g. S182G or G328R, lead to some residual activity and result in the milder type I phenotype either in homozygosity or in combination with a null allele.

α-Mannosidosis (gene: LAMAN; Chr. 19p13.2-q12; enzyme: α-D-mannosidase; EC 3.2.1.24)

α-Linked mannose residues occur in the core region of all N-linked glycans and in the branches of high-mannose and hybrid glycans. Therefore, the deficiency of lysosomal α-D-mannosidase in mannosidosis (Ockerman 1967) affects the catabolism of all N-linked glycans. Human cells contain at least 10 genetically distinct α-D-mannosidases with different sub-cellular locations, pH-optima, and substrate specificities (Daniel *et al.* 1994). The main lysosomal α-D-mannosidase hydrolyses the α-(1→2), α-(1→3), and α-(1→6) mannosidic linkages in N-linked glycans in a highly ordered manner at an acidic pH (Al Daher *et al.* 1991). Another lysosomal α-D-mannosidase with a narrow specificity towards the α(1→6)-linked mannose in the trimannosyl core of N-linked glycans acts in concert with the main α-D-mannosidase but is not affected in α-mannosidosis (Cenci di Bello *et al.* 1983). Its specificity explains the lack of α(1→6)-linked core mannose residues in the storage products in α-mannosidosis (Daniel *et al.* 1992). The main lysosomal α-D-mannosidase is synthesized as a precursor of 110 kDa (Pohlmann *et al.* 1983), which undergoes complex partial proteolysis during maturation to produce multiple forms of the active enzyme, all of which are deficient in α-mannosidosis (Nilssen *et al.* 1997). Cloning of the gene (Nebes and Schmidt 1994; Riise *et al.* 1997) and characterization of the recombinant enzyme (Berg *et al.* 2001) have shown that the gene encodes a polypeptide of 1011 amino acids, which is processed into five peptides in the mature enzyme. Over 60 disease-causing mutations have been found in patients, including three recurrent ones, R750W, L809P, and a splice-site mutation, IVS14 + 1G→C (Nilssen *et al.* 1997; Gotoda *et al.* 1998; Berg *et al.* 1999; Frostad Riise *et al.* 1999). R750W has been detected in 34 patients from Europe, Japan, Australia, and the USA and accounts for 21% of the disease alleles. Although there is a wide range of clinical severity in α-mannosidosis, no residual α-mannosidase activity was found in fibroblasts of patients and no correlation between clinical phenotype and genotype was evident. The 3-D structure of bovine lysosomal α-mannosidose has been elucidated, providing a basis for understanding the structure of the human enzymes (Heikinheimo *et al.* 2003).

β-Mannosidosis (gene; *MANBA*; Chr. 4q22–25; enzyme: β-D-mannosidase; EC 3.2.1.26)

β-Mannosidosis is a very rare and generally less severe disorder, which results from a deficiency of β-D-mannosidase (Cooper *et al.* 1986; Wenger *et al.* 1986). The enzyme catalyses the last step in the sequential breakdown of oligosaccharides released from glycoproteins, the cleavage of the core Manβ (1→4) GlcNAc bond. In consequence, Manβ (1→4) GlcNAc accumulates in the tissues of patients and is excreted into the urine together with a sialylated derivative and a urea conjugate (Dorland *et al.* 1988). The enzyme exists in at least two active forms and has a typical acidic pH-optimum (Guadalupi *et al.* 1996). The full-length cDNA for the human enzyme encodes a polypeptide of 879 amino acids (Alkhayat *et al.* 1998), which is processed to the mature active forms. There is tremendous clinical heterogeneity amongst the small number of patients, including intrafamilial variation. Two siblings, a severely affected girl and her less severely affected brother, were both homozygous for a splice-site mutation, IV2-A→G, which led to the activation of a cryptic splice site and exon skipping and the production of two abnormally spliced mutant mRNA species in both siblings (Alkhayat *et al.* 1998). Genotyping of further patients is necessary to see if there is a molecular basis for this clinical heterogeneity.

α-*N*-Acetylgalactosaminidase deficiency (Schindler or Kanzaki disease) (gene: *NAGA*; Chr. 22q13.1–13.2; enzyme; α-*N*-acetylgalactosaminidase (α-galactosidase B); EC 3.2.1.49)

A deficiency of α-*N*-acetylgalactosaminidase was first reported in a patient in 1987 (van Diggelen *et al.* 1987) and is still a very rare occurrence. α-*N*-Acetylgalactosaminidase was originally called α-galactosidase B because it can hydrolyse the α-galactosidic linkage in water-soluble synthetic substrates. It accounts for the residual activity measured with these substrates in plasma or cells from typical Fabry patients. The enzyme has very low activity *in vitro* and in fibroblasts towards globotriaosylceramide ($GbOse_3Cer$), the natural substrate for true α-galactosidase A, to which it is closely related structurally. However, it does hydrolyse the Forsmann antigen ($GbOse_5Cer$), which terminates in α-linked *N*-acetylgalactosamine, blood group A glycolipids, and synthetic α-*N*-acetylgalactosaminide substrates (Asfaw *et al.* 2002). This specificity accounts for the storage of glycopeptides containing the *O*-linked glycan core structure, GalNAcα1→OSer/Thr, and the blood group A trisaccharide, GalNAcα(1→3)Gal(2→1)αFuc. However, most excreted glycopeptides have galactose and sialic acids attached to the O-linked core. Immunoelectron microscopy showed that only GalNAcα1→OSer/Thr was stored in lysosomes of skin cells from patients, suggesting that secondary metabolic effects, such as disruption of the activity of the protective protein complex or transglycosylation, must occur in other cells (Kanda *et al.* 2002).

α-*N*-Acetylgalactosaminidase is synthesized as a precursor of 52 kDa, which is processed non-proteolytically to a mature enzyme of 49 kDa. This is consistent with the cDNA sequence, which predicts a polypeptide of 411 amino acids with a signal peptide of 17 residues (Wang *et al.* 1990*a*). It exists predominantly as a homodimer and is relatively stable. Three clinical phenotypes are recognized: infantile onset type 1 with severe neurodegeneration (Schindler), adult onset type II (Kanzaki), and intermediate and variable type III (Desnick and Schindler 2001). The recently published X-ray crystallographic structures of the free and ligand-bound enzyme provide a molecular basis for this clinical heterogeneity (Garman *et al.* 2002*a*). Patients in the original type I family were homozygous for a missense mutation, E325K (Wang *et al.* 1990*b*), which is in a highly conserved amino acid. Transient expression of this mutation did not produce any enzymic activity or cross-reacting protein. However, two siblings homozygous for the E325K mutation have been described recently, who are either very mildly affected at 3 years or asymptomatic at 7 years (Bakker *et al.* 2001). The two families with type II disease are homozygous for different mutations, substitution of a conserved arginine by tryptophan (R329W) (Wang *et al.* 1994), and a nonsense mutation, E193X (Keulemans *et al.* 1996). Patients from the two type III families are compound heterozygotes for the E325K mutation and either S160C (Keulemans *et al.* 1996) or E367K (Desnick and Schindler 2001), which are both in conserved amino acids. All patients have very low levels of α-*N*-acetylgalactosaminidase activity and protein and identical patterns of storage (Keulemans *et al.* 1996). None of the mutations is in the active site, and the loss of activity results from destabilization of the dimeric enzyme structure. Although blood group A status may affect severity, it is evident that factors other than the α-*N*-acetylgalactosaminidase genotype affect the phenotype.

Mucopolysaccharidoses

Glycosaminoglycans (GAGs or mucopolysaccharides) are broken down in the lysosomes in a sequential, stepwise manner from the non-reducing end (Fig. 4.4.) (Hopwood and Morris 1990; Winchester 1996; Neufed and Muenzer 2001). Five sulfatases, four exoglycosidases, a transferase, and endoglycosidases are involved in the pathways for the main classes of GAGs, heparan, dermatan, chondroitin and keratan sulfates, and hyaluronan. Defects in these enzymes lead to the lysosomal storage diseases, the MPSs. The linkages acted on by some of these enzymes occur in more than one pathway. Therefore, the storage products in some MPS disorders are heterogeneous, e.g. the accumulation of dermatan and heparan sulfates

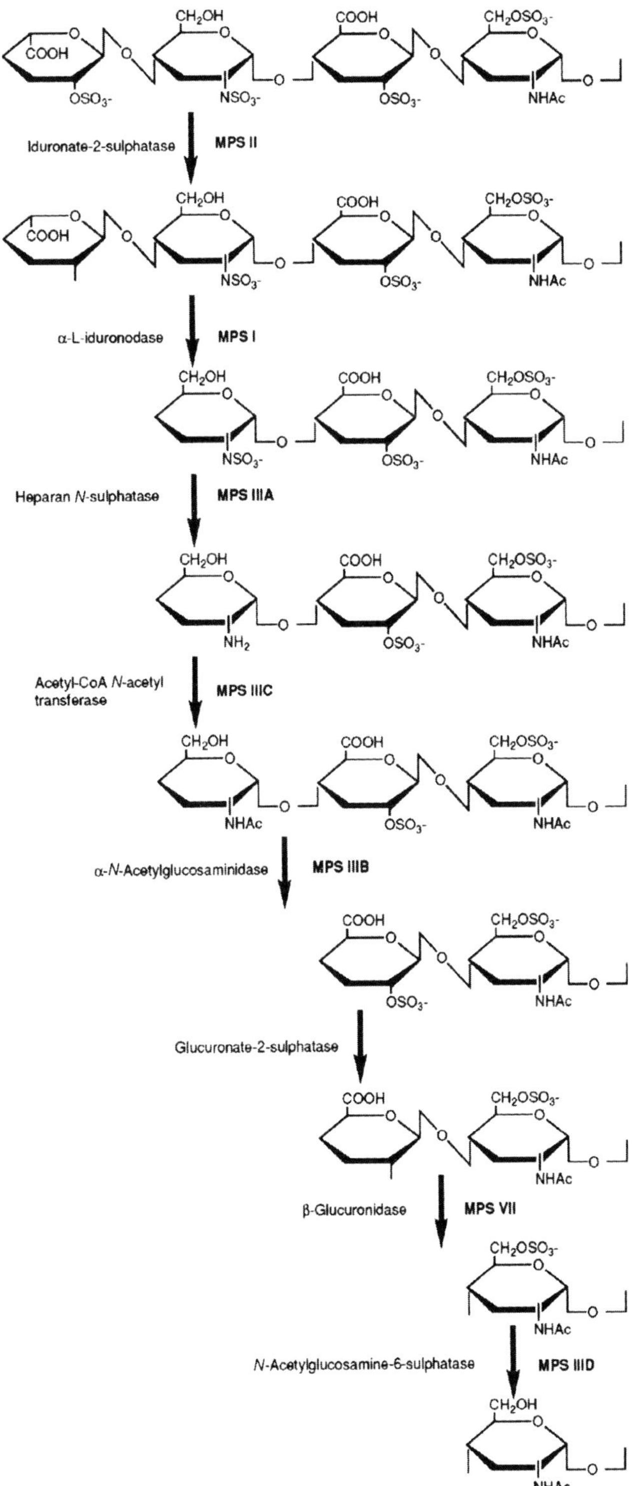

Fig. 4.4 Glycosaminoglycan catabolism in the lysosome.

with a deficiency of α-L-iduronidase (MPS I) or iduronidase 2-sulfatase (MPS II). MPS I and II share many clinical features, but the phenotypes in the severe infantile forms with complete deficiencies of enzymic activity are not identical. This indicates that in some cells the precise structure of the storage product affects the phenotype, by determining the use of an alternative pathway or depriving the cell of a specific digestion product, e.g. iduronic acid or sulfate, respectively. In contrast, where the enzymes are only essential in one pathway, a single type of GAG accumulates and deficiencies of different enzymes give rise to a similar phenotype, e.g. the four enzymic defects responsible for the Sanfilippo syndrome (MPS III). Although the MPSs share many clinical features, mental retardation is only a characteristic feature of MPS III and the most severe forms of MPS I and II. There is only a moderate involvement of the CNS in MPS VII, and patients with MPS IV and VI can have normal intelligence. The defective gene in MPS IX, *HYAL1*, which encodes the major lysosomal hyaluronidase, is not expressed in brain tissue (Frost *et al.* 1997). There is a wide variation in clinical severity in all the MPS, but the cloning of most of the genes for the enzymes deficient in MPS and elucidation of the mutations in individual patients are beginning to provide a molecular explanation for some of this variation.

MPS I (Hurler, Hurler/Scheie and Scheie syndrome) (gene: *IDUA*; Chr. 4p16.3; enzyme: α-L-iduronidase; EC. 3.2.1.76)

MPS I results from a deficiency of α-L-iduronidase, which catalyses the hydrolysis of non-reducing terminal α-L-iduronide bonds in dermatan and heparan sulfates. Three clinical phenotypes of decreasing severity and increasing age of onset are recognized: Hurler (MPS IH), Hurler/Scheie (MPS IH/S), and Scheie (MPS IS). They cannot be distinguished by routine enzyme assays or analysis of urinary GAGs, and there is a continuum of clinical presentation. However, careful measurement of residual activity using a natural substrate, immunodetection of protein, and measurement of GAG turnover in cells have shown that there is a good correlation between the biochemical phenotype, clinical course of the disease, and genotype (Bunge *et al.* 1998). The gene (*IDUA*) (Scott *et al.* 1992) encodes a precursor protein, which is processed via intermediates to a mature active monomer and is transported to the lysosomes by the mannose-6-phosphate pathway. No major gene rearrangements have been reported in MPS I patients, and the majority of patients have point mutations. Two nonsense mutations, W402X and Q70X, are prevalent in northern Europeans with the severe Hurler phenotype (Bunge *et al.* 1994). The frequency of these null alleles ranges from 84% in Scandinavia to only 24% in Italy, and they are absent from Japanese and Arab MPS IH patients. Patients homozygous or compound heterozygotes for these mutations have no detectable α-L-iduronidase enzyme or protein and accumulate GAGs rapidly (Bunge *et al.* 1998). Other stop codons or frameshifts give rise to the severe phenotype either in homozygosity or in combination with the common null alleles. Some of these are found in particular populations, e.g. 705ins5 in Japan (Yamagishi *et al.* 1996) and R628X in the Middle East (Beesley *et al.* 2001). Missense mutations result in severe or less severe phenotypes, depending on the effect of the amino acid substitution on the properties of the enzyme and on the other allele. Patients homozygous for A327P (or in combination Q70X) have the severe phenotype, whereas a compound heterozygote, A327P/1995del12, has the intermediate phenotype, suggesting that deletion of four amino acids in frame towards the end of the protein leads to some residual activity. Another in-frame deletion of four amino acids in the signal peptide leads to a severe phenotype in homozygotes but, paradoxically, to an attenuated phenotype when in combination with W402X (Scott *et al.* 1995*a*; Beesley *et al.* 2001). The missense mutation,

P533R, which is prevalent in the Western Mediterranean (Gatti *et al.* 1997; Gort *et al.* 1997; Alif *et al.* 1999), can produce a severe phenotype in homozygosity but also result in an atypical presentation and a milder phenotype (Gatti *et al.* 1997; Scott *et al.* 1992). Patients heterozygous for W402X and P533R have a less severe phenotype than W402X homozygotes, suggesting that the P533R allele may produce some residual α-L-iduronidase or that other factors must affect the phenotype. Two mutations are found commonly in patients with the milder forms of MPS I. The acceptor splice-site mutation, 678–7g→a (Moskowitz *et al.* 1993), leads to the use of a cryptic splice site 28 nucleotides upstream. However, the normal splice site is still used at a low level to produce some residual enzymic activity and the genotype, W402X/678–7g→a, results in the Scheie phenotype. The mutation, R89Q, produces an unstable and partially active mutant enzyme in expression studies and has been found in Caucasian and Japanese patients. In combination with a null allele, it gives the Hurler/Scheie phenotype and homozygotes have the Scheie phenotype (Scott *et al.* 1993). Two polymorphisms, A461T and V454I, which are in strong linkage disequilibrium, moderate the effect of R89Q on the enzyme. A second mutation R89W also leads to a milder form of the disease (Bunge *et al.* 1995). Modelling has suggested that Arg89 is in the active site of the enzyme and may play a role in the activation of the catalytic nucleophile (Durand *et al.* 2000). Glutamic acid residues 182 and 289 are also predicted to be involved in the catalytic mechanism. A patient, who is a compound heterozygote for W402X and E182X, has the severe MPS IH phenotype, demonstrating the importance of E182 for catalytic activity (Brooks *et al.* 2001). Over 30 polymorphisms have been found in the *IDUA* gene (Scott *et al.* 1995*b*), and their effect on phenotype is only just beginning to emerge. A pseudodeficiency of iduronidase due to the mutation A300T was discovered in a family afflicted with both MPS I and MPS II (Aronovich *et al.* 1996). There is a good correlation between the combination of alleles and the biochemical and clinical phenotype in MPS I, but other genetic factors can modify the phenotype.

MPS II (Hunter disease) (gene: *IDS*; Chr. Xq28; enzyme: iduronate-2-sulfatase; EC 3.1.6.13)

MPS II, which is the only X-linked MPS, presents with a wide range of clinical severity (Neufed and Muenzer 2001). It results from a deficiency of iduronate-2-sulfatase, which catalyses the removal of the sulfate from the 2′-position of iduronic acid at the non-reducing ends of heparan and dermatan sulfates. The investigation of iduronate-2-sulfatase, as the 'Hunter corrective factor', played a seminal role in the discovery of the mannose-6-phosphate pathway. The *IDS* gene has nine exons extending over 24 kb and encodes a protein of 550 amino acids (Flomen *et al.* 1993; Wilson *et al.* 1993), with five functional N-glycosylation sites (Di Natale *et al.* 2001). The enzyme is processed and transported to the lysosomes in the typical manner and has a high sequence homology with other sulfatases. A pseudogene (*IDS-2* locus) consisting of exons 2 and 3 and intron 7 occurs about 20 kb away. It probably arose through duplication, because the region between the two genes contains other repeated sequences (Rathman *et al.* 1995; Timms *et al.* 1995). The *IDS* gene occurs in a gene-rich region of the X-chromosome. These structural features account for some of the clinical and genetic heterogeneity in MPS II. About 10% of the over 280 different mutations that have been reported in the *IDS* gene are gross gene rearrangements or deletions, all of which lead to a severe form of the disease. Deletion of contiguous genes such as *FMR1* or *FMR2* as well as the *IDS* gene might explain the additional clinical features in some patients, who have large deletions and a particularly severe form of the disease (Wraith *et al.* 1991; Birot *et al.* 1996*a*; Timms *et al.* 1997).

Recombination between a sequence in intron 7 of the functional gene and an homologous sequence near exon 3 of the pseudogene has been found in many patients with the severe phenotype (Bondeson *et al.* 1995). It results from double-strand breaking and leads to the inversion of the intervening sequence (Lagerstedt *et al.* 1997). The presence of large duplicated sequences in the region of the *IDS* gene is responsible for other homologous (Birot *et al.* 1996*b*) and non-homologous (Karsten *et al.* 1997) recombinations that disrupt the *IDS* gene and lead to a severe phenotype.

Generally, nonsense and frameshift mutations produce the severe phenotype. However, two nonsense mutations, R443X and Q531X, have been found in patients with intermediate (Sukegawa *et al.* 1992) and mild phenotypes, respectively (Sukegawa *et al.* 1995; Froissart *et al.* 1998). Q531X results in a polypeptide lacking the last 19 C-terminal amino acids, which are normally removed by proteolytic processing, whereas R443X results in a protein lacking some amino acids present in the mature enzyme.

It is difficult to predict the effect of the missense mutations, most of which are family specific. Comparison of the sequences of sulfatases shows that certain residues are highly conserved and probably have an important functional role (Hopwood and Ballabio 2001). Cysteine 84 is predicted to be the essential active-site cysteine in the highly conserved CXPSR (84–88) sequence in iduronate-2-sulfatase. Mutation of cysteine 84 to alanine in a patient with the severe form of Hunter disease confirms the importance of this residue in the active site (Millat *et al.* 1997). Patients with mutations in proline 86 (P86L/R) and arginine 88 (R88C/G/H) are also severely affected, but mutation of the non-conserved alanine 85 can give rise to a mild/intermediate, A85T, or severe, A85S, phenotype. Missense mutations in other non-conserved amino acids, N63D and Y108S, give rise to milder forms of MPS II. Some recurrent missense mutations occur in mutation hotspots such as the CpG dinucleotides at codon 468 R, a non-conserved amino acid, e.g. R468W (CGG→TGG) and R468Q (CGG→CAG), which lead to a severe phenotype. Mutations occur more frequently in male meioses (Rathmann *et al.* 1996).

Female carriers of Hunter disease do not show clinical symptoms, but a few cases of Hunter disease in females have occurred. A balanced reciprocal chromosome translocation 46 XX t (X:5) disrupted the *IDS* gene and led to non-random inactivation of the normal X-chromosome in a severely affected girl (Mossman *et al.* 1983). The partial deletion of the long arm of the normal paternal X-chromosome resulting in its late replication and full expression of a mutated maternal X-chromosome was found in another severely affected female (Broadhead *et al.* 1986). Another cause of severe Hunter disease in a female was the combination of skewed inactivation of the normal maternal X-chromosome and a *de novo* rearrangement of the paternal chromosome (Cudry *et al.* 2000). Non-random inactivation of the normal X-chromosome has been found in karyotypically normal heterozygous females (Clarke *et al.* 1991; Sukegawa *et al.* 1997), including a girl whose identical carrier twin was unaffected (Winchester *et al.* 1992). A girl from a highly consanguineous family had a mild form of MPS II due to homozygosity for a novel mutation, L41P (Cudry *et al.* 2000).

MPS III (Sanfilippo syndrome)

Four different enzymic deficiencies occur in the Sanfillipo syndrome, but all patients are clinically very similar with severe CNS degeneration and mild somatic disease. There is, however, marked variation in severity within each disorder. MPS IIIA and B are more common than types C and D.

MPS IIIA (Sanfilippo A) (gene: MPS3A*; Chr. 17q25.3; enzyme: heparan N-sulphamidase; EC 3.10.1.1)*

Heparan *N*-sulphamidase hydrolyses the release of sulfate from the amino group of glucosamine at the non-reducing terminal of heparan sulfate. It possesses the structural and kinetic properties of a member of the sulfatase gene family and undergoes modification of an active-site cysteine to Cα-formylglycine. The native enzyme is a dimer of 115 kDa (Bielicki *et al.* 1998) and is transported to the lysosomes via the mannose-6-phosphate pathway. The sulphamidase gene, *MPS3A*, has been characterized (Scott *et al.* 1995*b*; Karageorgos *et al.* 1996), and over 60 different mutations have been reported, a majority of which are missense mutations (Weber *et al.* 2001). Some are in two highly conserved consensus sulfatase sequences, the active site (e.g. R74C and T79P) and residues 115–124 (G122R), and are predicted to destroy enzymic activity (Weber *et al.* 1997; Esposito *et al.* 2000). Certain mutations are found in high frequencies in particular populations—R245H (56.7%) in Dutch (Weber *et al.* 1997), R74C (56%) in Polish (Bunge *et al.* 1997), 1091delC in Spanish (Montfort *et al.* 1998), and S66W (33%) in Italian (Di Natale *et al.* 1998)—and are probably due to founder effects. Most genotypes are associated with the severe phenotype, but one patient, who is homozygous for I322S, has a milder phenotype despite no detectable heparan *N*-sulphamidase in leucocytes (Beesley *et al.* 2000). A correlation between the genotype/phenotype and amount of heparan *N*-sulphamidase protein and activity towards a natural substrate has been established (Perkins *et al.* 2001).

MPS IIIB (Sanfilippo B) (gene: NAGLU; Chr. 17q21; enzyme: α-N-acetylglucosaminidase; EC 3.2.1.50)

α-*N*-Acetylglucosaminidase catalyses the removal of terminal *N*-acetylglucosamine from heparan sulfate. The terminal *N*-acetylglucosamine is either a constituent of the original heparan sulfate or is generated by the action of acetyl-CoA-transferase on desulfated glucosamine during the catabolism of heparan sulfate. The biosynthesis of α-*N*-acetylglucosaminidase is typical of a lysosomal hydrolase, and it is active as a monomer or oligomer (von Figura *et al.* 1984). The cDNA predicts a protein of 743 amino acids with a signal peptide cleavage site at position 23 (Weber *et al.* 1996; Zhao *et al.* 1996). The two forms of human recombinant α-*N*-acetylglucosaminidase produced in CHO cells differed in their glycosylation but had similar kinetics and poor mannose-6-phosphate-mediated uptake (Weber *et al.* 2001). About 90 different mutations, mostly missense, have been found in the *NAGLU* gene, highlighting its genetic heterogeneity (Beesley *et al.* 1998; Schmidtchen *et al.* 1998; Zhao *et al.* 1998; Bunge *et al.* 1999; Weber *et al.* 1999; Tessitore *et al.* 2000; Weber *et al.* 2001). Most of the genotypes are associated with the severe phenotype even with two missense mutations. A few mutations have been found in more than one unrelated family, and there is some evidence of founder mutations in different populations. Three recurrent mutations, Y140C, R279X, and R626X, account for 36% of the mutations in the UK. Mutation of the CpG dinucleode of codon 643 gives rise to the recurrent mutations, R643H and R643C. The former is associated with a severe phenotype and the latter with an attenuated form, which is frequent in Dutch patients. Several other missense mutations have been implicated in the attenuated form, but very few expression studies have been carried out. However, the mutation, S534Y, which occurs in combination with an unknown allele in a patient with the attenuated disease does not give any activity on expression (Tessitore *et al.* 2000). It is assumed that the unidentified allele is responsible for the slower progression of the disease. Several polymorphisms have been described, but it is not known whether they modulate the effects of any mutations. The mutation or genetic factor responsible for the 'hyperactive allele' (Pericak-Vance *et al.* 1985) has not been isolated.

MPS IIIC (Sanfilippo C) (gene: MPS3C*; Chr.-; enzyme: acetyl-CoA (α-glucosamine-N-acetyltransferase); EC 2.3.1.3)*

α-Glucosamine-*N*-acetyltransferase is the only enzyme in lysosomal catabolism that is not a hydrolase. It catalyses the transfer of acetyl groups from acetyl-CoA generated in the cytosol across the lysosomal membrane to the desulfated 2-amino groups of glucosamine in the lumen of the lysosomes (Bame and Rome 1985). A deficiency of the transferase blocks the digestion of heparan sulfate because α-*N*-acetylglucosaminidase cannot release non-acetylated glucosamine (Klein *et al.* 1978). It is an integral lysosomal membrane protein, which accounts for its lack of complete purification (Freeman *et al.* 1983; Meikle *et al.* 1995). Although the enzyme has not been cloned, genetic studies have provided evidence for its mechanism of action (Bame and Rome 1986). The mutant enzyme in one group of patients has retained the ability to capture the acetyl group at neutral pH but cannot transfer it to glucosamine at an acidic pH in the lumen of the lysosome. In other patients, both steps in the reaction are defective.

MPS IIID (Sanfilippo D) (gene: MPS3D*; Chr. 12q14; enzyme: α-N-acetylglucosamine-6-sulfate sulfatase or N-acetylglucosamine-6-sulfatase; EC 3.1.6.14)*

N-Acetylglucosamine-6-sulfatase hydrolyses the release of sulfate from *N*-acetylglucosamine-6-sulfate in either the α-linkage or the β-linkage in heparan and keratan sulfates, respectively (Hopwood and Elliott 1983). As another member of the sulfatase family, it has the characteristic features of that family of enzymes. The cDNA predicts a protein of 552 amino acids (Robertson *et al.* 1988). The only reported mutation in the gene is a single base pair deletion (c1169delA), which is predicted to cause truncation of the protein and was found in a homozygous state in a child from a consainguineous marriage (Beesley *et al.* 2003). A model of human MPS IIID in Nubian goats has been studied extensively (Thompson *et al.* 1992).

MPS VII (Sly syndrome) (gene: GUSB*; Chr. 7q21-q22; enzyme: β-D-glucuronidase; EC 3.2.1.31)*

MPS VII results from a deficiency of β-D-glucuronidase, which catalyses the hydrolysis of the β-glucuronidic linkages in hyaluronan and in dermatan, heparan and chondroitin sulfates. The enzyme has been purified to homogeneity, and its three-dimensional structure has been obtained at 2.6 A resolution, allowing mutations to be related to the enzyme structure (Jain *et al.* 1996). It is synthesized as a precursor, which is processed in the usual manner to a mature subunit of 75 kDa, which aggregates to give an active tetramer. The cDNA encodes a protein of 651 amino acids (Oshima *et al.* 1987*b*). In addition to the functional gene (Miller *et al.* 1990), there are several pseudogenes (Shipley *et al.* 1993; Vervoort *et al.* 1993). About 40 mutations have been reported, mostly missense mutations, with some other small mutations but no large deletions or insertions. Patients with the severe neonatal MPS VII with hydrops fetalis have two null alleles (Vervoort *et al.* 1996), whereas patients with the intermediate or mild phenotype have combinations of missense mutations with nonsense mutations or frameshits (Shipley *et al.* 1993). One patient with a mild phenotype has a nonsense mutation and a 2 bp deletion. The deletion creates a strong 5′ cryptic splice site that leads to the inclusion of a new exon derived from an antisense Alu repeat in intron 8 and the skipping of exon 9 (IVS8 + 0.6kbdelTC) (Vervoort *et al.* 1998). These two events take place separately at low levels in normal mRNA. A pseudodeficiency allele D152N accelerates the turnover and decreases the secretion of β-D-glucuronidase from cells, probably through partial use of a newly created N-glycosylation sequon (Vervoort *et al.* 1995). A detailed analysis of the impact of over 20 point mutations on the tetrameric structure has been carried out using a bioinformatics approach (Durand *et al.* 2000). Some mutations are in active-site residues, H351Y, Y508C, and R382C/H. R382C has been shown to lower the enzymic activity and lead to a milder form of the disease (Tomatsu *et al.* 1991), whereas R382H gives a severe phenotype (Vervoort *et al.* 1996). Other mutations are postulated to affect the stability or formation of the tetramer (K606N, mild phenotype or R611W severe phenotype) or to affect the cavities in the core of the monomer (Y302C/S, severe phenotype). Expression studies of missense mutations are difficult to interpret, possibly because formation of tetramers might produce some activity (Wu *et al.* 1994).

Neuronal ceroid lipofuscinoses

The neuronal ceroid lipofuscinoses (NCLs or Batten disease) are collectively the most common neurodegenerative disorder of childhood. Although morphological and ultrastructural studies suggested that they were lysosomal storage diseases, analysis of the storage material did not reveal a simple enzymic defect—substrate storage product relationship. Neuronal ceroid lipofuscinosis is very heterogeneous clinically, and at least eight genetic forms of NCL, with different ages of onset, severity, and morphology of storage material, have been described (Hofmann and Peltonen 2001). It was the cloning of the *CLN1* gene and subsequent analysis of the encoded protein and the biochemical purification of the *CLN2* gene product that finally demonstrated that at least two forms of NCL are classic lysosomal enzyme deficiencies. The availability of specific enzyme assays and molecular diagnostic tests has enabled precise differential diagnosis of the major different childhood forms of NCL.

Infantile neuronal ceroid lipofuscinosis (INCL or NCL1) (gene: *CLN1*; Chr. 1p32; enzyme: palmitoyl protein thioesterase or PPT1; EC 3.1.2.22)

Mutations in the gene (*CLN1*) encoding the lysosomal enzyme, palmitoyl protein thioesterase or PPT1, are responsible for NCL1 (Vesa *et al.* 1995). A deficiency of PPT1 results in the accumulation in brain and other tissues of autofluorescent proteolipid storage material, which has the appearance of granular osmiophilic deposits (GROD) under the microscope (Elleder *et al.* 1999). There are elevated levels of sphingolipid activator proteins A and D in the storage material, but their relationship to the enzymic defect is not understood. Palmitoyl protein thioesterase-1 has a neutral pH-optimum *in vitro* but is a typical lysosomal enzyme and is transported to the lysosomes via the mannose-6-phosphate pathway (Verkryuse and Hofmann 1996). Palmitoyl protein thioesterase removes long-chain fatty acids, usually palmitate, from acylated cysteine residues at the carboxy terminal of membrane proteins. Such proteins are usually located at the inner surface of the plasma membrane and are transported to the lysosomes for degradation. Palmitoyl protein thioesterase-1 has been shown to remove palmitate from several neurospecific peptides (Cho *et al.* 2000) and may protect against apoptosis, which is increased in the brains of patients with NCL1 (Riikonen *et al.* 2000), indicating a special role in the CNS. The *CLN1* gene encodes a polypeptide of 306 amino acids with a 27-residue signal peptide and characteristic sequence motifs of thioesterases (Schriner *et al.* 1996). The bovine enzyme, which is 95% identical to the human enzyme, has been purified to homogeneity, and its crystal structure has been determined at 2.25 A resolution in the presence and absence of covalently bound palmitate (Bellizzi *et al.* 2000). It consists of a monomeric globular protein with α/β hydrolase fold, a catalytic triad composed of Ser115–His289–Asp233, and a deep hydrophobic groove along the surface in which the palmitate lies. A molecular explanation for the different phenotypes in INCL is possible by relating biochemical analysis of patients' cells and transient expression of mutations in mammalian cells to this structure (Mole *et al.* 1999; Bellizzi *et al.* 2000; Das *et al.* 2001). The crystal structure at the closely related human enzyme, PPT2, explains the difference in specify between PPT1 and PPT2 (Calero *et al.* 2003). No disease has yet been associated with a deficiency of PPT2. INCL is particularly prevalent in Finland (about 50% of cases), where the carrier frequency is 1 in 70. A single mutation, R122W, which accounts for 98% of the Finnish alleles, leads to a severe phenotype in the homozygous state. It completely abolishes PPT1 activity because the PPT1 protein is misfolded and rapidly degraded in the ER. Hydrogen bonding to Arg122 is important in maintaining the active conformation of PPT in the crystal structure. The loss of these bonds together with the introduction of the bulky and hydrophobic tryptophan residue disrupts the folding of the core and destabilizes the protein. Over 35 other mutations have been described. All patients with a combination of nonsense and frameshift alleles have a complete deficiency of PPT1 activity and the severe, early-onset, and rapidly progressive form of INCL. This is probably due to loss of the active-site His289, which is close to the C-terminal and would be deleted by most frameshift and nonsense mutations. The common R151X mutation resulted in no mRNA. Missense mutations may be associated with typical infantile NCL or with later onset phenotypes with GROD. Some missense mutations in the homozygous state or in combination with R122W or R151X lead to typical INCL with no residual activity in patient cells. They produce no activity after transient expression. Mutations associated with late infantile, e.g. Q177E, or juvenile, e.g. T75P, phenotypes had residual activity in patient cells or after transient expression. The former substitution disrupts the palmitate-binding site and increases K_m for palmitoylated substrates, whereas the latter does not alter the kinetic properties or mRNA level. The T75P substitution at the beginning of an a-helix altered the intracellular distribution of the enzyme in BHK cells but not in neurones (Salonen *et al.* 2001). This mutation probably originated in Scotland (Mitchison *et al.* 1998). A mutation in the methionine initiation codon (ATG→ATA) also leads to a late-onset phenotype. It was shown that this mutant was expressed to a significant extent in COS cells, suggesting that the ATA codon may be used *in vivo*. The age of onset of various symptoms varied markedly with genotype but closely resembled the pattern of onset of the symptoms in other NCLs, suggesting that the stage of development rather than the underlying defect is the main determinant of phenotype (Hofmann *et al.* 2001).

Late infantile neuronal ceroid lipofuscinosis (LINCL or NCL2) (gene: *CLN2*; Chr. 11p15; enzyme: tripeptidyl peptidase TPP-1; EC 1)

The underlying defect in classic late infantile NCL was initially identified biochemically as a deficiency of a typical lysosomal hydrolase, tripeptidyl peptidase 1 (TPP-1) (Sleat *et al.* 1997). The gene for the enzyme coincided with the site of the *CLN2* gene identified by linkage studies (Sharp *et al.* 1997). Tripeptidyl peptidase-1 is the human homologue of the TPP that had been purified from rat spleen (Vines and Warburton, 1998). Tripeptidyl peptidase-1 has significant sequence homology to two bacterial pepstatin-insensitive carboxyl peptidases and was originally thought to be the first human member of this sub-group of aspartyl proteases. Recently, the human recombinant enzyme has been shown to be a serine protease, which can be irreversibly inhibited by the serine protease inhibitor, di-isopropyl fluorophosphate (Lin *et al.* 2001). It is synthesized as an inactive precursor, which, after losing the signal peptide, can undergo proteolytic autoactivation at an acidic pH. Tripeptidyl peptidase 1 has been shown to have intrinsic endopeptidase as well as TPP activity (Ezaki *et al.* 2000*a*) and it can remove tripeptides from the N-terminus of peptides of up to 4.5–6 kDa with an extended, unstructured N-terminal domain (Bernardini and Warburton, 2001). The relationship of this substrate specificity to the characteristic curvilinear storage bodies containing subunit c of mitochondrial ATP synthase is unclear. Co-incubation of extracts of normal and CLN2 fibroblasts or addition of recombinant TPP-1 results in the breakdown of the subunit c in lysosomes from CLN2 fibroblasts, whereas inhibition of TPP-1 prevents the breakdown of subunit c (Ezaki *et al.* 2000*b*). This suggests that TPP-1 is involved in the lysosomal catabolism of subunit c. Over 30 mutations and 14 polymorphisms have been identified in the *CLN2* gene (Mole *et al.* 1999; Sleat *et al.* 1999; Wisniewski *et al.* 2001). Three mutations, R208X and IVS5–1G→A/C account for approximately 60% of the mutant alleles. Homozygotes or compound heterozygotes for these mutations had negligible TPP-1 activity in brain or fibroblasts and had the classic CLN2 phenotype. Very low levels of TPP-1 activity were also found in patients who were heterozygous or homozygous for missense mutations, indicating that these amino acid substitutions must be in functional regions of the enzyme structure. A patient with the genotype R447H/IVS5–1G→C had a small amount of TPP-1 activity in the lysosomal fraction of fibroblasts and a protracted form of CLN2. A full understanding of the genotype/phenotype correlation must await the elucidation of the three-dimensional structure of TPP-1. Neuronal ceroid lipofuscinosis illustrates very powerfully the value of biochemical and molecular genetic tests for the precise diagnosis of closely related disorders with overlapping ages of onset and clinical presentation.

Cathepsin D

Cathepsin D is deficient in an ovine form of neuronal ceroid lipofuscinosis (Tyynela *et al.* 2000), and a knockout mouse for cathepsin D has lysosomal storage of subunit c and ceroid lipofuscin in CNS neurones (Koike *et al.* 2000). A deficiency of cathepsin D has not been found in any of the human variants of NCL.

Summary

The rate of accumulation of storage products will depend upon the intralysosomal level of functional enzymic activity in cells that normally degrade the substrate of the defective enzyme. In those lysosomal storage diseases resulting directly from a deficiency of a lysosomal enzyme, the main factor determining the extent of the deficiency is the nature of the mutations in the structural gene for that enzyme. Mutations that prevent transcription or translation or lead to a severely truncated protein will produce null alleles. In rare cases, the mutation affects the regulation of expression and leads to overproduction of the enzyme. Most missense mutations affect the stability, folding, or intracellular transport of the enzyme, and a direct effect on a functional group in the catalytic site of the enzyme is relatively uncommon. Therefore, residual activity may have the same physicochemical properties and kinetics as the normal enzyme or it may be different. Polymorphisms in the gene may modify the effect of a mutation. Other genetic factors clearly affect the consequences of this decreased activity in specific cells. They include the level of ancillary catalytic proteins and proteins involved in the processing and transport of the enzyme, disruption of contiguous genes, and the influence of other genes on the expression of the affected gene. At the biochemical level, the existence of alternative pathways, genetic or environmental control of the substrate load presented to the cell, and the presence of stabilizing or inhibitory low-molecular weight molecules will affect the balance between catabolism and storage. Therefore, the phenotype resulting from mutations will depend upon the genetic makeup and environment of the individual patient.

References

Abrahamov, A., Elstein, D., Gross-Tsur, V. *et al.* (1995). Gaucher's disease varaint characterised by progressive calcification of heart valves and unique genotype. *Lancet*, **346**, 1000–3.

Achyuthan, K. E. and Achyuthan, A. M. (2001). Comparative enzymology, biochemistry and pathophysiology of human exo-α-sialidases (neuraminidases). *Comp Biochem Physiol B*, **129**, 29–64.

Aerts, J. M. F. G., Schram, A. W., Strijland, A. *et al.* (1988). Glucocerebrosidase, a lysosomal enzyme that does not undergo oligosaccharide phosphorylation. *Biochim Biophys Acta*, **964**, 303–8.

Ahn, V. E., Faull, K. F., Whitelegge, J. P., Fluhartz, A. L. and Prive, G. G. (2003). Crystal structure of saposin B reveals a dimeric shell for lipid binding. *PNAS*, **100**, 38–43.

Akagi, M., Inui, K., Nishigaki, T. *et al.* (1999). Mutation analysis of a Japanese patient with fucosidosis. *J Hum Genet*, **44**, 323–6.

Akerman, B. R., Natowicz, M. R., Kaback, M. M., Loyer, M., Campeau, E. and Gravel, R. A. (1997). Novel mutations and DNA-based screening in non-Jewish carriers of Tay–Sachs disease. *Am J Hum Genet*, **60**, 1099–106.

Akli, S., Chelly, J., Mezard, C., Gandy, S., Kahn, A. and Poenaru, L. (1990). A 'G' to 'A' mutation at position –1 of a 5' splice sire in a late infantile form of Tay–Sachs diease. *J Biol Chem*, **265**, 7324–30.

Akli, S., Chelly, J., Lacorte, J. M., Poenaru, L. and Kahn, A. (1991). Seven novel Tay–Sachs mutations detected by chemical mismatch cleavage of PCR-amplified cDNA fragments. *Genomics*, **11**, 124–34.

Al Daher, S., De Gasperi, R., Daniel, P., Hall, N., Warren, C. D. and Winchester, B. G. (1991). The substrate specificity of human lysosomal α-D-mannosidase in relation to genetic α-mannosidosis. *Biochem J*, **277**, 743–51.

Alif, N., Hess, K., Straczek, J. *et al.* (1999). Mucopolysaccharidosis type I: characterization of a common mutation that cause Hurler syndrome in Moroccan subjects. *Ann Hum Genet*, **63**, 9–16.

Alkhayat, A. H., Kraemer, S. A., Leipprandt, J. R., Macek, M., Kleijer, W. J. and Friderici, K. H. (1998). Human β-mannosidase cDNA characterization and first identification of a mutation associated with human β-mannosidosis. *Hum Mol Genet*, **7**, 75–83.

Aronovich, E. L., Pan, D. and Whitley, C. B. (1996). Molecular genetic defect underlying alpha-L-iduronidase pseudodeficiency. *Am J Hum Genet*, **58**, 75–85.

Aronson, N. N. Jr (1999). Aspartylglucosaminuria: biochemistry and molecular biology. *Biochem Biophys Acta*, **1455**, 139–54.

Asfaw, B., Ledvinova, J., Dobrovolny, R. *et al.* (2002). Defects in degradation of blood group A and B glycosphingolipids in Schindler and Fabry diseases. *J Lipid Res*, **43**, 1096–104.

Ashton-Prolla, P., Tong, B., Shabbeer, J., Astrin, K. H., Eng, C. M. and Desnick, R. J. (2000). Fabry disease: twenty two novel mutations in the α-galactosidase A gene and genotype/pheneotype correlations in severely and mildly affected hemizygotes and heterozygotes. *J Invest Med*, **48**, 227–35.

Aula, P., Jalanko, A. and Peltonen, L. (2001). Aspartylglucosaminuria. In *The metabolic and molecular bases of inherited disease* (Scriver, C. R., Beaudet, A. L., Sly, W. S., Valle, D., Childs, B., Kinzler, K. W. and Vogelstein, B., ed.), 8th edn, pp. 3535–50. New York: McGraw-Hill.

Bakker, H. D., de Sonnaville, M. L., Vreken, P. *et al.* (2001). Human alpha-*N*-acetylgalactosaminidase (alpha-NAGA) deficiency: no association with neuroaxonal dystrophy? *Eur J Hum Genet*, **9**, 91–6.

Baldwin, E. T., Bhat, T. N., Gulnik, S. *et al.* (1993). Crystal structures of native and inhibited forms of human cathepsin D: implications for lysosomal targeting and drug design. *Proc Natl Acad Sci USA*, **90**, 6796–800.

Bame, K. J. and Rome, L. H. (1985). Acetyl coenzyme A: alpha-glucosaminide *N*-acetyltransferase. Evidence for a transmembrane acetylation mechanism. *J Biol Chem*, **260**, 11293–9.

Bame, K. J. and Rome, L. H. (1986). Genetic evidence for a transmembrane acetylation by lysosomes. *Science* 233, 1087-X.

Barker, C., Dell, A., Rogers, M., Alhadeff, J. and Winchester, B. G. (1988). Canine α–L–fucosidase in relation to the enzymic defect and storage products in canine fucosidosis. *Biochem J*, **254**, 861–8.

Barth, M. L., Fensom, A. and Harris, A. (1993). Prevalence of common mutations in the arylsulfatase gene in metachromatic leukodystriophy patients diagnosed in Britain. *Hum Genet*, **91**, 73–7.

Bayleran, J., Hechtman, P., Kolodny, E. and Kaback, M. M. (1987). Tay–Sachs disease with hexosaminidase A characterization of the defective enzyme in two patients. *Am J Hum Genet*, **41**, 532–48.

Beesley, C. E., Burke, D., Jackson, M., Vellodi, A., Winchester, B. G. and Young, E. P. (2003). Sanfilippo syndrome type D: identification of the first mutation in the *N*-acetylglucosamine-6-sulfatase gene.

Beesley, C. E., Meaney, C. A., Greenland, G. *et al.* (2001). Mutational analysis of 85 mucopolysaccharidosis type I families: frequency of known mutations, identification of 17 novel mutations and *in vitro* expression of missense mutations. *J Hum Genet*, **109**, 503–11.

Beesley, C. E., Young, E. P., Vellodi, A. and Winchester, B. G. (1998). Identification of 12 novel mutations in the alpha-*N*-acetylglucosaminidase gene in 14 patients with Sanfilippo syndrome type B (mucopolysaccharidosis type IIIB). *J Med Genet*, **35**, 910–4.

Beesley, C. E., Young, E. P., Vellodi, A. and Winchester, B. G. (2000). Mutational analysis of Sanfilippo syndrome type A (MPS IIIA): identification of 13 novel mutations. *J Med Genet*, **37**, 704–7.

Beier, E. M., Kopishinskaia, S. V., Ploos van Amstel, J. K. and Tsvetkova, I. V. (1999). Mutation of the α-galactosidase gene in two unusual variations of Fabry's disease. *Vopr Med Khim*, **45**, 346–9.

Bellizzi, J. J. III, Widom, J., Kemp, C. *et al.* (2000). The crystal structure of palmitoyl protein thioesterase 1 and the molecular basis of infantile neuronal ceroid lipofuscinosis. *Proc Natl Acad Sci USA*, **97**, 4573–8.

Berg, T., Riise, H. M., Hansen, G. M. *et al.* (1999). Spectrum of mutations in alpha-mannosidosis. *Am J Hum Genet*, **64**, 77–88.

Berg, T., King, B., Meikle, P. J., Nilssen, O., Tollersrud, O. K. and Hopwood, J. J. (2001). Purification and characterization of recombinant human lysosomal α-mannosidase. *Mol Genet Metab*, **73**, 18–29.

Berger, A., Rosenthal, D. and Spiegel, S. (1995). Sphingosylphosphocholine, a signalling molecule which accumulates in Niemann–Pick disease type A, stimulates DNA-binding activity of the transcription activator protein AP-1. *Proc Natl Acad Sci USA*, **92**, 5885–9.

Berger, J., Loschl, B., Bernheimer, H. *et al.* (1997). Occurrence, distribution and phenotype of arylsulfatase A mutations in patients with metachromatic leukodystrophy. *Am J Med Genet*, **69**, 335–40.

Berg-Fussman, A., Grace, M. E., Ioannou, Y. and Grabowski, G. A. (1993). Human β-glucosidase: Nglycosylation site occupancy and the effect of glycosylation on enzymatic activity. *J Biol Chem*, **268**, 14861–6.

Bernardini, F. and Warburton, M. J. (2001). The substrate range of tripetidyl-peptidase I. *Eur J Paed Neurol*, **5**, 69–72.

Beutler, E. and Grabowski, G. A. (2001). Gaucher disease. In In *The metabolic and molecular bases of inherited disease* (Scriver, C. R., Beaudet, A. L., Sly, W. S., Valle, D., Childs, B., Kinzler, K. W. and Vogelstein, B., ed.), 8th edn, pp. 3733–74. New York: McGraw-Hill.

Bielicki, J., Hopwood, J. J., Melville, E. L. and Anson, D. S. (1998). Recombinant human sulphamidase: expression, amplification, purification and characterization. *Biochem J*, **1**, 145–50.

Birot, A. M., Delobel, B., Gronnier, P., Bonnet, V., Maire, I. and Bozon, D. (1996*a*). A 5-megabase familial deletion removes the IDS and FMR-1 genes in a male Hunter patient. *Hum Mutat*, **7**, 266–8.

Birot, A. M., Bouton, O., Froissart, R., Maire, I. and Bozon, D. (1996*b*). IDS gene-pseudogene exchange responsible for an intragenic deletion in a Hunter patient. *Hum Mutat*, **8**, 44–50.

Bishop, D. F., Calhoun, D. H., Bernstein, H. S., Hantzopoulos, P., Quinn, M. and Desnick, R. J. (1986). Human alpha-galactosidase A: nucleotide sequence of a cDNA clone encoding the mature enzyme. *Proc Nat Acad Sci USA*, **83**, 4859–63.

Boles, D. J. and Proia, R. L. (1995). The molecular basis of HEXA mRNA deficiency caused by the most common Tay–Sachs disease mutation. *Am J Hum Genet*, **56**, 716–24.

Bolhuis, P. A., Ponne, N. J., Bikker, H., Baas, F. and Vianney de Jong, J. M. (1993). Molecular basis of adult form of Sandhoff disease: substitution of glutamine for arginine at position 505 of the β-chain of β-hexosaminidase results in a labile enzyme. *Biochim Biophys Acta*, **1182**, 142–6.

Bond, C. S., Clements, P. R., Ashby, S. J. *et al.* (1997). Structure of a human lysosomal sulfatase. *Structure*, **5**, 277–89.

Bondeson, M.-L., Dahl, N., Malmgren, H. *et al.* (1995). Inversion of the IDS gene resulting from recombination with IDS-related sequences is a common cause of the Hunter syndrome. *Hum Mol Genet*, **4**, 615–21.

Bonten, E., van der Spoel, A. V., Fornerod, M. Grosveld, G. and d'Azzo S. (1996). Characterization of human lysosomal neuraminidase defines the molecular basis of the metabolic storage disorder sialidosis. *Genes Dev*, **10**, 3156–68.

Bonten, E. J., Arts, W. F., Beck, M. *et al.* (2000). Novel mutations in lysosomal neuraminidase identify functional domains and determine clinical severity in sialidosis. *Hum Mol Genet*, **9**, 2715–25.

Broadhead, D. M., Kirk, J. M., Burt, A. J., Gupta, V., Ellis, P. M. and Besley, G. T. N. (1986). Full expression of Hunter's disease in a female with an X-chromosome deletion leading to non-random inactivation. *Clin Genet*, **30**, 392–8.

Brooks, D. A., Fabrega, S., Hein, L. K. *et al.* (2001). Glycosidase active site mutations in human α-L-iduronidase. *Glycobiology*, **11**, 741–50.

von Bulow, R., Schmidt, B., Dierks, T. *et al.* (2002). Defective oligomerization of arylsulfatase A as a cause of its instability in lysosomes and metachromatic leukodystrophy. *J Biol Chem*, **277**, 9455–61.

Bunge, S., Kleijer, W. J., Steglich, C. *et al.* (1994). Mucopolysaccharidosis type I: identification of 8 novel mutations and determination of the frequency of the two common alpha-L-iduronidase mutations (W402X and Q70X) among European patients. *Hum Mol Genet*, **3**, 861–6.

Bunge, S., Kleijer, W. J., Steglich, C., Beck, M., Schwinger, E. and Gal, A. (1995). Mucopolysaccharidosis type I: identification of 13 novel mutations of the α-L-iduronidase gene. *Hum Mutat*, **6**, 91–4.

Bunge, S., Ince, H., Steglich, C. *et al.* (1997). Identification of 16 sulfamidase gene mutations including the common R74C in patients with mucopolysaccharidosis type IIIA (Sanfilippo A). *Hum Mutat*, **10**, 479–85.

Bunge, S., Clements, P. R., Byers, S., Kleijer, W. J., Brooks, D. and Hopwood, J. J. (1998). Genotype-phenotype correlations in mucopolysaccharidosis type I using enzyme kinetics, immuunoquantification and in vtiro turnover studies. *Biochim Biophys Acta*, **1407**, 249–56.

Bunge, S., Knigge, A., Steglich, C., Kleijer, W. J., van Diggelen, O. P., Beck, M. and Gal, A. (1999). Mucopolysaccharidosis type IIIB (Sanfilippo B): identification of 18 novel alpha-*N*-acetylglucosaminidase gene mutations. *J Med Genet*, **36**, 28–31.

Calero, G., Gupta, P., Nonato, M.C., *et al.* (2003). The crystal structure of palmitoyl protein thioesterase 2 reveals the basis for the divergent substrate specificities of the two lysosomal thioesterases (PPT1 and PPT2). *J. Biol Chem* (In Press).

Callahan, J. W. (1999). Molecular basis of GM1 gangliosidosis and Morquio disease, type B. Structure-function studies of lysosomal β-galactosidase and the non-lysosomal β-galactosidase-like protein. *Biochim Biophys Acta*, **1455**, 85–103.

Callebaut, I., Labesse, G., Durand, P. *et al.* (1997). Deciphering protein sequence information through hydrophobic cluster analysis (HCA): current status and perspectives. *Cellular Mol Life Sci*, **53**, 621–45.

Cao, Z., Petroulakis, E., Salo, T. and Triggs-Raine, B. (1997). Benign *HEXA* mutations, C739T (R247W) and C745T (R249W), cause β-hexosaminidase A pseudodeficiency by reducing the α-subunit protein levels. *J Biol Chem*, **272**, 14975–82.

Carritt, B. and Welch, H. N. (1987). An α-fucosidase pseudogene on human chromosome 2. *Hum Genet*, **2**, 248–50.

Cenci di Bello, I., Dorling, P. and Winchester, B. G. (1983). The storage products in genetic and swainsonine-induced human mannosidosis. *Biochem J*, **215**, 639–96.

Chakraborty, S., Rafi, M. A. and Wenger, D. A. (1994). Mutations in the lysosomal β-galactosidase that cause the adult form of GM1 gangliosidosis. *Am J Hum Genet*, **54**, 1004–13.

Chen, Y. Q., Rafi, M. A., de Gala, G. and Wenger, D. A. (1993). Cloning and expression of cDNA encoding human galactocerebrosidase, the enzyme deficient in globoid cell leukodystrophy. *Hum Mol Genet*, **2**, 1841–5.

Cho, S., Dawson, P. E. and Dawson, G. (2000). In vitro depalmitoylation of neurospecific peptides: implication for infantile neuronal croid lipofuscinosis. *J Neurosci Res*, **59**, 32–8.

Christomanou, H., Aignesberger, A. and Linke, R. P. (1986). Immunochemical characterization of two activator proteins stimulating enzyme sphingomyelin degradation in vitro. Absence of one of them in a human Gaucher disease variant. *H Seyler's J Biol Chem*, **367**, 879–90.

Clarke, J. T. R., Greer, W. L., Strasberg, P. M., Pearce, R. D., Skomorowski, M. A. and Ray, P. N. (1991). Hunter disease (mucopolysaccharidosis type II) associated with unbalanced inactivation of the X chromosomes in a karyotypically normal girl. *Am J Hum Genet*, **49**, 289–97.

Conzelmann, E. and Sandhoff, K. (1983). Partial enzyme deficiencies: residualactivities and and the development of neurological disorders. *Dev Neurosci*, **6**, 58–71.

Cooper, A., Sardharwalla, I. B. and Roberts, M. M. (1986). Human β-mannosidase deficiency. *N Engl J Med*, **315**, 1231.

Cormand, B., Diaz, A., Grinberg, D., Chabas, A. and Viageliu, L. (2000). A new gene-pseudogene fusion allele due to a recombination in intron 2 of the glucocerebrosidase gene causes Gaucher disease. *Blood Cell Mol Dis*, **26**, 409–16.

Coulombe, R., Grochulski, P., Sivaraman, J., Menard, R., Mort, J. S. and Cygler, M. (1996). Structure of human procathepsin L reveals the molecular basis of inhibition by the prosegment. *EMBO J*, **15**, 5492–503.

Cox, T. M. and Schofield, J. P. (1997). Gaucher disease: clinical features and natural history. *Bailliere's Clin Haematol*, **10**, 657–89.

Cudry, S., Tigaud, I., Froissart, R., Bonnet, V., Maire, I. and Bozon, D. (2000). MPS II in females: molecular basis of two different cases. *J Med Genet*, **37**, E29.

D'Azzo, A., Proia, R. L., Kolodny, E. H., Kaback, M. M. and Neufeld, E. F. (1984). Faulty association of the α- and β-subunits in some forms of β-hexosaminidase A deficiency. *J Biol Chem*, **259**, 11070–4.

Daniel, P. F., Evans, J. E., De Gasperi, R., Winchester, B. and Warren, C. D. (1992). A human lysosomal α (1–6)-mannosidase active on the branched trimannosyl core of complex glycans. *Glycobiology*, **2**, 327–36.

Daniel, P. E., Winchester, B. and Warren, C. D. (1994). Mammalian α-mannosidases – multiple forms but a common purpose. *Glycobiology*, **4**, 551–66.

Das, A. K., Lu, J.-Y. and Hofmann, S. L. (2001). Biochemical analysis of mutations in palmitoyl-proteinthioesterase causing infantile and late-onset forms of neuronal ceroid lipofuscinosis. *Hum Mol Genet*, **10**, 1431–9.

Desnick, R. J. and Schindler, D. (2001). α-*N*-Acetylgalactosaminidase deficiency: Schindler disease. In *The metabolic and molecular bases of inherited disease* (Scriver, C. R., Beaudet, A. L., Sly, W. S., Valle, D., Childs, B., Kinzler, K. W. and Vogelstein, B., ed.), 8th edn, pp. 3483–505. New York: McGraw-Hill.

Desnick, R. J., Ioannou, Y. A. and Eng, C. M. (2001). α-Galactosidase: Fabry disease deficiency. In *The metabolic and molecular bases of inherited disease* (Scriver, C. R., Beaudet, A. L., Sly, W. S., Valle, D., Childs, B., Kinzler, K. W. and Vogelstein, B., ed.), 8th edn, pp. 3733–74. New York: McGraw-Hill.

Di Natale, P., Balzano, N., Esposito, S. and Villani, G. R. (1998). Identification of molecular defects in Italian Sanfilippo A patients including 13 novel mutations. *Hum Mutat*, **11**, 313–20.

Di Natale, P., Vanacore, B., Daniele, A. and Esposito, S. (2001). *Biochem Biophys Res Commun*, **280**, 1251–7.

van Diggelen, O. P., Schindler, D., Kleijer, W. J. *et al.* (1987). Lysosomal α-*N*-acetylgalactosaminidase deficiency: a new inherited metabolic disease. *Lancet*, **2**, 804.

Dorland, L., Duran, M., Hoefnagels, F. E. T. *et al.* (1988). β-Mannosidosis in two brothers with hearing loss. *J Inher Metab Dis*, **11**, 255–8.

Dubois, G., Turpin, J. C. and Baumann, N. (1975). Absence of ASA activity in the healthy father of a patient with metachromatic leukodystrophy. *N Engl J Med*, **293**, 302.

Durand, P., Lehn, P., Callebaut, I., Fabrega, S., Henrissat, B. and Mornon, J.-P. (1997). Active-site motifs of lysosomal glycoside hydrolases: invariant feature of clan GH-A glycosyl hydrolases deduced from hydrophobic cluster analysis. *Glycobiology*, **7**, 277–84.

Durand, P., Fabrega, S., Henrissat, B., Mornon, J.-P. and Lehn, P. (2000). Structural features of normal and mutant lysosomal glycoside hydrolases deduced from bioinfomatics analysis. *Hum Mol Genet*, **9**, 967–77.

Dvir, H., Harel, M., McCarthy, A. A. *et al.* (2003). X-ray structure of human acid-β-glucosidase, the defective enzyme in Gaucher disease. *EMBO reports*, **4**, 704–9.

Eiberg, H., Mohr, J. and Nielsen, L. S. (1984). Linkage of plasma α-L-fucosidase (FUCA2) and the plasminogen (PLG) system. *Clin Genet*, **26**, 23–9.

Elleder, M., Lake, B. D., Goebel, H. H., Rapola, J., Haltia, M. and Carpenter, S. (1999). Definitions of the ultrastructural patterns found in NCL. In *The Neuronal Ceroid Lipofuscinoses (Batten Disease)* (Goebel, H. H. and Mole, S. E. and Lake, B. D., ed.), pp. 5–15. Amsterdam: IOS Press.

Elstein, D., Abrahamov, A., Hadas-Halpern, I. and Zimran, A. (2001). Gaucher's disease. *Lancet*, **358**, 324–7.

Erickson, A. H., Ginns, E. I. and Barranger, J. A. (1985). Biosnthesis of the lysosomal enzyme glucocerebrosidase. *J Biol Chem.*, **260**, 14319–24.

Esposito, S., Balzano, N., Daniele, A. *et al.* (2000). Heparan *N*-sulfatase gene: two novel mutations and transient expression of 15 defects. *Biochim Biophys Acta*, **1501**, 1–11.

Eto, Y., Kawame, H., Hasegawa, Y., Ohashi, T., Ida, H. and Tohoro, T. (1993). Molecular characteristics in Japanese patients with lipidosis: Novel mutations in metachromatic leukodystrophy and Gaucher disease. *Mol Cell Biochem*, **119**, 179–84.

Ezaki, J., Takeda-Ezaki, M., Oda, K. and Kominani, E. (2000*a*). Characterization of endopeptidase activity of tripeptidyl peptidase-I/CLN2 protein which is deficient in classical late infantile neuronal ceroid lipofuscinosis. *Biochem Biophys Res Comm*, **268**, 904–8.

Ezaki, J., Takeda-Ezaki, M. and Kominani, E. (2000*b*). Tripeptidyl peptidase I, the late infantile neuronal ceroid lipofuscinosis gene product, initiates the lysosomal degradation of subunit c of ATP synthase. *J Biochem*, **128**, 509–16.

Ferlinz, K., Hurwitz, R., Weiler, M., Suzuki, K., Sandhoff, K. and Vanier, M. T. (1995). Molecular analysis of the acid sphingomyelinase deficiency in a family with an intermediate form of Niemann–Pick disease. *Am J Hum Genet*, **56**, 1343–9.

Fernandes, M. J., Hechtman, P., Boulay, B. and Kaplan, F. (1997). A chronic GM2-gangliosidosis variant with a *HEXA* splicing defect: Quantitation of *HEXA* mRNAs in normal and mutant fibroblasts. *Eur J Hum Genet*, **5**, 129–36.

Fitzmaurice, T. F., Desnick, R. J. and Bishop, D. F. (1997). Human a-galactosidase A: high plasma activity expressed by the –30G?A allele. *J Inherit Metab Dis*, **20**, 643–57.

Fleming, C. J., Sinclair, D. U., White, E. J., Winchester, B., Whiteford, M. L. and Connor, J. M. (1998). A fucosidosis patient with relative longevity and a missense mutation in exon 7 of the α-fucosidase gene. *J Inherit Metab Dis*, **21**, 688–9.

Flomen, R. H., Green, E. P., Green, P. M., Bentley, D. R. and Giannelli, F. (1993). Determination of the organisation of coding sequences within the iduronate sulfate sulfatase (IDS) gene. *Hum Mol Genet*, **2**, 5–10.

Freeman, C., Clements, P. P. and Hopwood, J. J. (1983). Acetyl CoA: alpha-glucosaminide *N*-acetyltransferase. Partial purification from human liver. B*iochem Int* 6, 663-X.

Froissart, R., Maire, I., Millat, G. *et al.* (1998). Identification of iduronate sulfatase gene alterations in 70 unrelated Hunter patients. *Clin Genet*, **53**, 362–8.

Frost, G. I., Csoka, T. B., Wong, T. and Stern, R. (1997). Purification, cloning and expression of human plasma hyaluronidase. *Biochem Biophys Res Commun*, **236**, 10–5.

Frostad Riise, H. M., Hansen, G. M., Tollersrud, O. K. and Nilssen, O. (1999). Characterization of a novel alpha-mannosidosis-causing mutation and its use in leukocyte genotyping after bone marrow transplantation. *Hum Genet*, **104**, 106–7.

Fujimaru, M., Tanaka, A., Choeh, K., Wakamatsu, N., Sakuraba, H. and Isshki, G. (1998). Two mutations remote from an exon/intron junction in the β-hexosaminidase β-subunit gene affect-3′ splice site selection and cause Sandhoff disease. *Hum Genet*, **103**, 462–9.

Fujishima, A., Imai, Y., Nomura, T., Fujisawa, Y., Yamamoto, Y. and Sugawara, T. (1997). The crystal structure of human cathepsin L complexed with E-64. *FEBS Letters*, **407**, 47–50.

Garman, S. C., Hannick, L., Zhu, A. and Garboczi, D. N. (2002*a*). The 1.9 A structure of α-*N*-acetylgalactosaminidase: molecular basis of glycosidase deficiency diseases. *Structure (Camb)*, **10**, 425–34.

Garman, S. C. and Garboczi, D. N. (2002*b*). Structural basis of Fabry disease. *Molec. Genet Metab*, **7**, 3–11.

Gatti, R., Di Natale, P., Villani, G. R. D. *et al.* (1997). Mutations among Italian mucopolysaccharidosis type I patients. *J Inher Metab Dis*, **20**, 803–6.

Gelb, B. D., Shi, G. P., Chapman, H. A. and Desnick, R. J. (1996). Pycnodysostosis, a lysosomal disease caused by cathepsin K deficiency. *Science*, **273**, 1236–8.

Gieselmann, V. (1995). Lysosomal storage diseases. *Biochim Biophys Acta*, **1270**, 103–36.

Gieselmann, V., Polten, A., Kreysing, J. and von Figura, K. (1989). Arylsulphatse A pseudodeficiency: loss of a polyadenylation signal and *N*-glycosylation site. *Proc Natl Acad Sci USA*, **86**, 9436–40.

Gort, L., Chabas, A. and Coll, M. J. (1997). Analysis of five mutations in 20 mucopolysaccharidosis type I patients: prevalence of the W402X mutation. *Hum Mutat*, **11**, 332–3.

Gotoda, Y., Wakamatsu, N., Kawai, H., Nishida, Y. and Matsumoto, T. (1998). Missense and nonsense mutations in the lysosomal alpha-mannosidse gene (MANB) in severe and mild forms of alpha-mannosidosis. *Am J Hum Genet*, **63**, 1015–29.

Grabowski, G. A. and Horowitz, M. (1997). Gaucher's disease: molecular, genetic and enzymological aspects. *Bailliere's Clin Haematol*, **10**, 635–56.

Gravel, R. A., Kaback, M. M., Proia, R. L., Sandhoff, K., Suzuki, K. and Suzuki, K. (2001). The GM2 gangliosidoses. In *The metabolic and molecular bases of inherited disease* (Scriver, C. R., Beaudet, A. L., Sly, W. S., Valle, D., Childs, B., Kinzler, K. W. and Vogelstein, B., ed.), 8th edn, pp. 3827–76. New York: McGraw-Hill.

Guadalupi, R., Bernard, M., Orlacchio, A., Foglietti, M. J. and Emiliani, C. (1996). Purification and properties of human urinary β-D-mannosidase. *Biochem Biophys Acta*, **1293**, 9–16.

Guncar, G., Klemencic, I., Turk, B., Turk, V., Karaoglanovic-Carmona, A., Juliano, L. and Turk, D. (2000). Crystal structure of cathepsin X: a flip-flop of the ring of His23 allows carboxy-monopeptidase and carboxy-dipeptidase activity of the protease. *Structure-Fold-Des*, **8**, 305–13.

Handa, Y., Yotsumoto, S., Isobe, E. *et al.* (2000). A case of symptomatic heterozygous female Fabry disease without detectable mutation in the alpha-galactosidase gene. *Dermatology*, **200**, 262–5.

Harzer, K., Knoblich, R., Rolfs, A., Bauer, P. and Eggers, J. (2002). Residual galactosylsphingosine (psychosine) beta-galactosidase activities and associated GALC mutations in late and very late onset Krabbe disease. *Clin Chim Acta*, **317**, 77–84.

Heikinheimo, P., Helland, R., Leiros, H-K. S. *et al.* (2003). The structure of bovine lysosomal α-mannosidase suggests a novel mechanism for low pH-activation. *J Mol Biol*, **327**, 631–44.

Hepbildikler, S. T., Sandhoff, R., Kolzer, M., Proia, R. L. and Sandhoff, K. (2002). Physiological substrates for human β-hexosamindase S. *J Biol Chem*, **277**, 2562–72.

Hess, B., Kafert, S., Heinisch, U., Wenger, D. A., Zlotogora, J. and Gieselmann, V. (1996). Characterization of two arylsulfatase A missense mutations D335V and T274M causing late infantile metachromatic leukodystrophy. *Hum Mutat*, **7**, 311–7.

Hof, P., Mayr, L., Huber, R. *et al.* (1996). The 1.8 A crystal structure of human cathepsin G in complex with Suc-Val-Pro-Phe-(OPh) 2; a Janus-faced proteinase with two opposite specificities. *EMBO J*, **15**, 5481–91.

Hofmann, S. L. and Peltonen, L. (2001). The neuronal ceroid lipofuscinosis. In *The metabolic and molecular bases of inherited disease* (Scriver, C. R., Beaudet, A. L., Sly, W. S., Valle, D., Childs, B., Kinzler, K. W. and Vogelstein, B., ed.), 8th edn, pp. 3877–94. New York: McGraw-Hill.

Hofmann, S. L., Das, A. K., Lu, J.-Y., Wisniewski, K. E. and Gupta, P. (2001). Infantile neuronal ceroid lipofuscinosis: no longer just a 'Finnish' disease. *Eur J Paed*, **5**, 47–51.

Hong, C. M., Ohashi, T., Yu X. J., Weiler, S. and Barranger, J. A. (1990). Sequence of two alleles responsible for Gaucher disease. *DNA Cell Biol*, **9**, 223–41.

Hopwood, J. J. and Ballabio, A. (2001). Multiple sulfatase deficiency and the nature of the sulfatase family. The neuronal ceroid lipofuscinosis. In *The metabolic and molecular bases of inherited disease* (Scriver, C. R., Beaudet, A. L., Sly, W. S., Valle, D., Childs, B., Kinzler, K. W. and Vogelstein, B., ed.), 8th edn, pp. 3725–32. New York: McGraw-Hill.

Hopwood, J. J. and Elliott, H. (1983). N-acetylglucosamine 6-sulfate residues keratan and heparan are desulfated by the same enzyme. *Biochem. Int*, **6**, 141–X.

Hopwood, J. J. and Morris, C. P. (1990). The mucopolysaccharidoses: diagnosis, molecular genetics and treatment. *Mol Biol Med*, **7**, 381–404.

Hopwood, J. J., Bunge, S., Morris, C. P. *et al.* (1993). Molecular basis of mucopolysaccharidosis type II: mutations in the iduronate-2-sulfatase gene. *Hum Mutat*, **2**, 435–42.

Horowitz, M., Widre, S., Horowitz, Z., Reiner, O., Gelbart, T. and Beutler, E. (1989). The human glucocerebrosidase gene and pseudogene. Structure and evolution. *Genomics*, **4**, 87–96.

Ikonen, E., Julkunen, I. and Tollersrud, O.-K., Kalkkinen, N. and Peltonen L. . (1993). Lysosomal aspartylglucosaminidase is processed to the active subunit complex in the endoplasmic reticulum. *EMBO J*, **12**, 295–302.

Im, D.-S., Heise, C. E., Nguyen, T., O'Dowd, B. F. and Lynch, K. R. (2001). Identification of a molecular target of psychosine and its role in globoid cell formation. *JCell Biol*, **153**, 429–34.

Imai, K. (1985). Characterization of β-glucosidase as a peripheral enzyme of lysosomal membranesfrom mouse liver and purification. *J Biochem (Tokyo)*, **98**, 1405–16.

Ishii, S., Sakuraba, H. and Suzuki, Y. (1992). Point mutations in the upstream region of the alpha-galactosidase A gene exon 6 in an atypical variant of Fabry disease. *Hum Genet*, **89**, 29–32.

Islam, M. R., Vervoort, R., Lissens, W., Hoo, J. J., Valentino, L. A. and Sly, W. S. (1996). β-Glucuronidase P408S, P415L mutations: evidence that both mutations combine to produce an MPS VII allele in certain Mexican patients. *Hum Genet*, **98**, 281–4.

Itoh, K., Naganawa, Y., Matsuzawa, F. *et al.* (2002). Novel missense mutations in the human lysosomal sialidase gene in sialidosis patients and prediction of structural alterations of mutant enzymes. *J Hum Genet*, **47**, 29–37.

Jain, S., Drendel, W. B., Chen, Z. W., Mathews, F. S., Sly, W. S. and Grubb, J. H. (1996). Structure of human β-glucuronidase reveals candidiate lysosomal targeting and active site motifs. *Nat Struct Biol*, **3**, 375–81.

Kanda, A., Tsuyama, S., Murata, F., Kodama, K., Hirabayashi, Y. and Kanzaki, T. (2002). Immunoelectron microscopic analysis of lysosomal deposits in α-*N*-acetylgalactosaminidase deficiency with angiokeratoma corporis diffusum. *J Dermatol Sci*, **29**, 42–8.

Karageorgos, L. E., Guo, X. H., Blanch, L., Weber, B., Anson, D. S., Scott, H. S. and Hopwood, J. J. (1996). Structure and sequence of the human sulphamidase gene. *DNA Res*, **3**, 269–71.

Karsten, S. L., Lagerstedt, K., Carlberg, B.-M. *et al.* (1997). Two distinct deletions in the IDS gene and the gene W: a novel type of mutation associated with the Hunter syndrome. *Genomics*, **43**, 123–9.

Kase, R., Bierfreund, U., Klein, A., Kolter, T., Utsumi, K., Itoh, K., Sandhoff, K. and Sakuraba, H. (2000). Characterization of two alpha-galactosidase mutants (Q279E and R301Q) found in an atypical variant of Fabry disease. *Biochim Biophys Acta*, **1501**, 227–35.

Keulemans, J. L. M., Reuser, A. J. J. J., Kroos, M. A. *et al.* (1996). Human α-*N*-acetylgalactosaminidase deficiency: new mutations and the paradox between genotype and phenotype. *J Med Genet*, **33**, 458–64.

Klein, U., Kresse, H. and von Figura, K. (1978). Sanfilippo syndrome type C: Deficiency of acetyl CoA: alpha-glucosaminide *N*-acetyltransferase in skin fibroblasts. *Proc Natl Acad Sci USA*, **75**, 5185–9.

Knol, I. E., Ausems, M. G., Lindhout, D. *et al.* (1999). Different phenotypic expression in relatives with Fabry disease caused by a W226X mutation. *Am J Med Genet*, **82**, 436–9.

Koike, M., Nakanishi, H., Saftig, P. *et al.* (2000). Cathepsin D deficiency induces lysosomal storage with ceroid lipofuscin in mouse neurons. *J Neurosci*, **20**, 6898–906.

Kolodny, E. H. (2000). Niemann-Pick disease. *Curr Opin Hemat*, **7**, 48–52.

Kolter, T. and Sandhoff, K. (1999). Sphingolipids-their metabolic pathways and the pathobiochemistry of neurodegenerative diseases. *Angew Chem Int Ed*, **38**, 1532–68.

Koprivica, V., Stone, D. L., Park, J. K. *et al.* (2000). Analysis and classification of 304 mutant alleles in patients with Type 1 and Type 3 Gaucher disease. *Am J Hum Genet*, **66**, 1777–86.

Kornreich, R., Bishop, D. F. and Desnick, R. J. (1989). The gene encoding alpha-galactosidase A and gene rearrangements causing Fabry disease. *Trans Assoc Am Phys*, **102**, 30–43.

Kretz, K. A., Cripe, D., Carson, G. S., Fukushima, H. and O'Brien, J. S. (1992). Structure and sequence of the human α-L-fucosidase gene and pseudogene. *Genomics*, **12**, 276–80.

Kreysing, H. J., von Figura, K. and Gieselmann, V. (1990). The structure of the arylsulfatase gene. *Eur J Biochem*, **191**, 627–31.

Lagerstedt, K., Karsten, S. L., Carlberg, B. M., Kleijer, W. J., Tonnesen, T., Pettersson, U. and Bondeson, M. L. (1997). Double-strand breaks may initiate the inversion mutation causing the Hunter syndrome. *Hum Mol Genet*, **6**, 627–33.

Leistner, S., Young, E., Meaney, C. and Winchester, B. (1995). Pseudodeficiency of arylsulfatase A: a strategy for clarification of genotype in families of subjects with low ASA activity and neurological symptoms. *J Inher Metab Dis*, **18**, 710–6.

Lemansky, P., Bishop, D. F., Desnick, R. J., Hasilik, A. and von Figura, K. (1987). Synthesis and processing of α-galactosidase A in human fibroblasts. Evidence for different mutations in Fabry disease. *J Biol Chem*, **262**, 2062–5.

Lin, L., Sohar, I., Lackland, H. and Lobel, P. (2001). The human CLN2 protein/tripeptidyl-peptidase I is a serine protease that autoactivates at acidic pH. *J Biol Chem*, **276**, 2249–55.

Lowden, J. A. and O'Brien, J. S. (1979). Sialidosis: a review of human neuraminidase deficiency. *Am J Hum Genet*, **31**, 1–18.

Lukatela, G., Krauss, N., Theis, K. *et al.* (1998). Crystal structure of human arylsulfatase A: the aldehyde function and the metal ion at the active site suggest a novel mechanism for sulfate ester hydrolysis. *Biochemistry*, **37**, 3654–64.

Lukong, K. E., Elsliger, M.-A., Chang, Y. *et al.* (2000). Characterization of the sialidase molecular defects in sialidosis patients suggests the structural organization of the lysosomal multienzyme complex. *Hum Mol Genet*, **7**, 1075–85.

Lukong, K. E., Landry, K., Elsliger, M. A. *et al.* (2001). Mutations in sialidosis impair sialidase binding to the lysosomal multienzyme complex. *J Biol Chem*, **276**, 17286–90.

Mahuran, D. J. (1999). Biochemical consequences of mutations causing the GM2 gangliosidoses. *Biochim Biophys Acta*, **1455**, 105–38.

Maier, T., Strater, N., Schuette, C. G. *et al.* (2003). The X-ray crystal structure of human β-hexosaminidase B provides new insights into Sandhoff disease. *J Mol Biol*, **328**, 669–81.

Majer, P., Collins, J. R., Gulnik, S. V. and Erickson, J. W. (1997). Structure-based subsite specificity mapping of human cathepsin D using statine-based inhibitors. *Protein Sci*, **6**, 1458–66.

Mark, B. L., Mahuran, D. J., Cherney, M. M. *et al.* (2003). Crystal Structure of human hexosaminidase B: understanding the molecular basis of Sandhoff and Tay–Sachs disease. *J Mol Biol*, **327**, 1093–109.

McCarter, J. D., Burgoyne, D. L., Miao, S., Zhang, S., Callahan, J. W. and Withers, S. G. (1997). Identification of Glu-286 as the catalytic nucleophile of human lysosomal β-galactosidase precursor by mass spectrometry. *J Biol Chem*, **272**, 396–400.

McGrath, M. E., Klaus, J. L., Barnes, M. G. and Bromme, D. (1997). Crystal structure of human cathepsin K complexed with a potent inhibitor. *Nat Struct Biol*, **4**, 105–9.

McGrath, M. E., Palmer, J. T., Bromme, D. and Somoeo, J. R. (1998). Crystal structure of human cathepsin S. *Protein Sci*, **7**, 1294–302.

McInnes, B., Potier, M., Wakamatsu, N. *et al.* (1992). An unusual splicing mutationin the *HEXB* gene is associated with dramatically different phenotypes in patients from different racial backgrounds. *J Clin Invest*, **90**, 306–14.

Meikle, P. J., Whittle, A. M. and Hopwood, J. J. (1995). Human acetyl-coenzyme A alpha-glucosaminide *N*-acetyltransferase. Kinetic characterization and mechanistic interpretation. *Biochem J*, **308**, 327–33.

Meikle, P. J., Hopwood, J. J., Clague, A. E. and Carey, W. F. (1999). Prevalence of lysosomal storage diseases. *JAMA*, **281**, 249–54.

Michalski, J.-C. and Klein, A. (1999). Glycoprotein lysosomal storage disorders. α- and β-mannosidosis, fucosidosis and α-N-acetylgalactosaminidase deficiency. *Biochim Biophys Acta*, **1455**, 69–84.

Millat, G., Froissart, R., Maire, I. and Bozon, D. (1997). Characterization of iduronate sulfatase mutants affecting N-glycosylation sites and the cysteine-84 residue. *Biochem J*, **326**, 243–7.

Miller, R. D., Hoffmann, J. W., Powell, P. P., Kyle, J. W., Shipley, J. M., Bachinsky, D. and Rr, Sly, W. S. (1990). Cloning and characterization of the human beta-glucuronidase gene. *Genomics*, **7**, 280–3.

Mitchison, H. M., Hofmann, S. L., Becerra, C. H. *et al.* (1998). Mutations in the palmitoyl-protein thioesterase gene (PPT; CLN1) causing juvenile ceroid lipofuscinosis with granular osmiophilic deposits. *Hum Mol Genet*, **7**, 291–7.

Mole, S. E., Mitchison, H. M. and Munroe, P. B. (1999). Molecular basis of the neuronal ceroid lipofuscinoses: mutations in CLN1,CLN2,CLN3 and CLN5. *Hum Mutat*, **14**, 199–215.

Montfort, M., Vilageliu, L., Garcia-Giralt, N., Coll, M. J., Chabas, A. and Grinberg, D. (1998). Mutation 1091delC is highly prevalent in Spanish Sanfilippo syndrome type A patients. *Hum Mutat*, **12**, 274–9.

Morreau, H., Bonten, E., Zhou, X. Y. and d'Azzo A. (1991). Organization of the gene encoding human lysosomal β-galactosidase. *DNA Cell Biol*, **10**, 495–504.

Moskowitz, S. M., Tieu, P. T. and Neufeld, E. F. (1993). Mutation in Scheie syndrome (MPS IS): a G→A transition creates new splice site in intron 5 of one IDUA allele. *Hum Mutat*, **2**, 141–4.

Mossman, J., Blunt, S., Stephens, R., Jones, E. E. and Pembrey, M. (1983). Hunter's disease in a girl: association with X: 5 chromosomal translocation disrupting the Hunter gene. *Arch Dis Child*, **58**, 911–5.

Musil, D., Zucic, D., Turk, D. *et al.* (1991). The refined 2.15 A X-ray crystal structure of human liver cathepsin B: the structural basis for its specificity. *EMBO J*, **10**, 2321–30.

Naganawa, Y., Itoh, K., Shimmoto, M. *et al.* (2000). Molecular and structural studies of Japanese patients with sialidosis type 1. *J Hum Genet*, **45**, 241–9.

Nakano, T., Muscillo, M., Ohno, K., Hoffman, A. J. and Suzuki, K. (1988). A point mutation in the coding sequence of the β-hexosaminidase α-gene results in defective processing of the enzyme protein in an unusual GM2 gangliosidosis variant. *J. Neurochem*, **51**, 984–X.

Nebes, V. L. and Schmidt, M. C. (1994). Human lysosomal α-mannosidase. Isolation and nucleotide sequence of the full-length cDNA. *Biochem Biophys Res Commun*, **200**, 239–45.

Neote, K., McInnes, E., Mahuran, D. and Gravel, R. (1990). Structure and distribution of an Alu-type deletion mutation in Sandhoff disease. *J Clin Invest*, **86**, 1524–31.

Neufed, E. F. and Muenzer, J. (2001). The mucopolysaccharidoses. In *The metabolic and molecular bases of inherited disease* (Scriver, C. R., Beaudet, A. L., Sly, W. S., Valle, D., Childs, B., Kinzler, K. W. and Vogelstein, B., ed.), 8th edn, pp. 3421–52. New York: McGraw-Hill.

Nilssen, O., Berg, T., Riise, H. M. F. *et al.* (1997). α-Mannosidosis: functional cloning of the lysosomal α-mannosidase cDNA and identification of a mutation in two affected siblings. *Hum Mol Genet*, **6**, 717–26.

Noronkoski, T. and Mononen, I. (1997). Influence of 1-fucose attached α1?6 to asparagine-linked *N*-acetylglucosamine on the hydrolysis of the *N*-glycosidic linkage by human glycosylasparaginase. *Glycobiology*, **7**, 217–20.

Obenberger, J., Seidl, Z., Pavlu, H. and Elleder, M. (1999). MRI in an unusually protracted neuronopathic variant of acid sphingomyelinase deficiency. *Neuroradiology*, **41**, 182–4.

Ockerman, P. A. (1967). A generalised storage disorder resembling Hurler's syndrome. *Lancet*, **2**, 239–41.

Ohno, K. and Suzuki, K. (1988*a*). A splicing defect due to an exon–intron junctional mutation results in abnormal β-hexosaminidase alpha chain mRNAs in Ashkenazi Jewish patients with Tay–Sachs diseases. *Biochem Biophys Res Commun*, **153**, 463–9.

Ohno, K. and Suzuki, K. (1988*b*). Mutation in the GM2 gangliosidosis B1 variant. *J Neurochem*, **50**, 316–8.

Oinonen, C., Tikkanen, R., Rouvinen, J. and Peltonen, L. (1995). Three-dimensional structure of human lysosomal aspartylglucosaminidase. *Nat Struct Biol*, **2**, 1102–8.

Okumiya, T., Kawamura, O., Itoh, R. *et al.* (1998). Novel missense mutation (M72V) of α-galactosidase gene and its expression product in an atypical Fabry hemizygote. *Hum Mutat*, **S1**, S213–6.

Orvisky, E., Sidransky, E., Mckinney, C. E. *et al.* (2000). Glucosylsphingosine accumulation in mice and patients with type 2 Gaucher disease begins early in gestation. *Ped Res*, **48**, 233–7.

Oshima, A., Kyle, J. W., Miller, R. D. *et al.* (1987*a*). Cloning, sequencing, and expression of cDNA for human β-galalctosidase. *Biochem Biophys Res Commun*, **157**, 238–44.

Oshima, A., Tsuji, A., Nagao, Y., Sakuraba, H. and Suzuki, Y. (1987*b*). Cloning, sequencing, and expression of cDNA for human beta-glucuronidase. *Proc Natl Acad Sci USA*, **84**, 685–9.

Ott, R., Waye, S. and Chang, P. L. (1997). Evolutionary origins of two tightly linked mutations in arylsulfatase-A pseudodeficiency. *Hum Genet*, **101**, 135–40.

Parenti, G., Meroni, G. and Ballabio, A. (1997). The sulfatase gene family. *Curr Opin Genet Dev*, **7**, 386–91.

Paschke, E., Milos, I., Kreimer-Erlacher, H. *et al.* (2001). Mutation analyses in 17 patients with deficiency in acid β-galactosidase: three novel point mutations and high correlation of mutation W273L with Morquio disease type B. *Hum Genet*, **109**, 159–66.

Pavlu, H. and Elleder, M. (1997). Two novel mutations in patients with atypical phenotypes of acid sphingomyelinasr deficiency. *J Inher Metab Dis*, **20**, 615–6.

Paw, B. H., Moskowitz, S. M., Uhrhammer, N., Wright, N., Kaback, M. M. and Neufeld, E. F. (1990). Juvenile GM2 gangliosidosis caused by substitution of histidine for arginine at position 499 or 504 of the alpha subunit of beta-hexosaminidase. *J Biol Chem*, **265**, 9452–7.

Penzel, R., Uhl, J., Kopitz, J., Beck, M., Otto, H. F. and Cantz, M. (2001). Spllce donor site mutation in the lysosomal neuraminidase gene causing exon skipping and complete loss of enzymic activty in a sialidosis patient. *FEBS Letters*, **501**, 135–8.

Pericak-Vance, M. A., Vance, J. M., Elston, R. C., Namboodiri, K. K. and Fogle, T. A. (1985). Segregation and linkage analysis of alpha-*N*-acetyl-D-glucosaminidase (NAG) levels in a black family. *Am J Med Genet*, **20**, 295–306.

Perkins, K. J., Muller, V., Weber, B. and Hopwood, J. J. (2001). Prediction of Sanfilippo phenotype severity from immunoquantification of heparan-*N*-sulfamidase in cultured fibroblasts from mucopolysaccharidosis type IIIA patients. *Mol Genet Metab*, **73**, 306–12.

Pohlmann, R., Hasilik, A., Cheng, S., Pemble, S., Winchester, B. G. and von Figura, K. (1983). Synthesis of lysosomal α-D-mannosidase in normal and mannosidosis fibroblasts. *Biochem Biophys Res Comm*, **115**, 1083–9.

Polten, A., Fluharty, A. L., Fluharty, C. B., Kappler, J., von Figura, K. and Gieselmann, V. (1991). Molecular basis of different forms of metachromatic leukodystrophy. *NEngl J Med*, **324**, 18–22.

Pshezhetsky, A. V. and Ashmarina, M. (2001). Lysosomal multienzyme complex. biochemistry, genetics and molecular physiology. *Prog Nucl Acid Res Mol Biol*, **66**, 81–114.

Pshezhetsky, A. V., Richard, C., Michud, L. *et al.* (1997). Cloning expression and chromosomal mapping of human lysosomal sialidase and characterization of mutations in sialidosis. *Nat Genet*, **15**, 316–20.

Qi, X. and Grabowski, G. A. (2001). Molecular and cell biology of acid β-glucosidase and prosaposin. *Prog Nucl Acid Res Mol Biol*, **66**, 203–39.

Rafi, M. A., Luzi, P., Chen, Y. Q. and Wenger, D. A. (1995). A large deletion together with a point mutation in the GALC gene is a common mutant allele in patients with infantile Krabbe disease. *Hum Mol Genet*, **4**, 1285–9.

Rathmann, M., Bunge, S., Steglich, C., Schwinger, E. and Gal, A. (1995). Evidence for an iduronate-sulfatase pseudogene near the functional Hunter syndrome gene in Xq27.3-q28. *Hum Genet*, **95**, 34–8.

Rathmann, M., Bunge, S., Beck, M., Kresse, H., Tylki-Szymanska, A. and Gal, A. (1996). Mucopolysaccharidosis type II (Hunter syndrome): mutation 'hot spots' in the iduronate-2-sulfatase gene. *Am J Hum Genet*, **59**, 1202–9.

Redonnet-Vernhet, I., Ploos van Amstel, J. K., Jansen, R. P. *et al.* (1996). Uneven X-inactivation in a female monozygotic twin pair with Fabry disease and discordant expression of a novel mutation in the alpha-galactosidase A gene. *J Med Genet*, **33**, 682–8.

Regis, S., Corsolini, F., Stroppiano, M., Cusano, R. and Filocamo, M. (2002). Contribution of arylsulfatase A mutations located on the same allele to enzyme activity reduction and metachromatic leukodystrophy severity. *Hum Genet*, **110**, 351–5.

Ricketts, M. H., Goldman, D., Long, J. C. and Manowitz, P. (1996). Arylsulfatase A pseudodeficiency-associated mutations: population studies and identification of a novel haplotype. *Am J Med Genet*, **67**, 387–92.

Ricketts, M. H., Poretz, R. D. and Manowitz, P. (1998). The R496H mutation of arylsulfatase A does not cause metachromatic leukodystrophy. *Hum Mutat*, **12**, 238–9.

Riikonen, R., Vanhanen, S., Tyynela, J., Santavuori, P. and Turpeinen, U. (2000). CSF insulin-like growth factor-1 in infantile neuronal ceroid lipofuscinosis. *Neurology*, **54**, 1828–32.

Riise, H. M., Berg, T., Nillsen, O., Romeo, G., Tollersrud, O. K. and Ceccherii, I. (1997). Genomic structure of the human lysosomal alpha-mannosidase gene (MANB). *Genomics*, **42**, 200–7.

Robertson, D. A., Freeman, C., Nelson, P. V., Morris, C. P. and Hopwood, J. J. (1988). Human glucosamine-6-sulfatase cDNA reveals homology with steroid sulfatase. *Biochem Biophys Res Commun*, **157**, 218–24.

Rodriguez-Lafasse, C. and Vanier, M. T. (1999). Sphingosylphophorylcholine in Niemann-Pick disease brain: accumulation in type A but not type B. *Neurochem Res*, **24**, 199–208.

Roussel, A., Canaan, S., Egloff, M. P., Riviere, M., Dupuis, L., Verger, R. and Cambillau, C. (1999). Crystal structure of human gastric lipase and model of lysosomal acid lipase, two lipolytic enzymes of medical interest. *J Biol Chem*, **274**, 16995–7002.

Rudenko, G., Bonten, E., d'Azzo A and Hol WG. (1995). Three-dimensional structure of the human 'protective protein': structure of the precursor form suggests a complex activation mechanism. *Structure*, **3**, 1249–59.

Rudenko, G., Bonten, E., d'Azzo A and Hol WG. (1998). The atomic model of the human protective protein/cathepsin A suggests a structural basis for galactosialidosis *Proc Natl Acad Sci USA*, **95**, 621–5.

Saarela, J., Laine, M. Oinonen, C., vonSchantz C, Jalanko A, Rouvinen J and Peltonen L. (2001). Molecular pathogenesis of a disease: structural consequences of aspartyglucosaminuria mutations. *Hum Mol Genet*, **10**, 983–95.

Sakuraba, H., Oshima, A., Fukuhara, Y. *et al.* (1990). Identification of point mutations in the alpha-galactosidase A gene in classical and atypical hemizygotes with Fabry disease. *Am J Hum Genet*, **47**, 784–9.

Sakuraba, H., Matszawa, F., Aikawa, S. *et al.* (2002). Molecular and structural studies of the GM2 gangliosidosis O variant. *J Hum Genet*, **47**, 176–83.

Salonen, T., Heinonen-Kopra, O. and Jalanko, A. (2001). Neuronal trafficking of palmitoyl protein thioesterase provides an excellent model to study the effects of different mutations which cause infantile neuronal ceroid lipofuscinosis. *Mol Cell Neurosci*, **18**, 131–40.

Sandhoff, K. (2001). The GM2 gangliosidoses and the elucidation of the β-hexosaminidase system. *Adv Genet*, **44**, 67–91.

Sango, K., McDonald, M. P., Crawley, J. N. *et al.* (1996). Mice lacking both subunits of lysosomal β-hexosaminidase display gangliosidosis and mucopolysaccharidosis. *Nat Genet*, **14**, 348–52.

Schissel, S. L., Schuchman, E. H., Williams, K. J. and Tabas, I. (1996). Zn^{2+}-stimulated sphingomyelinase is secreted by many cell types and is a product of the acid sphingomyelnase gene. *J Biol Chem*, **271**, 1843–6.

Schmidtchen, A., Greenberg, D., Zhao, H. G. *et al.* (1998). NAGLU mutations underlying Sanfilippo syndrome type B. *Am J Hum Genet*, **62**, 64–9.

Schriner, J. E., Yi, W. and Hofmann, S. L. (1996). cDNA and genomic cloning of palmitoyl-protein thioesterase (PPT) the enzyme defective in infantile neuronal ceroid lipofuscinosi [pubished erratum appears in. *Genomics 38, 458*] *Genomics*, **34**, 317–22.

Schuchman, E. H., Suchi, M., Takahashi, T., Sandhoff, K. and Desnick, R. J. (1991). Human acid sphingomyelinase: Isolation, nucleotide sequence and expression of the full length and alternatively spliced c DNAs. *J Biol Chem*, **66**, 8531–9.

Schuchman, E. H., Levran, O., Pereira, L. V. and Desnick, R. J. (1992). Structural organization and complete nucleotide sequence of the gene encoding human acid sphingomyelinase. *Genomics*, **12**, 197–205.

Schuchman, E. H. and Desnick, R. J. (2001). Niemann–Pick disease types A and B: acid sphingomyelinase deficiencies. In *The metabolic and molecular bases of inherited disease* (Scriver, C. R., Beaudet, A. L., Sly, W. S., Valle, D., Childs, B., Kinzler, K. W. and Vogelstein, B., ed.), 8th edn, pp. 3589–610. New York: McGraw-Hill.

Scott, H. S., Guo, X.-H., Hopwood, J. J. and Morris, C. P. (1992). Structure and sequence of the human alpha-L-iduronidase gene. *Genomics*, **13**, 1311–3.

Scott, H. S., Bunge, S., Gal, A., Clarke, L. A., Morris, C. P. and Hopwood, J. J. (1995*a*). Molecular genetics of mucopolysaccharidosis type I: diagnostic, clinical and biological implications. *Hum Mutat*, **6**, 288–302.

Scott, H. S., Blanch, L., Guo, X. H. *et al.* (1995*b*). Cloning of the sulphamidase gene and identification of mutations in Sanfilippo A syndrome. *Nat Genet*, **11**, 465–7.

Scott, H. S., Litjens, T., Nelson, P. V. *et al.* (1993). Identification of mutations in the α-L-iduronidase gene (IDUA) that cause Hurler and Scheie syndromes. *Am J Hum Genet*, **53**, 973–86.

Shapiro, L. J., Aleck, K. A., Kaback, M. M. *et al.* (1979). Metachromatic leukodystrophy without arylsulfatase deficiency. *Pediatr Res*, **13**, 1179–81.

Sharp, J. D., Weeler, R. B., Lake, B. D. *et al.* (1997). Loci for classical and a varant late infantile neuronal ceroid lipofuscinosis map to chromosomes 11p15 and 15q21–23. *Hum Mol Genet*, **6**, 591–5.

Shipley, J. M., Klinkenberg, M., Wu, B. M., Bachinsky, D. R., Grubb, J. H. and Sly, W. S. (1993). Mutational analysis of a patient with mucopolysaccharidosis type VII, and identification of pseudogenes. *Am J Hum Genet*, **52**, 517–26.

Sivaraman, J., Lalumiere, M., Menard, R. and Cygler, M. (1999). Crystal structure of wild-type human procathepsin K. *Protein Sci*, **8**, 283–90.

Sleat, D. E., Donnelly, R. J., Lackland, H. *et al.* (1997). Association of mutations in a lysosomal protein with classical late-infantile neuronal ceroid lipofuscinosis. *Science*, **277**, 1802–5.

Sleat, D. E., Gin, R. M., Sohar, I. *et al.* (1999). Mutational analysis of the defective protease in classic late-infantile neuronal ceroid lipofuscinosis, a neurodegenerative lysosomal storage disorder. *Am J Hum Genet*, **64**, 1511–23.

Somoza, J. R., Zhan, H., Bowman, K. K. *et al.* (2000). Crystal structure of human cathepsin V. *Biochemistry*, **39**, 12543–51.

Somoza, J. R., Palmer, J. T. and Ho, J. D. (2002). The crystal structure of human cathepsin F and its implications for the development of novel immunomodulators. *J Molec Biol*, **322**, 559–68.

Sorge, J., West, C., Westwood, B. and Beutler, E. (1985). Molecular cloning and nucleotide sequence of human beteglucocerebrosidase. *Proc Natl Acad Sci USA*, **82**, 7289–93.

Stone, D. L., Tayebi, N., Orvisky, E., Stubblefield, B., Madike, V. and Sidransky, E. (2000). Glucocerebrosidase gene mutations in patients with type 2 Gaucher disease. *Hum Mutat*, **15**, 181–8.

Strasberg, P. M. and Callahan, J. (1998). Lysosphingolipid and mitochondrial function. II. Deleterious effect of sphingosylphosphorylcholine. *Biochem Cell Biol*, **66**, 1322–32.

Sukegawa, K., Tomatsu, S., Tama, K. *et al.* (1992). Intermediate form of mucopolysaccharidosis type II (Hunter disease): a C-1327 to T substitution in the iduronate sulfatase gene. *Biochem Biophys Res Commun*, **183**, 809–13.

Sukegawa, K., Tomatsu, S., Fukao, T. *et al.* (1995). Mucopolysaccharidosis type II (Hunter disease): identification and characterization of eight point mutations in the iduronate-2-sulfatase gene in Japanese patients. *Hum Mutat*, **6**, 136–43.

Sukegawa, K., Song, X.-Q., Masuno, M. *et al.* (1997). Hunter disease in a girl caused by R468Q mutation in the iduronate-2-sulfatase gene and skewed inactivation of the X chromosome carrying the normal allele. *Hum Mutat*, **10**, 361–7.

Sukegawa, K., Nakamura, H., Kato, Z. *et al.* (2000). Biochemical and structural analysis of missense mutations in *N*-acetylgalactosamine-6-sulfate sulfatase causing mucopolysaccharidosis IVA phenotypes. *Hum Mol Genet*, **9**, 1283–90.

Suzuki, K. (1998). Twenty five years of the 'psychosine hypothesis': a personal perspective of its history and present status. *Neurochem Res*, **23**, 251–9.

Suzuki, Y., Oshima, A. and Nanba, E. (2001). β-Galactosidase deficiency (β-galactosidosis). GM1 gangliosidosis and Morquio B disease. In *The metabolic and molecular bases of inherited disease* (Scriver, C. R., Beaudet, A. L., Sly, W. S., Valle, D., Childs, B., Kinzler, K. W. and Vogelstein, B., ed.), 8th edn, pp. 3775–809. New York: McGraw-Hill.

Tayebi, N., Park, P., Madiike, V. and Sidransky, E. (2000). Gene rearrangement on 1q21 introducing a duplication of the glucocerbrosidase pseudogene and a metaxin fusion gene. *Hum Genet*, **107**, 400–3.

Terp, B. N., Cooper, D. N., Christensen, I. T. *et al.* (2002). Assessing the relative importance of the biophysical properties of amino acid substitutions associated with human genetic disease. *Hum Mutat*, **20**, 98–109.

Tessitore, A., Villani, G. R. D., Di Domenico, C., Filocamo, M., Gatti, R. and Di Natale, P. (2000). Molecular defects in the alpha-*N*-acetylglucosaminidase gene in Italian Sanfilippo type B patients. *Hum Genet*, **107**, 568–76.

Thomas, G. H. (1994). 'Pseudodeficiencies' of lysosomal hydrolases. *Am J Hum Genet*, **54**, 934–40.

Thomas, G. H. (2001). Disorders of glycoprotein degradation: α-mannosidosis, β-mannosidosis, fucosidosis and sialidosis. In *The metabolic and molecular bases of inherited disease* (Scriver, C. R., Beaudet, A. L., Sly, W. S., Valle, D., Childs, B., Kinzler, K. W. and Vogelstein, B., ed.), 8th edn, pp. 3507–33. New York: McGraw-Hill.

Thompson, J. N., Jones, M. Z., Dawson, G. and Huffman, P. S. (1992). *N*-acetylglucosamine 6-sulfatase deficiency in a Nubian goat: a model of Sanfilippo syndrome type D (mucopolysaccharidosis IIID). *J Inherit Metab Dis*, **15**, 760–8.

Tikkanen, R., Rouvinen, J., Torronen, A., Kalkkinen, N. and Peltonen, L. (1996). Large-scale purification and preliminary X-ray diffraction studies of human aspartyl- glucosaminidase. *Proteins*, **24**, 253–8.

Timms, K. M., Lu, F., Shen, Y. *et al.* (1995). 130kb of DNA sequence reveals two new genes and a regional duplication distal to the human iduronate-2-sulfatase sulfatase locus. *Genome Res*, **5**, 71–7.

Timms, K. M., Bondeson, M.-L., Ansari-Lari, M. A. *et al.* (1997). Molecular and phenotypic variation in patients with severe Hunter syndrome. *Hum Mol Genet*, **6**, 479–86.

Tomatsu, S., Fukuda, S., Sukegawa, K. *et al.* (1991). Mucopolysaccharidosis type VII: characterization of mutations and molecular heterogeneity. *Am J Hum Genet*, **48**, 89–96.

Toomes, C., James, J., Wood, A. J. *et al.* (1999). Loss of function mutations in the cathepsin C gene result in peridontal disease and palmoplantar keratosis. *Nat Genet*, **23**, 421–4.

Trop, I., Kaplan, F., Brown, C., Mahuran, D. and Hechtman, P. (1992). A glycine 250→aspartate substitution in the α-subunit of hexosaminidase A causes juvenile onset Tay–Sachs diseases in a Lebanese-Canadian family. *Hum Mutat*, **1**, 35–9.

Tsuji, S., Choudray, P. V., Martin, B. M., Winfield, S., Barranger, J. A. and Ginns, E. I. (1986). Nucleotide sequence of cDNA containing the complete coding sequence for human lysosomal glucocerebrosidase. *J Biol Chem*, **261**, 50–3.

Tyynela, J., Sohar, I., Sleat, D. E. (2000). A mutation in the ovine cathepsin D gene causes a congenital lysosomal storage disease with profound neurodegeneration. *EMBO J*, **19**, 2786–92.

Ulrich-Bott, B., Klem, B., Kaiser, R., Spranger, J. and Cantz, M. J. (1987). Lysosomal sialidase deficiency: Increased ganglioside content in autopsy tissues of a sialidosis patient. *Enzyme*, **38**, 262–6.

Vanier, M. T., Ferlinz, K., Rousson, R., Duthel, S., Louisot, P., Sandhoff, K. and Suzuki, K. (1993). Deletion of arginine (608) in acid sphingomyelinase is the prevalent mutation among Niemann–Pick disease type B patients from northern Africa. *Hum Genet*, **92**, 325–30.

Verkryuse, L. A. and Hofmann, S. L. (1996). Lysosomal targeting of palmitoyl-protein thioesterase. *J Biol Chem*, **271**, 15831–6.

Vervoort, R., Lissens, W. and Liebaers, I. (1993). Molecular analysis of a patient with hydrops fetalis caused by beta-glucuronidase deficiency, and evidence for additional pseudogenes. *Hum Mutat*, **2**, 443–5.

Vervoort, R., Islam, M. R., Sly, W. *et al.* (1995). A pseudodeficiency allele (D152N) of the human beta-glucuronidase gene. *Am J Hum Genet*, **57**, 798–804.

Vervoort, R., Islam, M. R., Sly, W. S. *et al.* (1996). Molecular analysis of patients with beta-glucuronidase deficiency presenting as hydrops fetalis or as early mucopolysaccharidosis VII. *Am J Hum Genet*, **58**, 457–71.

Vervoort, R., Gitzelmann, R., Lissens, W. and Liebaers, I. (1998). A mutation (IVS8 + 0.6kbdelTC) creating a new donor splice site activates a cryptic exon in an Alu-element in intron 8 of the human beta-glucuronidase gene. *Hum Genet*, **103**, 686–93.

Vesa, J., Hellsten, E., Verkruyse, L. A. *et al.* (1995). Mutations in t palmitoyl protein thioesterase gene causing infantile neuronal ceroid lipofuscinosis. *Nature*, **376**, 584–7.

Vidgoff, J., Buist, N. and O'Brien, J. (1973). Absence of β-*N*-acetyl-D-hexosaminidase A activity in a healthy woman. *Am J Hum Genet*, **25**, 372–81.

Vines, D. J. and Warburton, M. J. (1998). Purification and characterisation of a tripeptidyl aminopeptidase-I from rat spleen. *Biochim Biophys Acta*, **1384**, 145–54.

Von Bulow, R., Schmidt, B., Dierks, T., von Figura, K. and Uson, I. (2001). Crystal structure of an enzyme-substrate complex provides insight into the interaction between human arylsulfatase A and its substrate during catalysis. *J Mol Biol*, **305**, 269–77.

von Figura, K., Hasilik, A., Steckel, F. and van de Kamp, J. (1984). Biosynthesis and maturation of alpha-*N*-acetylglucosaminidase in normal and Sanfilippo B-fibroblasts. *Am J Hum Genet*, **36**, 93–100.

von Figura, K., Gieselmann, G. and Jaeken, J. (2001). Metachromatic leukodystrophy. In *The metabolic and molecular bases of inherited disease* (Scriver, C. R., Beaudet, A. L., Sly, W. S., Valle, D., Childs, B., Kinzler, K. W. and Vogelstein, B., ed.), 8th edn, pp. 3695–724. New York: McGraw-Hill.

Wakamatsu, N., Kobayashi, H. and Miyatake, T. (1992). Tsuji S. A novel exon mutation in the human β-hexosaminidase subunit gene affects 3′ splice site selection. *J Biol Chem*, **267**, 2406–13.

Wang, A. M. and Desnick, R. J. (1991). Structural organization and complete sequence of the human α-*N*-acetylgalactosaminidase gene: Homology with the α-galactosidase gene provides evidence for evolution from a common ancestral gene. *Genomics*, **10**, 133–42.

Wang, A. M., Bishop, D. F. and Desnick, R. J. (1990*a*). Human α-*N*-acetylgalactosaminidase—molecular cloning, nucleotide sequence, and expression of a full-length cDNA. *J Biol Chem*, **265**, 21859–66.

Wang, A. M., Schindler, D. and Desnick, R. J. (1990*b*). The molecular lesion in the α-*N*-acetylgalactosaminidase gene that causes an infantile neuroaxonal dystrophy. *J Clin Invest*, **86**, 1752–6.

Wang, A. M., Kanzaki, T. and Desnick, R. J. (1994). The molecular lesion in the α-*N*-acetylgalactosaminidase gene that causes angiokratoma corporis diffusum with glycopeptiduria. *J Clin Invest*, **94**, 839–45.

Weber, B., Blanch, L., Clements, P. R., Scott, H. S. and Hopwood, J. J. (1996). Cloning and expression of the gene involved in Sanfilippo B syndrome (mucopolysaccharidosis IIIB). *Hum Mol Genet*, **5**, 771–7.

Weber, B., Guo, X. H., Wraith, J. E., Cooper, A., Kleijer, W. J., Bunge, S. and Hopwood, J. J. (1997). Novel mutations in Sanfilippo A syndrome: implications for enzyme function. *Hum Mol Genet*, **6**, 1573–9.

Weber, B, van de Kamp, J. J., Kleijer, W. J. *et al.* (1998). Identification of a common mutation (R245H) in Sanfilippo A patients from The Netherlands. *J Inherit Metab Dis*, **21**, 416–22.

Weber, B., Guo, X.-H., Kleijer, W. J., van de Kamp, J. J. P., Poorthuis, B. J. H. M. and Hopwood, J. J. (1999). Sanfilippo type B syndrome (mucopolysaccharidosis III B): allelic heterogeneity corresponds to the wide spectrum of clinical phenotypes. *Eur J Hum Genet*, **7**, 34–44.

Weber, B., Hopwood, J. J. and Yogalingam, G. (2001). Expression and characterization of human recombinant α-N-acetylglucosaminidase. *Protein Expr Purif*, **21**, 251–9.

Wenger, D. A., Sujansky, E., Fennessey, P. V. and Thompson, J. N. (1986). Human β-mannosidase deficiency. *N Engl J Med*, **315**, 1201–5.

Wenger, D. A., Rafi, M. A., Luzi, P., Datto, J. and Costatino-Ceccarini, E. (2000). Krabbe disease: genetic aspects and progress towards therapy. *Mol Genet Metab*, **70**, 1–9.

Wenger, D. A., Suzuki, K., Suzuki, Y. and Suzuki, K. (2001). Galactosylceramide lipidosis. Globoid Cell Leukodystrophy (Krabbe disease). In *The metabolic and molecular bases of inherited disease* (Scriver, C. R., Beaudet, A. L., Sly, W. S., Valle, D., Childs, B., Kinzler, K. W. and Vogelstein, B., ed.), 8th edn, pp. 3669–94. New York: McGraw-Hill.

White, W. J., Schray, K. J., Legler, G. and Alhadeff, J. A. (1987). Further studies on the catalytic mechanism of human liver α-L-fucosidase. *Biochem Biophys Acta*, **912**, 132–8.

Whybra, C., Kampmann, C., Willers, I. *et al.* (2001). Fabry disease: clinical manifestation in carriers. *J Inher Metab Dis* [in press].

Willems, P. J., Gatti, R., Darby, J. K., Romeo, G., Durand, P., Dumon, J. E. and O'Brien, J. S. (1991). Fucosidosis revisited: a review of 77 patients. *Am J Med Genet*, **38**, 111–31.

Willems, P. J., Seo, H. C., Coucke, P., Tonlorenzi, R. and O'Brien, J. S. (1999). Spectrum of mutations in fucosidosis. *Eur J Hum Genet*, **7**, 60–7.

Wilson, P. J., Meaney, C. A., Hopwood, J. J. and Morris, C. P. (1993). Sequence of the human iduronate 2-sulfatase (IDS) gene. *Genomics*, **17**, 773–5.

Winchester, B. (1996). Lysosomal metabolism of glycoconjugates. In *Subcellular biochemistry: biology of the lysosome* (Lloyd, J. B. and Mason, R. W., ed.), Vol. 27, pp. 191–238. New York: Plenum Press.

Winchester, B., Young, E., Geddes, S. *et al.* (1992). Female twin with Hunter disease due to non-random inactivation of the X-chromosome: a consequence of twinning. *Am J Med Genet*, **44**, 834–8.

Winchester, B., Barker, C., Baines, S., Jacob, G. S., Namgoong, S. K. and Fleet, G. (1990). Inhibition of α-L-fucosidase. by derivatives of deoxyfuconojirimycin and deoxymannonojirimycin. *Biochem J*, **265**, 277–82.

Wisniewski, K., Kida, E., Walus, M., Wujek, P., Kaczmarski, W. and Golabek, A. A. (2001). Tripeptidyl peptidase I in neuronal ceroid lipofuscinoses and other lysosomal storage diseases. *Eur J Paed Neurol*, **5**, 73–9.

Wraith, J. E., Cooper, A., Thornley, M. *et al.* (1991). The clinical phenotype of two patients with a complete deletion of the iduronate-2-sulfatase gene (mucopolysaccharidosis II–Hunter syndrome). *Hum Genet*, **87**, 205–6.

Wright, C. S., Li, S-C., and Rashinejad, F. (2000). Crystal structure of human GM2 activator protein with a novel β-cup topology. *J Molec Biol*, **304**, 411–22.

Wu, B. M., Tomatsu, S., Fukuda, S., Sukegawa, K., Orii, T. and Sly, W. S. (1994). Overexpression rescues the mutant phenotype of L176F mutation causing β-glucuronidase deficiency in mucopolysaccharidosis in two Menonite siblings. *J Biol Chem*, **269**, 23681–8.

Yamagishi, A., Tomatsu, S. Fukuda S. *et al.* (1996). Mucopolysaccharidosis type I: identification of common mutations that cause Hurler and Scheie syndromes in Japanese populations. *Hum Mutat*, **7**, 23–9.

Yoshitama, T., Nakao, S., Takenaka, T. *et al.* (2001). Molecular genetic, biochemical, and clinical studies in three families with cardiac Fabry's disease. *Am J Cardiol*, **87**, 71–5.

Zhao, H. G., Li, H. H., Bach, G., Schmidtchen, A. and Neufeld, E. F. (1996). The molecular basis of Sanfilippo syndrome type B. *Proc Nat Acad Sci*, **93**, 6101–5.

Zhao, B., Janson, C. A., Amegadzie, B. Y. *et al.* (1997). Crystal structure of human osteoclast cathepsin K complex with E-64. *Nat Sruct Biol*, **4**, 109.

Zhao, H. G., Aronovich, E. L. and Whitley, C. B. (1998). Genotype-phenotype correspondence in Sanfilippo syndrome type B. *Am J Hum Genet*, **62**, 53–63.

Zimmer, K. P., LeCoutre, P., Aerts, H. M. F. G., Harzer, K., Fukuda, M. O., Brien, J. S. and Naim, H. Y. (1999). Intracellular transport of acidic β-glucosidase and lysosome-associated membrane proteins is affected in Gaucher's disease (G202R mutation). *J Pathol*, **188**, 407–14.

Zlotogora, J. and Bach, G. (1985). Pseudodeficiencies in lysosomal storage disorders. *Lancet*, **2**, 1296.

Chapter 5

Defects in lysosomal enzyme modification for catalytic activity

Kurt von Figura, Ljudmila V. Borissenko, Jens Fey, Jianhe Peng, Bernhard Schmidt and Thomas Dierks

Introduction

So far, two types of modifications are known that are required for catalytic activity of lysosomal enzymes. The first type represents the conversion of the catalytically inactive pro-form of cysteinyl- and aspartyl-proteinases into the catalytically active mature form by limited proteolysis. Disorders caused by the lack of this activation step, other than by loss-of-function mutations in genes encoding the proteinase executing the limited proteolysis, are presently not known. This chapter focuses on the second type of modification, which is represented by the posttranslational generation of a Cα-formylglycine (FGly) residue in the catalytic centre of sulfatases (for review see von Figura *et al.* 1998). Deficiency of this modification is the molecular cause of multiple sulfatase deficiency (MSD).

Clinical and biochemical background of multiple sulfatase deficiency

Two years after the description of arylsulfatase A (ASA) deficiency as a cause of metachromatic leukodystrophy in 1963, which represented the first description of a single sulfatase deficiency, Austin *et al.* (1965) reported on the deficiency of three sulfatases in two siblings. In addition to ASA, arylsulfatase B (ASB) and arylsulfatase C were found to be deficient and an accumulation of both sulfated glycolipids and sulfated glycosaminoglycans was noted. Since then it has become apparent that MSD is a rare lysosomal storage disorder that is transmitted in an autosomal-recessive mode and presents as a clinically and biochemically heterogeneous disease. Depending on the onset and severity of the disease, the rare neonatal and juvenile forms can be distinguished from the classical infantile form. The clinical picture combines the signs of mental regression, gait disturbances, and progressive polyneuropathy with signs of an ichthyosis and mild mucopolysaccharidosis, such as stiff joints, mild facial coarsening, and hepatosplenomegaly. Biochemically, a marked reduction of the activity of all known sulfatases is the key diagnostic parameter. The residual activities of the sulfatases are variable but generally less than 15%. The residual activity of ASB (*N*-acetylgalactosamine 4-sulfatase) tends to be higher than that of other sulfatases (Steckel *et al.* 1985).

Early investigations had established that the structural genes of several sulfatases are normal in MSD. The hypothesis was put forward that the molecular defect in multiple sulfatases either abolishes or impairs a posttranslational modification that is common to all sulfatases and required for their catalytic activity and stability, or that it causes the lack of an activator or induces an inhibitor common to sulfatases. When induced to express cDNAs encoding sulfatases, MSD fibroblasts produce sulfatase polypeptides, which are inactive and remain inactive also after purification to homogeneity, while expression of the same cDNAs in non-MSD fibroblasts yields catalytically active sulfatases that remain active also after purification to homogeneity (Rommerskirch *et al.* 1992). This led to the conclusion that the molecular defect in MSD is not linked to the presence of an inhibitor or the lack of an activator but is likely to cause the loss of a posttranslational modification which renders sulfatases catalytically active.

Cα-Formylglycine in sulfatases

Based on the hypothesis that sulfatases carry a posttranslational modification that ensures their catalytic activity, ASA was purified from the medium of eukaryotic cells which secrete the bulk of newly synthesized lysosomal enzymes and overexpress human ASA as an active enzyme. The purified ASA was fragmented with trypsin. Comparison of the molecular mass of the tryptic fragments with their mass predicted from the cDNA sequence revealed that the peptide comprising amino acid residues 59–73 had a lower mass than predicted. A combination of amino acid sequencing and tandem mass spectrometry in a glycerol matrix suggested that this peptide carried in position 69 instead of the predicted cysteine a derivative in which the thiol group was replaced by an aldehyde group (Schmidt *et al.* 1995). This derivative, an FGly or 2-amino-3-oxopropanoic acid, allowed the formation of a Schiff base with *p*-nitroaniline, of a hydrazone with dinitrophenylhydrazine, and of a semiacetal with glycerol and could be converted to serine by reduction with $NaBH_4$ (Fig. 5.1) (Schmidt *et al.* 1995; Dierks *et al.* 1997). These properties allowed the identification of this residue and of FGly-containing peptides by reverse phase high-performance liquid chromatography (RP-HPLC), Edman degradation, and mass spectrometry.

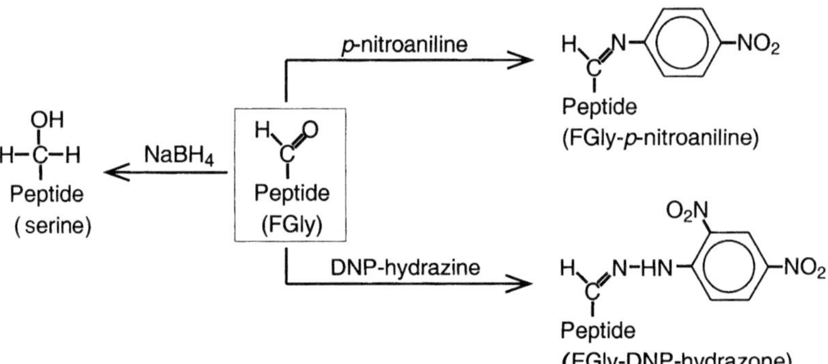

Fig. 5.1 Detection of Cα-formylglycine (FGly) in tryptic sulfatase peptides. Cα-formylglycine-containing peptides undergo specific reactions with $NaBH_4$ (reduction to serine), *p*-nitroaniline (Schiff base formation), and dinitrophenyl (DNP)-hydrazine (formation of the corresponding hydrazone). The reaction products can be detected by Edman sequencing or MALDI mass spectrometry (Schmidt *et al.* 1995; Dierks *et al.* 1997).

	Sequence (↓ = C)	Position	Length (residues)	Accession No.
Arylsulfatase A	L C T P S R A A L L T G R	(Pos. 68–80)	507	X52151
Arylsulfatase B	L C T P S R S Q L L T G R	(Pos. 90–102)	533	J05225
Arylsulfatase C (steroid sulfatase)	L C T P S R A A F M T G R	(Pos. 82–94)	583	J04964
Arylsulfatase D	L C T P S R A A F L T G R	(Pos. 88–100)	593	X83572
Arylsulfatase E	L C T P S R A A F L T G R	(Pos. 85–97)	589	X83573
Arylsulfatase F	L C S P S R S A F L T G R	(Pos. 78–90)	591	X97868
N-Acetylgalactosamine 6-sulfatase	L C S P S R A A L L T G R	(Pos. 78–90)	522	U06088
N-Acetylglucosamine 6-sulfatase	L C C P S R A S I L T G K	(Pos. 90–102)	552	Z12173
Iduronate sulfatase	V C A P S R V S F L T G R	(Pos. 83–95)	550	M58342
Sulfamidase	S C S P S R A S L L T G L	(Pos. 69–81)	502	U30894

Fig. 5.2 Human sulfatases: sequence conservation in the region determining Cα-formylglycine (FGly) modification. The cysteine to be modified (*arrow*) is surrounded by several fully or highly conserved amino acid residues (boxed in dark or light grey, respectively). Most of these residues are conserved also in lower eukaryotic or prokaryotic sulfatases (not shown) (Dierks *et al.* 1999) or putative sulfatases found in the genomes of various species. Cα-formylglycine modification has been shown for human arylsulfatases A and B, and for the arylsulfatases from *Volvox carteri*, *Pseudomonas aeruginosa*, and *Klebsiella pneumoniae* (Schmidt *et al.* 1995; Selmer *et al.* 1996; Dierks *et al.* 1998*a*; Miech *et al.* 1998). All biochemically characterized sulfatases comprise 500–650 amino acid residues, with the key cysteine being located in the *N*-terminal fifth of the polypeptide, as indicated.

The cysteine 69 in ASA represents a residue which is conserved among all known eukaryotic sulfatases (von Figura *et al.* 1998; Dierks *et al.* 1999). Moreover, it is located in a 13-mer sequence that represents the peptide with the highest degree of sequence conservation within the family of sulfatase proteins (Fig. 5.2). In fact the CXPSR pentapeptide, which in ASA contains cysteine 69, can be used as a signature for eukaryotic sulfatases (with the exception of *Neurospora crassa* sulfatase containing CCPAR). Analysis of human ASB and of an arylsulfatase, which is secreted by the green alga *Volvox carteri* under conditions of sulfur starvation, confirmed that also in these sulfatases an FGly residue is found in the position of the cysteine in the respective CXPSR motif (Schmidt *et al.* 1995; Selmer *et al.* 1996). Prokaryotic sulfatases fall into two classes. In one class the genomic DNA predicts a cysteine as in eukaryotic sulfatases, while in the other class a serine is predicted at the corresponding position. However, in both classes of prokaryotic sulfatases, an FGly residue is found in the polypeptides (Dierks *et al.* 1998*a*; Miech *et al.* 1998; Szameit *et al.* 1999). Thus it appears that the FGly residue is present in all pro- and eukaryotic sulfatases and that it can be generated from either a serine (prokaryotes) or a cysteine (pro- and eukaryotes).

Interestingly, the catalytically inactive ASA and ASB expressed in fibroblasts from MSD patients retain the predicted cysteine residue in their CXPSR motifs (Schmidt *et al.* 1995). This supports the notion that it is the absence of this modification which is responsible for the inactivity of sulfatases produced in cells from MSD patients.

Functional role of Cα-formylglycine

The crystal structure of ASA and ASB established that FGly is located in the active site of these two sulfatases (Bond *et al.* 1997; Lukatela *et al.* 1998). Owing to the modest resolution of the two structures, 2.1 Å for ASA and 2.5 Å for ASB, the nature of the side chain of the FGly could not be established unequivocally. Cα-formylglycine was proposed to be present as a hydrated aldehyde or as a free aldehyde, respectively. Accordingly, two different reaction mechanisms were proposed. The aldehyde hydrate could start the reaction by a nucleophilic attack of one of the geminal hydroxyls (O_γ) on the sulfate sulfur, leading to a pentacoordinated sulfur intermediate from which the substrate alcohol would be released. The aldehyde hydrate would be regenerated from the sulfated enzyme intermediate by elimination of the sulfate and addition of water (Lukatela *et al.* 1998). On the contrary, the free aldehyde could initiate sulfate ester cleavage through an electrophilic attack of the aldehyde C_β on a sulfate oxygen, resulting in a sulfate diester which could then be hydrolysed by an unspecified nucleophile (Bond *et al.* 1997).

Structural and enzymatic studies of ASA mutants, in which the FGly was replaced by a serine or alanine, and the recent solution of the X-ray structure of a bacterial sulfatase at 1.3 Å have provided clarification (Recksiek *et al.* 1998; Boltes *et al.* 2001; von Bülow *et al.* 2001). The resting state of the key catalytic residue FGly in sulfatases is a FGly hydrate (Fig. 5.3, state A). One of the two O_γ of the geminal diol, the $O_\gamma2$, is oriented towards the core of the protein, while the $O_\gamma1$ is positioned close enough towards the sulfate sulfur atom to start a nucleophilic attack on the substrate (Fig. 5.3, state B). The nucleophilicity of the $O_\gamma1$ in the diol is enhanced by its coordination to a calcium cation and by the possibility of a proton transfer to an aspartate carboxyl group. On the other hand, the electrophilicity of the sulfur in the substrate is enhanced by interaction of the sulfate oxygens with positively charged side chains of histidines and lysines and with the calcium cation. An S_N2 substitution reaction with a pentacoordinated sulfur intermediate and heterolytic cleavage of the S–O ester bond results in a covalently sulfated enzyme intermediate (Fig. 5.3, state C).

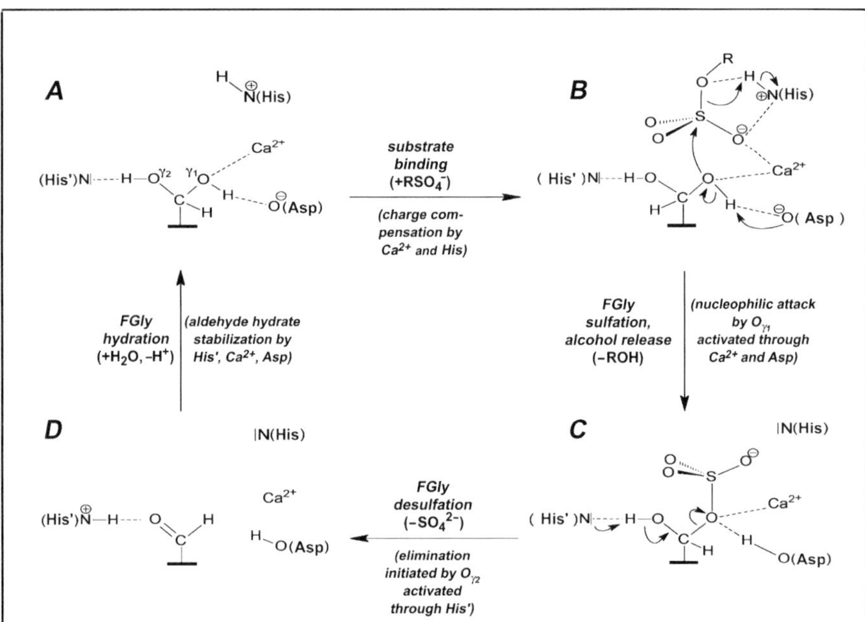

Fig. 5.3 Catalytic mechanism of Cα-formylglycine (FGly)-mediated sulfate ester hydrolysis. In the active site of sulfatases, an FGly hydrate with two geminal hydroxyls is the key residue during the catalytic cycle. (*A*) Upon binding of the sulfate ester, (*B*) $O_\gamma1$ attacks the substrate's sulfur atom, leading to the release of the substrate's alcohol component and concomitant FGly sulfation. (*C*) $O_\gamma2$ initiates FGly desulfation and aldehyde reformation. (*D*) Addition of water regenerates the aldehyde hydrate ground state of the enzyme (*A*).

This mechanism is predicted to result in the inversion of the sulfate tetrahedron. Regeneration of the FGly requires elimination of the sulfate. This is proposed to start with deprotonation of the $O_{\gamma}2$ of the geminal diol, facilitated by the close proximity of a histidine residue acting as a proton acceptor (Fig. 5.3, state D). Finally, an incoming water molecule regenerates the aldehyde hydrate. The mechanism, as described, is based on the structural analyses of sulfatases and their substrate complexes (Bond *et al.* 1997; Lukatela *et al.* 1998; Boltes *et al.* 2001; von Bülow *et al.* 2001), and was also confirmed by kinetic studies of numerous active-site mutants (Knaust *et al.* 1998; Recksiek *et al.* 1998; Waldow *et al.* 1999). The ASA-C69S and the corresponding ASB-C91S mutants allowed the sulfated FGly intermediate to be trapped (Fig. 5.3, state C). The sulfate could no longer be eliminated from this intermediate, since the $O_{\gamma}2$ hydroxyl was absent in these mutants (Recksiek *et al.* 1998).

The structural similarity of sulfatases and in particular of the geometry of their active site regions, which are equal within the experimental error for the two human and the bacterial sulfatases, strongly suggests that the proposed catalytic mechanism holds true for all sulfatases. The key function of the FGly residue in this mechanism explains the critical role of the posttranslational generation of this residue in the biogenesis of enzymatically active sulfatases.

Generation of Cα-formylglycine in the endoplasmic reticulum

The majority of human sulfatases are found in lysosomes as soluble proteins. As for most soluble lysosomal proteins, a small fraction is found also in secretions of cells and thereby in body fluids such as plasma, cerebrospinal fluid, urine, and tears. Arylsulfatase C (steroid sulfatase) is a membrane-anchored protein and is found as such also at the plasma membrane. For none of the human sulfatases a cytosolic location has been reported. This made it likely that the generation of FGly residues, if it occurs posttranslationally, takes place in the endoplasmic reticulum or a more distal compartment of the secretory route.

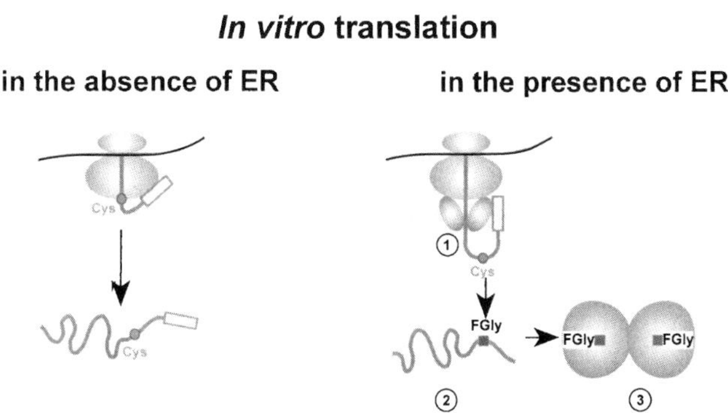

Fig. 5.4 Cα-Formylglycine (FGly) formation in the endoplasmic reticulum. *Left panel*: *In vitro* translation of arylsulfatase A (ASA) cDNAs leads to polypeptides carrying an N-terminal signal peptide (open box) and a cysteine in position 69. *Right panel*: In the presence of transport-competent endoplasmic reticulum-derived microsomes (ER), the polypeptides are imported and processed by signal peptidase and the FGly-modifying enzyme at the lumenal side of the ER membrane. Early translocation intermediates retaining the signal peptide still carry the cysteine (1), while the FGly is found after the completion of translocation and signal peptide cleavage (2). Cα-formylglycine modification occurs before folding of the polypeptide to its native structure and dimerization (3).

In vitro translation of ASA and ASB demonstrated that the primary translation products contain the predicted cysteine at the position where the FGly residue is found in the active sulfatase (Dierks *et al.* 1997, 1998*b*). When the *in vitro* translation was carried out in the presence of endoplasmic reticulum-derived microsomes, to allow import of secretory proteins, a fraction of the translocated sulfatase polypeptides contained FGly residues. This clearly established the existence of an FGly-generating system in the endoplasmic reticulum (Fig. 5.4).

Translocation intermediates of sulfatases did not contain FGly residues. Thus, conversion of cysteine to FGly occurs after translocation or at a late stage of translocation. For generation of FGly partial sulfatase sequences were sufficient, indicating that FGly formation does not depend on folding of sulfatases to their native conformation (Dierks *et al.* 1997, 1998*b*, 1999). It rather implies that formation of FGly residues occurs as long as newly synthesized sulfatase polypeptides are in an unfolded or partially folded stage (Fig. 5.4). It is therefore temporally closely linked to translocation.

Structural determinants controlling Cα-formylglycine formation

The modification of truncated forms of ASA during coupled *in vitro* translation/translocation suggested that a linear sequence motif rather than a conformational motif is critical for the conversion of the specific cysteine into an FGly residue. To identify the structural determinants that are necessary and sufficient to direct the formation of FGly 69 in ASA, cDNAs encoding progressively shorter ASA peptides were placed into a neutral background represented by a preprolactin fragment. It turned out that an ASA peptide of 16 amino acid residues (PVSLCTPSRAALLTGR) containing the cysteine 69 was sufficient to allow the formation of FGly 69 in the fusion polypeptide (Fig. 5.5). In a subsequent series of experiments, the requirement of the individual 16 residues for FGly formation was determined by

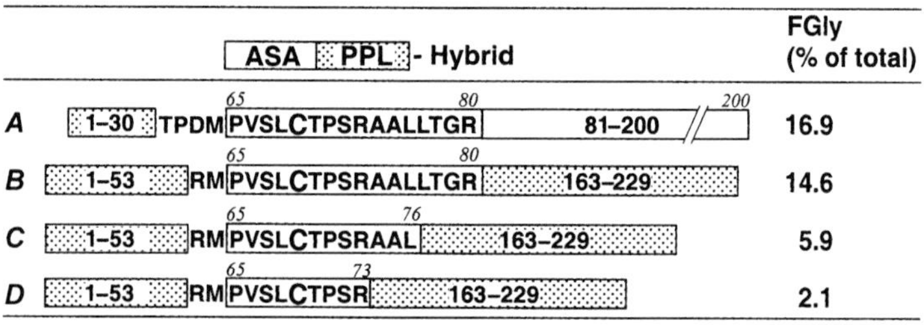

	ASA PPL - Hybrid	FGly (% of total)
A	1–30 TPDM [65] PVSLCTPSRAALLTGR [80] 81–200 [200]	16.9
B	1–53 RM [65] PVSLCTPSRAALLTGR [80] 163–229	14.6
C	1–53 RM [65] PVSLCTPSRAAL [76] 163–229	5.9
D	1–53 RM [65] PVSLCTPSR [73] 163–229	2.1

Fig. 5.5 Residues 65–80 of arylsulfatase A (ASA) comprise an autonomous signal directing Cα-formylglycine (FGly) modification. *In vitro* translation of ASA (residues 65–200), equipped with the signal peptide of preprolactin (PPL, residues 1–30), in the presence of transport-competent endoplasmic reticulum (ER) membranes led to FGly formation in 16.9% of polypeptides (construct *A*). Residues 65–80 of arylsulfatase A (ASA) (PVSLCTPSRAALLTGR) were inserted into the preprolactin sequences, as indicated by the stippled bars. Translation of this hybrid also led to efficient FGly modification (*B*). Significant reduction of modification efficiency was observed after progressive C-terminal shortening of the ASA sequence (*C, D*). Elongation of the ASA fragments at their *N*-terminal side did not improve FGly modification efficiency (not shown). *B–D*: The dipeptide RM was inserted at the N-terminal junction of the ASA sequence to preprolactin to provide a tryptic cleavage site (arginine) and to introduce a [^{35}S]methionine label into the relevant tryptic peptide during *in vitro* translation. *A*: The TPD sequence ensured correct cleavage of the preprolactin signal peptide.

an alanine/glycine scanning mutagenesis. This analysis revealed that the cysteine 69 and the proline and arginine in positions +2 and +4 (relative to cysteine 69) are essential (Dierks *et al.* 1999). Surprisingly, substitution of the threonine and serine in positions +1 and +3, which are highly conserved among eukaryotic sulfatases (50 and 94%, respectively), did not (or only moderately) affect(ed) the FGly formation. This also held true for the highly conserved threonine/glycine pair in position +9/+10. Removal (Fig. 5.5) or substitution of two or more residues within the 16-mer sequence by alanine revealed, however, that apart from the essential core CXPXR motif, the conserved LTGR motif in position +8 to +11 greatly enhances the modification efficiency, suggesting that it functions as an auxiliary element, possibly by establishing a critical secondary structure (Dierks *et al.* 1999).

In vitro assay for Cα-formylglycine formation

Based on the information that translation of a 16-mer ASA sequence in a neutral polypeptide background and its translocation into the endoplasmic reticulum allows the generation of FGly, an *in vitro* assay for the FGly formation was established (Fig. 5.6). A detergent-solubilized extract from canine pancreas microsomes served as a source for the modifying enzyme. A fragment of ASA labelled during *in vitro* translation in the presence of [^{35}S]methionine was used as a substrate. This fragment was synthesized as a fusion polypeptide consisting of the *N*-terminal heptapeptide MGLRMPD, providing the initiator methionine and a tryptic cleavage site at position 4, followed by the ASA sequence 64–158 in which the three naturally occurring methionines, 85, 87, and 120, were mutated. Labelling of the fusion polypeptide by *in vitro* translation in the presence of [^{35}S]methionine and tryptic cleavage yields a single [^{35}S]-labelled peptide of 13 residues representing the MPD tripeptide

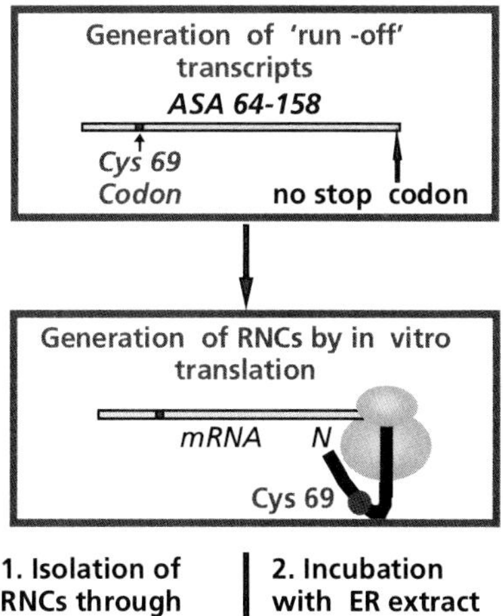

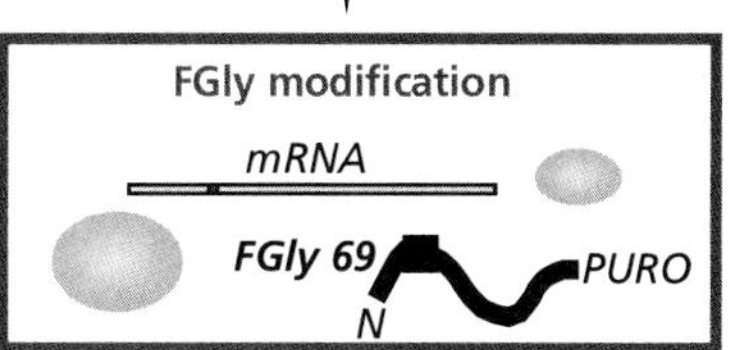

Fig. 5.6 Cα-formylglycine (FGly) formation by endoplasmic reticulum (ER) extract. A 'run-off' transcript encoding residues 64–158 of arylsulfatase A (ASA) but lacking a stop codon is translated *in vitro* leading to ribosome-nascent chain complexes (RNCs). Ribosome-associated polypeptides are isolated from the translation mixture through a sucrose cushion and used as a substrate for FGly modification catalysed by a detergent ER extract. Puromycin is added to the incubation mixture to release the nascent polypeptides from the ribosomes as peptidyl-puromycin.

followed by the ASA sequence 64–73. This peptide is the only [^{35}S]-labelled peptide in the tryptic digest, as the initiator methionine is removed by methionine aminopeptidase present in the translation system. After incubation of the translation product with the microsomal extract and tryptic digestion, the labelled peptide contains in position 69 of the ASA sequence either cysteine or, if modified, FGly. The cysteine and FGly containing forms of the peptide can be separated by RP-HPLC, and the formyl group can be detected after conversion of the FGly into a hydrazone derivative. Using this procedure, about one fifth of the Cys69 was found to be converted into FGly. The efficiency of conversion was about doubled when the *in vitro*-translated ASA fragment was added to the incubation mixture as a ribosome-nascent chain complex rather than as a terminated translation product that is released from the ribosomes (Fig. 5.6). For this purpose, an mRNA construct lacking a stop codon was translated *in vitro* and the translation product was released from the ribosomes by adding puromycin together with the microsomal extract to the assay. After optimizing the reaction conditions, conversion of up to 85% of the Cys69 in the ASA fragment into FGly was observed (Fey *et al.*, 2001).

Characterization of the Cα-formylglycine-generating system

Using the *in vitro* assay system, we determined whether the components of the FGly-generating machinery are part of the microsomal membrane or of the lumenal content of microsomes or of both. Gentle extraction of microsomes with increasing concentrations of detergent solubilized increasing amounts of the FGly-forming activity. Under conditions that extract the lumenal proteins but leave membrane proteins such as Sec61α in the membrane fraction, essentially all FGly-forming activity was recovered in the soluble fraction (Fey *et al.*, 2001).

Kinetic characterization of the FGly-forming activity in fractions containing the lumenal proteins of the endoplasmic reticulum revealed that the *in vitro* assay can be performed under conditions where the fraction of substrate cysteine 69 converted into FGly is proportional to the amount of enzyme and the time of incubation at 37°C. The activation energy for FGly formation is 61.3 kJ/mol. The activity is sensitive to the −SH/−SS equilibrium and is stimulated by 15 μM Ca^{2+}. A rather unusual pH dependence was observed. The reaction rate was fastest at a high alkaline pH of 10 with about 50% activity at pH 7.0 and 30% activity at pH 11.9. A synthetic ASA 16-mer peptide, representing the sequence that was found to be sufficient for FGly formation in the coupled translation/translocation assay (see Fig. 5.5), inhibits the FGly formation in the *in vitro* assay with a K_i of 100–200 nM (Fey *et al.*, 2001).

Purification of the Cα-formylglycine-generating system

Using the *in vitro* assay and matrix proteins of pancreas microsomes we established several chromatographic procedures that separate the FGly-forming system from the bulk of proteins with a reasonable yield. The successful chromatographic matrices included Superdex 200, Mono Q, Phenylsepharose, Concanavalin A-Sepharose, and an affinity matrix based on the immobilized 16-mer ASA peptide that acts as a competitive inhibitor. Presently, we are establishing the conditions for optimal combination of the individual chromatographic steps. In parallel, a much faster *in vitro* assay is worked out that is based on the identification of the FGly-containing product by mass spectrometry rather than by the time-consuming separation of [^{35}S]-labelled peptides by RP-HPLC and their quantitation by scintillation counting.

Summary

The new developments in detecting and purifying the FGly-forming system should in the near future allow the identification of critical polypeptides and cofactors involved in the modification reaction. These data will pave the way for accessing the molecular defects that cause the inactivity of the FGly-forming system in MSD. The clinical and biochemical heterogeneity of MSD suggests that the molecular cause of MSD also is heterogeneous.

Acknowledgements

Work in the authors' laboratories was made possible through the continuous support of the Deutsche Forschungsgemeinschaft and the Fonds der Chemischen Industrie. A number of students and technicians have contributed to the identification of FGly in various sulfatases and the characterization of the FGly-forming system. They include M. Balleininger, I. Boltes, R. von Bülow, A. Kahnert, M. R. Lecca, C. Marquordt, C. Miech, P. Schlotterhose, N. Schwabauer, K. Unthan-Hermeling, A. Waldow, Q. Fang, A. Knaust, K. Neifer, M. Recksiek, and T. Selmer. The fruitful collaboration with Dr. W. Saenger (Berlin), Dr. I. Usón (Göttingen), and Dr. M. Kertesz (Manchester) is gratefully acknowledged.

References

Austin, J., Armstrong, D. and Shearer, L. (1965). Metachromatic form of diffuse cerebral sclerosis. V. The nature and significance of low sulfatase activity: a controlled study of brain, liver and kidney in four patients with metachromatic leukodystrophy (MLD). *Arch Neurol*, **13**, 593–614.

Boltes, I., Czapinski, H., von Kahnert, A., von Bülow, R., Dierks, T., Schmidt, B. *et al.* (2001). 1.3 Å Crystal structure of arylsulfatase from *Pseudomonas aeruginosa* establishes the catalytic mechanism for sulfate ester cleavage in the sulfatase family. *Structure*, **9**, 483–91.

Bond, C. S., Clements, P. R., Ashby, S. J., Collyer, C. A., Harrop, S. J., Hopwood, J. J. *et al.* (1997). Structure of a human lysosomal sulfatase. *Structure*, **5**, 277–89.

von Bülow, R., Schmidt, B., Dierks, T., von Figura, K. and Usón, I. (2001). Crystal structure of an enzyme-substrate complex provides insight into the interaction between human arylsulfatase A and its substrates during catalysis. *J Mol Biol*, **305**, 269–77.

Dierks, T., Lecca, M. R., Schlotterhose, P., Schmidt, B. and von Figura, K. (1999). Sequence determinants directing conversion of cysteine to formylglycine in eukaryotic sulfatases. *EMBO J*, **18**, 2084–91.

Dierks, T., Lecca, M. R., Schmidt, B. and von Figura, K. (1998b). Conversion of cysteine to formylglycine in eukaryotic sulfatases occurs by a common mechanism in the endoplasmic reticulum. *FEBS Lett*, **423**, 61–5.

Dierks, T., Miech, C., Hummerjohann, J., Schmidt, B., Kertesz, M. A. and von Figura, K. (1998a). Posttranslational formation of formylglycine in prokaryotic sulfatases by modification of either cysteine or serine. *J Biol Chem*, **273**, 25560–4.

Dierks, T., Schmidt, B. and von Figura, K. (1997). Conversion of cysteine to formylglycine: a protein modification in the endoplasmic reticulum. *Proc Natl Acad Sci USA*, **94**, 11963–8.

Fey, J., Balleininger, M., Borissenko, L. V., Schmidt, B., von Figura, K. and Dierks, T. (2001) Characterization of posttranslational formylglycine formation by luminal components of the endoplasmic reticulum, *J Biol Chem*, **276**, 47021–28.

von Figura, K., Schmidt, B., Selmer, T. and Dierks, T. (1998). A novel protein modification generating an aldehyde group in sulfatases: its role in catalysis and disease. *Bioessays*, **20**, 505–10.

Knaust, A., Schmidt, B., Dierks, T., von Bülow, R. and von Figura, K. (1998). Residues critical for formylglycine formation and/or catalytic activity of arylsulfatase A. *Biochemistry*, **37**, 13941–6.

Lukatela, G., Krauss, N., Theis, K., Selmer, T., Gieselmann, V., von Figura, K. *et al.* (1998). Crystal structure of human arylsulfatase A: The aldehyde function and the metal ion at the active site suggest a novel mechanism for sulfate ester hydrolysis. *Biochemistry*, **37**, 3654–64.

Miech, C., Dierks, T., Selmer, T., von Figura, K. and Schmidt, B. (1998). Arylsulfatase from *Klebsiella pneumoniae* carries a formylglycine generated from a serine. *J Biol Chem*, **273**, 4835–7.

Recksiek, M., Selmer, T., Dierks, T., Schmidt, B. and von Figura, K. (1998). Sulfatases: Trapping of the sulfated enzyme intermediate by substituting the active site formylglycine. *J Biol Chem*, **273**, 6096–103.

Rommerskirch, W. and von Figura, K. (1992). Multiple sulfatase deficiency: catalytically inactive sulfatases are expressed from retrovirally introduced cDNAs. *Proc Natl Acad Sci USA*, **89**, 2561–5.

Schmidt, B., Selmer, T., Ingendoh, A. and von Figura, K. (1995). A novel amino acid modification in sulfatases that is defective in multiple sulfatase deficiency. *Cell*, **82**, 271–8.

Selmer, T., Hallmann, A., Schmidt, B., Sumper, M. and von Figura, K. (1996). The evolutionary conservation of a novel protein modification, the conversion of cysteine to serinesemialdehyde in arylsulfatase from *Volvox carteri*. *Eur J Biochem*, **238**, 341–5.

Steckel, F., Hasilik, A. and von Figura, K. (1985). Synthesis and stability of arylsulfatase A and B in fibroblasts from multiple sulfatase deficiency. *Eur J Biochem*, **151**, 141–5.

Szameit, C., Miech, C., Balleininger, M., Schmidt, B., von Figura, K. and Dierks, T. (1999). The iron sulfur protein AtsB is required for posttranslational formation of formylglycine in the *Klebsiella* sulfatase. *J Biol Chem*, **274**, 15375–81.

Waldow, A., Schmidt, B., Dierks, T., von Bülow, R. and von Figura, K. (1999). Amino acid residues forming the active site of arylsulfatase A: role in catalytic activity and substrate binding. *J Biol Chem*, **274**, 12284–8.

Note

The molecular nature of the FGLY-generating enzyme, encoded by the *SUMFI* gene (accession no. AY 208752), and numerous MSD-causing mutations have very recently been identified (Dierks, T., Schmidt, B., Borissenko, L. V., Peng, J., Preusser, A., Mariappan, M. and von Figura, K. (2003) Multiple Sulfatase Deficiency is caused by mutations in the gene encoding the human C_α-formylglycine generating enzyme. *Cell* **113**, 435–44; Cosma, M. P., Pepe, S., Annunziata, I., Newbold, R. F., Grompe, M., Parenti, G. and Ballabio, A. (2003) The Multiple Sulfatase Deficiency gene encodes an essential and limiting factor for the activity of sulfatases. *Cell* **113**, 445–56).

Chapter 6

Defects in lysosomal enzyme trafficking

Andrej Hasilik and Peter Lemansky

Introduction

Most known lysosomal enzymes are soluble proteins that are localized in the lysosomal matrix (Chapter 1 and 4). After biosynthesis, these proteins are targeted to lysosomes by a combination of mechanisms operating to different extents in different tissues. This allows for finely and individually tuning the proportion of lysosomal targeting and secretion. A detailed knowledge is available on the synthesis of mannose-6-phosphate (M6P)-recognition markers on soluble lysosomal enzymes and their M6P-dependent targeting as well as on sorting of M6P receptors and several proteins associated with lysosomal membranes. In humans, defects in the synthesis of M6P residues in lysosomal enzymes present as mucolipidosis (ML) II, in which the phosphorylation is missing completely, and as its milder form, ML III, in which a residual phosphorylation is present. This chapter focuses on the synthesis and sorting of the M6P-bearing soluble lysosomal enzymes. Alternatives for lysosomal targeting of soluble proteins are insufficiently understood and will be mentioned only briefly.

At the beginning of studies that eventually led to the elucidation of the M6P-dependent targeting pathway of lysosomal enzymes, two important phenomena were recognized: (i) accumulation of non-degradable materials in cultured cells that were obtained from persons affected with lysosomal storage disorders and (ii) an experimental correction of the lysosomal storage in cultured cells. After mixing cultured fibroblasts from patients with different mucopolysaccharidoses, the degradation resumed (Fratantoni *et al.* 1968). Subsequently, it was demonstrated that correction was due to enzymes secreted by the cells. These enzymes could also be obtained from urine, platelets, and other sources. It was observed that lysosomal enzymes occur in the so-called low- and high-uptake forms, the latter being endowed with a recognition marker that mediates binding onto and endocytosis by the cells. The uptake of lysosomal enzymes was then explained by the process of adsorptive endocytosis, and this implicated the presence of specific receptors on the surface of cells in addition to the recognition marker (reviewed by Neufeld *et al.* 1975). Not knowing about the nature of the receptor yet, in 1977, Kaplan *et al.* using a high-uptake β-glucuronidase showed that the enzyme is taken up in a M6P-sensitive manner and that its high-uptake property was abolished after a treatment with alkaline phosphatase. These inhibitory effects are characteristic of the uptake of soluble lysosomal enzymes in general (Ullrich *et al.* 1978*b*). Later, M6P residues were identified in β-glucuronidase (Natowicz *et al.* 1979) and β-hexosaminidase (Hasilik and Neufeld 1980*b*). These results extended a previous finding by Hickman *et al.* (1974) on the sensitivity of the recognition marker to periodate, revealing the carbohydrate nature of the recognition marker. Subsequently, this field witnessed the elucidation of the biosynthesis and structure of lysosomal enzymes and their recognition marker, characterization of two M6P receptors (MPRs) and their cycling between three or more subcellular compartments, of genes encoding these various proteins and the molecular bases of lysosomal enzyme defects. Many laboratories contributed to research on lysosomes and lysosomal storage diseases that culminated in successful treatment procedures for some of the patients. Impressive health improvements were observed in non-neuropathic Gaucher disease patients after multiple infusions of purified β-glucosidase with carbohydrate side chains specifically tailored for uptake in macrophages (reviewed by Beck 2002; Zhao and Grabowski 2002). Today, this so-called enzyme replacement therapy shows promising results also in patients with Anderson–Fabry disease (Beck 2002; Mehta 2002; Schiffman and Brady 2002), mucopolysaccharidoses I, II, and VI (Kakkis *et al.* 2001; Anon 2002; Kakkis 2002), and Pompe disease (Van den Hout *et al.* 2001; Raben *et al.* 2002) (Chapter 13). Unfortunately, the enzyme replacement therapy is currently not applicable to lysosomal defects that affect brain and requires life-long substitution of the missing enzyme. As discussed, for example, by Poenaru (2001) and Cabrera-Salazar *et al.* (2002), and in Chapter 16, gene transfer and gene therapy are anticipated to provide more widely applicable protocols and more durable therapeutical effects. In this chapter, we highlight some findings on the targeting of soluble lysosomal enzymes and its defects. We start with the biosynthesis of the recognition marker that is elaborated in two reactions.

Synthesis of *N*-acetylglucosamine-1-phospho-6-mannose diester groups in lysosomal enzymes

Identification of phosphodiester groups in metabolically labelled lysosomal enzymes (Hasilik *et al.* 1980; Varki and Kornfeld 1980*a*) indicated that the synthesis of M6P residues in lysosomal enzymes proceeds in two steps. The first enzyme involved is UDP-*N*-acetylglucosamine: lysosomal enzyme *N*-acetylglucosamine-1-phosphotransferase (EC 2.7.8.17). It will be referred to as GlcNAc-phosphotransferase in this Chapter. The properties of this enzyme and other proteins participating in the targeting are compiled in Table 6.1.

Initially, an enzyme activity transferring GlcNAc-phosphoryl groups to glycopeptides (Reitman and Kornfeld 1981*a*) and to dephosphorylated lysosomal enzyme precursors (Hasilik *et al.* 1981; Waheed *et al.* 1981*b*) was demonstrated. This activity was shown to be missing in fibroblasts from ML II (Hasilik *et al.* 1981; Reitman *et al.* 1981) and diminished in those from ML III patients (Reitman *et al.* 1981; Hasilik *et al.* 1982). Subsequently, numerous cell biological and enzymological studies on GlcNAc-phosphotransferase were conducted. Briefly, it should be mentioned that the enzyme is localized in the ERGIC (endoplasmic reticulum (ER)–Golgi intermediate compartment) and *cis*-Golgi (Dittmer and von Figura 1999). This presence in the proximal part of the secretory route establishes phosphorylation of selected mannose-rich oligosaccharides in lysosomal enzymes before these are encountered by the trimming mannosidases in the Golgi apparatus (reviewed by Herscovics 1999). Using arylsulfatase A (ASA), it was shown that the phosphorylation occurs in the *cis*-Golgi both proximally and distally of the KDEL retrieval site (KDEL is an amino acid sequence motif in soluble proteins that is responsible for retention in the ER and retrieval from more distal compartments; this motif consists of four amino acids that are represented in the single-letter code in its name.) However, extending the C-terminus with the KDEL signal does not

1 GlcNAc-phosphotransferase

UDP-*N*-acetylglucosamine: lysosomal enzyme *N*-acetylglucosamine-1-phosphotransferase (EC 2.7.8.17).

Subcellular location: ERGIC and *cis*-Golgi.

The enzyme forms a $\alpha_2\beta_2\gamma_2$ hexameric complex (M_r = 540 kDa), consisting of two α-chains (M_r = 166 kDa; chromosome 12p), β-chains (M_r = 51 kDa; chromosome 12p) and γ-chains (M_r = 56 kDa; chromosome 16p).

2 Uncovering enzyme

N-acetylglucosamine-1-phosphodiester α-N-acetylglucosaminidase (EC 3.1.4.45)

Subcellular location: TGN and plasma membrane

The enzyme is a type I transmembrane protein (M_r = 272 kDa) and forms homotetramers of 68 kDa-subunits, two of which are linked via disulfide-bridges.

3 Mannose-6-phosphate receptors (MPRs)

(a) Cation-dependent (CD)-MPR

Subcellular location: TGN, plasma membrane, endosomes.

The receptor is a type I transmembrane di- and tetramerizing (monomer M_r = 46 kDa) protein, that is palmitoylated at the C-terminus. Binding to M6P-bearing ligands is enhanced by divalent cations. It has a binding optimum between pH 5.5 and 6.5. This receptor is unable to mediate endocytic uptake of M6P-bearing ligands.

(b) Cation independent (CI)-MPR (identical with the M6P/ IGF II-receptor)

Subcellular location: TGN, plasma membrane, endosomes.

The receptor is a type I transmembrane protein (M_r = 275 kDa) and is palmitoylated. Binding to M6P-bearing ligands occurs in the third and ninth of fifteen lumenal homologous domains, is independent of divalent cations, stable at neutral and disrupted at acidic (< 5.5) pH. Another domain binds insulin like growth factor (IGF) II independent of M6P. CI-MPR mediates endocytic uptake of M6P-bearing ligands, IGF II, TGFβ1 precursor and others. It forms mono- and dimers and is downregulated in certain tumours such as hepatocellular carcinoma.

4 Proteins of vesicular traffic, interacting with cytosolic domains of MPRs

(a) Diversion from the secretory route at the TGN

This involves the Golgi-localized, γ-ear-containing, Arf-binding protein-1 (GGA-1), that is a monomeric, multidomain protein. It is recruited to membrane-associated Arf-1 and binds to the acidic-cluster-dileucine motif of MPR cytosolic domains and to clathrin. Also the heterotetrameric adaptor protein (AP)-1 complex is considered to be involved in the segregation in the TGN, either in parallel or in sequence with GGA-1. The binding of AP-1 to membranes depends on the GTPase Arf-1. This adaptor can interact with both the cytosolic domains of MPRs and with clathrin.

(b) Endocytic uptake at the plasma membrane

The heterotetrameric adaptor protein complex AP-2 mediates association of MPRs with clathrin in coated pits and coated vesicles.

(c) Recycling from endosomes to TGN

Currently, among others, AP-1/clathrin, rab9, and TIP 47 are implicated in this process.

ERGIC, endoplasmic reticulium–Golgi intermediate compartment; IGF, insulin-like growth factor; TGN, trans-Golgi network enhance the frequency of phosphorylation, although it significantly prolongs the retention of ASA in the early synthetic compartments (Dittmer and von Figura 1999).

Recently, GlcNAc-phosphotransferase was purified from bovine liver 480,000-fold by immunoaffinity as a hexameric complex ($\alpha_2\beta_2\gamma_2$) of 540 kDa. Its three homodimer moieties consist of 166, 51, and 56 kDa subunits (Bao *et al.* 1996*a, b*). Cloning of the cDNA of the human γ-subunit was described by Raas-Rothschild *et al.* (2000). This protein is coded on chromosome 16p, whereas the precursor of the α-and β-subunits by a single gene on chromosome 12p (Canfield *et al.* 1998).

GlcNAc-phosphotransferase can modify up to two mannose residues in a single oligosaccharide (Varki and Kornfeld 1980*b*). The enzyme preferentially phosphorylates native lysosomal enzymes (Reitman and Kornfeld 1981*b*; Lang *et al.* 1984). The simplest substrate is α-methyl mannoside. However, artificial substrates mimicking the lysosomal enzymes are not known. The determinant that is bound by the enzyme in natural substrates is not defined by a linear peptide structure. Rather, it consists of patches of amino acids shaping the protein surface. A sophisticated study on these structures was performed with pepsinogen. This precursor of pepsin is elaborated in chief cells of the stomach as a secreted non-glycosylated dormant aspartic proteinase. Owing to the known structural homology between pepsin and cathepsin D, Kornfeld and co-workers constructed chimeras of the two. When certain sequence segments in pepsinogen were replaced with the homologous portions of cathepsin D, phosphorylation and lysosomal targeting were observed (Baranski *et al.* 1990; Baranski *et al.* 1992; Cantor *et al.* 1992). Lysine residues displayed at distinct surface locations appeared to be the major determinants. Other studies confirmed and extended these results (Cuozzo and Sahagian 1994; Cuozzo *et al.* 1995; Nishikawa *et al.* 1997; Tikkanen *et al.* 1997; Cuozzo *et al.* 1998; Nishikawa *et al.* 1999). Based on these results, a model of GlcNAc-phosphotransferase with an active centre and a site binding lysosomal enzyme precursors was proposed. Using a different approach, a similar conclusion was drawn from a study on the phosphorylation of ASA. Schierau *et al.* (1999) examined the interacting surface of ASA with a panel of monoclonal anti-ASA antibody Fab fragments. The results confirmed the importance of lysine residues and indicated the existence of additional areas directing the phosphorylation. Careful analysis of ASA mutants with impaired glycosylation consensus sites indicated that polypeptides bearing a single oligosaccharide at asparagine residue number 158, 184, or 350 can all be phosphorylated. However, at the first two sites, the phosphorylation is mutually exclusive (Gieselmann *et al.* 1992).

In simple eukaryotes, for example in slime molds (Temesvari *et al.* 1996) and baker's yeast (Rothman *et al.* 1989), lysosomal targeting is not directed by M6P residues, although it still makes use of a pH-sensitive mechanism and of receptors. A well-studied example is the Vps10p receptor in *Saccharomyces cerevisiae* that binds various protein motifs and segregates carboxypeptidase Y and several other vacuolar proteins from the secretory into the lysosomal pathway (Jorgensen *et al.* 1999). The evolution of the M6P recognition marker in higher eukaryotes probably coincided with the early development of vertebrates. The formidable task of introducing a recognition site for the *N*-acetylglucosaminylphosphoryl transfer into a group of lysosomal proteins may have been facilitated by the rather modest requirement for binding of glycosylated substrate proteins to GlcNAc-phosphotransferase: two basic residues at a proper distance from the modified carbohydrate side chain (Warner *et al.* 2002). The results of these authors indicated that the requirements for a basal phosphorylation or binding to GlcNAc-phosphotransferase are rather simple. A possible explanation is that basic residues were common in digestive enzymes or defence proteins and played a role in an attachment of these proteins to the surface of cells. Once a basic patch was started to be utilized as a signal for phosphorylation, an evolutionary stage was set up for adjustments in other moieties of the signal. These considerations are supported by results in which the phosphorylation of the carbohydrate in non-lysosomal proteins such as renin (Faust *et al.* 1987) and pancreatic DNase (Nishikawa *et al.* 1999) or the non-mammalian vacuolar proteinase A from *S. cerevisiae* (Faust and Kornfeld 1989) was enhanced upon introducing basic residues at the surface of these glycoproteins or even after fusing a normally non-phosphorylated glycoprotein to cathepsin D (Horst *et al.* 1993). This result indicated that the enzyme can reach and phosphorylate several oligosaccharides, while attached to a substrate protein.

In some proteins, phosphorylation of oligosaccharides does not necessarily result in lysosomal targeting. Thus, targeting of myeloperoxidase to azurophilic granules, the specialized lysosomes of neutrophils, is independent of this modification, although a portion of the enzyme becomes phosphorylated (Hasilik *et al.* 1984; Strömberg *et al.* 1986, Lemansky *et al.* 2003). A few other glycoproteins, such as renin, thyroglobulin, and clusterin (Faust *et al.* 1987; Herzog *et al.* 1987; Lemansky *et al.* 1999), are secreted in spite of a phosphorylation. The efficacy of the lysosomal targeting depends on several factors, including the number of M6P residues in the individual oligosaccharide side chains (Munier-Lehmann *et al.* 1996) that is known to vary with their localization (Cantor *et al.* 1992). Therefore, it is assumed that during evolution, the phosphorylation signals in lysosomal enzymes were adjusted to individual targeting needs. It may be speculated that interactions of the oligosaccharides with the side chains of amino acids on the surface of the protein are likely to support or interfere with their recognition or processing. It is also known that an M6P-bearing protein can abstain from the intracellular lysosomal targeting and be subjected to endocytosis still using the M6P-dependent recognition. Thus, M6P recognition plays an important role in the uptake and activation of the latent form of transforming growth factor-β1 (TGF-β1) (Purchio *et al.* 1988; Kovacina *et al.* 1989; Jirtle *et al.* 1991; Liu *et al.* 1999; Yang *et al.* 2000). Obviously, distinct cells may be responsible for the elaboration and the uptake of the latent factor. Finally, uteroferrin should be mentioned as a good substrate of GlcNAc-phosphotransferase. However, as will be discussed below, a major portion of this protein is subject to secretion, while its M6P recognition signal remains covered (Baumbach *et al.* 1984; Saunders *et al.* 1985).

The uncovering

The discovery of the biosynthesis of M6P residues via a phosphodiester precursor resulted in the prediction of a novel enzyme that is able to hydrolyse the carbohydrate phosphodiester moiety and, thus, to uncover the lysosomal recognition marker. Subsequent to demonstrating the activity of this enzyme (Hasilik *et al.* 1980; Varki and Kornfeld 1980*a*), it was recognized as a specific α-*N*-acetylglucosaminidase rather than a phosphodiesterase (Varki *et al.* 1983). Now, it is referred to as *N*-acetylglucosamine-1-phosphodiester α-*N*-acetylglucosaminidase (EC 3.1.4.45) or, briefly, the uncovering enzyme. *In vitro*, its activity can conveniently be determined with UDP-*N*-acetylglucosamine as a substrate. The manifestation of its activity in cultured cells is revealed by the presence of uncovered residues in a lysosomal enzyme(s). This can be detected by metabolic labelling with [^{32}P]phosphate, isolation by immunoprecipitation, and treatment of the solubilized precipitate with alkaline phosphatase (Isidoro *et al.* 1991). The loss of radioactivity associated with the lysosomal enzyme is a measure of mono- and the remainder of diester groups.

The uncovering enzyme was purified 7000-fold from human lymphoblasts (Page *et al.* 1996), 600,000-fold from human serum (Lee and Pierce 1995), and 670,000-fold from bovine liver (Kornfeld *et al.* 1998). Subsequently, human cDNA and the mouse gene were cloned and the respective amino acid sequences were deduced (Kornfeld *et al.* 1999). Early results on the subcellular localization suggested that the uncovering enzyme resides in the *cis*-Golgi. However, Rohrer and Kornfeld (2001) demonstrated convincingly that the bulk of the enzyme is confined to the *trans*-Golgi network (TGN). Consistent with this finding is the presence of sialylated oligosaccharides in its extracytosolic domain and of internalization signals in its C-terminal domain (Rohrer and Kornfeld 2001; Lee *et al.* 2002). These observations are consistent with previous reports on strong inhibition by brefeldin A of the uncovering of either cathepsin D-associated (Radons *et al.* 1990) or the total cellular oligosaccharides (Sampath *et al.* 1992). The phosphorylation was much less inhibited than the uncovering. The confinement of the uncovering to the distal portions of the biosynthesis and segregation path is ensured by synthesizing the uncovering enzyme as an inactive precursor that must be clipped by furin for activation (Do *et al.* 2002). Furin is a subtilisin-like proteinase that is synthesized as an inactive precursor and can be activated autocatalytically (Leduc *et al.* 1992). Synthesis of the uncovering enzyme as an inactive precursor form seems to be mandatory owing to the ability of the mature enzyme to hydrolyse UDP-*N*-acetylglucosamine and its transport through the Golgi cisternae, in which this glycoside should not be endangered (Lee *et al.* 2002).

The uncovering enzyme is a type I transmembrane protein with several potential glycosylation sites (Kornfeld *et al.* 1999). This contrasts with sugar transferases in the Golgi apparatus that are type II transmembrane proteins. In agreement with its localization in the TGN, the oligosaccharides in the uncovering enzyme are sialylated. In its C-terminal sequence it contains internalization signals, indicating that it may reside, at least temporarily, in the plasma membrane. Apparently, it is shed off the cell surface by proteinolysis, since it is present in blood plasma (Lee and Pierce 1995). The uncovering enzyme is a tetramer of 272 kDa, containing two pairs of internally disulfide-bridged 68 kDa subunits (Kornfeld *et al.* 1998).

Uteroferrin is a paradigm of a phosphorylated lysosomal enzyme with rather incomplete uncovering of M6P residues. It is identical with the lysosomal tartrate-resistant 'purple' acid phosphatase (TRAP) (Ling and Roberts 1993*b*; Fleckenstein *et al.* 1996). It is an iron transport protein that is expressed in the epithelia of various visceral organs and in histiocytic cells (Hayman *et al.* 2001). In various animals, uteroferrin is secreted by glandular epithelial cells of the uterine endometrium and placenta and participates in iron transport through the placenta and into fetal liver (Saunders *et al.* 1985; Michel *et al.* 1992). In Gaucher disease uteroferrin expression is increased. In Gaucher cells from a spleen biopsy, TRAP immunostaining revealed a conspicuous vacuolar staining (Schindelmeiser *et al.* 1991). Serum uteroferrin phosphatase activity was established to monitor responses to enzyme replacement in Gaucher disease.

The basis of the low rate of uncovering of M6P residues in uteroferrin has not been elucidated. Ling and Roberts (1993*a*) examined the uncovering in uteroferrin expressed at a varied rate in CHO cells and concluded that high rates of synthesis and partial masking of the phosphodiester groups may contribute to the incomplete uncovering and hypersecretion of the iron transport protein.

A varied amount of any phosphorylatable lysosomal enzyme can escape the phosphorylation, uncovering, and targeting. As a result, the secreted forms of lysosomal enzyme precursors are enriched in complex oligosaccharides, as determined by their resistance to endoglucosaminidase H (Hasilik and von Figura 1981) or a characteristic binding to lectins (den Tandt 1980). When phosphorylation occurs merely in the α1-6-linked branch of the oligosaccharide, or when phosphorylation is absent altogether, as in I-cell disease (see below), lysosomal enzymes become endowed with phosphorylated hybrid and complex-type oligosaccharides, respectively (den Tandt 1980; Miller *et al.* 1981; Vladutiu 1983). In ASA that is secreted by normal cells, oligosaccharides bearing two phosphate residues are in the minority and most of the phosphate groups are covered (Dittmer and von Figura 1999). Such molecules avoid the packaging that is described in the subsequent section and are secreted by the so-called default pathway. Serum lysosomal enzymes contain little, if any, uncovered M6P groups (Sleat *et al.* 1996) and are assumed to originate from cells by default secretion.

Mannose-6-phosphate-dependent packaging

Mannose-6-phosphate receptors, which are present in the TGN, selectively bind with high-affinity newly synthesized lysosomal enzymes that display their just uncovered M6P residues and that are responsible for their segregation from the secretory route and transport into prelysosomal compartments. A few M6P-bearing glycoproteins such as renin and thyroglobulin are thought to possess a low affinity for MPRs. These proteins are secreted (Faust *et al.* 1987; Lemansky and Herzog 1992). However, the bulk of the phosphorylated lysosomal enzymes attach to the receptors as soon as their M6P residues become uncovered. A scheme depicting this and the other major steps in the modification and segregation of lysosomal enzymes and their receptors is shown in Fig. 6.1. Traditionally, vesicular transport is envisioned between the TGN and endosomes. Alternatively, the cargo may be channeled through a tubulo-vesicular network in an association with the cytoskeleton (Waguri *et al.* 2003). The molecular machinery involved in this process will be discussed further below.

In the TGN, two distinct MPRs are engaged in the sorting of phosphorylated lysosomal enzyme precursors (Table 6.1) and both are needed for the normal targeting (Kasper *et al.* 1996). Initially, an MPR was isolated from bovine liver (Sahagian *et al.* 1981). The primary structure of the human receptor was described by Oshima *et al.* (1988). Soon, it was recognized that it is identical with a previously cloned insulin-like growth factor II (IGF II) receptor (Morgan *et al.* 1987; Braulke *et al.* 1988; Kiess *et al.* 1988; MacDonald *et al.* 1988). Therefore, it is commonly referred to as the M6P/IGF II receptor. This receptor has an apparent molecular mass of 275 kDa and consists of a large extracytosolic N-terminal, a hydrophobic transmembrane, and a relatively short cytosolic domain. Recently, Byrd *et al.* (2000) reported that it forms monomers and dimers with distinct binding properties for M6P-containing ligands. Its unique property is a strong binding of M6P-bearing ligands at neutral pH in the absence of divalent cations. Here, it will be referred to as the cation-independent M6P receptor, CI-MPR. This receptor is responsible for the high uptake of lysosomal enzymes and the cross-correction phenomenon described in the introductory section.

The lumenal moiety of the CI-MPR contains 15 internal homologous domains. Two of them, number 3 and number 9, bind M6P ligands with distinct characteristics (Marron-Terada *et al.* 1998; Hancock *et al.* 2002); the others as a group bind an astonishingly diverse collection of highly potent molecules. The M6P-binding domains are involved not only in lysosomal targeting, but also in an activation of latent TGF-β (mentioned above) and in cytotoxic T-cell- and granzyme B-mediated apoptosis of target cells (Motyka *et al.* 2000). Interestingly, the targeting of at least a portion of granzyme B itself, into the NK granules, is M6P dependent (Burkhardt *et al.* 1989). Another M6P-bearing ligand of CI-MPR is proliferin (Lee and Nathans 1988); an essential role of CI-MPR in a proliferin-induced angiogenesis was indicated by the results of Volpert *et al.* (1996). Cation-independent M6P receptor binds (without signalling) several cytokines that bear M6P residues (Blanchard *et al.* 1999). With another domain, this receptor participates in the regulation of the extracellular level of

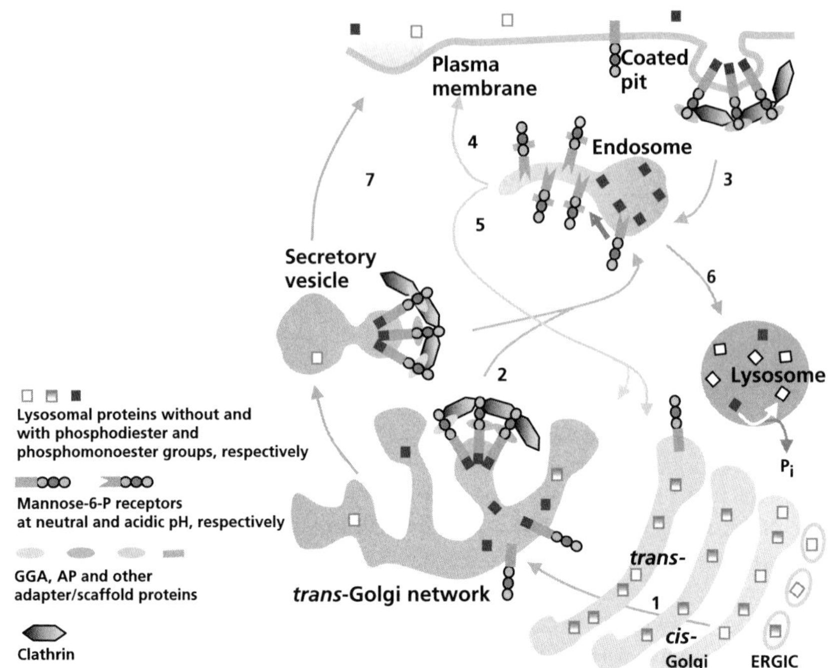

Fig. 6.1 Modification and transport of soluble lysosomal proteins into lysosomes. **1**: After synthesis, glycosylation and folding in the RER proteins are transported into and through the ERGIC and Golgi cisternae; most of the soluble lysosomal enzymes that bear a recognition signal for N-acetyl-glucosaminyl phosphotransferase become phosphorylated. **2**: The phosphorylated glycoproteins leaving the *trans*-Golgi cisternae bear covered mannose 6-phosphate residues. In the *trans*-Golgi network (TGN) uncovering takes place and the uncovered M6P-residues mediate binding to M6P-receptors. In the TGN and possibly the secretory vesicles phosphatidyl inositol-bisphosphate and Arf-1 initiate the formation of a protein scaffold, in which the cytosolic domains of the receptors, Rab, GGA, AP-1 and coat (clathrin) proteins promote budding of vesicles. A vesicle detachment is assisted by dynamin and followed by uncoating and fusion with early and/or late endosomes. **3**: Phosphorylated lysosomal enzymes that escape sorting and become secreted may be captured by the original or a remote cell bearing the CI-MPR at the plasma membrane. The formation of coated pits and endocytic vesicles involves besides CI-MPR, Arf-6, AP-1, clathrin also dynamin that facilitates the detachment. Following uncoating, these vesicles fuse with early endosomes. In the acidic interior of endosomes phosphorylated lysosomal enzymes dissociate from their receptors and their proteolytic processing is initiated. **4** and **5**: In early and late endosomes cargo-free receptors interact with a retrieval machinery that mediates their return to the plasma membrane and *trans*-Golgi. For the sake of brevity the scheme does not differentiate between the recycling, early and late endosomes that have their characteristic sets of proteins facilitating the recycling. **6**: The contents of the late endosomes are delivered to lysosomes, where a dephosphorylation and even a partial deglycosylation of lysosomal enzymes may proceed and the proteolytic maturation is completed. **7**: Default secretion of lysosomal proteins that have escaped segregation into the lysosomal pathway. **See Plate 5**.

IGF II, as will be discussed later. Furthermore, CI-MPR binds retinoic acid and may mediate some of its antiproliferative effects (Kang *et al.* 1997). Finally, Nykjaer *et al.* (1998) described a CI-MPR-dependent targeting of urokinase receptors to lysosomes.

The cation-dependent M6P receptor, CD-MPR, was first described by Hoflack and Kornfeld (1985). As implicated by the nomenclature, the binding of M6P-containing ligands by this receptor is enhanced in the presence of divalent cations. It forms dimers and tetramers with an apparent subunit molecular mass of 46 kDa (Waheed and von Figura 1990). Thus, binding to both receptor subunits may be enhanced, when lysosomal enzymes or their aggregates bear two or more phosphorylated oligosaccharides at a proper distance from each other. A comparison of the deduced primary structure of the CI-MPR (Oshima *et al.* 1988) with that of the CD-MPR (Dahms *et al.* 1987; Pohlmann *et al.* 1987) reveals that all binding domains in the two receptors have a common origin. Besides the cation dependence, the distinctions of the CD-MPR are: (i) it cannot endocytose phosphorylated lysosomal enzymes and (ii) under certain conditions it can promote secretion of newly synthesized phosphorylated lysosomal enzymes (Chao *et al.* 1990).

The two receptors are transporting distinct sets of lysosomal enzymes (Ludwig *et al.* 1994; Pohlmann *et al.* 1995; Kasper *et al.* 1996; Munier-Lehmann *et al.* 1996; Dittmer *et al.* 1998, 1999; Sohar *et al.* 1998) and, thus, in lysosomal targeting they perform non-redundant functions and complement each other. A selectivity in binding the phosphorylated ligands is likely to occur due to the multiplicity of the binding sites in the oligomerizing receptors and, often, of multiple recognition markers on the surface of the precursors of lysosomal enzymes. Owing to the oligomeric nature of many lysosomal enzymes and a multiplicity of the oligosaccharides bearing the recognition marker, incomplete phosphorylation or uncovering of the phosphate residues is likely to have a distinct modulatory effect on the lysosomal targeting depending on the availability of either receptor. Complementarily, alterations in the amounts, oligomerization, and subcellular localization of MPRs may selectively affect the rate of secretion of certain lysosomal enzymes.

The intracellular distribution of the two receptors is similar, though not identical to each other (Klumperman *et al.* 1993). It depends mainly on the interactions of the cytosolic domains of the receptors with vesicle scaffold proteins and the directionality of the vesicular traffic. In early studies, a possible involvement of CI-MPR in signal transduction via G-proteins was examined (reviewed in Kornfeld 1992). Currently, it is established that the binding of IGF II by this receptor plays a decisive role in the degradation of the hormone. Interestingly, in mouse and human, the expression of *IGF II* gene and, in mouse, that of CI-MPR gene is regulated by genomic imprinting (O'Dell and Day 1998). Cation-independent M6P receptor is absent in astrogliotic plaques in multiple sclerosis (Wilczak *et al.* 2000). Since this receptor shows a characteristic distribution in distinct areas of the brain (Hill *et al.* 1988), further studies on the expression of both the receptor and IGF II should be of interest in relation to the physiology and pathology of the central nervous system.

Mannose-6-phosphate receptors represent type I membrane integral proteins with a large glycosylated lumenal N-terminal portion that contains the ligand-binding site(s), a membrane-spanning region, and a short C-terminal cytosolic domain. The three-dimensional structure of the extracytoplasmic CD-MPR domain including the M6P-binding pocket was characterized by X-ray crystallography at 1.8 Å resolution (Roberts *et al.* 1998). Both MPRs are palmitoylated. This modification seems to be important for their recycling or stabilization (Westcott and Rome 1988; Schweizer *et al.* 1996; Breuer and Braulke 1998).

At various intracellular locations, MPRs are packaged into transport vesicles by virtue of their cytosolic domains. Multiple short amino acid sequence motifs in these domains are responsible for interactions of the receptor with a variety of proteins at distinct subcellular locations. Multimeric adapter proteins (APs) and monomeric multidomain Golgi-localized, γ-ear-containing, Arf-binding (GGA) proteins appear to be major players in the packaging of the receptors into vesicles. Through their different domains, these proteins bind Arf and Rab G-proteins, the phosphatidylinositol 3-phosphate (PI-3P)-responsive proteins TIP47 and EEA-1, and clathrin or other coat proteins. Earlier studies implicated the adaptor protein AP-1 in the packaging of the lysosomal cargo into clathrin-coated vesicles in the TGN (reviewed by Le Borgne and Hoflack 1998). More recent results indicate that in this packaging a major role is played by the GGA proteins (Costaguta *et al.* 2001; Meyer *et al.* 2001; Puertollano *et al.* 2001; Zhu *et al.* 2001; reviewed in Dell' Angelica and Payne 2001; Doray *et al.* 2002; Reusch *et al.* 2002). AP-1 adaptin-dependent receptor packaging is likely to be involved in the retrograde transport of MPRs from endosomes to the TGN rather than in the export from the TGN (Meyer *et al.* 2000). According to Doray *et al.* (2002), however, GGAs are needed for transfer of MPRs to AP-1 adaptins at the TGN-budding sites. More experiments are needed to clarify the role of the different scaffold proteins in the budding of vesicles and tubules from different compartments.

The GAT/H, VHS, and GAE domains in GGA proteins mediate their recruitment to membrane-associated activated Arf proteins, binding to acidic-cluster-dileucine motifs in the cytosolic domains of the MPRs, and binding to clathrin, respectively. The structure of the GGA-1 (Shiba *et al.* 2002) and GGA-3 (Misra *et al.* 2002) VHS domains complexed with acidic-cluster-dileucine motifs of the MPRs was recently resolved by X-ray crystallography. Multiple interactions between Arf, Rabs, various effector, and scaffold proteins and distinct motifs in the cytosolic domains of the receptors stabilize a combinatorial assembly of receptors for a particular destination. Concomitant interactions with PI-3P (reviewed in Cullen *et al.* 2001) ensure a rapid orchestration of the budding from a distinct membrane area of vesicles filled with a cargo chosen by the receptors. The importance of the synthesis of PI-3P in targeting of lysosomal proteins is illustrated by the fact that an overexpression of an activity-deficient mutant of the PI-3-kinase Vps34p impairs the maturation of cathepsin D (Row *et al.* 2001).

Depending on the cell type, 10–40% of newly synthesized lysosomal enzymes may become secreted. A portion of these molecules bears the uncovered recognition marker. Molecules originating from the very same cell or a distant source can be delivered to lysosomes and, thus, recaptured or cross-fed, respectively. Such an uptake suggested the presence of MPRs at the cell surface. Indeed, a small fraction of the MPRs, approximately 10%, are localized to the plasma membrane. Both M6P receptors are subject to packaging into clathrin-coated pits and vesicles that is organized by the adaptor protein AP-2. Owing to its ability to bind M6P-bearing ligands at neutral pH, CI-MPR, but not the CD-MPR, is a good cellular tool for the uptake of lysosomal enzymes from the medium. Uptake of MPRs with these ligands depends on the interaction of the μ2- and β-chains of the AP-2 adaptor complex with specific motifs in their cytosolic domains and with clathrin, respectively (Johnson *et al.* 1990; Canfield *et al.* 1991; Jadot *et al.* 1992). Several other proteins participate in the formation of a scaffold on the cytosolic aspect of the membrane. An AP-2-associated protein kinase phosphorylates a threonine residue in the μ2-chain and strongly enhances its affinity to MPRs (Ricotta *et al.* 2002).

The endocytic and the intracellular biosynthetic transport pathways merge within the acidic endocytic compartments, in which the majority of the MPRs are present. As MPRs bind their ligands best at neutral (CI-MPR) or weakly acidic pH (CD-MPR) and release them below pH 5.5, acidification of endosomes leads to a detachment of the phosphorylated ligands from their receptors. In the presence of chloroquine or ammonia, the acidification is impaired and the secretion of phosphorylated enzymes is strongly enhanced (Gonzalez-Noriega *et al.* 1980; Hasilik and Neufeld 1980*a*).

After the dissociation in the acidified compartments, MPRs are returned to the TGN or plasma membrane to be engaged in new transport rounds, whereas the soluble ligands are delivered to lysosomes. Returning MPRs to the TGN from endosomes was shown to depend in part on the heterotetrameric adaptor AP-1, its μ1A-chain (Meyer *et al.* 2001), and the phosphofurin-binding protein PACS1. These two proteins are present in early endosomes and bind each other as well as the CI-MPR. The transfer of CI-MPR from the endosomes to the TGN proceeds via vesicles (Barbero *et al.* 2002), and this recycling requires the presence of Rab9 and TIP47 proteins. These bind CI-MPR synergistically (Diaz and Pfeffer 1998; Carroll *et al.* 2001). In the presence of a dominant negative Rab9 mutant, the recycling of MPRs is impaired and thus so is the sorting of lysosomal enzymes (Riederer *et al.* 1994). TIP47 binds to recycling motifs in both MPRs (Orsel *et al.* 2000). In the scaffold of the recycling vesicles, TIP47 may play the role of a coat protein (Barbero *et al.* 2002). A reduction in its level impairs the recycling of CI-MPR and enhances the turnover of the latter. Among the Rab7- and Rab9-positive domains of the late endosomes, the latter are relatively enriched in CI-MPR (Barbero *et al.* 2002). Based on these results, it was proposed that AP-1 facilitates recycling of MPRs from the early endosomes, whereas Rab9 and TIP47 proteins are needed for recycling from the late endosomes. Alternatively, the transfer may occur in two steps with scaffolds containing AP-1 and TIP47 proteins, respectively (reviewed in Dell'Angelica and Payne 2001).

Defects and alterations in mannose-6-phosphate-dependent targeting

Defects in M6P-dependent targeting may result in two changes. One is a deficiency of lysosomal enzymes with lysosomal accumulation of undegraded materials and the other an elevated secretion of lysosomal enzyme precursors. By the second of these two criteria, the targeting defects differ from deficiencies that are caused by mutations in structural genes of lysosomal enzymes.

Two enzymes encoded by three genes, further two receptors and numerous adaptor and other vesicular scaffold, targeting, docking, and fusion proteins participate in the M6P-dependent transport of lysosomal enzymes. This suggests that diseases resulting from general impairments of this pathway can be caused by defects in numerous genes. However, the number of genes known to be responsible for inherited defects in M6P-dependent targeting in humans is defined by merely three complementation groups representing the known ML II and III patients, while the number of affected proteins identified to date is just one (Chapter 3). This protein is GlcNAc-phosphotransferase. Defects in other proteins that participate in the lysosomal targeting such as μ1A-adaptin (Meyer *et al.* 2000) were shown to impair this process in an experimental setting but did not surface among natural mutations as yet.

Complete and partial absence of the activity of GlcNAc-phosphotransferase is the cause of ML II (I-cell disease, ML II, MIM 252 500) and ML III (pseudo-Hurler polydystrophy, ML III, MIM 252 600), respectively (Chapter 3). With a combined birth prevalence of less than 1 in 100,000, ML II and ML III belong to the most rare lysosomal storage diseases. ML II patients suffer from a severe psychomotor retardation and gross skeletal abnormalities. Coarse, gargoylic facial features and gingival hyperplasia are two of many signs of connective tissue impairments. Similar to other lysosomal storage diseases is the progressive course of the disease. Life expectation of ML II patients is between 5 and 8 years (Chapter 3).

The first description of ML II was presented by Leroy and DeMars (1967) who noticed a similarity to Hurler syndrome as well as major distinct features such as lack of mucopolysacchariduria, an earlier clinical onset, and conspicuous inclusions in cultured skin fibroblasts. The name I-cell disease refers to these inclusions. The elucidation of the biochemical and the genetic bases and the pathophysiological sequelae of the disease make up an impressive chapter in modern molecular medicine.

ML III is a milder form of the same disease with an onset of symptoms at 2–4 years, slower progression and survival into adulthood (Spranger and Weidemann 1970). An excellent biomedical review on the two MLs was prepared by Kornfeld and Sly (2001). In both diseases, primarily mesenchymal cells and tissues including the skeleton and cartilage are affected. In peripheral nerves, alterations can hardly be found, while Schwann cells may contain enlarged vacuoles. In the central nervous system, few alterations such as lamellar bodies in spinal ganglia neurones were described. In brain, inclusion bodies, though not numerous, were found in both neurones and astrocytes (Tondeur *et al.* 1971). The nervous system seems to be less involved than other tissues, and mental development is less retarded than motor functions (Okada *et al.* 1985).

Cells from patients with ML II or ML III show a defective phosphorylation of lysosomal enzymes. The activity of the GlcNAc-phosphotransferase is absent or very low in ML II, while in ML III higher residual activity is found. The enzymatic defect is manifest in all tissues, although in liver, histiocytes, and other tissues of non-mesenchymal origin delivery of synthesized enzymes to lysosomes is still possible. Two genes contribute to the hexameric complex $\alpha_2\beta_2\gamma_2$ of the GlcNAc-phosphotransferase, and cDNA clones of both polypeptide products were isolated. One of these genes localizes to chromosome 12p and encodes a single polypeptide precursor of the α- and β-subunits (Canfield *et al.* 1998). It is this gene in which mutations are found in ML II patients. The γ-subunit is encoded on chromosome 16p, and mutations in its gene are the cause of type C ML III (Raas-Rothschild *et al.* 2000). The corresponding normal cDNA was expressed in COS cells, and the protein product resembled the γ-subunit of the purified bovine GlcNAc-phosphotransferase. The enzyme containing the mutation identified by Raas-Rothschild *et al.* (2000) was shown to be active with a subset of substrates such as α-methyl mannoside and inactive towards lysosomal enzymes. Enzymatic characterization of GlcNAc-phosphotransferase activity in cells carrying the same mutation, an insertion of cytosine at codon 167 (Varki *et al.* 1981), showed that the transferase has a catalytic and a recognition site which localize to the α, β-subunits and to the γ-subunit, respectively. I-Cell disease was also described in cats (Hubler *et al.* 1996 (Chapter 11)). In these animals, the activity of GlcNAc-phosphotransferase is missing and the levels of many lysosomal enzymes in serum are elevated. However, the genes and the mutations involved in this model are not known.

No disease has yet been described with a defect in the transport of lysosomal enzymes due to defects in their receptors or beyond this step. However, mouse models were constructed (knockouts of MPRs) that result in an enhanced rate of secretion of lysosomal enzymes (Ludwig *et al.* 1994; Munier-Lehmann *et al.* 1996; Dittmer *et al.* 1998; Sohar *et al.* 1998). Mice lacking both MPRs show a phenotype strongly resembling human ML II (Dittmer *et al.* 1998). From mouse models with a loss of adaptor proteins, it is further known that segregation of the receptors in the TGN or their AP-1-dependent recycling from endosomes (Meyer *et al.* 2000) is required for normal targeting of soluble lysosomal enzymes such as cathepsin D. In mouse embryonic fibroblasts, deficiency in μ1A-adaptin enhanced the secretion of procathepsin D to 60% of synthesized molecules. The remainder was subjected to proteolytic processing that suggested that the precursor was also targeted to endosomes or lysosomes.

This residual targeting of procathepsin D (Meyer *et al.* 2000) indicated that in these cells, in the absence of μ1A-adaptin, either the recycling of the receptors is not completely abolished or the transport of procathepsin D is mediated by an alternative mechanism.

Of further interest is the phenotype of human colon carcinoma LoVo cells that lack furin. Owing to this defect, the uncovering enzyme is not activated and M6P residues cannot be uncovered. Consequently, the targeting of lysosomal enzymes in LoVo cells is impaired and the enzymes are secreted (Do *et al.* 2002). Thus, examples are known of targeting defects and an enhancement of secretion in cells unable to transfer glucosaminyl phosphate residues, uncover the resulting phosphodiester groups (this is the case in cells lacking either the uncovering enzyme or furin), or incorporate MPRs into the coat protein scaffolds during vesicle budding from the TGN or during their recycling from endocytic compartments. In these reports, the findings refer to different kinds of organs and somatic cells. Further investigations are needed to see whether these effects can be generalized to all tissues, including brain cells.

Individuals with an elevated activity of lysosomal enzymes in serum were described and claimed to have a reduced activity of the uncovering enzyme (Alexander *et al.* 1986). In a later study, it was found, however, that in fibroblasts from a subject belonging to the collective studied by Alexander *et al.* (1986), the secretion of cathepsin D was enhanced while the secreted protein was phosphorylated and its recognition marker uncovered (Faulhaber *et al.* 1998). Apart from the conflict in the interpretation of an increase in the rate of the secretion of lysosomal enzyme precursors, the two reports point to a substantial variation between individuals in this respect. The variation could be caused by an increase in targeting CD-MPRs to the plasma membrane or a deficiency in one of the numerous scaffold proteins. It should be of interest to monitor the level of serum lysosomal enzyme activities in a larger group of clinically normal persons.

In Alzheimer's disease, an increase in the level of lysosomal enzymes and of the CD-MPR in early endosomes was observed. Overexpression of this receptor in mouse brain resulted in an increase in the production of amyloid β (Mathews *et al.* 2002). These and other results implicated MPRs and lysosomal enzymes such as cathepsin D (Haas and Sparks 1996) in the pathogenesis of Alzheimer's disease.

Several experimental models on defects in the M6P-dependent lysosomal path deal with MPRs and the Rab protein-dependent transport of phosphorylated lysosomal proteins. Mice lacking MPRs were mentioned above to resemble the ML II phenotype. In cultured cells, mutations in Rab5a (Rosenfeld *et al.* 2001) and Rab7 (Press *et al.* 1998) were shown to perturb the endosomal compartments. A mutant of Rab5 with a low GTPase activity (Q79L) induces a fusion of endocytic compartments and formation of giant vacuoles. The delivery of cathepsin D and lysosomal membrane-associated protein-1 (LAMP1) and LAMP2 proteins into these organelles is not however impaired (Rosenfeld *et al.* 2001).

A GTPase-negative mutant of Rab22 (a G-protein known to interact with the early endosomal marker EEA-1) caused an accumulation of aspartylglucosaminidase (a lysosomal enzyme known to be targeted by the M6P-dependent pathway) in abnormal vesicles harbouring markers of both early and late endosomes (Kauppi *et al.* 2002). In fibroblasts deficient in the μ1A-chain of AP-1, the retrograde endosome to TGN transport of MPRs was impaired, while endocytosis of CI-MPR was strongly enhanced (Meyer *et al.* 2001). In yeast, disruptions in the AP-1 β-subunit and in a GGA protein inhibited the maturation of the α-factor and the vacuolar targeting of carboxypeptidase S (Costaguta *et al.* 2001).

In numerous reports, enhancement in synthesis and secretion of various lysosomal proteinases was described to occur during tumour progression and metastasis (Tao *et al.* 2001).

No unifying explanation of this phenomenon is available so far. In hepatocellular carcinoma, a down-regulation of CI-MPR was frequently observed in the affected tissue (reviewed in Scharf *et al.* 2001). The loss of these receptors may result in the lowering of the rate of IGF II breakdown, thus accelerating cell growth. In various tumours and during their progression towards metastases, increased secretion of lysosomal enzymes was observed. In the case of cathepsin D, an enhanced secretion was correlated with altered glycosylation and an enhanced growth at distant sites (Garcia *et al.* 1996). A correlation between defects in the binding of IGF II by CI-MPR and proliferation of cells suggests that the gene of this receptor represents a tumour-suppressor gene (Devi *et al.* 1999). In conclusion, an increase in extracellular levels of both the IGF II and the lysosomal enzymes may be relevant for neoplastic growth.

As mentioned further above, the M6P-dependent targeting of lysosomal enzymes can be disrupted by agents that cause an elevation of pH in the endosomal/lysosomal compartments. These effects demonstrate that unloading and reutilization of MPRs is necessary to maintain the lysosomal transport of phosphorylated lysosomal enzymes.

Mannose-6-phosphate-independent lysosomal targeting

Characteristic sequence signals, adaptors such as AP-3, Rab, and other proteins are involved in M6P-independent targeting of membrane proteins to lysosomes (Karlsson and Carlsson 1998; reviewed in Rouille *et al.* 2000). Findings on these pathways and their defects are not discussed here, nor are specialized lysosomal pathways that are important in phagocytic cells and defence mechanisms that are impaired in Chédiak–Higashi, Hermansky–Pudlak and Griscelli's syndromes (reviewed in Dell'Angelica *et al.* 2000; Huizing *et al.* 2001; Stinchcombe and Griffiths 2001). Nevertheless, it should be mentioned that the classical lysosomal marker, lysosomal acid phosphatase (LAP), is synthesized as a precursor with transmembrane and cytosolic domains. Initially, the precursor is targeted to early endosomes and cycles between this compartment and the plasma membrane. Its non-lumenal domains are removed during or after its transport to late endosomes (reviewed by Peters and von Figura 1994; Obermüller *et al.* 2002). Similarly, the lysosomal sialidase (neuraminidase I) appears to be transported to lysosomes via the plasma membrane. Its internalization signal consists of the amino acid sequence YGTL that is localized near the C-terminus on the cytosolic side of the membrane (Lukong *et al.* 2001).

Varied M6P-independent mechanisms seem to be involved in lysosomal targeting of soluble proteins. The existence of such mechanisms was predicted from the observation that in I-cell disease lysosomal storage is manifest in fibroblasts (Hickman and Neufeld 1972; Martin *et al.* 1975) but not in non-mesenchymal cells and organs such as liver. The chondroitin sulfate-containing proteoglycan serglycin and an as yet unknown receptor appear to be responsible for targeting of basic proteins such as lysozyme and myeloperoxidase to lysosomes and to related organelles in U937 and HL-60 cells (Lemansky and Hasilik 2001). Several basic proteins from leucocytes and platelets were found to associate with the chondroitin sulfate moiety of serglycin (Kolset *et al.* 1996). It is likely that this proteoglycan mediates the packaging and retention of basic molecules in cells and the extracellular matrix, respectively.

Little is known about alternatives to M6P-dependent targeting that appear to be effective in non-mesenchymal cells and tissues, although numerous reports on phenomena related to this issue can be found in the literature. At present, there is no unifying base and it seems that any of the protein, carbohydrate, and lipid moieties may be involved in targeting alternatives. To name just a few enzyme examples, we have compiled a paradigmatic list: β-hexosaminidase binds to cells and membranes from liver tissue in a complex manner that is sensitive to different sugars (Ullrich *et al.* 1978*a*; Kato and Suzuki 1985). In fibroblasts, a fraction of β-hexosaminidase B associates with the plasma membrane in a M6P-independent manner (Orlacchio *et al.* 1998). Tsuji *et al.* (1988) examined the binding of precursors of β-hexosaminidase and α-glucosidase to membranes from fibroblasts and concluded that the binding of the former was sensitive to M6P, whereas that of the latter was not. Binding of β-glucosidase to membranes is independent of carbohydrates (Imai 1988; Leonova and Grabowski 2000) and persists from the ER through lysosomes (Rijnboutt *et al.* 1991). In bovine liver a 78 kDa receptor is present that may mediate M6P-independent uptake of β-glucuronidase from the same species (Gonzalez-Noriega and Michalak 2001). A fraction of *ASA* is transported into lysosomes even in I-cell fibroblasts, i.e. in the absence of phosphorylation in cells with grossly impaired lysosomal functions (Waheed *et al.* 1988). Procathepsin S can be phosphorylated and targeted by the M6P pathway; non-glycosylated procathepsin S is targeted to lysosomes also, indicating the presence of an additional sorting motif (Nissler *et al.* 1998). Procathepsin B in tumour cells is targeted to lysosomes by both MPR-dependent and MRP-independent pathways (Moin *et al.* 2000). In HepG2 cells, procathepsin D and prosaposin and their intermediate processing forms associate with membranes in an M6P-dependent and—independent manner (Rijnboutt *et al.* 1991). Procathepsin D was found to be included in a complex with another protein (Grässel and Hasilik 1992) that turned out to be identical with prosaposin (Zhu and Conner 1994). Prosaposin (reviewed in Schuette *et al.* 2001) can be phosphorylated and targeted via MPRs. However, it can be endocytosed by the low-density lipoprotein receptor-related protein and delivered to lysosomes independently of phosphorylation (Hiesberger *et al.* 1998). Interestingly, both prosaposin (Vaccaro *et al.* 1999; Qi and Grabowski 2001) and procathepsin D (Heinrich *et al.* 1999, 2000) bind to membrane lipids and, therefore, are likely to form quaternary complexes. Lefrancois *et al.* (2002) reported that the targeting signal in prosaposin is associated with domain D of the precursor. This targeting may be directed by the lipid composition of membranes, since it depends on an interaction with sphingomyelin. Regulation of the synthesis, targeting, and secretion of these proteins is of great interest owing to implications of cathepsins in apoptosis and pathogenesis of Alzheimer's disease (reviewed in Nixon 2000) and to possible extracellular functions of prosaposin that was shown to be a potential source of a neurotrophic factor (O' Brien *et al.* 1995; Qi *et al.* 1996) and to associate with the neuronal plasma membrane (Fu *et al.* 1994).

Infantile neuronal ceroid lipofuscinosis is caused by mutations in the thioesterase gene (Chapters 3 and 4). In various cells, the enzyme is targeted to lysosomes in an M6P-dependent manner. For example, in COS cells, the enzyme is synthesized with endoglycosidase H-sensitive phosphorylated oligosaccharides and its uptake from the medium is sensitive to M6P (Verkruyse and Hofmann 1996). However, in neurones, this thioesterase appears to be localized to the synaptic vesicles (Lehtovirta *et al.* 2001). If this finding is confirmed, it will be of interest to explain the role of the enzyme in this location and the principle of its extralysosomal targeting.

Dephosphorylation and degradation of lysosomal enzymes

Dephosphorylation of oligosaccharides in lysosomal enzymes may occur after delivery of the enzymes into lysosomes by either an intracellular route or endocytosis. However, the rate and the extent of dephosphorylation vary considerably from case to case. This depends on the storage compartment, the cell type, and the external conditions.

The final stage in the itinerary of a lysosomal enzyme is its own destruction. This may proceed in several steps, in which a few exposed bonds become cleaved until the remaining structure cannot resist continued attempts of fellow hydrolases to destroy any destabilized proteins. Little is known about the destruction scenarios of lysosomal enzymes. However, mutations were described that reduced the stability of these proteins. In pulse-chase labelling experiments, it was shown that ASA has a shorter half-life in multiple sulfatase deficiency fibroblasts as compared with controls (Waheed *et al.* 1981*a*). While at present we know that in this disorder a specific post-translational modification of ASA is missing (Chapter 5), it is not known whether the modification is needed for normal stability of the enzyme. In numerous lysosomal storage disease cases, decreased enzyme activity was shown to be paralleled by a decrease in enzyme stability. As an example referring to ASA, in fibroblasts from several late-onset metachromatic leukodystrophy patients, the enzyme was shown to be stabilized in the presence of inhibitors of cysteine proteinases such as leupeptin (von Figura *et al.* 1986). In a culture dish, the mutant enzyme could be rescued by including 10 mM NH_4Cl in the medium. Owing to inhibited acidification of the endosomal/lysosomal compartments, unloading of MPR cargo was impaired and strong secretion of the newly synthesized ASA resulted. Thus, its delivery into and degradation in lysosomes were avoided. The question is whether drugs will be found that inhibit the degradation of vulnerable mutant lysosomal enzymes without unduly impeding the general lysosomal proteinolysis. Recently, this question was revived following the discovery that in adult metachromatic leukodystrophy, a mutant (P426L) enzyme is unable to form octamers upon delivery to lysosomes (von Bülow *et al.* 2002). It appears that at acidic pH in lysosomes, ASA becomes a prey of cathepsin L and possibly other lysosomal cysteine proteinases, unless octamers are formed.

An obvious possibility resulting from the initiation of degradation in lysosomes is the removal of N- or C-terminal amino acids or of carbohydrate residues. These residues may interact with groups in their vicinity such that the structure is resistant to both proteinases and glycosidases. A striking difference was observed between the oligosaccharides from rat liver cathepsins B and H. Both enzymes contain a single N-linked side chain. In the former, most molecules contained just one α-mannose residue, while in the latter the number of these residues varied between 4 and 8 (Taniguchi *et al.* 1985). The absence of shorter oligosaccharides in cathepsin H suggests that in this enzyme either the oligosaccharide is protected by the protein or vice versa. In human fibro-blasts, the oligosaccharides of cathepsin D present in the small chain differ from those in the large chain by their apparent size as well as by their sensitivity to endoglucosaminidase H (Hasilik and von Figura 1981). In porcine spleen cathepsin D, a significant difference in the structures of the oligosaccharides attached to the two lobes of the enzyme was reported (Takahashi *et al.* 1983). This heterogeneity indicates the existence of selective interactions between the carbohydrate and protein moieties. Furthermore, heterogeneity was reported to occur at the N-termini of both the small and the large mature polypeptides of cathepsin D from human placenta, U937 promonocytes, or transfected CHO cells (Horst and Hasilik 1991). It is conceivable that loss of a critical terminal residue is followed by rapid degradation.

Carbohydrate side chains of many glycoproteins were shown to turn over faster than the protein backbone (Tauber *et al.* 1989; Porwoll *et al.* 1998). Similarly, in lysosomal glycoproteins, the carbohydrate chains are likely to be degraded prior to the protein backbone. Thus, the oligosaccharides may be considered as protectants impeding proteinolysis. Heavy glycosylation of LAMPs was postulated to protect them from proteinolysis similar to oligosaccharides in the mucous coatings protecting the digestive tract (Carlsson *et al.* 1988). Indeed, Kundra and Kornfeld (1999) reported that deglycosylation of LAMPs in living cells with endoglucosaminidase H initiates rapid proteinolytic degradation of these proteins. Impaired N-glycosylation is known to occur in congenital disorders of glycosylation (reviewed by Freeze 2001). Impairment of lysosomal functions seems to play a minor, if any, role in these disorders.

In ASA pseudodeficiency (see below), an altered enzyme, N350S, with decreased stability was found (Shen *et al.* 1993; Barth *et al.* 1994; Leistner *et al.* 1995). Since the mutant is lacking the oligosaccharide that is normally attached to N350, the decrease in the concentration of the enzyme may result from proteinolysis of vulnerable bonds that become exposed in the absence of carbohydrates or from a secondary effect such as a change in the oligomerization of ASA.

One of the first residues to become cleaved off the oligosaccharides in lysosomal enzymes is the phosphate group in the recognition marker, M6P. Obviously, a LAP is needed for the hydrolysis. This enzyme, however, has not been identified yet. As far as the compartment is concerned, it appears that the dephosphorylation is confined to lysosomes and possibly late endosomes. In BHK cells, lysosomal enzymes endocytosed at 20°C reach early endosomes and remain phosphorylated as long as the temperature is not elevated and the transport to lysosomes is prevented.

In a few systems, the dephosphorylation is slow or incomplete and phosphorylated enzymes are present in endosomal/lysosomal organelles or even dense bodies. Such systems are excellent sources of lysosomal enzymes with a high proportion of uncovered M6P residues, i.e. of the high-uptake forms. They include platelets (Brot *et al.* 1974) and human urine (Neufeld *et al.* 1975), as was already mentioned in the introduction. The high-uptake properties of such enzymes are destroyed by a treatment with alkaline phosphatase (Kaplan *et al.* 1977; Ullrich *et al.* 1978*b*; Neufeld 1980). Corticomedullar boundary tubule cells in kidney were reported to be the source of urinary lysosomal enzymes (Brandt *et al.* 1975). It is possible that in these cells lysosomal enzymes are stored in secretory lysosomes resembling granules in leucocytes (Blott and Griffiths 2002).

Sleat *et al.* (1996) examined different rat tissues for the presence of phosphorylated lysosomal enzymes with uncovered M6P residues. Brain contained two to eight times more glycoproteins binding to immobilized MPRs than other tissues. In contrast, liver and serum contained hardly any M6P-bearing glycoproteins. In liver cells, uncovered phosphorylated lysosomal enzymes were found mainly in endosomal/prelysosomal compartments. In brain, however, the bulk of the uncovered M6P groups were associated with neuronal lysosomes (Jadot *et al.* 1999). The persistence of uncovered phosphate groups in lysosomal enzymes in brain tissue was observed also in human. In juvenile neuronal ceroid lipofuscinosis, the rate of the synthesis of several lysosomal enzymes is enhanced and the total amount of the M6P-containing glycoproteins, especially of tripeptidylpeptidase I, is increased several fold (Sleat *et al.* 1998).

Lysosomes contain several phosphatases that were considered to hydrolyse the recognition marker. Recent work with transfected cell and transgene models excluded both a tartrate-sensitive and a tartrate-insensitive acid phosphatase as candidates for dephosphorylation. Bresciani *et al.* (1992) used mouse L cells, in which the dephosphorylation is proceeding rather slowly. The rate of the dephosphorylation was not enhanced, when it was examined with either endogenous or endocytosed lysosomal enzymes in cells overexpressing the tartrate-sensitive LAP (or Acp2 according to Mouse Genome Informatics). Thus, this classical lysosomal marker protein that is related to the secretory phosphatase of the prostate (PAP) is not responsible for dephosphorylation. Another candidate for hydrolysis of M6P residues might be the lysosomal tartrate-resistant phosphatase type 5. However, dephosphorylation of lysosomal enzymes was not impaired in mice doubly deficient in Acp2 and Acp5 (Suter *et al.* 2001). Physiologically, any remaining LAP(s) is not substituting for the knocked-out enzyme, since in the transgenic animals alterations in soft and mineralized tissues, in growth plates, and in tissue macrophages become manifest. In the liver of these animals, vacuolated hepatocytes and Kupffer cells are found, indicating lysosomal storage. Currently, the best candidate for the hydrolysis of M6P residues in lysosomes is uteroferrin (Bresciani and von Figura 1996), the TRAP that was described above.

Sequelae of targeting defects

Unfortunately, little is known about the pathogenesis of lysosomal storage diseases in general and even less about the problems ensuing from targeting defects (Chapter 12). A par excellence targeting defect impairing the lysosomal organelles and their functions is manifest in ML II (Chapter 3). Biochemically, it was elucidated more than 20 years ago, and yet, the path from storage of the undegraded material to the clinical sequelae in this disorder is poorly understood. Primarily, as in any lysosomal deficiency, cells are affected by undegraded materials that originate from both external and internal compartments. Secondarily, many cells may suffer from inflammatory reactions in the affected tissue that seem to be induced by the storage. In a single enzyme deficiency, the clinical problems unfold from storage of undegraded materials. In a targeting defect, such as in I-cell disease, an additional problem may arise from abnormal secretion. Often it is assumed that lysosomal enzyme precursors are inactive, but this is not always the case. Thus, β-hexosaminidase precursors are active. Outside of cells, a plethora of proteolytic enzymes are found. It should be of interest to examine the capacity of metalloproteinases to activate lysosomal enzyme precursors. Metalloproteinases are produced by monocytes and infiltrating macrophages as well as local cells such as microglia (Rosenberg 2002) and are candidates for such a function. However, to our knowledge, this possibility was not examined. Another handicap for an extracellular role of lysosomal enzymes is their dependence on an acidic pH. There are exceptions to this rule, however. Some lysosomal enzymes such as cathepsin S are active at either acidic or neutral pH, and therefore, secretion of mistargeted lysosomal enzyme precursors may result in the degradation of molecules at the surface of cells and in the intercellular matrix. It is of interest that in macrophages and microglia, cathepsin S is subjected to regulation by neurotrophic factors (Liuzzo *et al.* 1999*a*) and inflammatory mediators (Liuzzo *et al.* 1999*b*).

Since inflammatory reactions in the central nervous system are contributing to the pathogenesis of lysosomal storage diseases, the role of secreted lysosomal enzymes deserves thorough consideration. Mouse models seem to provide important information on the interplay of neurones and glial cells. In Tay–Sachs (Wada *et al.* 2000; Myerowitz *et al.* 2002) and Sanfilippo type B (Li *et al.* 2002) disease knockout mice (Chapter 11), upregulation of inflammatory proteins and activation of microglia and astrocytes were observed along with a loss of neurones. The expansion of inflammatory cells and the loss of neurones were suppressed in Sandhoff disease model mice after transplantation of normal bone marrow, although decrease in the storage of GM1 ganglioside could not be detected (Wada *et al.* 2000).

Summary

This chapter describes the targeting of proteins to lysosomes, their modifications, and recognition. It summarizes our knowledge on receptors of lysosomal proteins, on their vesicular transport, and recycling. It discusses I-cell disease as a paradigm of a targeting defect. It points out the basic difference between this defect that results in abnormal secretion, in addition to lysosomal deficiency, in a whole group of soluble lysosomal enzymes on the one side, and loss of lysosomal enzyme activity due to mutations in the genes of particular lysosomal enzymes on the other.

References

Alexander, D., Deeb, M. and Talj, F. (1986). Heterozygosity for phosphodiester glycosidase deficiency: a novel human mutation of lysosomal enzyme processing. *Hum Genet*, **73**, 53–9.

Anon. (2002). Laronidase. *Bio Drugs*, **16**, 316–8.

Bao, M., Booth, J. L., Elmendorf, B. J. and Canfield, W. M. (1996*a*). Bovine UDP-*N*-acetylglucosamine: Lysosomal-enzyme *N*-acetylglucosamine-1-phosphotransferase. I. Purification and subunit structure. *J Biol Chem*, **271**, 31437–45.

Bao, M., Elmendorf, B. J., Booth, J. L., Drake, R. R. and Canfield, W. M. (1996*b*). Bovine UDP-*N*-acetylglucosamine: Lysosomal-enzyme *N*-acetylglucosamine-1-phosphotransferase. II. Enzymatic characterization and identification of the catalytic subunit. *J Biol Chem*, **271**, 31446–51.

Baranski, T. J., Faust, P. L. and Kornfeld, S. (1990). Generation of a lysosomal targeting signal in the secretory protein pepsinogen. *Cell*, **63**, 281–91.

Baranski, T. J., Cantor, A. B. and Kornfeld, S. (1992). Lysosomal enzyme phosphorylation. *J Biol Chem*, **267**, 23342–48.

Barbero, P., Bittova, L. and Pfeffer, S. R. (2002). Visualization of Rab9-mediated vesicle transport from endosomes to the trans-Golgi in living cells. *J Cell Biol*, **156**, 511–8.

Barth, M. L., Ward, C., Harris, A., Saad, A. and Fensom, A. (1994). Frequency of arylsulfatase A pseudodeficiency associated mutations in a healthy population. *J Med Genet*, **31**, 667–71.

Baumbach, G. A., Saunders, P. T., Bazer, F. W. and Roberts, R. M. (1984). Uteroferrin has *N*-asparagine-linked high-mannose-type oligosaccharides that contain mannose 6-phosphate. *Proc Natl Acad Sci USA*, **81**, 2985–9.

Beck, M. (2002). Agalsidase alfa – a preparation for enzyme replacement therapy in Anderson–Fabry disease. *Expert Opin Investig Drugs*, **11**, 851–8.

Blanchard, F., Duplomb, L., Raher, S., Vusio, P., Hoflack, B., Jacques, Y. *et al.* (1999). Mannose 6-phosphate/insulin-like growth factor II receptor mediates internalization and degradation of leukemia inhibitory factor but not signal transduction. *J Biol Chem*, **274**, 24685–93.

Blott, E. J. and Griffiths, G. M. (2002). Secretory lysosomes. *Nat Rev Mol Cell Biol*, **3**, 122–31.

Brandt, E. J., Elliott, R. W. and Swank, R. T. (1975). Defective lysosomal enzyme secretion in kidneys of Chédiak–Higashi (beige) mice. *J Cell Biol*, **67**, 774–88.

Braulke, T., Causin, C., Waheed, A., Junghans, U., Hasilik, A., Maly, P. *et al.* (1988). Mannose 6-phosphate/insulin-like growth factor II receptor: distinct binding sites for mannose 6-phosphate and insulin-like growth factor II. *Biochem Biophys Res Commun*, **157**, 1287–93.

Bresciani, R., Peters, C. and von Figura, K. (1992). Lysosomal acid phosphatase is not involved in the dephosphorylation of mannose 6-phosphate containing lysosomal proteins. *Eur J Cell Biol*, **58**, 57–61.

Bresciani, R. and von Figura, K. (1996). Dephosphorylation of the mannose-6-phosphate recognition marker is localized in later compartments of the endocytic route. Identification of purple acid phosphatase (uteroferrin) as the candidate phosphatase. *Eur J Biochem*, **238**, 669–74.

Breuer, P. and Braulke, T. (1998). Stabilization of mutant 46-kDa mannose 6-phosphate receptors by proteasomal inhibitor lactacystin. *J Biol Chem*, **273**, 33254–8.

Brot, F. E., Glaser, J. H., Roozen, K. J. and Sly, W. S. (1974). *In vitro* correction of deficient human fibroblasts by β-glucuronidase from different human sources. *Biochem Biophys Res Commun*, **57**, 1–8.

von Bülow, R., Schmidt, B., Dierks, T., Schwabauer, N., Schilling, K., Weber, E. *et al.* (2002). Defective oligomerization of arylsulfatase A as a cause of its instability in lysosomes and metachromatic leukodystrophy. *J Biol Chem*, **277**, 9455–61.

Burkhardt, J. K., Hester, S. and Argon, Y. (1989). Two proteins targeted to the same lytic granule compartment undergo very different posttranslational processing. *Proc Natl Acad Sci USA*, **86**, 7128–32.

Byrd, J. C., Park, J. H., Schaffer, B. S., Garmroudi, F. and MacDonald, R. G. (2000). Dimerization of the insulin-like growth factor II/mannose 6-phosphate receptor. *J Biol Chem*, **275**, 18647–56.

Cabrera-Salazar, M. A., Novelli, E. and Barranger, J. A. (2002). Gene therapy for the lysosomal storage disorders. *Curr Opin Mol Ther*, **4**, 349–58.

Canfield, W. M., Johnson, K. F., Ye, R. D., Gregory, W. and Kornfeld, S. (1991). Localization of the signal for rapid internalization of the bovine cation-independent mannose 6-phosphate/insulin-like growth factor-II receptor to amino acids 24–29 of the cytoplasmic tail. *J Biol Chem*, **266**, 5682–8.

Canfield, W., Bao, M., Pan, J., D'Souza, A., Brewer, K., Pan, H. *et al.* (1998). Mucolipidosis II and mucolipidosis IIIA are caused by mutations in the GlcNAc-phosphotransferase αβ gene on chromosome 12. *Am J Hum Genet*, **63**, A15.

Cantor, A. B., Baranski, T. J. and Kornfeld, S. (1992). Lysosomal enzyme phosphorylation. *J Biol Chem*, **267**, 23349–56.

Carlsson, S. R., Roth, J., Piller, F. and Fukuda, M. (1988). Isolation and characterization of human lysosomal membrane glycoproteins, h-LAMP-1 and h-LAMP-2. Major sialoglycoproteins carrying polylactosaminoglycan. *J Biol Chem*, **263**, 18911–9.

Carroll, K. S., Hanna, J., Simon, I., Krise, J., Barbero, P. and Pfeffer, S. R. (2001). Role of Rab9 GTPase in facilitating receptor recruitment by TIP47. *Science*, **292**, 1373–6.

Chao, H. H., Waheed, A., Pohlmann, R., Hille, A. and von Figura, K. (1990). Mannose 6-phosphate receptor dependent secretion of lysosomal enzymes. *EMBO J*, **9**, 3507–13.

Costaguta, G., Stefan, C. J., Bensen, E. S., Emr, S. D. and Payne, G. S. (2001). Yeast Gga coat proteins function with clathrin in Golgi to endosome transport. *Mol Biol Cell*, **12**, 1885–96.

Cullen, P. J., Cozier, G. E., Banting, G. and Mellor, H. (2001). Modular phosphoinositide-binding domains—their role in signalling and membrane trafficking. *Curr Biol*, **11**, R882–93.

Cuozzo, J. W. and Sahagian, G. G. (1994). Lysine is a common determinant for mannose phosphorylation of lysosomal proteins. *J Biol Chem*, **269**, 14490–6.

Cuozzo, J. W., Tao, K., Cygler, M., Mort, J. S. and Sahagian, G. G. (1998). Lysine-based structure responsible for selective mannose phosphorylation of cathepsin D and cathepsin L defines a common structural motif for lysosomal targeting. *J Biol Chem*, **273**, 21067–76.

Cuozzo, J. W., Tao, K., Wu, Q. L., Young, W. and Sahagian, G. G. (1995). Lysine-based structure in the proregion of procathepsin L is the recognition site for mannose phosphorylation. *J Biol Chem*, **270**, 15611–9.

Dahms, N. M., Lobel, P., Breitmeyer, J., Chirgwin, J. M. and Kornfeld, S. (1987). 46 kd mannose 6-phosphate receptor: cloning, expression, and homology to the 215 kd mannose 6-phosphate receptor. *Cell*, **50**, 181–92.

Dell'Angelica, E. C. and Payne, G. S. (2001). Intracellular cycling of lysosomal enzyme receptors: cytoplasmic tails' tales. *Cell*, **106**, 395–8.

Dell'Angelica, E. C., Mullins, C., Caplan, S. and Bonifacino, J. S. (2000). Lysosome-related organelles. *FASEB J*, **14**, 1265–78.

Devi, G. R., De Souza, A. T., Byrd, J. C., Jirtle, R. L. and MacDonald, R. G. (1999). Altered ligand binding by insulin-like growth factor II/mannose 6-phosphate receptors bearing missense mutations in human cancers. *Cancer Res*, **59**, 4314–9.

Diaz, E. and Pfeffer, S. R. (1998). TIP47: a cargo selection device for mannose 6-phosphate receptor trafficking. *Cell*, **93**, 433–43.

Dittmer, F. and von Figura, K. (1999). Phosphorylation of arylsulfatase A occurs through multiple interactions with the UDP-*N*-acetylglucosamine-1-phosphotransferase proximal and distal to its retrieval site by the KDEL receptor. *Biochem J*, **340**, 729–36.

Dittmer, F., Hafner, A., Ulbrich, E. J., Moritz, J. D., Schmidt, P., Schmahl, W. *et al.* (1998). I-Cell disease-like phenotype in mice deficient in mannose 6-phosphate receptors. *Transgenic Res*, **7**, 473–83.

Dittmer, F., Ulbrich, E. J., Hafner, A., Schmahl, W., Meister, T., Pohlmann, R. *et al.* (1999). Alternative mechanisms for trafficking of lysosomal enzymes in mannose 6-phosphate receptor-deficient mice are cell type-specific. *J Cell Sci*, **112**, 1591–7.

Do, H., Lee, W. S., Ghosh, P., Hollowell, T., Canfield, W. and Kornfeld, S. (2002). Human mannose 6-phosphate-uncovering enzyme is synthesized as a proenzyme that is activated by the endoprotease furin. *J Biol Chem*, **277**, 29737–44.

Doray, B., Bruns, K., Ghosh, P. and Kornfeld, S. (2002). Interaction of the cation-dependent mannose 6-phosphate receptor with GGA proteins. *J Biol Chem*, **277**, 18477–82.

Faulhaber, J., Fensom, A. and Hasilik, A. (1998). Abnormal lysosomal sorting with an enhanced secretion of cathepsin D precursor molecules bearing monoester phosphate groups. *Eur J Cell Biol*, **77**, 134–40.

Faust, P. L. and Kornfeld, S. (1989). Expression of the yeast aspartyl protease, proteinase A. Phosphorylation and binding to the mannose 6-phosphate receptor are altered by addition of cathepsin D sequences. *J Biol Chem*, **264**, 479–88.

Faust, P. L., Chirgwin, J. M. and Kornfeld, S. (1987). Renin, a secretory glycoprotein, acquires phosphomannosyl residues. *J Cell Biol*, **105**, 1947–55.

von Figura, K., Steckel, F., Conary, J., Hasilik, A. and Shaw, E. (1986). Heterogeneity in late-onset metachromatic leukodystrophy. Effect of inhibitors of cysteine proteinases. *Am J Hum Genet*, **39**, 371–82.

Fleckenstein, E., Dirks, W., Dehmel, U. and Drexler, H. G. (1996). Cloning and characterization of the human tartrate-resistant acid phosphatase (TRAP) gene. *Leukemia*, **10**, 637–43.

Fratantoni, J. C., Hall, C. W. and Neufeld, E. F. (1968). Hurler and Hunter syndromes: Mutual correction of the defect in cultured fibroblasts. *Science*, **162**, 570–2.

Freeze, H. (2001). Update and perspectives on congenital disorders of glycosylation. *Glycobiology*, **11**, 129R–43R.

Fu, Q., Carson, G. S., Hiraiwa, M., Grafe, M., Kishimoto, Y. and O'Brien, J. S. (1994). Occurrence of prosaposin as a neuronal surface membrane component. *J Mol Neurosci*, **5**, 59–67.

Garcia, M., Platet, N., Liaudet, E., Laurent, V., Derocq, D., Brouillet, J. P. *et al.* (1996). Biological and clinical significance of cathepsin D in breast cancer metastasis. *Stem Cells*, **14**, 642–50.

Gieselmann, V., Schmidt, B. and von Figura, K. (1992). *In vitro* mutagenesis of potential N-glycosylation sites of arylsulfatase A. Effects on glycosylation, phosphorylation, and intracellular sorting. *J Biol Chem*, **267**, 13262–6.

Gonzalez-Noriega, A. and Michalak, C. (2001). Mannose 6-phosphate-independent endocytosis of beta-glucuronidase. II. Purification of a cation-dependent receptor from bovine liver. *Biochim Biophys Acta*, **1538**, 152–61.

Gonzalez-Noriega, A., Grubb, J. H., Talkad, V. and Sly, W. S. (1980). Chloroquine inhibits lysosomal enzyme pinocytosis and enhances lysosomal enzyme secretion by impairing receptor recycling. *J Cell Biol*, **85**, 839–52.

Grässel, S. and Hasilik, A. (1992). Human cathepsin D precursor is associated with a 60 kDa glycosylated polypeptide. *Biochem Biophys Res Commun*, **182**, 276–82.

Haas, U. and Sparks, D. L. (1996). Cortical cathepsin D activity and immunolocalization in Alzheimer's disease, critical coronary artery disease, and aging. *Mol Chem Neuropathol*, **29**, 1–14.

Hancock, M. K., Yamani, R. D. and Dahms, N. M. (2002). Localization of the carbohydrate recognition sites of the insulin-like growth factor II/mannose 6-phosphate receptor to domains 3 and 9 of the extracytoplasmic region. *J Biol Chem*, 277, 47205–12.

Hasilik, A. and Neufeld, E. F. (1980*a*). Biosynthesis of lysosomal enzymes in fibroblasts synthesis as precursors of higher molecular weight. *J Biol Chem*, **255**, 4937–45.

Hasilik, A. and Neufeld E. F. (1980*b*). Biosynthesis of lysosomal enzymes. Phosphorylation of mannose residues. *J Biol Chem*, **255**, 4946–50.

Hasilik, A. and von Figura, K. (1981). Oligosaccharides in lysosomal enzymes. *Eur J Biochem*, **121**, 125–9.

Hasilik, A., Klein, U., Waheed, A., Strecker, G. and von Figura, K. (1980). Phosphorylated oligosaccharides in lysosomal enzymes: identification of α-*N*-acetylglucosamine(1)phospho(6)mannose diester groups. *Proc Natl Acad Sci USA*, **77**, 7074–8.

Hasilik, A., Waheed, A. and von Figura, K. (1981). Enzymatic phosphorylation of lysosomal enzymes in the presence of UDP-*N*-acetylglucosamine. Absence of the activity in I-cell fibroblasts. *Biochem Biophys Res Commun*, **98**, 761–7.

Hasilik, A., Waheed, A., Cantz, M. and von Figura, K. (1982). Impaired phosphorylation of lysosomal enzymes in fibroblasts of patients with mucolipidosis III. *Eur J Biochem*, **122**, 119–23.

Hasilik, A., Pohlmann, R., Olsen, R. L. and von Figura, K. (1984). Myeloperoxidase is synthesized as larger phosphorylated precursor. *EMBO J*, **3**, 2671–6.

Hayman, A. R., Macary, P., Lehner, P. J. and Cox, T. M. (2001). Tartrate-resistant acid phosphatase (Acp 5): identification in diverse human tissues and dendritic cells. *J Histochem Cytochem*, **49**, 675–84.

Heinrich, M., Wickel, M., Schneider-Brachert, W., Sandberg, C., Gahr, J., Schwandner, R. *et al.* (1999). Cathepsin D targeted by acid sphingomyelinase-derived ceramide. *EMBO J*, **18**, 5252–63.

Heinrich, M., Wickel, M., Winoto-Morbach, S., Schneider-Brachert, W., Weber, T., Brunner, J. *et al.* (2000). Ceramide as an activator lipid of cathepsin D. *Adv Exp Med Biol*, **477**, 305–15.

Herscovics, A. (1999). Importance of glycosidases in mammalian glycoprotein biosynthesis. *Biochim Biophys Acta*, **1473**, 96–107.

Herzog, V., Neumüller, W. and Holzmann, B. (1987). Thyroglobulin, the major and obligatory exportable protein of thyroid follicle cells, carries the lysosomal recognition marker mannose-6-phosphate. *EMBO J*, **6**, 555–60.

Hickman, S. and Neufeld, E. F. (1972). A hypothesis for I-cell disease: defective hydrolases that do not enter lysosomes. *Biochem Biophys Res Commun*, **49**, 992–9.

Hickman, S., Shapiro, L. J. and Neufeld, E. F. (1974). A recognition marker required for uptake of a lysosomal enzyme by cultured fibroblasts. *Biochem Biophys Res Commun*, **57**, 55–61.

Hiesberger, T., Huttler, S., Rohlmann, A., Schneider, W., Sandhoff, K. and Herz, J. (1998). Cellular uptake of saposin (SAP) precursor and lysosomal delivery by the low density lipoprotein receptor-related protein (LRP). *EMBO J*, **17**, 4617–25.

Hill, J. M., Lesniak, M. A., Kiess, W. and Nissley, S. P. (1988). Radioimmunohistochemical localization of type II IGF receptors in rat brain. *Peptides*, **9**, Suppl. 1, 181–7.

Hoflack, B. and Kornfeld, S. (1985). Purification and characterization of a cation-dependent mannose 6-phosphate receptor from murine P388D1 macrophages and bovine liver. *J Biol Chem*, **260**, 12008–14.

Horst, M. and Hasilik, A. (1991). Expression and maturation of human cathepsin D in baby-hamster kidney cells. *Biochem J*, **273**, 355–61.

Horst, M., Mares, M., Zabe, M., Hummel, M., Wiederanders, B., Kirschke, H. *et al.* (1993). Synthesis of phosphorylated oligosaccharides in lysozyme is enhanced by fusion to cathepsin D. *J Biol Chem*, **268**, 19690–6.

Hubler, M., Haskins, M. E., Arnold, S., Kaser-Hotz, B., Bosshard, N. U., Briner, J. *et al.* (1996). Mucolipidosis type II in a domestic shorthair cat. *J Small Anim Pract*, **37**, 435–41.

Huizing, M., Anikster, Y. and Gahl, W. A. (2001). Hermansky–Pudlak syndrome and Chédiak–Higashi syndrome: disorders of vesicle formation and trafficking. *Thromb Haemost*, **86**, 233–45.

Imai, K. (1988). A macrophage receptor for liver lysosomal beta-glucosidase. *Cell Struct Funct*, **13**, 325–32.

Isidoro, C., Grässel, S., Baccino, F. M. and Hasilik, A. (1991). Determination of the phosphorylation, uncovering of mannose 6-phosphate groups and targeting of lysosomal enzymes. *Eur J Clin Chem Clin Biochem*, **29**, 165–71.

Jadot, M., Canfield, W. M., Gregory, W. and Kornfeld, S. (1992). Characterization of the signal for rapid internalization of the bovine mannose-6-phosphate/insulin-like growth factor II receptor. *J Biol Chem*, **267**, 11069–77.

Jadot, M., Lin, L., Sleat, D. E., Sohar, I., Hsu, M. S., Pintar, J. *et al.* (1999). Subcellular localization of mannose 6-phosphate glycoproteins in rat brain. *J Biol Chem*, **274**, 21104–13.

Jirtle, R. L., Carr, B. I. and Scott, C. D. (1991). Modulation of insulin-like growth factor-II/mannose 6-phosphate receptors and transforming growth factor-beta 1 during liver regeneration. *J Biol Chem*, **266**, 22444–50.

Johnson, K. F., Chan, W. and Kornfeld, S. (1990). Cation-dependent mannose 6-phosphate receptor contains two internalization signals in its cytoplasmic domain. *Proc Natl Acad Sci USA*, **87**, 10010–4.

Jorgensen, M. U., Emr, S. D. and Winther, J. R. (1999). Ligand recognition and domain structure of Vps10p, a vacuolar protein sorting receptor in *Saccharomyces cerevisiae*. *Eur J Biochem*, **260**, 461–9.

Kakkis, E. D. (2002). Enzyme replacement therapy for the mucopolysaccharide storage disorders. *Expert Opin Investig Drugs*, **11**, 675–85.

Kakkis, E. D., Muenzer, J., Tiller, G. E., Waber, L., Belmont, J., Passage, M. *et al.* (2001). Enzyme-replacement therapy in mucopolysaccharidosis I. *N Engl J Med*, **2001**, 182–8.

Kang, J. X., Li, Y. and Leaf, A. (1997). Mannose-6-phosphate/insulin-like growth factor-II receptor is a receptor for retinoic acid. *Proc Natl Acad Sci USA*, **94**, 13671–6.

Kaplan, A., Achord, D. T. and Sly, W. S. (1977). Phosphohexosyl components of a lysosomal enzyme are recognized by pinocytosis receptors on human fibroblasts. *Proc Natl Acad Sci USA*, **74**, 2026–30.

Karlsson, K. and Carlsson, S. R. (1998). Sorting of lysosomal membrane glycoproteins LAMP-1 and LAMP-2 into vesicles distinct from mannose 6-phosphate receptor/gamma-adaptin vesicles at the trans-Golgi network. *J Biol Chem*, **273**, 18966–73.

Kasper, D., Dittmer, F., von Figura, K. and Pohlmann, R. (1996). Neither type of mannose 6-phosphate receptor is sufficient for targeting of lysosomal enzymes along intracellular routes. *J Cell Biol*, **134**, 615–23.

Kato, G. and Suzuki, Y. (1985). Membrane-bound *N*-acetyl-beta-glucosaminidase. Different binding specificity in control and I-cell disease livers. *FEBS Lett*, **193**, 222–6.

Kauppi, M., Simonsen, A., Bremnes, B., Vieira, A., Callaghan, J., Stenmark, H. *et al.* (2002). The small GTPase Rab22 interacts with EEA1 and controls endosomal membrane trafficking. *J Cell Sci*, **115**, 899–911.

Kiess, W., Blickenstaff, G. D., Sklar, M. M., Thomas, C. L., Nissley, S. P. and Sahagian, G. G. (1988). Biochemical evidence that the type II insulin-like growth factor receptor is identical to the cation-independent mannose 6-phosphate receptor. *J Biol Chem*, **263**, 9339–44.

Klumperman, J., Hille, A., Veenendaal, T., Oorschot, V., Stoorvogel, W., von Figura, K. *et al.* (1993). Differences in the endosomal distributions of the two mannose 6-phosphate receptors. *J Cell Biol*, **121**, 997–1010.

Kolset, S. O., Mann, D. M., Uhlin-Hansen, L., Winberg, J. O. and Ruoslahti, E. (1996). Serglycin-binding proteins in activated macrophages and platelets. *J Leukoc Biol*, **59**, 545–54.

Kornfeld, S. (1992). Structure and function of the mannose 6-phosphate/insulin like growth factor II receptors. *Annu Rev Biochem*, **61**, 307–30.

Kornfeld, S. and Sly, W. S. (2001). I-Cell disease and pseudo-Hurler polydystrophy: Disorders of lysosomal enzyme phosphorylation and localization. In *The metabolic & molecular bases of inherited disease* (Scriver, C. R., Beaudet, A. L., Sly, W. S. and Valle, D., ed.) Vol. III, pp. 3469–82. New York: McGraw-Hill.

Kornfeld, R., Bao, M., Brewer, K., Noll, C. and Canfield, W. M. (1998). Purification and multimeric structure of bovine *N*-acetylglucosamine-1-phosphodiester alpha-*N*-acetylglucosaminidase. *J Biol Chem*, **273**, 23203–10.

Kornfeld, R., Bao, M., Brewer, K., Noll, C. and Canfield, W. (1999). Molecular cloning and functional expression of two splice forms of human *N*-acetylglucosamine-1-phosphodiester α-*N*-acetylglucosaminidase. *J Biol Chem*, **274**, 32778–85.

Kovacina, K. S., Steele-Perkins, G., Purchio, A. F., Lioubin, M., Miyazono, K., Heldin, C. H. *et al.* (1989). Interactions of recombinant and platelet transforming growth factor-beta 1 precursor with the insulin-like growth factor II/mannose 6-phosphate receptor. *Biochem Biophys Res Commun*, **160**, 393–403.

Kundra, R. and Kornfeld, S. (1999). Asparagine-linked oligosaccharides protect LAMP-1 and LAMP-2 from intracellular proteolysis. *J Biol Chem*, **274**, 31039–46.

Lang, L., Reitman, M., Tang, J., Roberts, R. M. and Kornfeld, S. (1984). Lysosomal enzyme phosphorylation. Recognition of a protein-dependent determinant allows specific phosphorylation of oligosaccharides present on lysosomal enzymes. *J Biol Chem*, **259**, 14663–71.

Le Borgne, R. and Hoflack, B. (1998). Protein transport from the secretory to the endocytic pathway in mammalian cells. *Biochim Biophys Acta*, **1404**, 195–209.

Leduc, R., Molloy, S. S., Thorne, B. A. and Thomas, G. J. (1992). Activation of human furin precursor processing endoprotease occurs by an intramolecular autoproteolytic cleavage. *J Biol Chem*, **267**, 14304–8.

Lee, S. J. and Nathans, D. (1988). Proliferin secreted by cultured cells binds to mannose 6-phosphate receptors. *J Biol Chem*, **263**, 3521–7.

Lee, J. K. and Pierce, M. (1995). Purification and characterization of human serum *N*-acetylglucosamine-1-phosphodiester α-*N*-acetylglucosaminidase. *Arch Biochem Biophys*, **319**, 413–25.

Lee, W. S., Rohrer, J., Kornfeld, R. and Kornfeld, S. (2002). Multiple signals regulate trafficking of the mannose 6-phosphate-uncovering enzyme. *J Biol Chem*, **277**, 3544–51.

Lefrancois, S., May, T., Knight, C., Bourbeau, D. and Morales, C. R. (2002). The lysosomal transport of prosaposin requires the conditional interaction of its highly conserved D domain with sphingomyelin. *J Biol Chem*, **277**, 17188–99.

Lehtovirta, M., Kyttala, A., Eskelinen, E. L., Hess, M., Heinonen, O. and Jalanko, A. (2001). Palmitoyl protein thioesterase (PPT) localizes into synaptosomes and synaptic vesicles in neurons: implications for infantile neuronal ceroid lipofuscinosis (INCL). *Hum Mol Genet*, **10**, 69–75.

Leistner, S., Young, E., Meaney, C. and Winchester, B. (1995). Pseudodeficiency of arylsulfatase A: strategy for clarification of genotype in families of subjects with low ASA activity and neurological symptoms. *J Inherit Metab Dis*, **18**, 710–6.

Lemansky, P. and Hasilik, A. (2001). Chondroitin sulfate is involved in lysosomal transport of lysozyme in U937 cells. *J Cell Sci*, **114**, 345–52.

Lemansky, P., Gerecitano-Schmidek, M., Das, R. C., Schmidt, B. and Hasilik, A. (2003). Targeting of myeloperoxidase to azurophilic granules in HL-60 cells. *J Leukoc Biol* (in press).

Lemansky, P. and Herzog, V. (1992). Endocytosis of thyroglobulin is not mediated by mannose-6-phosphate receptors in thyrocytes. *Eur J Biochem*, **209**, 111–9.

Lemansky, P., Brix, K. and Herzog, V. (1999). Subcellular distribution, secretion, and posttranslational modifications of clusterin in thyrocytes. *Exp Cell Res*, **251**, 147–55.

Leonova, T. and Grabowski, G. A. (2000). Fate and sorting of acid beta-glucosidase in transgenic mammalian cells. *Mol Genet Metab*, **70**, 281–94.

Leroy, J. G. and DeMars, R. I. (1967). Mutant enzymatic and cytological phenotypes in cultured human fibroblasts. *Science*, **157**, 804–6.

Li, H. H., Zhao, H. Z., Neufeld, E. F., Cai, Y. and Gomez-Pinilla, F. (2002). Attenuated plasticity in neurons and astrocytes in the mouse model of Sanfilippo syndrome type B. *J Neurosci Res*, **69**, 30–8.

Ling, P. and Roberts, R. M. (1993*a*). Overexpression of uteroferrin, a lysosomal acid phosphatase found in porcine uterine secretions, results in its high rate of secretion from transfected fibroblasts. *Biol Reprod*, **49**, 1317–27.

Ling, P. and Roberts, R. M. (1993*b*). Uteroferrin and intracellular tartrate-resistant acid phosphatases are the products of the same gene. *J Biol Chem*, **268**, 6896–902.

Liu, Q., Grubb, J. H., Huang, S. S., Sly, W. S. and Huang, J. S. (1999). The mannose 6-phosphate/insulin-like growth factor-II receptor is a substrate of type V transforming growth factor-beta receptor. *J Biol Chem*, **274**, 20002–10.

Liuzzo, J. P., Petanceska, S. S. and Devi, L. A. (1999*a*). Neurotrophic factors regulate cathepsin S in macrophages and microglia: a role in the degradation of myelin basic protein and amyloid beta peptide. *Mol Med*, **5**, 334–43.

Liuzzo, J. P., Petanceska, S. S., Moscatelli, D. and Devi, L. A. (1999*b*). Inflammatory mediators regulate cathepsin S in macrophages and microglia: a role in attenuating heparan sulfate interactions. *Mol Med*, **5**, 320–33.

Ludwig, T., Munier-Lehmann, H., Bauer, U., Hollinshead, M., Ovitt, C., Lobel, P. *et al.* (1994). Differential sorting of lysosomal enzymes in mannose 6-phosphate receptor-deficient fibroblasts. *EMBO J*, **13**, 3430–7.

Lukong, K. E., Seyrantepe, V., Landry, K., Trudel, S., Ahmad, A., Gahl, W. A. *et al.* (2001). Intracellular distribution of lysosomal sialidase is controlled by the internalization signal in its cytoplasmic tail. *J Biol Chem*, **49**, 46172–81.

MacDonald, R. G., Pfeffer, S. R., Coussens, L., Tepper, M. A., Brocklebank, C. M., Mole, J. E. *et al.* (1988). A single receptor binds both insulin-like growth factor II and mannose-6-phosphate. *Science*, **239**, 1134–7.

Marron-Terada, P. G., Brzycki-Wessell, M. A. and Dahms, N. M. (1998). The two mannose 6-phosphate binding sites of the insulin-like growth factor-II/mannose 6-phosphate receptor display different ligand binding properties. *J Biol Chem*, **273**, 22358–66.

Martin, J. J., Leroy, J. G., Farriaux, J. P., Fontaine, G., Desnick, R. J. and Cabello, A. (1975). I-Cell disease (mucolipidosis II): a report on its pathology. *Acta Neuropathol*, **30**, 285–305.

Mathews, P. M., Guerra, C. B., Jiang, Y., Grbovic, O. M., Kao, B. H., Schmidt, S. D. *et al.* (2002). Alzheimer's disease-related overexpression of the cation-dependent mannose 6-phosphate receptor increases Abeta secretion: role for altered lysosomal hydrolase distribution in beta-amyloidogenesis. *J Biol Chem*, **277**, 5299–307.

Mehta, A. (2002). New developments in the management of Anderson-Fabry disease. *QJM*, **95**, 647–53.

Meyer, C., Zizioli, D., Lausmann, S., Eskelinen, E.-L., Hamann, J., Saftig, P. *et al.* (2000). μ1A-adaptin-deficient mice: lethality, loss of AP-1 binding and rerouting of mannose 6-phosphate receptors. *EMBO J*, **19**, 2193–203.

Meyer, C., Eskelinen, E. L., Guruprasad, M. R., von Figura, K. and Schu, P. (2001). Mu 1A deficiency induces a profound increase in MPR300/IGF-II receptor internalization rate. *J Cell Sci*, **114**, 4469–76.

Michel, F. J., Fliss, M. F., Bazer, F. W. and Simmen, R. C. (1992). Characterization and developmental expression of binding sites for the transplacental iron transport protein, uteroferrin, in fetal hematopoietic tissues. *Biol Neonate*, **61**, 82–91.

Miller, A. L., Kress, B. C., Stein, R., Kinnon, C., Kern, H., Schneider, J. A. *et al.* (1981). Properties of *N*-acetyl-beta-D-hexosaminidase from isolated normal and I-cell lysosomes. *J Biol Chem*, **256**, 9352–62.

Misra, S., Puertollano, R., Kato, Y., Bonifacino, J. S. and Hurley, J. H. (2002). Structural basis for acidic-cluster-dileucine sorting-signal recognition by VHS-domains. *Nature*, **415**, 933–7.

Moin, K., Demchik, L., Mai, J., Duessing, J., Peters, C. and Sloane, B. F. (2000). Observing proteases in living cells. *Adv Exp Med Biol*, **477**, 391–401.

Morgan, D. O., Edman, J. C., Standring, D. N., Fried, V. A., Smith, M. C., Roth, R. A. *et al.* (1987). Insulin-like growth factor II receptor as a multifunctional binding protein. *Nature*, **329**, 301–7.

Motyka, B., Korbutt, G., Pinkoski, J., Heibein, J. A., Caputo, A., Hobman, M. *et al.* (2000). Mannose 6-phosphate/insulin-like growth factor II receptor is a death receptor for granzyme B during cytotoxic T cell-induced apoptosis. *Cell*, **103**, 491–500.

Munier-Lehmann, H., Mauxion, F., Bauer, U., Lobel, P. and Hoflack, B. (1996). Re-expression of the mannose 6-phosphate receptors in receptor-deficient fibroblasts. Complementary function of the two mannose 6-phosphate receptors in lysosomal enzyme targeting. *J Biol Chem*, **271**, 15166–74.

Myerowitz, R., Lawson, D., Mizukami, H., Mi, Y., Tifft, C. J. and Proia, R. L. (2002). Molecular pathophysiology in Tay–Sachs and Sandhoff diseases as revealed by gene expression profiling. *Hum Mol Genet*, **11**, 1343–50.

Natowicz, M. R., Chi, M. M. Y., Lowry, O. H. and Sly, W. S. (1979). Enzymatic identification of mannose 6-phosphate on the recognition marker for receptor-mediated pinocytosis of β-glucuronidase by human fibroblasts. *Proc Natl Acad Sci USA*, **76**, 4322–6.

Neufeld, E. F. (1980). The uptake of enzymes into lysosomes: An overview. *Birth Defects* orig Artic sec. 16, 77–84.

Neufeld, E. F., Lim, T. W. and Shapiro, L. J. (1975). Inherited disorders of lysosomal metabolism. *Annu Rev Biochem*, **44**, 357–76.

Nishikawa, A., Gregory, W., Frenz, J., Cacia, J. and Kornfeld, S. (1997). The phosphorylation of bovine DNase I Asn-linked oligosaccharides is dependent on specific lysine and arginine residues. *J Biol Chem*, **272**, 19408–12.

Nishikawa, A., Nanda, A., Gregory, W., Frenz, J. and Kornfeld, S. (1999). Identification of amino acids that modulate mannose phosphorylation of mouse DNase I, a secretory glycoprotein. *J Biol Chem*, **274**, 19309–15.

Nissler, K., Kreusch, S., Rommeskirch, W., Strubel, W., Weber, E. and Wiederanders, B. (1998). Sorting of non-glycosylated human procathepsin S in mammalian cells. *Biol Chem*, **379**, 219–24.

Nixon, R. A. (2000). A "protease activation cascade" in the pathogenesis of Alzheimer's disease. *Ann N Y Acad Sci*, **924**, 117–31.

Nykjaer, A., Christensen, E. I., Vorum, H., Hager, H., Petersen, C. M., Roigaard, H. *et al.* (1998). Mannose 6-phosphate/insulin-like growth factor-II receptor targets the urokinase receptor to lysosomes via a novel binding interaction. *J Cell Biol*, **141**, 815–28.

O'Brien, J. S., Carson, G. S., Seo, H. C., Hiraiwa, M., Weiler, S., Tomich, J. M. *et al.* (1995). Identification of the neurotrophic factor sequence of prosaposin. *FASEB J*, **9**, 681–5.

O'Dell, S. D. and Day, I. N. (1998). Insulin-like growth factor II (IGF-II). *Int J Biochem Cell Biol*, **30**, 767–71.

Obermüller, S., Kiecke, C., von Figura, K. and Honing, S. (2002). The tyrosine motifs of LAMP1 and LAP determine their direct targeting to lysosomes. *J Cell Sci*, **115**, 185–94.

Okada, S., Owada, M., Sakiyama, T., Yutaka, T. and Ogawa, M. (1985). I-Cell disease: clinical studies of 21 Japanese cases. *Clin Genet*, **28**, 207–15.

Orlacchio, A., Martino, S., Sarchielli, P., Gallai, V. and Emiliani, C. (1998). Beta-*N*-acetylhexosaminidase in peripheral blood lymphocytes and monocytes in the different forms and stages of multiple sclerosis. *J Neurochem*, **71**, 1168–76.

Orsel, J. G., Sincock, P. M., Krise, J. P. and Pfeffer, S. R. (2000). Recognition of the 300-kDa mannose 6-phosphate receptor cytoplasmic domain by 47-kDa tail-interacting protein. *Proc Natl Acad Sci USA*, **97**, 9047–51.

Oshima, A., Nolan, C. M., Kyle, J. W., Grubb, J. H. and Sly, W. S. (1988). The human cation-independent mannose 6-phosphate receptor. Cloning and sequence of the full-length cDNA and expression of functional receptor in COS cells. *J Biol Chem*, **263**, 2553–62.

Page, T., Zhao, K. W., Tao, L. and Miller, A. L. (1996). Purification and characterization of human lymphoblast *N*-acetylglucosamine-1-phosphodiester alpha-*N*-acetylglucosaminidase. *Glycobiology*, **6**, 619–26.

Peters, C. and von Figura, K. (1994). Biogenesis of lysosomal membranes. *FEBS Lett*, **346**, 108–14.

Poenaru, L. (2001). From gene transfer to gene therapy in lysosomal storage diseases affecting the central nervous system. *Ann Med*, **33**, 28–36.

Pohlmann, R., Nagel, G., Schmidt, B., Stein, M., Lorkowski, G., Krentler, C. *et al.* (1987). Cloning of a cDNA encoding the human cation-dependent mannose 6-phosphate-specific receptor. *Proc Natl Acad Sci USA*, **84**, 5575–5579.

Pohlmann, R., Boeker, M. W. and von Figura, K. (1995). The two mannose 6-phosphate receptors transport distinct complements of lysosomal proteins. *J Biol Chem*, **270**, 27311–8.

Porwoll, S., Loch, N., Nuck, R., Grunow, D., Reutter, W. and Tauber, R. (1998). Cell surface glycoproteins undergo postbiosynthetic modification of their N-glycans by stepwise demannosylation. *J Biol Chem*, **273**, 1075–85.

Press, B., Feng, Y., Hoflack, B. and Wandinger-Ness, A. (1998). Mutant Rab7 causes the accumulation of cathepsin D and cation-independent mannose 6-phosphate receptor in an early endocytic compartment. *J Cell Biol*, **140**, 1075–89.

Puertollano, R., Aguilar, R. C., Gorshkova, I., Crouch, R. J. and Bonifacino, J. S. (2001). Sorting of mannose 6-phosphate receptors mediated by the GGAs. *Science*, **292**, 1712–6.

Purchio, A. F., Cooper, J. A., Brunner, A. M., Lioubin, M. N., Gentry, L. E., Kovacina, K. S. *et al.* (1988). Identification of mannose 6-phosphate in two asparagine-linked sugar chains of recombinant transforming growth factor-beta 1 precursor. *J Biol Chem*, **263**, 14211–5.

Qi, X. and Grabowski, G. A. (2001). Differential membrane interactions of saposins A and C: implications for the functional specificity. *J Biol Chem*, **276**, 27010–7.

Qi, X., Qin, W., Sun, Y., Kondoh, K. and Grabowski, G. A. (1996). Functional organization of saposin C. Definition of the neurotrophic and acid beta-glucosidase activation regions. *J Biol Chem*, **271**, 6874–80.

Raas-Rothschild, A., Cormier-Daire, V., Bao, M., Genin, E., Salomon, R., Brewer, K. *et al.* (2000). Molecular basis of variant pseudo-Hurler polydystrophy (mucolipidosis IIIC). *J Clin Invest*, **105**, 673–81.

Raben, N., Plotz, P. and Byrne, B. J. (2002). Acid alpha-glucosidase deficiency (glycogenosis type II, Pompe disease). *Curr Mol Med*, **2**, 145–66.

Radons, J., Isidoro, C. and Hasilik, A. (1990). Brefeldin A prevents uncovering but not phosphorylation of the recognition marker in cathepsin D. *Biol Chem*, **371**, 567–73.

Reitman, M. L. and Kornfeld, S. (1981*a*). UDP-*N*-Acetylglucosamine: glycoprotein *N*-acetylglucosamine-1-phosphotransferase. *J Biol Chem*, **256**, 4275–81.

Reitman, M. L. and Kornfeld, S. (1981*b*). Lysosomal enzyme targeting. *N*-Acetylglucosaminyl-phosphotransferase selectively phosphorylates native lysosomal enzymes. *J Biol Chem*, **256**, 11977–80.

Reitman, M. L., Varki, A. and Kornfeld, S. (1981). Fibroblasts from patients with I-cell disease and pseudo-Hurler polydystrophy are deficient in uridine 5′-diphosphate-*N*-acetylglucosamine: glycoprotein *N*-acetylglucosaminylphosphotransferase activity. *J Clin Invest*, **67**, 1574–9.

Reusch, U., Bernhard, O., Koszinowski, U. and Schu, P. (2002). AP-1A and AP-3A lysosomal sorting functions. *Traffic*, **10**, 752–61.

Ricotta, D., Conner, S. D., Schmid, S. L., von Figura, K. and Honing, S. (2002). Phosphorylation of the AP2 μ subunit by AAK1 mediates high affinity binding to membrane protein sorting signals. *J Cell Biol*, **156**, 791–5.

Riederer, M. A., Soldati, T., Shapiro, A. D., Lin, J. and Pfeffer, S. R. (1994). Lysosome biogenesis requires Rab9 function and receptor recycling from endosomes to the trans-Golgi network. *J Cell Biol*, **125**, 573–82.

Rijnboutt, S., Aerts, H. M., Geuze, H. J., Tager, J. M. and Strous, G. J. (1991). Mannose 6-phosphate-independent membrane association of cathepsin D, glucocerebrosidase, and sphingolipid-activating protein in HepG2 cells. *J Biol Chem*, **266**, 4862–8.

Roberts, D. L., Weix, D. J., Dahms, N. M. and Kim, J.-J. P. (1998). Molecular basis of lysosomal recognition: three-dimensional structure of the cation-dependent mannose 6-phosphate receptor. *Cell*, **93**, 639–48.

Rohrer, J. and Kornfeld, R. (2001). Lysosomal hydrolase mannose 6-phosphate uncovering enzyme resides in the trans-Golgi network. *Mol Biol Cell*, **12**, 1623–31.

Rosenberg, G. A. (2002). Matrix metalloproteinases in neuroinflammation. *Glia*, **39**, 279–91.

Rosenfeld, J. L., Moore, R. H., Zimmer, K. P., Alpizar-Foster, E., Dai, W., Zarka, M. N. *et al.* (2001). Lysosome proteins are redistributed during expression of a GTP-hydrolysis-defective rab5a. *J Cell Sci*, **114**, 4499–508.

Rothman, J. H., Yamashiro, C. T., Raymond, C. K., Kane, P. M. and Stevens, T. H. (1989). Acidification of the lysosome-like vacuole and the vacuolar H^+-ATPase are deficient in two yeast mutants that fail to sort vacuolar proteins. *J Cell Biol*, **109**, 93–100.

Rouille, Y., Rohn, W. and Hoflack, B. (2000). Targeting of lysosomal proteins. *Semin Cell Dev Biol*, **11**, 165–71.

Row, P. E., Reaves, B. J., Domin, J., Luzio, J. P. and Davidson, H. W. (2001). Overexpression of a rat kinase-deficient phosphoinositide 3-kinase, Vps34p, inhibits cathepsin D maturation. *Biochem J*, **353**, 655–61.

Sahagian, G. G., Distler, J. and Jourdian, G. W. (1981). Characterization of a membrane-associated receptor from bovine liver that binds phosphomannosyl residues of bovine testicular beta-galactosidase. *Proc Natl Acad Sci USA*, **78**, 4289–93.

Sampath, D., Varki, A. and Freeze, H. H. (1992). The spectrum of incomplete N-linked oligosaccharides synthesized by endothelial cells in the presence of brefeldin A. *J Biol Chem*, **267**, 4440–55.

Saunders, P. T., Renegar, R. H., Raub, T. J., Baumbach, G. A., Atkinson, P. H., Bazer, F. W. *et al.* (1985). The carbohydrate structure of porcine uteroferrin and the role of the high mannose chains in promoting uptake by the reticuloendothelial cells of the fetal liver. *J Biol Chem*, **260**, 3658–65.

Scharf, J. G., Dombrowski, F. and Ramadori, G. (2001). The IGF axis and hepatocarcinogenesis. *Mol Pathol*, **54**, 138–44.

Schierau, A., Dietz, F., Lange, H., Schestag, F., Parastar, A. and Gieselmann, V. (1999). Interaction of arylsulfatase A with UDP-*N*-acetylglucosamine: Lysosomal enzyme-*N*-acetylglucosamine-1-phosphotransferase. *J Biol Chem*, **274**, 3651–8.

Schiffmann, R. and Brady, R. O. (2002). New prospects for the treatment of lysosomal storage diseases. *Drugs*, **62**, 733–42.

Schindelmeiser, J., Radzun, H. J. and Munstermann, D. (1991). Tartrate-resistant, purple acid phosphatase in Gaucher cells of the spleen. Immuno- and cytochemical analysis. *Pathol Res Pract*, **187**, 209–13.

Schuette, C. G., Pierstorff, B., Huettler, S. and Sandhoff, K. (2001). Sphingolipid activator proteins: proteins with complex functions in lipid degradation and skin biogenesis. *Glycobiology*, **11**, 81R–90R.

Schweizer, A., Kornfeld, S. and Rohrer, J. (1996). Cysteine 34 of the cytoplasmic tail of the cation-dependent mannose 6-phosphate receptor is reversibly palmitoylated and required for normal trafficking and lysosomal enzyme sorting. *J Cell Biol*, **132**, 577–84.

Shen, N., Li, Z. G., Waye, J. S., Francis, G. and Chang, P. L. (1993). Complications in the genotypic molecular diagnosis of pseudo arylsulfatase A deficiency. *Am J Med Genet*, **45**, 631–7.

Shiba, T., Takatsu, H., Nogi, T., Matsugaki, N., Kawasaki, M., Igarashi, N. *et al.* (2002). Structural basis for recognition of acidic-cluster dileucine sequence by GGA1. *Nature*, **415**, 937–41.

Sleat, D. E., Sohar, I., Lackland, H., Majercak, J. and Lobel, P. (1996). Rat brain contains high levels of mannose-6-phosphorylated glycoproteins including lysosomal enzymes and palmitoyl-protein thioesterase, an enzyme implicated in infantile neuronal lipofuscinosis. *J Biol Chem*, **271**, 19191–8.

Sleat, D. E., Sohar, I., Pullarkat, P. S., Lobel, P. and Pullarkat, R. K. (1998). Specific alterations in levels of mannose 6-phosphorylated glycoproteins in different neuronal ceroid lipofuscinoses. *Biochem J*, **334**, 547–51.

Sohar, I., Sleat, D., Gong Liu, C., Ludwig, T. and Lobel, P. (1998). Mouse mutants lacking the cation-independent mannose 6-phosphate/insulin-like growth factor II receptor are impaired in lysosomal enzyme transport: Comparison of cation-independent and cation-dependent mannose 6-phosphate receptor-deficient mice. *Biochem J*, **330**, 903–8.

Spranger, J. W. and Weidemann, H. R. (1970). The genetic mucolipidoses. *Hum Genet*, **9**, 113–39.

Stinchcombe, J. C. and Griffiths, G. M. (2001). Normal and abnormal secretion by haemopoietic cells. *Immunology*, **103**, 10–16.

Strömberg, K., Persson, A.-M. and Olsson, I. (1986). The processing and intracellular transport of myeloperoxidase—modulation by lysosomotropic agents and monensin. *Eur J Cell Biol*, **39**, 424–31.

Suter, A., Everts, V., Boyde, A., Jones, S. J., Lullmann-Rauch, R., Hartmann, D. *et al.* (2001). Overlapping functions of lysosomal acid phosphatase (LAP) and tartrate-resistant acid phosphatase (Acp5) revealed by doubly deficient mice. *Development*, **128**, 4899–910.

Takahashi, T., Schmidt, P. G. and Tang, J. (1983). Oligosaccharide units of lysosomal cathepsin D from porcine spleen. Amino acid sequence and carbohydrate structure of glycopeptides. *J Biol Chem*, **258**, 2819–30.

den Tandt, W. R. (1980). Affinity chromatography of lysosomal enzymes in plasma, urine and fibroblasts of patients with mucolipidosis (ML) II and III. *Clin Chim Acta*, **28**, 199–205.

Taniguchi, T., Mizuochi, T., Towatari, T., Katunuma, N. and Kobata, A. (1985). Structural studies on the carbohydrate moieties of rat liver cathepsins B and H. *J Biochem (Tokyo)*, **97**, 973–6.

Tao, K., Li, J., Warner, J., MacLeod, K., Miller, F. R. and Sahagian, G. G. (2001). Multiple lysosomal trafficking phenotypes in metastatic mouse mammary tumor cell lines. *Int J Oncol*, **19**, 1333–9.

Tauber, R., Park, C. S., Becker, A., Geyer, R. and Reutter, W. (1989). Rapid intramolecular turnover of N-linked glycans in plasma membrane glycoproteins. *Eur J Biochem*, **186**, 55–62.

Temesvari, L. A., Rodriguez-Paris, J. M., Bush, J. M., Zhang, L. and Cardelli, J. A. (1996). Involvement of the vacuolar proton-translocating ATPase in multiple steps of the endo-lysosomal system and in the contractile vacuole system of *Dictyostelium discoideum*. *J Cell Sci*, **109**, 1479–95.

Tikkanen, R., Peltola, M., Oinonen, C., Rouvinen, J. and Peltonen, L. (1997). Several cooperating binding sites mediate the interaction of a lysosomal enzyme with phosphotransferase. *EMBO J*, **16**, 6684–93.

Tondeur, M., Vamos-Hurwitz, E., Mockel-Pohl, S., Dereume, J. P., Cremer, N. and Loeb, H. (1971). Clinical, biochemical, and ultrastructural studies in a case of chondrodystrophy presenting the I-cell phenotype in tissue culture. *J Pediatr*, **79**, 366–78.

Tsuji, A., Omura, K. and Suzuki, Y. (1988). Intracellular transport of acid alpha-glucosidase in human fibroblasts: evidence for involvement of phosphomannosyl receptor-independent system. *J Biochem*, **104**, 276–8.

Ullrich, K., Mersmann, G., Fleischer, M. and von Figura, K. (1978*a*). Epithelial rat liver cells have cell surface receptors recognizing a phosphorylated carbohydrate on lysosomal enzymes. *Hoppe Seylers Z Physiol Chem*, **359**, 1591–8.

Ullrich, K., Mersmann, G., Weber, E., and von Figura, K. (1978*b*). Evidence for lysosomal enzyme recognition by human fibroblasts via a phosphorylated carbohydrate moiety. *Biochem J*, **170**, 643–50.

Vaccaro, A. M., Salvioli, R., Tatti, M. and Ciaffoni, F. (1999). Saposins and their interaction with lipids. *Neurochem Res*, **24**, 307–14.

Van den Hout, J. M., Reuser, A. J., De Klerk, J. B., Arts, W. F., Smeitink, J. A. and Van der Ploeg, A. T. (2001). Enzyme therapy for Pompe disease with recombinant human alpha-glucosidase from rabbit milk. *J Inherit Metab Dis*, **24**, 266–74.

Varki, A. and Kornfeld, S. (1980*a*). Identification of a rat liver alpha-*N*-acetylglucosaminyl phosphodiesterase capable of removing "blocking" alpha-*N*-acetylglucosaminyl residues from phosphorylated high mannose oligosaccharides of lysosomal enzymes. *J Biol Chem*, **255**, 8398–401.

Varki, A. and Kornfeld, S. (1980*b*). Structural studies of phosphorylated high mannose-type oligosaccharides. *J Biol Chem*, **255**, 10847–58.

Varki, A. P., Reitman, M. L. and Kornfeld, S. (1981). Identification of a variant of mucolipidosis III (pseudo-Hurler polydystrophy): a catalytically active *N*-acetylglucosaminylphosphotransferase that fails to phosphorylate lysosomal enzymes. *Proc Natl Acad Sci USA*, **78**, 7773–7.

Varki, A., Sherman, W. and Kornfeld, S. (1983). Demonstration of the enzymatic mechanisms of α-*N*-acetyl-D-glucosamine-1-phosphodiester *N*-acetylglucosaminidase (formerly called α-*N*-acetylglucosaminylphosphodiesterase) and lysosomal α-*N*-acetylglucosaminidase. *Arch Biochem Biophys*, **222**, 145–9.

Verkruyse, L. A. and Hofmann, S. L. (1996). Lysosomal targeting of palmitoyl-protein thioesterase. *J Biol Chem*, **271**, 15831–6.

Vladutiu, G. D. (1983). Effect of the co-existence of galactosyl and phosphomannosyl residues on beta-hexosaminidase on the processing and transport of the enzyme in mucolipidosis I fibroblasts. *Biochim Biophys Acta*, **760**, 363–70.

Volpert, O., Jackson, D., Bouck, N. and Linzer, D. I. (1996). The insulin-like growth factor II/mannose 6-phosphate receptor is required for proliferin-induced angiogenesis. *Endocrinology*, **137**, 3871–6.

Wada, R., Tifft, C. J. and Proia, R. L. (2000). Microglial activation precedes acute neurodegeneration in Sandhoff disease and is suppressed by bone marrow transplantation. *Proc Natl Acad Sci USA*, **20**, 10954–9.

Waguri, S., Dewitte, F., Le Borgne, R., Rouillé, Y., Uchiyama, Y., Dubremetz, J.-F., and Hoflack, B. (2003). Visualization of TGB to endosome trafficking through fluorescently labeled MPR and AP-1 in living cells. *Mol Biol Cell*, **14**, 142–55.

Waheed, A. and von Figura, K. (1990). Rapid equilibrium between monomeric, dimeric and tetrameric forms of the 46-kDa mannose 6-phosphate receptor at 37 degrees C. Possible relation to the function of the receptor. *Eur J Biochem*, **193**, 47–54.

Waheed, A., Hasilik, A. and von Figura, K. (1981*a*). Enhanced breakdown of arylsulfatase A in multiple sulfatase deficiency. *Eur J Biochem*, **123**, 317–21.

Waheed, A., Pohlmann, R., Hasilik, A. and von Figura, K. (1981*b*). Subcellular location of two enzymes involved in the synthesis of phosphorylated recognition markers in lysosomal enzymes. *J Biol Chem*, **256**, 4150–2.

Waheed, A., van Etten, R. L., Koob, R. and Drenkhahn, D. (1988). Targeting of phosphomannosyl-deficient arylsulfatase A to lysosomes of I-cell fibroblasts. *Eur J Cell Biol*, **45**, 262–7.

Warner, J. B., Thalhauser, C., Tao, K. and Sahagian, G. G. (2002). Role of *N*-linked oligosaccharide flexibility in mannose phosphorylation of lysosomal enzyme cathepsin L. *J Biol Chem*, **277**, 41897–905.

Westcott, K. R. and Rome, L. H. (1988). Cation-independent mannose 6-phosphate receptor contains covalently bound fatty acid. *J Cell Biochem*, **38**, 23–33.

Wilczak, N., De Bleser, P., Luiten, P., Geerts, A., Teelken, A. and De Keyser, J. (2000). Insulin-like growth factor II receptors in human brain and their absence in astrogliotic plaques in multiple sclerosis. *Brain Res*, **863**, 282–8.

Yang, L., Tredget, E. E. and Ghahary, A. (2000). Activation of latent transforming growth factor-beta1 is induced by mannose 6-phosphate/insulin-like growth factor-II receptor. *Wound Repair Regen*, **8**, 538–46.

Zhao, H. and Grabowski, G. A. (2002). Gaucher disease: Perspectives on a prototype lysosomal disease. *Cell Mol Life Sci*, **59**, 694–707.

Zhu, Y. and Conner, G. E. (1994). Intermolecular association of lysosomal protein precursors during biosynthesis. *J Biol Chem*, **269**, 3846–51.

Zhu, Y., Doray, B., Poussu, A., Lehto, V.-P. and Kornfeld, S. (2001). Binding of GGA2 to the lysosomal sorting motif of the mannose 6-phosphate receptor. *Science*, **292**, 1716–8.

Chapter 7

Defects in lysosomal enzyme protection: galactosialidosis

Alessandra d'Azzo

Introduction

Galactosialidosis (GS) is a neurodegenerative lysosomal storage disorder of glycoprotein metabolism. This disease is unique among storage diseases in that it is caused by a primary defect in a protease, the protective protein/cathepsin A (PPCA), although its biochemical hallmark remains the combined secondary deficiency of the two glycosidases, neuraminidase (NEU1, sialidase) and β-galactosidase (β-GAL) (d'Azzo *et al.* 2001). The reason for the triple deficiency lies in the pleiotropic nature of the primary enzyme defect. Protective protein/cathepsin A is a member of the serine carboxypeptidase family of proteases and in this capacity exerts carboxypeptidase, deamidase, and esterase activities on a selected number of neuropeptides (McDonald and Barrett 1986; Jackman *et al.* 1990; Galjart *et al.* 1991; Jackman *et al.* 1992). It also binds to β-GAL and NEU1, forming one of the best-characterized lysosomal multi-enzyme complexes (Verheijen *et al.* 1985; van der Spoel *et al.* 1998). Association with PPCA assures the efficient transport of the glycosidases to the lysosome and their intralysosomal activation/stability (vander Spoel *et al.* 1998). This function identifies PPCA as a novel intracellular transport protein and explains the complete deficiency of NEU1 activity and partial deficit of β-GAL secondary to a PPCA defect (van der Spoel *et al.* 1998). Loss of NEU1 activity is mostly responsible for the type of storage products found in patients' tissues and body fluids, which are probably the primary cause of the pathogenesis. Although the catalytic and protective functions of PPCA are completely separable (Galjart *et al.* 1991), so far only null mutations or mutations that interfere with both the protective and the catalytic activity of the protein have been identified in humans (d'Azzo *et al.* 2001). To date, no patients have been described who have an isolated deficiency of cathepsin A. Mutations at the PPCA locus give rise to a prototypical lysosomal disease with heterogeneous clinical manifestations affecting both systemic organs and the nervous system. It is, however, not known to what extent loss of cathepsin A activity contributes to the clinical manifestations in GS patients. The mouse model of GS mimics closely the human severe phenotype and represents a valuable tool for studying the pathogenesis of the disease and developing and implementing therapy (Zhou *et al.* 1995) (Chapter 11). Here, I review what we have learned so far about the enzyme and how this knowledge may help to understand the disease.

Protective protein/cathepsin A is a component of a lysosomal multi-enzyme complex

The name protective protein relates to the protective function of PPCA towards β-GAL and NEU1. Prior to the discovery of the protein's catalytic activity, its biological function was assayed by supplementing conditioned medium from normal fibroblasts, containing the PPCA precursor, to deficient fibroblasts from GS patients. Internalization of the PPCA precursor restored both β-GAL and NEU1 activities in these cells—proof that loss of PPCA was responsible for the combined deficiency of the two glycosidases and that PPCA was indispensable for their activities (d'Azzo *et al.* 1982). These initial data were in line with enzyme purification studies that showed that the three proteins physically associate to form a multi-enzyme complex, and that they co-purify on β-GAL or PPCA affinity chromatography columns (Verheijen *et al.* 1982, 1985; Yamamoto and Nishimura 1987; Scheibe *et al.* 1990; Hiraiwa *et al.* 1997). While both PPCA and β-GAL are active as oligomeric free forms, NEU1 is only found in an approximately 1200-kDa complex, which includes only 1–2% of the total amounts of PPCA and β-GAL. This is indicative of the strict dependence of NEU1 on the association with PPCA for maintaining its activity. Although the role of PPCA in the multi-enzyme complex is pivotal, the mutual advantage of the three enzymes from being in complex is not yet fully understood. In mammalian cells, PPCA associates with NEU1 and β-GAL in an early biosynthetic compartment and thereby promotes the timely and efficient transport of these enzymes to the lysosome (van der Spoel *et al.* 1998). Once in the lysosome, a pool of PPCA remains in the complex and hence activates NEU1 and stabilizes β-GAL (Heyworth *et al.* 1981; Verheijen *et al.* 1985; Yamamoto and Nishimura 1986; van der Horst *et al.* 1989). These events are accomplished by oligomerization of the two glycosidases. In the absence of PPCA, the enzyme complex is not formed because NEU1 is retained in the endosomal compartment and the pool of β-GAL that reaches the lysosomes is rapidly degraded (van Diggelen *et al.* 1981, 1982; van der Spoel *et al.* 1998). The stoichiometry and composition of the multi-enzyme complex remains unclear; purification studies have shown that at least one other lysosomal enzyme, *N*-acetylgalactosamine-6-sulfate sulfatase, is loosely associated with the complex (Pshezhetsky and Potier 1996). A partial deficiency of this enzyme was detected in GS patients (Pshezhetsky and Potier 1996). The most plausible scenario is that complex formation is a dynamic event that depends on the cell type, animal species, and types of substrates to be catabolized.

Molecular, biochemical, and structural properties of protective protein/cathepsin A

The human and murine PPCA loci on chromosome 20q13.1 and 2H, respectively, are situated in a complex genomic region, which is highly conserved both in organization and in sequence (Wiegant *et al.* 1991; Rottier *et al.* 1998*a*). In both species, the 5′ and 3′ ends of the PPCA gene overlap two other genes both transcribed from the antisense strand relative to PPCA. The gene at the 3′ end encodes a previously described phospholipid transfer protein (Day *et al.* 1994; Whitmore *et al.* 1995); the gene at the 5′ end is transcribed from the constitutive PPCA promoter, which has bi-directional activity (Rottier and d'Azzo 1997) and encodes a novel protein expressed exclusively in striated muscle, whose function is under investigation. Considering the distinct tissue distribution of PPCA and this muscle-specific protein, it may be crucial to investigate how these two genes are regulated both at the transcriptional and at the translational levels, since genetic lesions affecting the PPCA gene may also disturb the expression of the 5′ neighbouring gene and may contribute to some of the phenotypic manifestations of GS patients.

Human and murine PPCA proteins are 87% identical at their amino acid level and share similar biochemical and catalytic properties (Galjart *et al.* 1990). In fact the murine enzyme can substitute its human counterpart in correcting β-GAL and NEU1 activity in PPCA-deficient human fibroblasts (Galjart *et al.* 1990). Both enzymes are synthesized as precursors containing a conventional hydrophobic signal peptide, two N-linked glycosylation sites, and nine cysteines (Galjart *et al.* 1988, 1990) (Chapter 4). The glycosylated precursor of 54 kDa dimerizes soon after synthesis and acquires the mannose-6-phosphate (M6P) recognition marker (Zhou *et al.* 1991). Both events are essential for the intracellular transport and lysosomal localization of the precursor molecule. A small pool of the phosphorylated precursor is also found extracellularly, but this secreted form can be taken up via M6P receptor-mediated endocytosis and be routed to the lysosomes (Galjart *et al.* 1991). As it is the case for other proteases, the PPCA precursor is a zymogen. In the endosomal/lysosomal compartment, the one-chain precursor undergoes a two-step proteolytic maturation: an initial endoproteolytic cleavage gives rise to a 34- and a 20-kDa inactive intermediate; this is followed by the removal of a 2-kDa 'linker' or 'excision' peptide from the C-terminus of the large 34-kDa domain (Bonten *et al.* 1995; Rudenko *et al.* 1995). The mature and functional protein present in lysosomes consists of two chains of 32 and 20 kDa, held together by disulfide bridges.

Mammalian PPCAs belong to the serine protease family of enzymes. Their primary structures share a 30% identity to wheat and yeast serine carboxypeptidases (CPW and CPY respectively) and the yeast KEX1 and sxa2^{+} gene products (Breddam and Svendsen 1984; Dmochowska *et al.* 1987; Valls *et al.* 1987). The active site Ser at position 150 in human PPCA is embedded in a domain of six amino acids (GE*S*YA(G)G) found in all family members (Brenner 1988); the essential Ser residue in exo- and endo-serine proteases is activated by the coordinated action of two other residues, a histidine and an aspartic acid. These three amino acids form the catalytic triad. Based on sequence alignment, the crystal structure, and mutagenesis studies (Galjart *et al.* 1991; Rudenko *et al.* 1995), it was determined that the catalytic triad of PPCA is composed of residues Ser150, His429, and Asp372.

The three-dimensional structure of the 108-kDa dimer of the PPCA precursor has been solved by a combination of molecular replacement and two-fold density averaging (Rudenko *et al.* 1995). The protein fold consists of two large domains, a 'core' domain and a 'cap' domain. The core domain houses the catalytic triad and resembles a domain found in CPW and CPY and other proteases and lipases with different catalytic properties that are members of the hydrolase fold family (Liao *et al.* 1992; Ollis and Goldman 1992; Endrizzi *et al.* 1994). The cap domain includes a helical subdomain and a maturation subdomain that fills the active-site cleft and includes the 'excision' peptide. The mode of activation of PPCA is unique among proteases with known structure. The active site is structurally already poised for catalysis in the zymogen, but it is blocked by the maturation subdomain, which is not removed during enzyme activation; instead, it refolds after cleavage of the excision peptide to render the catalytic cleft substrate accessible. The conformation of the enzymatic machinery remains unaffected (Rudenko *et al.* 1995).

Protective protein/cathepsin A is a multifunctional protein

Aside from its protective function, PPCA has cathepsin A/carboxypeptidase activity at acidic pH and can function as a deamidase and esterase at neutral pH (Jackman *et al.* 1990; Hanna *et al.* 1994). *In vitro*, the enzyme catabolizes a selected number of neuropeptides: it deamidates substance P and neurokinin and removes the C-terminal amino acid from oxytocin-free acid, bradykinin, and endothelin I (Jackman *et al.* 1990; Jackman *et al.* 1992; Itoh *et al.* 1995; Skidgel and Erdos 1998; Itoh *et al.* 2000). Mature PPCA is released from thrombin-stimulated human platelets and from ionophore B-stimulated natural killer cells, and is detected in granules of human interleukin-2 (IL-2)-activated killer cells (Jackman *et al.* 1990; Hanna *et al.* 1994). All three activities are severely reduced in cells from patients with GS (Kase *et al.* 1990). Furthermore, the hydrolysis of the C-terminus of endothelin I by the cathepsin A activity of PPCA was found to be deficient in tissues from a GS patient (Itoh *et al.* 2000). These authors have implicated PPCA as the major endothelin-degrading enzyme present in human tissues. Thus, PPCA functions may extend to metabolic processes like the inactivation of bioactive peptides or granzyme-mediated cellular cytotoxicity (Skidgel and Erdos 1998).

The enzyme is, however, still referred to as PPCA because catalytically inactive variants maintain the capacity to associate with β-GAL and NEU1 and correct both enzyme activities when taken up by GS fibroblasts (Galjart *et al.* 1991). The distinct and separable functions of PPCA may relate to the presence of different pools of the protein, free or in complex, that may vary among cell types and differentially catabolize a broad spectrum of substrates. Hence, although it is PPCA's protective function, and not its enzymatic function, that is the main cause of lysosomal dysfunction in GS patients, the possibility remains that some of their phenotypic features are due to the loss of cathepsin A activity. A full understanding of the functions of PPCA may come from the identification of substrates that are the *in vivo* targets of the enzyme. *In vitro*, PPCA has a substrate preference for hydrophobic residues in the P1 and P1′-binding pocket (Kawamura *et al.* 1977). N-Blocked acylated dipeptides, like Z-Phe-Ala or Z-Phe-Leu, are commonly used to assay cathepsin A activity in cultured cells and tissues, as well as in GS material (Galjart *et al.* 1991). The cathepsin A activity is now routinely assayed together with β-GAL and NEU1 in chorionic villi and amniocytes for carrier detection and prenatal diagnosis (d'Azzo *et al.* 2001).

Human protective protein/cathepsin A deficiency

Galactosialidosis can be suspected in children with features typical of a lysosomal disorder, such as coarse facies, macular cherry-red spots, vertebral changes, foam cells in the bone marrow (BM), and vacuolated lymphocytes in peripheral blood (d'Azzo *et al.* 2001) (Chapter 3). Three phenotypic subtypes are recognized among GS patients based on the age of onset and severity of the symptoms (Andria *et al.* 1981; Spranger 1981; d'Azzo *et al.* 2001). The early infantile form has a poor prognosis and rapid course (Kleijer *et al.* 1979; Kyllerman *et al.* 1993; Landau *et al.* 1995; Zammarchi *et al.* 1996; Groenen *et al.* 2000). Affected children show signs at birth of non-immune hydrops fetalis, neonatal oedema, and ascites (Stone and Sidransky 1999). Common features include severe kidney involvement with proteinuria, coarse facies, inguinal hernias, and telangiectasias. The patients develop visceromegaly, severe psychomotor delay, and skeletal dysplasia. Heart involvement consists of cardiomegaly, thickened septum, and cardiac failure. Ocular abnormalities such as corneal clouding and fundal changes have been described in a few infants. Death occurs at an average age of 7–8 months, mostly as a result of renal and cardiac failure. The early infantile type of GS may be associated with fetal loss (Kleijer *et al.* 1979; Landau *et al.* 1995).

Late (mild) infantile patients develop symptoms in the first year of life (d'Azzo *et al.* 2001). The clinical picture at onset is generally characterized by coarse facies, hepatosplenomegaly, and dysostosis multiplex, affecting especially the spine (Chapter 3). In most patients, severe neurologic manifestations, such as myoclonus or ataxia, are absent. Mild or very mild mental retardation have been diagnosed in only few patients, while progressive neurologic course has been reported in only one case (Pinsky *et al.* 1974; Andria *et al.* 1981; Yuce *et al.* 1996; Zhou *et al.* 1996; Richard *et al.* 1998). Instead, the patients develop a progressive heart disease, characterized by thickened mitral and aortic valves resulting in valvular insufficiency. All patients but one are alive; however, growth disturbance partly due to the spine involvement and often associated with muscular atrophy has become apparent in the majority of these patients.

The largest number of patients with GS is of the juvenile/adult subtype and is mainly of Japanese origin. In spite of the late onset of the symptoms (average 16 years), these patients develop very severe neurologic manifestations which include myoclonus, cerebellar ataxia, generalized seizures, and mental retardation (Orii *et al.* 1972; Wenger *et al.* 1978; Takano *et al.* 1991; d'Azzo *et al.* 2001). Angiokeratoma, corneal clouding, bilateral cherry-red spot, absence of visceromegaly, and long survival are distinctive of this subtype.

Pathology

Only a few autopsy reports of patients with GS have been reported in the literature, most of which are of Japanese juvenile/adult variants. The overall findings point to a disease affecting primarily cells of the reticuloendothelial system. Immunohistochemical and ultrastructural examination of a few cases have revealed major swelling of the endothelial cells of blood vessels and foamy macrophages/histiocytes in visceral organs and the peripheral, enteric, and central nervous systems (CNS) (Yoshino *et al.* 1990; Oyanagi *et al.* 1991; Nordborg *et al.* 1997). Focusing on the neuropathology of a severe early-onset case, Arai *et al.* (1999) have described extensive vacuolation of endothelial cells in brain specimens that was accompanied by loss of CD31 reactivity and breakdown of vascular cell adhesion molecules—these authors have speculated that these phenomena could promote the development of brain infarctions and various degree of axonal damage in cerebral and cerebellar white matter. Similar neuropathological features were observed in post-mortem brain of a 14-month-old girl, which included multiple cortical–subcortical infarctions due to a compromised circulation as a consequence of endothelial luminal encroachment (Nordborg *et al.* 1997). Semithin sections revealed a considerable loss of Purkinje cells and an increase in the Bergmann astroglia. Prominent cytoplasmic vacuolation was detected by electron microscopy in the endothelial cells lining the cerebral blood vessels and in neurones and glial cells of the cerebrum, the cerebellum, and the spinal cord (Nordborg *et al.* 1997). The vacuoles were mostly empty or contained finely granular or membranous material, as expected from a primary storage consisting of soluble glycoproteins or oligosaccharides. Notably, Purkinje cells also included zebra bodies in addition to vacuoles, while granule neurones were devoid of storage. Gliosis was confined to cerebrovascular regions in the grey matter but was widespread in the white matter, presumably induced by loss of nerve fibres and vasogenic oedema, suggesting a condition of hypertension. Since endothelial vacuolation and focal cerebrovascular lesions were never described before, these authors have suggested that these features could be specific for the severe early infantile form of the disease (Nordborg *et al.* 1997). Other neuropathological findings in this patient were similar to those reported in a few juvenile/adult-onset cases of GS.

Neuropathologic analysis of the CNS and peripheral nervous system was performed in post-mortem tissues from a patient with the juvenile form of GS (Yoshino *et al.* 1990; Oyanagi *et al.* 1991). Mental retardation, visual disturbance, cerebellar ataxia, myoclonus, and epilepsy developed at the age of 10 years and the patient died 3 years later. Macroscopic examination revealed marked atrophy of the thalamus, globus pallidus, lateral geniculate body, dentate nucleus, cerebellar vermis, and optic nerve. Light microscopy indicated a severe neuronal loss with fibrillary gliosis in the globus pallidus, thalamus, dentate nucleus, and cerebellum. Loss of Purkinje cells and granule neurones was prominent in the superior vermis. Abundant storage materials were seen in Betz cells and neurones of the basal forebrain and motor nuclei of the spinal cord and brainstem (Oyanagi *et al.* 1991). Histochemical evaluation of storage material indicated that it was heterogeneous and differed in the neurones from various anatomic regions with respect to reactivity to staining with Sudan black B and periodic acid–Schiff (PAS), as well as with respect to autofluorescence (Oyanagi *et al.* 1991). Ultrastructural examination revealed a variety of inclusions, such as membranous cytoplasmic bodies, lamellar structures, lipofuscin-like pleomorphic bodies, and cytoplasmic vacuoles with fine granules. Gross assessment of the retina and optic nerve in the same patient revealed extensive loss of ganglion cells in the retina and myelinated nerve fibres (Usui *et al.* 1991). The remaining ganglion cells were filled with vacuoles, which contained proteinaceous material, lipofuscin-like substances, and phospholipids based on histological staining.

These neuropathologic findings were similar to those described in an adult Japanese patient characterized by coarse facies, cerebellar ataxia, myoclonus, retinal degeneration, and cortical blindness (Amano *et al.* 1983). The brain had diffuse cerebral atrophy with enlargement of the lateral ventricles and greyish discoloration of the white matter. Extensive loss of neurones was observed in the cerebral cortex especially at the level of the third, fifth, and sixth layers. The remaining neurones in nuclei of the midbrain, brainstem, cerebellum, and spinal cord contained numerous cytoplasmic vacuoles with heterogeneous material and lipofuscin-like granules. Ultrastructurally, the neuronal inclusions consisted of membranous lamellar structures, like zebroid bodies, multilamellar structures and granular material similar to lipofuscin. The type of storage varied among neuronal nuclei (Amano *et al.* 1983). Similar histopathological and ultrastructural findings were described in a 20-year-old woman and a 48-year-old man with mental retardation, bilateral macular cherry-red spots, corneal clouding, cerebellar ataxia, myoclonus, and seizures (Kobayashi *et al.* 1979; Miyatake *et al.* 1979*b*). Biopsies of the sural nerve or peripheral nerve bundles of the dermis revealed membrane-bound vacuoles containing fine granular material in the Schwann cells and perineurial and endoneurial epithelium. The neurones in the paravertebral sympathetic ganglia and myenteric plexus of the rectum contained concentric lamellar inclusions.

Molecular and biochemical defects

Clinical heterogeneity among GS patients is paralleled by molecular and biochemical heterogeneity. Depending on the genetic lesion, PPCA mRNA levels range from undetectable to normal in different patients, even belonging to the same subtype (Galjart *et al.* 1988; d'Azzo *et al.* 2001) (Chapter 4). This, in turn, affects the quality and quantity of immunoprecipitable PPCA protein and the percentage of residual cathepsin A activity (Palmeri *et al.* 1986; Galjart *et al.* 1988; Nanba *et al.* 1988; Strisciuglio *et al.* 1988; d'Azzo *et al.* 2001). Most of the patient are either homozygous or compound heterozygous for point mutations resulting in single-amino acid substitutions, but splicing defects and small deletions have also been described (d'Azzo *et al.* 2001). Using Z-Phe-Ala as the substrate, Kleijer *et al.* (1996) have surveyed 20 GS patients and their parents, and made a clear correlation between levels of residual cathepsin A activity and severity of the clinical phenotypes. In addition, several amino acid substitutions found in defective PPCA from different phenotypic variants of GS have been modelled onto the three-dimensional structure (Rudenko *et al.* 1998). There appears to be a significant correlation between the effect of each mutation on the integrity of the protein structure and the general severity of the clinical phenotype. Thus, even though the two functions of PPCA are completely separable, in all GS patients so far identified there is a combined loss of catalytic activity and protective function of PPCA because of aberrant folding of the mutant protein.

Sialyloligosacchariduria is diagnostic of the disease, but it is indistinguishable from that observed in patients with sialidosis, a glycoproteinosis caused by an isolated deficiency of NEU1 (d'Azzo *et al.* 2001; Thomas 2001). Essentially, the same collection of α(2,6)- and α(2,3)-sialylated oligosaccharides has been isolated from urine and fibroblasts of these patients, as well as from the placenta of a GS fetus (van Pelt *et al.* 1988*a*, *b*, 1991). In addition, increased amounts of the gangliosides GM3, GM2, GM1, and GD1a were detected in sympathetic and spinal ganglia and the grey matter of the spinal cord of GS patients (Miyatake *et al.* 1979*a*; Yoshino *et al.* 1990). Thus, primary or secondary deficiency of lysosomal NEU1 might result in impaired ganglioside catabolism, especially GM3 and GD1a desialylation.

Overall, many of the clinical, biochemical, and pathologic features of patients with GS resemble those described in GM1 gangliosidosis, a glycolipidosis caused by deficiency of β-GAL, and especially sialidosis. This reiterates the contribution of the secondary loss of NEU1 activity in the pathogenesis of GS. However, understanding the unique role played by the loss of cathepsin A activity in the disease phenotype will be a challenging task that may be tackled only by the generation of mouse models lacking only the cathepsin A activity.

Mouse model of galactosialidosis

Mice homozygous for a null mutation at the PPCA locus develop a GS-like phenotype, resembling human patients with the severe form of the disease (Zhou *et al.* 1995). Mutant mice excrete excessive amounts of sialylated oligosaccharides in the urine, which is diagnostic of the disease in children and is consistent with the severe reduction of NEU1 activity coupled to the cathepsin A deficiency in all tissues tested (Zhou *et al.* 1995). Although viable and fertile, $PPCA^{-/-}$ mice weigh 25–40% less than their normal littermates, and they have a noticeably flattened snout, disheveled coat, and shorter lifespan (approximately 10 months). Their overall gross appearance progressively worsens with age: at 7–10 months of age the mice give a debilitating impression (Fig. 7.1). Diffuse oedema with swelling of the eyelids often accompanied by inflammation, swelling of the subcutaneous tissue, and limbs is accompanied by progressive loss of coordination, ataxic movements, and tremor, which are features indicative of severe cerebellar dysfunction. As observed in GS patients, newborn $PPCA^{-/-}$ mice show signs of lysosomal storage primarily in the reticuloendothelial system of most organs, including the nervous system (Zhou *et al.* 1995;

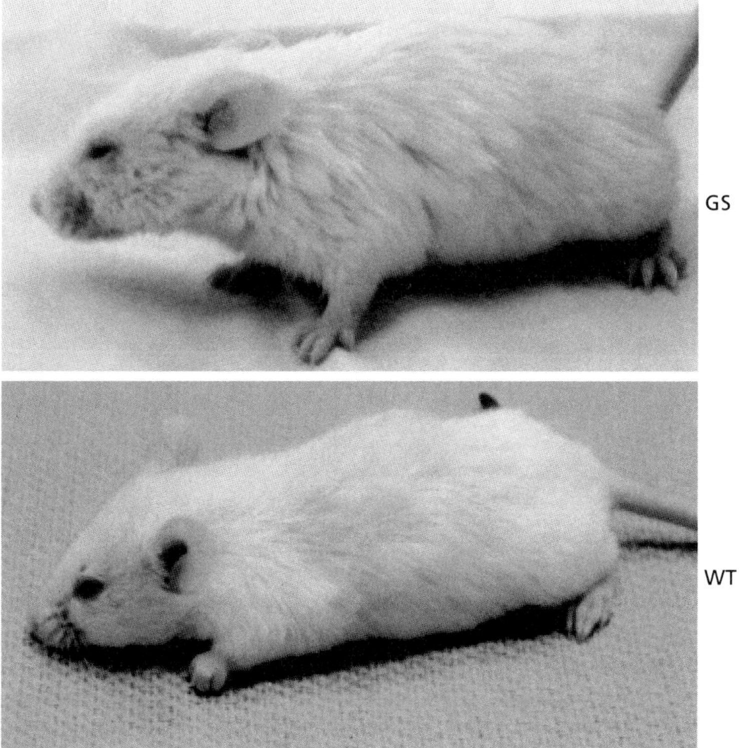

Fig. 7.1 Gross phenotypic appearance of a PPCA$^{-/-}$ mouse [*upper panel*: at 8 months of age compared to a wild-type littermate (*lower panel*)]. The affected mouse has a flattened snout, disheveled coat, and swollen limbs and eyelids.

Rottier *et al.* 1998*b*). Nephropathy, which is a major complication and cause of death in early infantile patients, is also the most apparent cause of physical deterioration in affected mice. Histopathology of the brain of mutant mice killed at different time points during disease progression has revealed a significant variation in the distribution of accumulating cells that mostly parallel the sites of expression of PPCA mRNA and protein (Rottier *et al.* 1998*b*). Perivascular and leptomeningeal macrophages and microglia, often juxtaposed to degenerating neurones (Fig. 7.2, SO), are the primary and most affected cells. Extensive storage is also apparent in the epithelial and stromal cells of the choroid plexi (Fig. 7.2, CP), the trigeminal ganglia, and the pituitary gland. Neurones of different brain nuclei are affected to a variable extent. Storage appears to be most pronounced in the cells of the limbic system, namely the anterior olfactory and subolfactory nuclei (Fig. 7.2, OL and SO), the amygdala, the entorhinal cortex, and pyriform cortex. On toluidine blue-stained sections, metachromatic, lipofuscin-like granules are occasionally encountered (Fig. 7.2, SO). In the hippocampus and dentate gyrus, only a few vacuolated neurones are distinguished mostly in the CA3 region (Fig. 7.2, HIP). In older mice, also the large neurones of the brainstem appear vacuolated (Fig. 7.2, BS). The most overt consequence of the disease in the brain of $^{-/-}$ mice is seen in the cerebellum—a phenotypic manifestation which seems consistent with GS patients. Purkinje cells degenerate in a time- and site-dependent

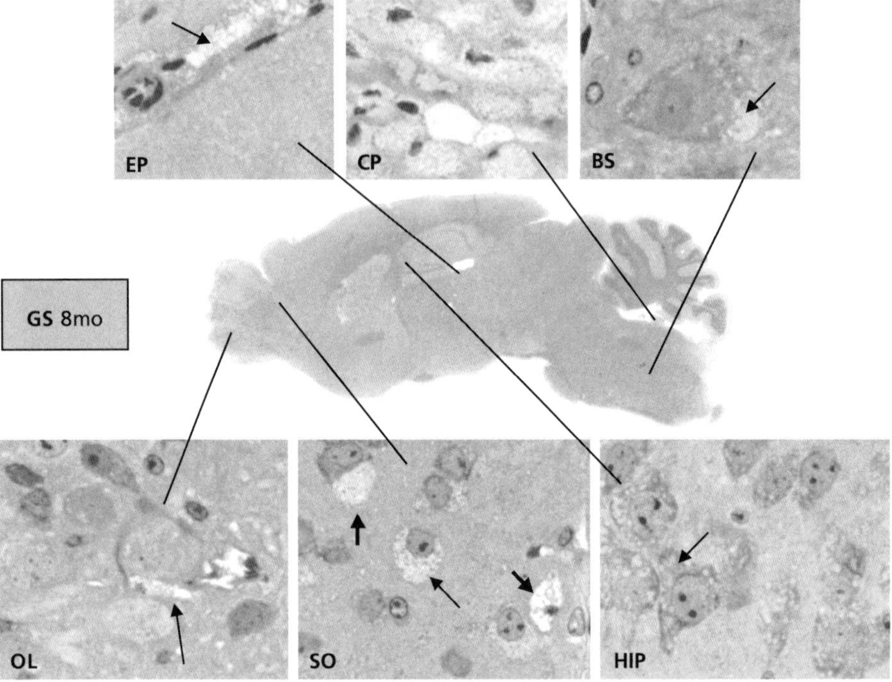

Fig. 7.2 The brain of a galactosialidosis (GS) mouse aged 8 months was fixed in 10% neutral-buffered formalin and embedded in glycol methacrylate. Sections of 1 μm thickness were stained with toluidine blue. The different regions of the brain that were photographed are indicated in the parasagittal section in the middle panel. *Top row*: ependyma (EP), choroid plexus (CP), and brainstem (BS). *Bottom row*: anterior olfactory (OL), subolfactory (SO), and hippocampus (HIP). **See Plate 6**.

manner: these cells die in clusters, following an anteroposterior and lateromedial pattern, the anterior lobes being the ones that are affected sooner and to a greater extent (Hahn *et al.* 1998; Leimig *et al.* 2002). At the age of 3–4 months, only about 20–25% of the total Purkinje cells are lost. In the anterior lobes, signs of cell degeneration begin to appear at this age and some Purkinje cells are missing (Fig. 7.3, GS 3mo). By the age of 8–10 months, a dramatic loss of these cells becomes apparent: In the paravermis at the point where the lateral cerebellar nuclei first become obvious (medial), the average total loss reaches approximately 80%, but it is clearly more severe in the anterior lobes (Fig. 7.3, GS 8mo) than in the posterior lobes (approximately 90% and approximately 60% loss, respectively). The remaining Purkinje cells contain storage vacuoles in their perikarya that appear filled with granular or membranous material in electron micrographs (Fig. 7.4, GS-PC and EM GS panel). The granule neurones seem to be well preserved. The Purkinje cell degeneration in PPCA$^{-/-}$ mice is reminiscent of that observed in the sphingomyelinase knockout mouse model (Sarna *et al.* 2001). In addition to the neuronal involvement, influx of macrophages in the Purkinje cell layer at the site of degeneration, as well as vacuolated basket cells and Bergmann astroglia is visible (Fig. 7.4, GS-PC). In the deep cerebellar nuclei, storage vacuoles are evident in the large neurones as well as in perivascular macrophages and endothelial cells (Fig. 7.4, GS-CbN).

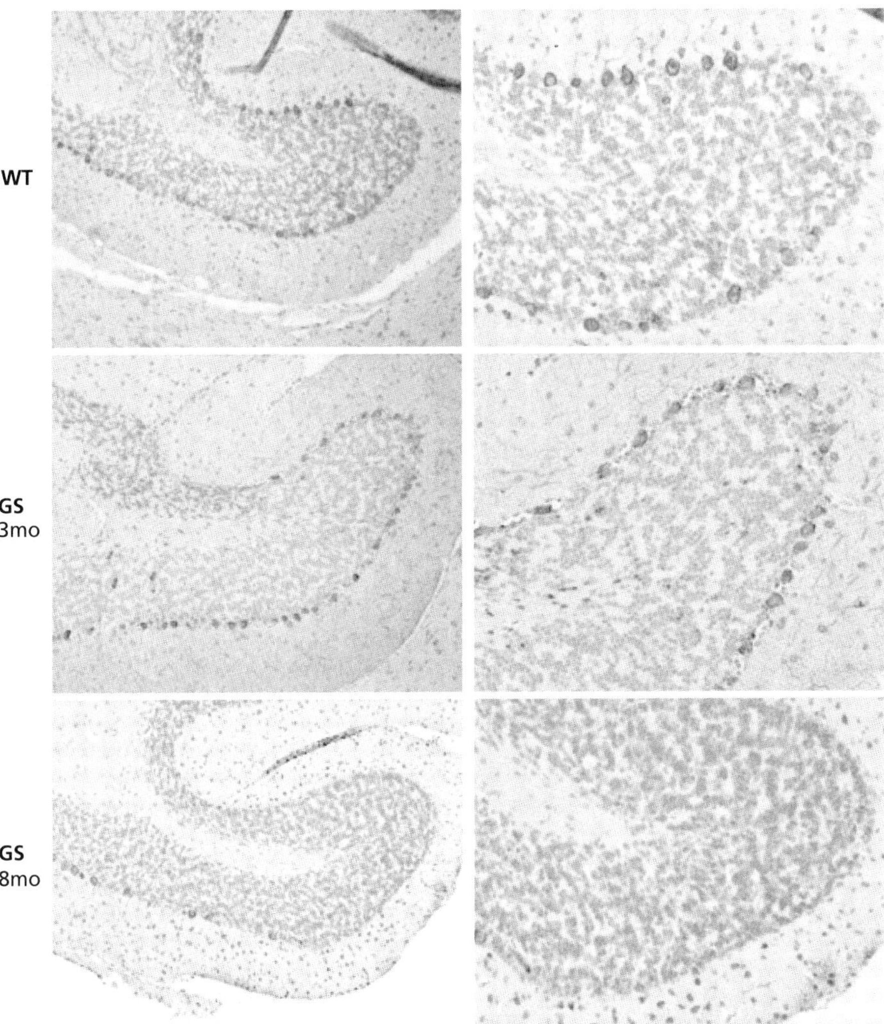

Fig. 7.3 Wild-type (WT), 3-month-old PPCA$^{-/-}$ (GS, 3 months) and 8-month-old PPCA$^{-/-}$ mice were perfused with 4% paraformaldehyde and the brains were fixed in 10% neutral-buffered formalin, processed, and embedded in paraffin. 10 μm sections were stained with an anti-PEP19 antibody, recognizing preferentially Purkinje cells, and counterstained with haematoxylin. The anterior lobes of the cerebellum are shown. **See Plate 7**.

As in GS patients, in PPCA$^{-/-}$ mice, the numerous membrane-bound vacuoles in cells throughout the CNS appear either empty or filled with sparse fibrillar and membranous structures, reflecting lysosomal accumulation of low-molecular weight compounds, like oligosaccharides or glycopeptides (Zhou *et al.* 1995; Rottier *et al.* 1998*b*). However, contrary to what was observed in some GS patients (see above), there is no evidence of ganglioside or glycolipid accumulation in knockout mice (A. d'Azzo, unpublished data). In general, this mouse model has provided a powerful means to study the pathogenesis and pathophysiology of the disease and to evaluate therapies that could be eventually useful for treating patients.

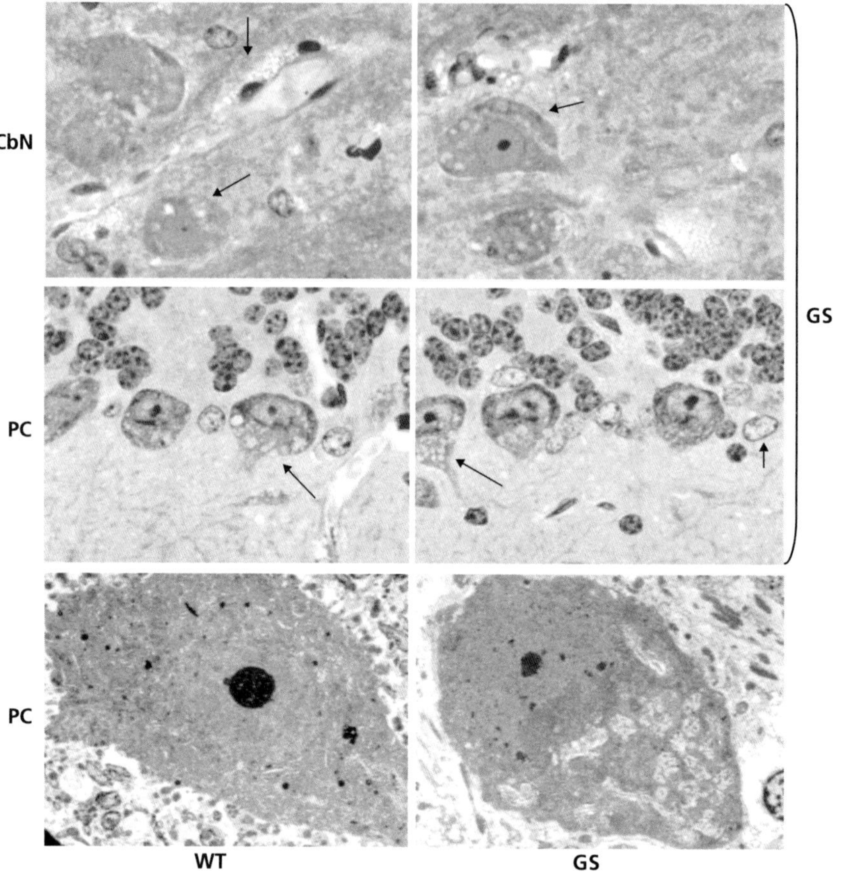

Fig. 7.4 *Upper panels*: The brain of a GS mouse aged 8 months was fixed and embedded in plastic. Sections of 1 μm thickness were stained in toluidine blue. *Top row* (GS): deep cerebellar nucleus (CbN). *Bottom row* (GS): Purkinje cells (PC). *Lower panels*: The brains of two mice, PPCA$^{-/-}$ and wild type of 7 months of age, were fixed in 4% buffered glutaraldehyde, postfixed in OsO_4, dehydrated, and embedded in Spurr. The ultrathin sections (80 nm) were stained with uranyl acetate and lead citrate. **See Plate 8**.

In recent studies, both cathepsin A and NEU1 activity in knockout mice were restored after transplantation with BM from either normal mice or transgenic mice that overexpress PPCA exclusively in erythroid cells or in the monocyte/macrophage lineage (Zhou *et al.* 1995; Hahn *et al.* 1998). Accordingly, most of the pathological symptoms were prevented by this treatment. Overexpressing BM afforded a better and more-timely correction of the phenotype: Transplanted mice had a gross appearance identical to wild-type mice and outlived the untreated knockout animals (Hahn *et al.* 1998). Complete correction of systemic organ pathology was accompanied by a delayed onset of Purkinje cell degeneration in inter-crosses between the mutant and the transgenic mice (Hahn *et al.* 1998). These results have encouraged the use of genetically modified BM cells for *ex vivo* gene therapy of the GS model (Leimig *et al.* 2002). PPCA$^{-/-}$ mice that received haematopoietic progenitors transduced with a retroviral vector overexpressing PPCA showed complete correction of the systemic organs up to 10 months after transplantation. Protective protein/cathepsin A expression in the CNS, albeit mainly localized to perivascular areas, was apparently sufficient to delay the onset of Purkinje cell degeneration and to correct the ataxic phenotype (Leimig *et al.* 2002). The overall outcome of these therapeutic interventions in the PPCA$^{-/-}$ mice supports the future use of a gene therapy approach for the treatment of GS in humans.

Summary

Protective protein/cathepsin A is a pleiotropic lysosomal enzyme, whose full range of activities may not have been discovered yet. Its function(s) appears to be determined by its association state, either in the multi-enzyme complex or as a free dimer. *In vivo*, the localization of PPCA must also play a role in determining its activity with regard to the substrates that the enzyme hydrolyses. The protective function of the protein is pivotal in view of the fact that its loss leads to a neurodegenerative lysosomal disorder. Thus, formation of the multi-enzyme complex with NEU1 and β-GAL not only seems to control the intracellular routing and lysosomal activity of the two glycosidases, but may also influence their substrate specificity. The availability of pools of free and assembled PPCA molecules that are committed to different functions, which could potentially be targeted differentially, creates a very dynamic degradation system. It is noteworthy that sialidase-deficient mice do not undergo Purkinje cell loss to the extent that the GS mice do (De Geest *et al.* 2002). This opens the possibility that the cathepsin A activity of PPCA may play a central role in cerebellar degeneration. In line with this hypothesis is the observation by Itoh *et al.* (2000) that endothelin 1, a potential natural substrate of cathepsin A, was markedly increased and abnormally distributed in the cerebellum, hippocampus, and spinal cord of an autopsied GS patient (Itoh *et al.* 2000). These authors have implicated the loss of cathepsin A activity of PPCA and consequent lack of degradation of endothelin 1 as the potential cause of some of the neurological abnormalities of this disease. A full knowledge of how PPCA functions *in vivo* may help in the identification of the molecular pathways controlled directly or indirectly by this enzyme and its partners, and may impact the way we diagnose and treat the patients with a PPCA deficiency.

Acknowledgements

The author wishes to thank Erik Bonten for his useful comments on the manuscript and for his help in editing the references and Angela Ingrassia, Linda Mann, and Huimin Hu for their assistance in making the figures. The work discussed in this chapter was supported in part by grants DK52025 and GM60950 from the National Institutes of Health, the Assisi Foundation of Memphis, and the American Lebanese Syrian Associated Charities (ALSAC) of St. Jude Children's Research Hospital.

References

Amano, N., Yokoi, S., Akagi, M., Sakai, M., Yagishita, S. and Nakata, K. (1983). Neuropathological findings of an autopsy case of adult β-galactosidase and neuraminidase deficiency. *Acta Neuropathol*, **61**, 283–90.

Andria, G., Strisciuglio, P., Pontarelli, G., Sly, W. S. and Dodson, W. E. (1981). Infantile neuraminidase and β-galactosidase deficiencies (galactosialidosis) with mild clinical courses. In *Sialidases and sialidoses* (ed.p. Durand, P., Tettamanti, G. and DiDonato, S., ed.), pp. 379–95. Milan: Edi. Ermes.

Arai, Y., Edwards, V., Takashima, S. and Becker, L. E. (1999). Vascular pathology in galactosialidosis. *Ultrastruct Pathol*, **23**, 369–74.

d'Azzo, A., Hoogeveen, A., Reuser, A. J., Robinson, D. and Galjaard, H. (1982). Molecular defect in combined beta-galactosidase and neuraminidase deficiency in man. *Proc Natl Acad Sci USA*, **79**, 4535–9.

d'Azzo, A., Andria, G., Strisciuglio, P. and Galjaard, H. (2001). Galactosialidosis. In *The metabolic and molecular bases of inherited disease* (Scriver, C., Beaudet, A., Sly, W. S. and Valle, D., ed.), pp. 3811–26. New York: McGraw-Hill.

Bonten, E. J., Galjart, N. J., Willemsen, R., Usmany, M., Vlak, J. M. and d'Azzo, A. (1995). Lysosomal protective protein/cathepsin A: Role of the 'linker' domain in catalytic activation. *J Biol Chem*, **270**, 26441–5.

Breddam, K. and Svendsen, I. (1984). Identification of methionyl and cysteinyl residues in the substrate binding site of carboxypeptidase Y. *Carlsberg Res Commun*, **49**, 639–45.

Brenner, S. (1988). The molecular evolution of genes and proteins: a tale of two serines. *Nature*, **334**, 528.

Day, J., Albers, J., Lofton-Day, C., Ching, A., Grant, F., O'Hara, P. *et al.* (1994). Complete cDNA encoding human phospholipid transfer protein from human endothelial cells. *J Biol Chem*, **269**, 9388–91.

De Geest, N., Bonten, E., Mann, L., De Sousa-Hitzler, J., Hahn, C. and d'Azzo, A. (2002). Systemic and neurologic abnormalities distinguish the lysosomal disorders sialidosis and galactosialidosis in mice. *Hum Mol Genet*, **11**, 1455–64.

van Diggelen, O. P., Schram, A. W., Sinnott, M. L., Smith, P. J., Robinson, D. and Galjaard, H. (1981). Turnover of beta-galactosidase in fibroblasts from patients with genetically different types of beta-galactosidase deficiency. *J Biol Chem*, **200**, 143–51.

van Diggelen, O. P., Hoogeveen, A. T., Smith, P. J., Reuser, A. J. and Galjaard, H. (1982). Enhanced proteolytic degradation of normal beta-galactosidase in the lysosomal storage disease with combined beta-galactosidase and neuraminidase deficiency. *Biochim Biophys Acta*, **703**, 69–76.

Dmochowska, A., Dignard, D., Henning, D., Thomas, D. Y. and Bussey, H. (1987). Yeast KEX1 gene encodes a putative protease with a carboxypeptidase B-like function involved in killer toxin and alpha-factor precursor processing. *Cell*, **50**, 573–84.

Endrizzi, J., Breddam, K. and Remington, S. (1994). 2.8-Å structure of yeast serine carboxypeptidase. *Biochemistry*, **33**, 11106.

Galjart, N. J., Gillemans, N., Harris, A., van der Horst, G. T. J., Verheijen, F. W., Galjaard, H. *et al.* (1988). Expression of cDNA encoding the human "protective protein" associated with lysosomal beta-galactosidase and neuraminidase: Homology to yeast proteases. *Cell*, **54**, 755–64.

Galjart, N. J., Gillemans, N., Meijer, D. and d'Azzo, A. (1990). Mouse "protective protein." cDNA cloning, sequence comparison, and expression. *J Biol Chem*, **265**, 4678–84.

Galjart, N. J., Morreau, H., Willemsen, R., Gillemans, N., Bonten, E. J. and d'Azzo, A. (1991). Human lysosomal protective protein has cathepsin A-like activity distinct from its protective function. *J Biol Chem*, **266**, 14754–62.

Groener, J., Maaswinkel-Mooy, P., Smit, V., Hoeven, M., Bakker, J., Campos, Y., d'Azzo, A. (2003). New mutations in two Dutch patients with early infantile galactosialidosis. *Mol Genet Metab*, **78**: 222–8.

Hahn, C., Martin, M., Zhou, X.-Y., Mann, L. and d'Azzo, A. (1998). Correction of murine galactosialidosis by bone marrow-derived macrophages overexpressing human protective protein/cathepsin A under control of the colony-stimulating factor-1 receptor promoter. *Proc Natl Acad Sci USA*, **95**, 14880–5.

Hanna, W. L., Turbov, J. M., Jackman, H. L., Tan, F. and Froelich, C. J. (1994). Dominant chymotrypsin-like esterase activity in human lymphocyte granules is mediated by the serine carboxypeptidase called cathepsin A-like protective protein. *J Immunol*, **153**, 4663–72.

Heyworth, C., Neumann, E. and Wynn, C. (1981). The stability and aggregation properties of human liver acid β-D-galactosidase. *Biochem J*, **193**, 773.

Hiraiwa, M., Saitoh, M., Arai, N., Shiraishi, T., Odani, S., Uda, Y. *et al.* (1997). Protective protein in the bovine lysosomal beta-galactosidase complex. *Biochim Biophys Acta*, **1341**, 189–99.

van der Horst, G., Galjart, N. J., d'Azzo, A., Galjaard, H. and Verheijen, F. W. (1989). Identification and in vitro reconstitution of lysosomal neuraminidase from human placenta. *J Biol Chem*, **264**, 1317–22.

Itoh, K., Kase, R., Shimmoto, M., Satake, A., Sakuraba, H. and Suzuki, Y. (1995). Protective protein as an endogenous endothelin degradation enzyme in human tissues. *J Biol Chem*, **270**, 515–8.

Itoh, K., Oyanagi, K., Takahashi, H., Sato, T., Hashizume, Y., Shimmoto, M. and Sakuraba, H. (2000). Endothelin-1 in the brain of patients with galactosialidosis: its abnormal increase and distribution pattern. *Ann Neurol*, **47**, 122–6.

Jackman, H. L., Tan, F. L., Tamei, H., Buerling-Harbury, C., Li, X. Y., Skidgel, R. A. *et al.* (1990). A peptidase in human platelets that deamidates tachykinins. Probable identity with the lysosomal "protective protein". *J Biol Chem*, **265**, 11265–72.

Jackman, H. L., Morris, P. W., Deddish, P. A., Skidgel, R. A. and Erdos, E. G. (1992). Inactivation of endothelin I by deamidase (lysosomal protective protein). *J Biol Chem*, **267**, 2872–5.

Kase, R., Itoh, K., Takiyama, N., Oshima, A., Sakuraba, H. and Suzuki, Y. (1990). Galactosialidosis: Simultaneous deficiency of esterase, carboxy-terminal deamidase and acid carboxypeptidase activities. *Biochem Biophys Res Commun*, **172**, 1175–9.

Kawamura, Y., Matoba, T., Hata, T. and Doi, E. (1977). Substrate specificities of cathepsin A, L and A, S from pig kidney. *J Biochem*, **81**, 435.

Kleijer, W. J., Hoogeveen, A., Verheijen, F. W., Niermeijer, M. F., Haljaard, H., O'Brien, J. S. *et al.* (1979). Prenatal diagnosis of sialidosis with combined neuraminidase and β-galactosidase deficiency. *Clin Genet*, **16**, 60–1.

Kleijer, W. J., Geilen, G. C., Janse, H. C., van Diggelen, O. P., Zhou, X.-Y., Galjart, N. J. *et al.* (1996). Cathepsin A deficiency in galactosialidosis: Studies of patients and carriers in 16 families. *Pediatr Res*, **39**, 1067–71.

Kobayashi, T., Ohta, M., Goto, I., Tanaka, Y. and Kuroiwa, Y. (1979). Adult type mucolipidosis with β-galactosidase and sialidase deficiency. *J Neurol*, **221**, 137.

Kyllerman, M., Månsson, L., Westphal, O., Conradi, N. and Nellström, H. (1993). Infantile galactosialidosis with congenital adrenal hyperplasia and renal hypertension. *Pediatr Neurol*, **9**, 318.

Landau, D., Zeigler, M., Shinwell, E., Meisner, I. and Bargal, R. (1995). Hydrops fetalis in four siblings caused by galactosialidosis. *Isr J Med Sci*, **31**, 321.

Leimig, T., Mann, L., Martin, M. d. P., Bonten, E., Persons, D., Knowles, J. *et al.* (2002). Functional amelioration of murine galactosialidosis by genetically modified bone marrow hematopoietic progenitor cells. *Blood*, **99**, 3169–78.

Liao, D., Breddam, K., Sweet, B., Bullock, T. and Remington, S. (1992). Refined atomic model of wheat serine carboxypeptidase II at 2.2 Å resolution. *Biochemistry*, **31**, 9796.

McDonald, J. and Barrett, A. (1986). Lysosomal carboxypeptidase A. In *Mammalian proteases: a glossary and bibliography*, pp. 186. New York: Academic Press.

Miyatake, T., Atsumi, T., Obayashi, T., Mizuno, Y., Ando, S., Ariga, T. *et al.* (1979*a*). Adult type neuronal storage disease with neuraminidase deficiency. *Ann Neurol*, **6**, 232.

Miyatake, T., Yamada, T., Suzuki, M., Pallmann, B., Sandhoff, K., Ariga, T. *et al.* (1979*b*). Sialidase deficiency in adult-type neuronal storage disease. *FEBS Lett*, **97**, 257.

Nanba, E., Tsuji, A., Omura, K. and Suzuki, Y. (1988). Galactosialidosis: Molecular heterogeneity in biosynthesis and processing of protective protein for β-galactosidase. *Hum Genet*, **80**, 329–32.

Nordborg, C., Kyllerman, M., Conradi, N. and Månsson, J. (1997). Early infantile galactosialidosis with multiple brain infarctions: morphological, neuropathological and neurochemical findings. *Acta Neuropathol*, **93**, 24.

Ollis, D. and Goldman, A. (1992). The alpha/β hydrolase fold. *Protein Eng*, **5**, 197–211.

Orii, T., Minami, R., Sukegawa, K., Sato, S., Tsugawa, S., Horino, K. *et al.* (1972). A new type of mucolipidosis with β-galactosidase deficiency and glycopeptiduria. *Tohoku J Exp Med*, **107**, 303.

Oyanagi, K., Ohama, E., Miyashita, K., Yoshino, H., Miyatake, T., Yamazaki, M. *et al.* (1991). Galactosialidosis: neuropathological findings in a case of the late-infantile type. *Acta Neuropathol*, **82**, 331.

Palmeri, S., Hoogeveen, A. T., Verheijen, F. W. and Galjaard, H. (1986). Galactosialidosis: Molecular heterogeneity among distinct clinical phenotypes. *Am J Hum Genet*, **38**, 137–48.

van Pelt, J., Kamerling, J. P., Vliegenthart, J. F., Hoogeveen, A. T. and Galjaard, H. (1988*a*). A comparative study of the accumulated sialic acid-containing oligosaccharides from cultured human galactosialidosis and sialidosis fibroblasts. *Clin Chim Acta*, **174**, 325–35.

van Pelt, J., van Kuik, J. A., Kamerling, J. P., Vliegenthart, J. F., van Diggelen, O. P. and Galjaard, H. (1988*b*). Storage of sialic acid-containing carbohydrates in the placenta of a human galactosialidosis fetus. Isolation and structural characterization of 16 sialyloligosaccharides. *Eur J Biol Chem*, **177**, 327–38.

van Pelt, J., Bakker, H., Kamerling, J. and Vliegenthart, J. (1991). A comparative study of sialyloligosaccharides isolated from sialidosis and galactosialidosis urine. *J Inherit Metab Dis*, **14**, 730.

Pinsky, L., Miller, J., Shanfield, B., Watters, G. and Wolfe, L. S. (1974). GM1 gangliosidosis in skin fibroblast culture: Enzymatic difference between types 1 and 2 and observations on a third variant. *Am J Hum Genet*, **26**, 563–77.

Pshezhetsky, A. and Potier, M. (1996). Association on *N*-acetylgalactosamine-6-sulfate sulfatase with the multienzyme lysosomal complex of β-galactosidase, cathepsin A, and neuraminidase. *J Biol Chem*, **271**, 28359–65.

Richard, C., Tranchemontague, J., Elsliger, M., Mitchell, G., Potier, M. and Pshezhetsky, A. (1998). Molecular pathology of galactosialidosis in a patient affected with two new frameshift mutations in the cathepsin A/protective protein gene. *Hum Mutat*, **11**, 461.

Rottier, R. and d'Azzo, A. (1997). Identification of the promoters for the human and murine protective protein/cathepsin A genes. *DNA Cell Biol*, **16**, 599–610.

Rottier, R., Bonten, E. and d'Azzo, A. (1998*a*). A point mutation in the *neu-1* locus causes the neuraminidase defect in the SM/J mouse. *Hum Mol Genet*, **7**, 313–21.

Rottier, R., Hahn, C., Mann, L., Martin, M., Smeyne, R., Suzuki, K. *et al.* (1998*b*). Lack of PPCA expression does not always correlate with lysosomal storage: a possible requirement for the catalytic function of PPCA in galactosialidosis. *Hum Mol Genet*, **7**, 1787–94.

Rudenko, G., Bonten, E., d'Azzo, A. and Hol, W. G. J. (1995). Three-dimensional structure of the human "protective protein": Structure of the precursor form suggests a complex activation mechanism. *Structure*, **3**, 1249–59.

Rudenko, G., Bonten, E., Hol, W. and d'Azzo, A. (1998). The atomic model of the human protective protein/cathepsin A suggests a structural basis for galactosialidosis. *Proc Natl Acad Sci USA*, **95**, 621–25.

Sarna, J., Miranda, S. R., Schuchman, E. H. and Hawkes, R. (2001). Patterned cerebellar Purkinje cell death in a transgenic mouse model of Niemann Pick type A/B disease. *Eur J Neurosci*, **13**, 1873–80.

Scheibe, R., Hein, K. and Wenzel, K. W. (1990). Lysosomal beta-galactosidase from rat liver: Purification, molecular forms and association with neuraminidase. *Biomed Biochim Acta*, **49**, 547–56.

Skidgel, R. and Erdos, E. (1998). Cellular carboxypeptidases. *Immunol Rev*, **161**, 129–41.

van der Spoel, A., Bonten, E. and d'Azzo, A. (1998). Transport of human lysosomal neuraminidase to mature lysosomes requires protective protein/cathepsin A. *EMBO J*, **17**, 1588–97.

Spranger, J. (1981). Mucolipidosis I: phenotype and nosology. In *Sialidases and sialidoses* (Durand, P., Tettamanti, G. and DiDonato, S., ed.), pp. 379. Milan: Edi. Ermes.

Stone, D. and Sidransky, E. (1999). Hydrops fetalis: lysosomal storage disorders in extremis. *Adv Pediatr*, **46**, 409–40.

Strisciuglio, P., Parenti, G., Giudice, C., Lijoi, S., Hoogeveen, A. T. and d'Azzo, A. (1988). The presence of a reduced amount of 32-kd "protective" protein is a distinct biochemical finding in late infantile galactosialidosis. *Hum Genet*, **80**, 304–6.

Takano, T., Shimmoto, M., Fukuhara, Y., Itoh, K., Kase, R., Takiyama, N. *et al.* (1991). Galactosialidosis: Clinical and molecular analysis of 19 Japanese patients. *Brain Dysfunct*, **4**, 271–80.

Thomas, G. H. (2001). Disorders of glycoprotein degradation and structure: α-mannosidosis, β-mannosidosis, fucosidosis, and sialidosis. In *The metabolic and molecular bases of inherited disease* (Scriver, C., Beaudet, A., Sly, W. S. and Valle, D., ed.), pp. 3507–34. New York: McGraw-Hill.

Usui, T., Sawaguchi, S., Abe, H., Iwata, K. and Oyanagi, K. (1991). Late-infantile type galactosialidosis—Histopathology of the retina and optic nerve. *Arch Ophthalmol*, **109**, 542–6.

Valls, L., Hunter, C., Rothman, J. and Stevens, T. (1987). Protein sorting in yeast: the localization determinant of yeast vacuolar carboxypeptidase. *Cell*, **48**, 887.

Verheijen, F., Brossmer, R. and Galjaard, H. (1982). Purification of acid beta-galactosidase and acid neuraminidase from bovine testis: Evidence for an enzyme complex. *Biochem Biophys Res Commun*, **108**, 868–75.

Verheijen, F. W., Palmeri, S., Hoogeveen, A. T. and Galjaard, H. (1985). Human placental neuraminidase. Activation, stabilization and association with beta-galactosidase and its protective protein. *Eur J Biochem*, **149**, 315–21.

Wenger, D. A., Tarby, T. J. and Wharton, C. (1978). Macular cherry-red spots and myoclonus with dementia: Coexistent neuraminidase and β-galactosidase deficiencies. *Biochem Biophys Res Commun*, **82**, 589–95.

Whitmore, T., Day, J. and Albers, J. (1995). Localization of the human phospholipid transfer protein gene to chromosome 20q12-q13.1. *Genomics*, **28**, 599–600.

Wiegant, J., Galjart, N. J., Raap, A. K. and Dazzo, A. (1991). The gene encoding human protective protein (PPGB) is on chromosome-20. *Genomics*, **10**, 345–9.

Yamamoto, Y. and Nishimura, K. (1986). Aggregation–dissociation and stability of acid β-galactosidase purified from porcine spleen. *Int Biochem*, **4**, 327.

Yamamoto, Y. and Nishimura, K. (1987). Copurification and separation of β-galactosidase and sialidase from porcine testis. *J Biol Chem (Tokyo)*, **19**, 435–42.

Yoshino, H., Miyashita, K., Miyatani, N., Ariga, T., Hashimoto, Y., Tsuji, S. *et al.* (1990). Abnormal glycosphingolipid metabolism in the nervous system of galactosialidosis. *J Neurol Sci*, **97**, 53–65.

Yuce, A., Kocak, N. and Besley, G. (1996). Galactosialidosis in two siblings. *Turk J Pediatr*, **38**, 85.

Zammarchi, E., Donati, M. A., Marrone, A., Donzelli, G., Zhou, X.-Y. and d'Azzo, A. (1996). Early infantile galactosialidosis: Clinical, biochemical, and molecular observations in a new patient. *Am J Med Genet*, **64**, 453–8.

Zhou, X.-Y., Galjart, N. J., Willemsen, R., Gillemans, N., Galjaard, H. and d'Azzo, A. (1991). A mutation in a mild form of galactosialidosis impairs dimerization of the protective protein and renders it unstable. *EMBO J*, **10**, 4041–8.

Zhou, X.-Y., Morreau, H., Rottier, R., Davis, D., Bonten, E., Gillemans, N. *et al.* (1995). Mouse model for the lysosomal disorder galactosialidosis and correction of the phenotype with over-expressing erythroid precursor cells. *Genes Dev*, **9**, 2623–34.

Zhou, X.-Y., van der Spoel, A., Rottier, R., Hale, G., Willemsen, R., Berry, G. T. *et al.* (1996). Molecular and biochemical analysis of protective protein/cathepsin A mutations: Correlation with clinical severity in galactosialidosis. *Hum Mol Genet*, **5**, 1977–87.

Chapter 8

Defects in activator proteins and other soluble proteins of the lysosome

Oliver Macheleidt, Thomas Kolter and Konrad Sandhoff

Introduction

In 1909, the physicochemist Wolfgang Ostwald was awarded the Nobel Prize for chemistry. One of his contributions to science was the description of kinetics and catalysis of chemical reactions. He was the first to provide the definition of a catalyst still used today. The catalyst, in biochemistry usually an enzyme, is a substance that increases the rate of a chemical reaction without being consumed in the overall reaction and without influencing the reaction equilibrium. Substances that participate directly in an enzyme-catalysed reaction, but are not able to carry it out themselves, are called activators. Activators are involved in many physiological processes, and there are different mechanisms by which activators work. The requirement of activator proteins is a characteristic feature in lysosomal glycolipid catabolism which takes place at the membrane—water interfacial region where the reactants are not in the same phase: enzymes dissolved in the lysosol have to degrade their membrane-bound glycolipid and sphingolipid substrates at the interface. In this chapter we report on enzymatically inactive proteins that play a part in two areas of endosomal–lysosomal membrane lipid metabolism. Some are involved in binding and transfer processes that assist lysosomal sphingolipid catabolism and others appear to regulate cholesterol transport from these acidic compartments back to the plasma membrane and the endoplasmic reticulum (ER). These activator-mediated processes are of physiological relevance since defects in activator function can lead to fatal human diseases.

Glycosphingolipid structure, function, and biosynthesis

Glycosphingolipids (GSLs) are amphiphilic components of eukaryotic cell membranes. They are composed of a hydrophobic ceramide moiety which anchors the molecules in the membrane and an extracellular hydrophilic oligosaccharide headgroup (Merrill and Sweely 1996). Variations in number, identity, and linkage of the carbohydrates lead to the wide range of naturally occurring GSLs. Together with other glycolipids, glycoproteins, and glycosaminoglycans, they contribute to the extracellular glycocalix. On the cell surface, GSLs are involved in adhesion processes (Varki 1993) and serve as binding sites for toxins, viruses, and bacteria (Karlsson 1989). They can segregate into glycolipid-enriched microdomains and thereby alter the functional properties of membrane proteins (Brown and London 2000). Furthermore, they influence physiological processes like embryogenesis, neuronal cell and leukocyte differentiation, as well as signal transduction (Zeller and Marchase 1992). The cellular GSL composition is dependent on species, on cell type, and on the cellular state of differentiation.

Glycosphingolipids are synthesized at intracellular membranes of the ER and the Golgi apparatus (Kolter and Sandhoff 1999). The first steps leading to ceramide, the membrane anchor of most glycolipids, occur at the cytosolic face of the ER membrane (Merrill 2002). Glucosylceramide is formed on the cytosolic face of the Golgi membrane and is subsequently translocated to the luminal face by an unknown mechanism. Further glycosylation reactions are catalysed by glycosyltransferases in the Golgi apparatus. These are membrane-bound enzymes and operate within the same membrane as their substrates. Therefore, the reactions should show two-dimensional enzyme kinetics (Scheel *et al.* 1982). After their biosynthesis, GSLs reach the plasma membrane through vesicular exocytotic flow. Participation of activator proteins in GSL biosynthesis is not known.

Lysosomal glycosphingolipid catabolism

Sphingolipids are degraded by the action of exohydrolases, in many cases in combination with sphingolipid-activator proteins (SAPs) (Fig. 8.1). Five SAPs are known so far, the GM2 activator protein (GM2 AP) and SAP-A to -D, also called saposins A–D. Defects in either degrading enzymes or activator proteins give rise to a group of human-inherited diseases, the sphingolipidoses (Kolter and Sandhoff 1998).

Topology

Glycosphingolipids and other components of the plasma membrane—lipids and proteins—reach the lysosome by endocytotic vesicular flow. Parts of the plasma membrane enriched in GSLs bud into coated pits that are internalized and uncoated, and subsequently fuse with early endosomes (Chapter 1). Therefore, sphingolipids derived from the cell surface should become part of the limiting membrane of endosomes and lysosomes and should be somehow degraded there without impairment of lysosomal integrity. This is rather unlikely since the leaflet of the lysosomal perimeter membrane that faces the lysosol is covered with a thick glycocalix that protects the membrane from the attack by the lipid-degrading enzymes present in the lysosol (Peters and von Figura 1994). This glycocalyx, visible in the microscope, is essentially composed of the carbohydrate part of LIMPs (lysosomal integral membrane proteins) and LAMPs (lysosomal associated membrane proteins) (Carlsson *et al.* 1988) which are highly N-glycosylated with lactosamine units. The enzyme/activator system required for degradation cannot be expected to reach their substrates through this glycocalix. And indeed, glycolipids of the perimeter membrane are much more resistant towards degradation than plasma membrane-derived GSLs (Henning and Stoffel 1973).

The question of selectivity and how the integrity of the limiting lysosomal membrane is preserved led us to the assumption that the major part of GSL catabolism cannot take place within the limiting lysosomal membrane (Fürst and Sandhoff 1992). Instead, we assume that vesicles from the plasma membrane fuse with endosomes in a way that glycolipids from the cell surface reach the lumen of the digesting organelles as small intraendosomal and intralysosomal vesicles (Sandhoff and Kolter 1996). This assumption will be of decisive importance for the understanding of the molecular bases of glycolipid degradation. It means that parts of the

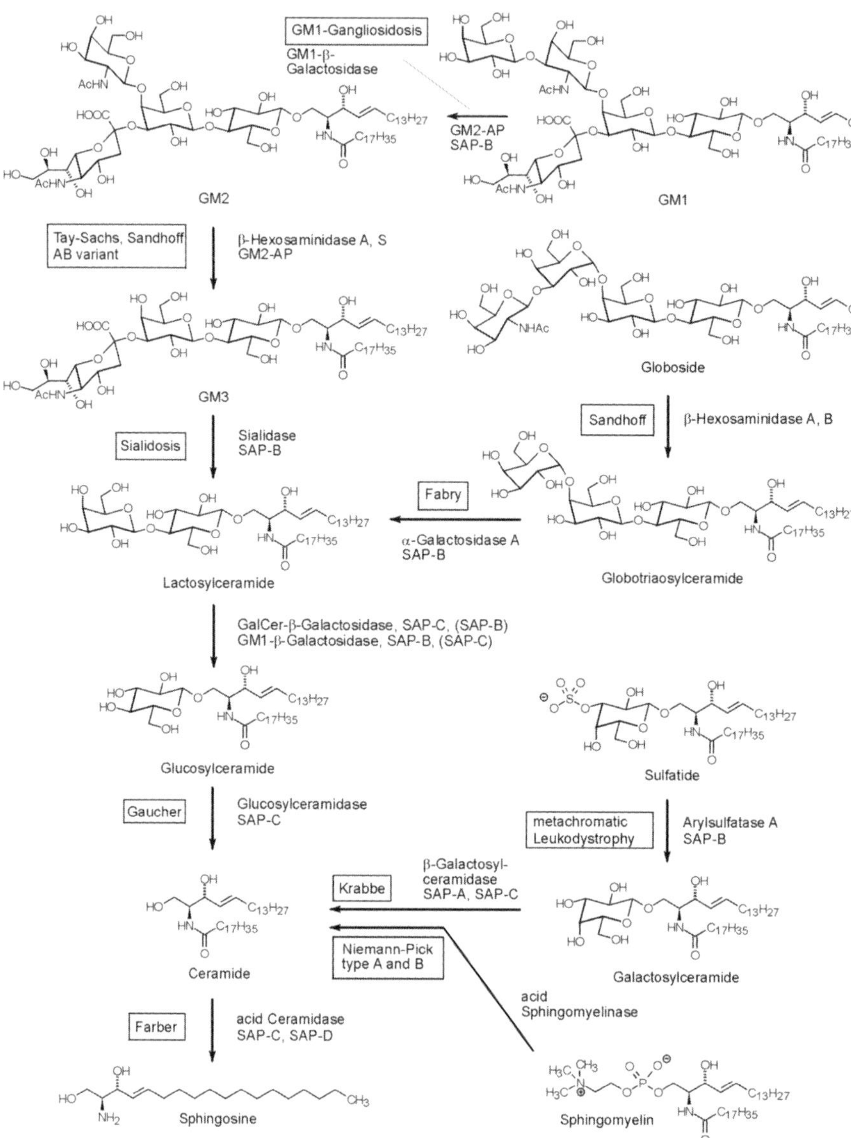

Fig. 8.1 Lysosomal degradation of glycosphingolipids. The eponyms of known metabolic diseases and those of sphingolipid activator proteins necessary for *in vivo* degradation are indicated. Heterogeneity in the lipid part of the sphingolipids is not indicated. AB variant = variant AB of GM2 gangliosidosis, deficiency of GM2 activator protein (GM2 AP), SAP = sphingolipid activator protein (modified from Kolter and Sandhoff 1999).

endosomal membrane, enriched in components derived from the plasma membrane, invaginate and bud into the endosomal lumen. Therefore, GSLs originating from the outer leaflet of the plasma membrane face the lumen of the endosomes on the surface of intraendosomal vesicles or other lipid aggregates and not as parts of the perimeter membrane. In this way they are exposed to the proteins of the digesting system. The topology is strictly determined since endogenous glycolipids are not able to undertake an uncatalysed transversal membrane translocation to change their orientation. One of the observations leading to the proposal of the model was that multivesicular structures accumulate in cells of sphingolipidosis patients, especially in cells with a simultaneous deficiency of SAPs A–D. Later, it could be shown that they refer to the late endosomal-lysosomal compartment (Burkhardt *et al.* 1997). Additional evidence for the proposed route came from experiments in human fibroblasts: biotin-labelled ganglioside GM1 derived from the plasma membrane is targeted to intralysosomal structures and not to the lysosomal perimeter membrane (Möbius *et al.* 1999). If degradation occurs on the surface of these intralysosomal membrane structures, their respective size, lipid composition, and lateral pressure should influence the degradation process. Analysis of these molecular details supports the initial hypothesis of GSL degradation at intralysosomal membrane structures.

Enzymology

Glycosphingolipids of the plasma membrane are degraded after endocytosis in late endosomes and lysosomes (Kolter and Sandhoff 1999). The terminal sugars are sequentially split off by different water-soluble acid exohydrolases. According to the model discussed above, these enzymes degrade substrates that are embedded in intralysosomal membrane structures. It turned out that in the absence of detergents that solubilize the lipids, GSLs with carbohydrate chains of one to four residues (Wilkening *et al.* 2000) are hardly or not accessible to the hydrolases. Their degradation requires the additional presence of an activator protein.

In the case of ganglioside degradation, ganglioside GM1 (four sugar residues in a row) is degraded to ganglioside GM2 by a β-galactosidase which cleaves the terminal neutral sugar, a β-linked galactose residue, in the presence of either the GM2 AP or SAP-B (Wilkening *et al.* 2000). The resulting ganglioside GM2 (three sugar residues in a row) is then decomposed to ganglioside GM3 and *N*-acetyl-galactosamine mainly by β-hexosaminidase A (HexA). Both enzymes are resident within the lumen of the lysosomes. HexA is a heterodimer (α,β) with two active sites that differ in their substrate specificity (Kytzia and Sandhoff 1985). The other subunit combinations in the hexosaminidases are HexB (β,β-homodimer) and HexS (α,α-homodimer). The catalytic centre of the β-subunit cleaves predominantly neutral sugar chains with terminal *N*-acetyl-β-*D*-galactosaminyl and *N*-acetyl-β-*D*-glucosaminyl residues. Towards uncharged substrates, the active site on the α-subunit is less active than the β-unit but cleaves sugars from negatively charged substrates (Hepbildikler *et al.* 2002) In addition to the β-hexosaminidase A or S, degradation of ganglioside GM2 requires the GM2 AP (see section *GM2 Activator Protein*). This activator is essential for the *in vivo* degradation of this ganglioside (Sandhoff *et al.* 2001). Historically, this was the first example for the absolute requirement of an activator for the *in vivo* degradation of a glycolipid. Its absence leads to the so called AB variant of the GM2 gangliosidoses (Conzelmann and Sandhoff 1978, 1979). In the absence of additional factors like detergents or activator proteins, the enzyme is only able to degrade water-soluble substrates or such membrane-bound substrates with sugar chains that reach sufficiently far from the lipid core into the aqueous space (Meier *et al.* 1991).

A sialidase cleaves ganglioside GM3 into lactosylceramide and sialic acid, before the galactose is split off by either galactosylceramide-β-galactosidase or GM1-β-galactosidase to yield glucosylceramide. The stepwise cleavage of the hydrophilic headgroups from these glycolipids finally leads to ceramide (Fig. 8.1) which is cleaved by acid ceramidase in the presence of SAP-C or -D (Linke *et al.* 2001*b*) into sphingosine and a fatty acid. Together with the other cleavage products, these two metabolites are able to leave the lysosome.

For the non-glycosylated sphingolipids like ceramide and sphingomyelin, also non-lysosomal degradation steps are known which apparently do not need the assistance of an activator protein. Sphingomyelin is cleaved to ceramide and phosphorylcholine. Ceramide later on is degraded into sphingosine and a fatty acid by ceramidases of different subcellular localization. In the cytosol, sphingosine can be phosphorylated to sphingosine-1-phosphate or can be re-acylated to ceramide. These highly regulated degradation processes occur at several subcellular places to produce various signalling molecules (Huwiler *et al.* 2000; Pyne and Pyne 2000; Hannun *et al.* 2001; Hannun and Obeid 2002; Spiegel and Milstien 2002).

GM2 Activator protein

The GM2 AP was identified during the analysis of a patient with massive storage of ganglioside GM2 and glycolipid GA2 in the brain, in spite of the presence of hexosaminidases A and B (Sandhoff 1977). In the presence of a surfactant, the isolated enzymes from the patient were able to cleave the storage material *in vitro*. The search for the essential '*in vivo* detergent' defective in the tissues of the patient led to the discovery of the GM2 AP (Conzelmann and Sandhoff 1978). This activator has been purified and structurally and functionally characterized (Conzelmann and Sandhoff 1979; Fürst and Sandhoff 1992). It turned out to be a lysosomal glycoprotein of 17.6 kDa in the deglycosylated form. It bears an N-glycosidically bound oligosaccharide chain (Fürst *et al.* 1990) and contains four disulfide bridges (Schütte *et al.* 1998) that contribute to its stability towards heat and proteases. Recently, the crystal structure of the human GM2 AP recombinantly expressed in *Escherichia coli* has been solved (Wright *et al.* 2000). According to the structure of the non-glycosylated protein, it contains a cavity for the ceramide moiety and an adjacent possible recognition site for the oligosaccharide chain. It also has a flexible hydrophobic loop which may facilitate two functions discussed below, the interaction with the membrane and the extraction of the GM2 ganglioside. The cDNA and the gene on chromosome 5 are known (Klima *et al.* 1991; Swallow *et al.* 1993; Schepers *et al.* 2000). A non-functional pseudogene was mapped to chromosome 3 (Xie *et al.* 1992) and an alternatively spliced variant was found (Wu *et al.* 1996). Until now, five different mutations in the gene of the GM2 activator have been identified. Point mutations (Schröder *et al.* 1991, 1993) lead to the exchange of one amino acid and to the complete deficiency of the protein. The mutated activator proteins are of limited stability and the mutations cause premature degradation (Schepers *et al.* 1996).

Functional properties of the GM2 activator protein

The GM2 AP is essential for the degradation of ganglioside GM2 and of glycolipid GA2 *in vivo* (Conzelmann and Sandhoff 1979). After binding of the membrane-active GM2 AP to the substrate-carrying membranes, a water-soluble ganglioside-activator protein complex might be formed. The GM2 AP can be regarded as a weak detergent with high selectivity or, in other words, as a 'liftase'. It lifts ganglioside GM2 or related GSLs (e.g. GM1; Wilkening *et al.* 2000) out of the membrane so that they become accessible for the active site of the degrading enzyme (Fig. 8.2). GM2 Activator proteins can insert into and disturb intralysosomal vesicle membranes. It can also bind to glycolipids such as ganglioside GM2. Hexosaminidase A recognizes the complex of ganglioside GM2 and GM2 AP, hydrolyses

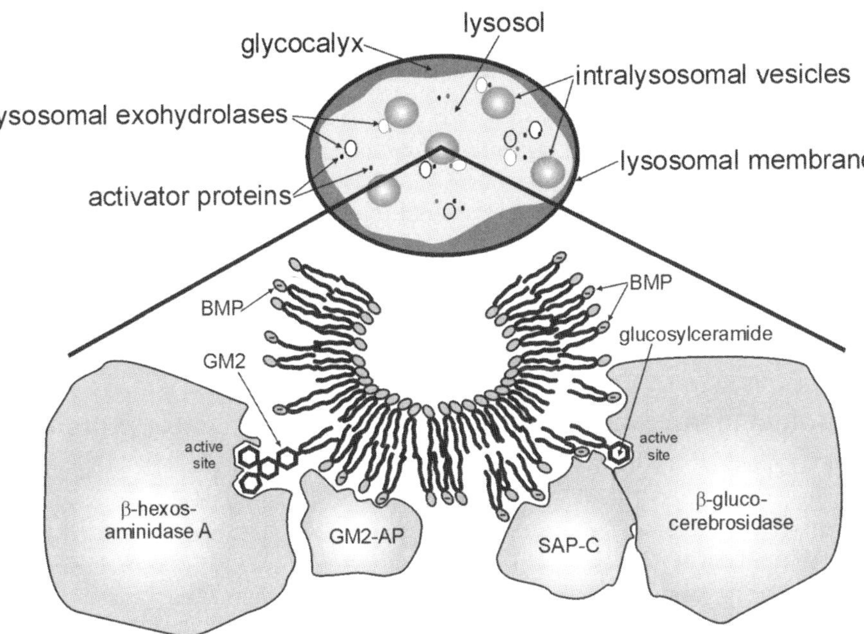

Fig. 8.2 Lysosomal glycosphingolipid catabolism. Model for the lysosomal degradation of membrane-bound glycosphingolipids by lysosomal exohydrolases and activator proteins. Given are two examples: GM2 degradation by β-hexosaminidase A and the GM2 activator protein (GM2 AP); glucosylceramide-degradation by β-glucocerebrosidase and sphingolipid activator protein C (SAP-C). The model emphasizes the topology of degradation, the properties of the intralysosomal membrane structure, and the interactions between membrane surface, activator protein, hydrolytic enzyme, and substrate. BMP = bis-(monoacylglycero)-phosphate (modified from Wilkening *et al.* 2000).

ganglioside GM2, and releases ganglioside GM3. The enzymatic process may occur at the interface of the membrane aggregates or even in free solution in the lysosome. Lifting the ganglioside just a few angstroms out of the membrane might be sufficient to present the substrate in an enzyme-accessible form. This is supported by the fact that synthetic analogues of ganglioside GM2 with shortened fatty acid chains and therefore of higher water solubility are degraded by HexA already in the absence of the GM2 AP or detergents (Meier *et al.* 1991). GM2 Activator Proteins recognizes the hydrophobic ceramide moiety (Conzelmann *et al.* 1982), the sialic acid, and the *N*-acetyl-galactosamine moiety of ganglioside GM2 (Smiljanic-Georgijev *et al.* 1997) and might also cleave an intramolecular hydrogen bond between the terminal sugar residues to facilitate the degradation of the ganglioside (Wu *et al.* 1994). This hypothesis, however, does not explain that the degradation of short-chain analogues of ganglioside GM2 and of ganglioside GD1aGalNAc by HexA already occurs in the absence of GM2 AP. The cleavage of two glycolipids which apparently do not contain such an intramolecular hydrogen bond is also stimulated by GM2 AP: GM2 AP stimulates the HexA- and HexS-catalysed degradation of sulfoglycolipid SM2 (Hepbildikler *et al.* 2002; Sandhoff *et al.* 2002), and glycolipid GA2 accumulates in patients (Sandhoff *et al.* 1971) and knockout mice deficient in the GM2 AP (Liu *et al.* 1997).

Besides its function in the hydrolysis of ganglioside GM2, further physiological roles have been attributed to GM2 AP (Mahuran 1998). It is suggested to act as a factor that stimulates phospholipase D activity through enhancing the association between the enzyme and enzyme activators (Nakamura *et al.* 1998; Sarkar *et al.* 2001). Another potential role of the GM2 AP is the regulation of proton pumps in intercalated cells of the kidney (Mundel *et al.* 1999). Because a cytosolic localization of the GM2 AP has not been convincingly demonstrated to date, functional roles within the cytosol, as mentioned above, remain ambiguous.

Taken together, the GM2 AP recognizes, binds, and releases a subgroup of membrane-bound GSL. Its inherited deficiency leads to the AB variant of GM2 gangliosidosis, in which the lipid accumulation in neuronal cells leads to early death of the patients.

Lysosomal membrane structures and the GM2 activator protein

In this chapter, we discuss other factors that influence the digestion of glycolipids on intralysosomal vesicles. The diameter of these vesicles has to be taken into account. As determined in tissues from SAP-deficient patients, it is in the range of 50–100 nm (Bradova *et al.* 1993) and can be mimicked in *in vitro* experiments by vesicles of a comparable size. The convex curvature favours spreading of the GSL headgroups and makes them more easily accessible for exohydrolases in the presence of activator proteins (Fig. 8.2). The geometry of the membrane vesicles depends on their lipid composition (Kobayashi *et al.* 1998), the chain length, and the degree of saturation of the amphiphilic lipids. Owing to steric and electrostatic repulsion, lipids with large and negatively charged hydrophilic headgroups favour a strong curvature and a smaller size of the vesicles. This should result in a relatively low lateral pressure of such membrane structures.

For recognition and binding of a GSL, such as ganglioside GM2, the GM2 AP should insert into the membrane. Physicochemical measurements with lipid monolayers show that the GM2 AP protein inserts only if the lateral pressure of the monolayer is below a critical value of 15–25 m/Nm, depending on the lipid composition (Giehl *et al.* 1999). Therefore, we assume that the GM2 AP cannot penetrate into biological membranes like the perimeter membrane of the lysosome. Their lateral pressure is in the range between 30 and 35 m/Nm (Marsh 1996). Albeit there are no data on the lateral pressure of intralysosomal vesicles available, we expect it to be below the critical value of 25 m/Nm.

In addition to size, curvature, and lateral pressure, the lipid composition of the inner membranes of late endosomes and lysosomes appears to be unique. They contain bis-(monoacylglycero)-phosphate (BMP, in the literature also erroneously known as LBPA, lysobisphosphatidic acid), as analysed by immunogold electron microscopy (Kobayashi *et al.* 1998) and subcellular fractionation (Becker, PhD Thesis, University of Bonn, 2000). Bis-(monoacylglycero)-phosphate is an anionic phospholipid with a lysolipid structure and is synthesized in the acidic compartment of the cell (Amidon *et al.* 1996). It has been described as a marker lipid of lysosomes (Brotherus and Renkonen 1977). Owing to its unusual sn1,sn1′-configuration, it is more resistant to the action of phospholipases than normal phospholipids (Matsuzawa and Hostetler 1979). Bis-(monoacylglycero)-phosphate is presumably formed during the degradation of phosphatidylglycerol and cardiolipin which are derived from mitochondria that enter the lysosomal compartment by autophagy. During this degradation process, BMP should be formed on intralysosomal vesicles and distinguishes these membranes from the perimeter membrane. Besides BMP, smaller amounts of phosphatidylinositol (Kobayashi *et al.* 1998) and dolicholphosphate (Chojnacki and Dallner 1988) have been found as anionic lipids within the lysosomal compartment.

Bis-(monoacylglycero)-phosphate and other anionic lysosomal phospholipids dramatically stimulate the interfacial hydrolysis of membrane-bound glycolipids by their water-soluble exohydrolases in the presence of GM2 AP; ganglioside GM2 by HexA (Werth *et al.* 2001), ganglioside GM1 by β-galactosidase (Wilkening *et al.* 2000), and the sulfated gangliotriaosylceramide SM2 by HexA and HexS (Hepbildikler *et al.* 2002). Bis-(monoacylglycero)-phosphate did not enhance the binding of the GM2 AP to the membrane but increased its ability to solubilize lipids. This ability should lead to a destabilization of the membranes and facilitate the attack of water-soluble exohydrolases.

In vitro, glucosylceramide degradation is drastically enhanced by the presence of negatively charged lipids such as phosphatidylserine, phosphatidylglycerol, and phosphatidic acid (Berent and Radin 1981; Sarmientos *et al.* 1986; Salvioli *et al.* 2000).

Sphingolipid activator proteins derived from prosaposin

Besides the GM2 AP, four additional enzymatically inactive proteins are required for the degradation of GSLs with short oligosaccharide chains. These proteins are called SAPs (Mehl and Jatzkewitz 1964) or saposins (Morimoto *et al.* 1988). Having different specificity, they facilitate the degradation of membrane-bound sphingolipids by water-soluble exohydrolases.

All four saposins or SAPs A–D are derived from a single protein, SAP precursor or prosaposin, by proteolytic processing (Fürst *et al.* 1988; O'Brien *et al.* 1988; Nakano *et al.* 1989). The SAP precursor is synthesized in the ER and transported through the Golgi stacks, where it is glycosylated to a 70 kDa protein. It is secreted to the extracellular space and can be endocytosed by the low-density lipoprotein receptor (LDL)-related protein, LRP (Hiesberger *et al.* 1998). The SAP precursor itself is reported to have neurotrophic and neuroprotective properties of its own (Hiraiwa *et al.* 1997). It is found in several body fluids, including human milk and semen (Hineno *et al.* 1991; Kondoh *et al.* 1991).

In the acidic compartment of the cell, the individual domains of the precursor protein are proteolytically processed to the individual SAPs A–D (Vielhaber *et al.* 1997). The four SAPs show homology to each other and have similar properties but differ in their specificity and their mode of action. Their sequences (all about 80 amino acids) contain six highly conserved cysteines and a conserved N-glycosylation site (Kishimoto *et al.* 1992). The disulfide bridges are essential for the activity and might account for the unusual stability of the proteins (Vaccaro *et al.* 1995*b*). A structural motif known as saposin-like domain has been identified in several proteins (Munford *et al.* 1995). It is characterized by three intradomain disulfide linkages and a subset of conserved amino acid residues with hydrophobic side chains. 'Saposin-like proteins' (SAPLIP) carry out diverse functions on a common backbone structure. The three-dimensional structure of one SAP-like domain has been solved by NMR spectroscopy (Liepinsh *et al.* 1997). In the so-called 'swaposins', carboxy- and aminoterminal halves of the domains have been swapped (Ponting and Russell 1995). There is evidence that the precursor of pulmonary surfactant protein B contains three SAP-like domains (Zaltash and Johansson 1998). All proteins of this group share a lipid-binding and a membrane-perturbing property.

The first SAP was discovered in 1964 by Mehl and Jatzkewitz. They identified the sulfatide-activator protein (SAP-B or saposin B), which is required for the degradation of sulfatide (galactosylceramide-3-sulfate) by the lysosomal enzyme arylsulfatase A. Sphingolipid-activator protein B is a small lysosomal glycoprotein with one N-glycosidically linked oligosaccharide chain and three disulfide bridges (Fischer and Jatzkewitz 1975; Fürst *et al.* 1990). These cross linkages might account for the unusual stability against pH (1.5–12), heat (up to 95°C), and proteases (Gärtner *et al.* 1983). Until now, five point mutations on the SAP-B domain of the SAP precursor gene have been identified (Wrobe *et al.* 2000).

Like the GM2 AP, SAP-B behaves like a physiological detergent and stimulates sulfatide degradation by solubilizing the membrane-bound substrate. *In vitro*, it was found to be a transport protein for sulfatides and other GSLs (Vogel *et al.* 1991). The inherited defect of SAP-B leads to the accumulation of sulfatides, digalactosylceramides, and globotriao sylceramides (Sandhoff *et al.* 2001). The phenotype of the patients resembles a variant form of metachromatic leukodystrophy (MLD) with late infantile or juvenile onset (Kretz *et al.* 1990).

Sphingolipid-activator protein C or saposin C is required for the lysosomal degradation of glucosylceramide by glucosylceramide-β-glucosidase. Sphingolipid-activator protein C is a 20 kDa protein, obviously in homodimeric structure, and has been first isolated from spleen of Gaucher patients (Ho and O'Brien 1971). In contrast to SAP-B, it binds not only to lipids and membranes but interacts also with glucosylceramide-β-glucosidase and stimulates the enzyme directly (Berent and Radin 1981; Fabbro and Grabowski 1991). The β-glucosidase is a water-soluble lysosomal enzyme that can associate with membranes. *In vitro*, it requires detergents or negatively charged phospholipids for its full enzymatic activity (Wilkening *et al.* 1998). The activator enhances the activity against the natural lipid substrate as well as against synthetic water-soluble substrates *in vitro* (Sarmientos *et al.* 1986; Vaccaro *et al.* 1997). Sphingolipid-activator protein C apparently does not bind glucosylceramide but the degrading enzyme. Kinetic data suggest an allosteric activation of the enzyme (Morimoto *et al.* 1990). Under acidic pH, the affinity of SAP-C to membranes is strongly increased (Vaccaro *et al.* 1995*a*). At these pH values, SAP-C (and SAP-D) also destabilizes phospholipid membranes of large unilamellar vesicles *in vitro* (Wilkening *et al.* 1998). This could facilitate the association of glucosylceramide-β-glucocerebrosidase with membranes, which favours the degradation of glucosylceramide (Vaccaro *et al.* 1999). *In vitro*, SAP-C also stimulates the degradation of galactosylceramide by galactosylceramide-β-galactosidase (Wenger *et al.* 1982), sphingomyelin by acid sphingomyelinase (Tayama *et al.* 1993; Linke *et al.* 2001*a*), and ceramide by acid ceramidase (Linke *et al.* 2001*b*). The deficiency of SAP-C leads to an abnormal juvenile form of Gaucher disease and an accumulation of glucosylceramide (Christomanou *et al.* 1986; Schnabel *et al.* 1991) (Chapter 3). Feeding of purified SAP-C to patients fibroblasts reduces the level of glucosylceramide storage, whereas SAP-A, -B, and -D were not effective (Klein *et al.* 1994).

Until now, no human disease is known which is based on the isolated defect of SAP-A (Morimoto *et al.* 1989) or SAP-D (Fürst *et al.* 1988). *In vitro*, SAP-A can bind to gangliosides GM1 and GM2 (Hiraiwa *et al.* 1992) and stimulate to some extent the enzyme-catalysed hydrolysis of glucosyl- and galactosylceramide (Morimoto *et al.* 1990). *In vivo*, it is required for the degradation of galactosylceramide: mice carrying a mutation in the SAP-A domain of the SAP precursor accumulate galactosylceramide and suffer from a late-onset form of Krabbe disease (Matsuda *et al.* 2001).

Sphingolipid-activator protein D contains 78 amino acids and one N-linked oligosaccharide chain. It stimulates lysosomal ceramide degradation by acid ceramidase in cultured cells (Klein *et al.* 1994) as well as *in vitro* (Linke *et al.* 2001*b*). An activating effect is also described for the acid sphingomyelinase, but this seems not to be necessary for the *in vivo* degradation of sphingomyelin (Morimoto *et al.* 1988; Linke *et al.* 2001*a*). At the appropriate pH, SAP-D binds to vesicles containing negatively charged lipids and solubilizes membranes (Ciaffoni *et al.* 2001).

A lipidosis patient with a pleiotrophic sphingolipid accumulation, but without an enzyme defect, showed a complete lack of the whole SAP precursor protein. The patient died within 16 weeks (Harzer *et al.* 1989). The molecular analysis revealed a homoallelic mutation in the start codon of the SAP precursor protein from ATG to TTG (Schnabel *et al.* 1992). This led to the complete loss of SAPs A–D. Neutral glycolipids were stored in the liver, in the kidney, and in cultured skin fibroblasts (Bradova *et al.* 1993). Sulfatide was stored in the kidney and free ceramide was accumulated in the liver and kidney. The levels of gangliosides GM2 and GM3 were elevated in the liver but not in the brain, while sphingomyelin and phospholipids were not affected.

The *in vivo* role of the different SAPs A–D in sphingolipid degradation was investigated in cultured fibroblasts from this patient in metabolic labelling studies (Klein *et al.* 1994). Accumulation of lactosylceramide could be normalized by feeding SAP-B (stimulating GM1-β-galactosidase-catalysed reaction) as well as SAP-C (stimulating galactosylceramide-β-galactosidase-catalysed reaction); this was likewise confirmed *in vitro* (Zschoche *et al.* 1994). Sphingolipid-activator protein D also reduces the accumulation of ganglioside GM3 and glucosylceramide. The exogenous addition of SAP-D stimulates ceramide degradation in cultured cells and *in vitro* (Linke *et al.* 2001*b*). Recently, a second case with complete deficiency of the SAP precursor and the mature SAPs has been reported. Here, a deletion within the SAP-B domain leads to a frameshift and a premature stop codon (Hulkova *et al.* 2001).

Clinical aspects of activator protein deficiencies

The inherited dysfunction of one or more GSL degradation steps leads to the accumulation of the nondegradable lipid material. The resulting diseases are usually named according to the identity of the storage material in these sphingolipidoses (Kolter and Sandhoff 1998; Suzuki and Vanier 1999) (Chapters 2 and 3). Ganglioside storage leads to neuronal disease. Defects are known for nearly every GSL degradation step. Most GSLs are not toxic themselves, with the exception of some lyso-compounds, such as galactosylsphingosine in Krabbe disease, which is also a ligand of an orphan receptor (Im *et al.* 2001). The amphiphilic storage compounds are not excreted by the affected cells, and the growing amount of accumulating material might initially lead to a mechanical damage of the cell and subsequently to apoptosis (e.g. Taniike *et al.* 1999; Finn *et al.* 2000). The clinical manifestations of the sphingolipidoses depend on the cell-type-specific expression of the glycolipid and the residual activity of the degrading system (Chapters 3 and 4) (Kolter and Sandhoff 1999).

The variant forms of GM2 gangliosidosis (Sandhoff *et al.* 1971) are Tay–Sachs disease (deficient HexA α-subunit), Sandhoff disease (deficient β-subunit), and the AB variant. This is a GM2 gangliosidosis in which both, α- and β-chains, are intact, but the polypeptide chain for the GM2 AP is deficient. In spite of the presence of functional HexA and -B, a massive storage of ganglioside GM2 occurs in the brain. The clinical and pathological findings of these patients resemble Tay–Sachs disease. At the age of 3–8 months, motor abilities start to decrease. At about 1 year of age, psychomotoric regression and dementia become evident. Compared with Tay–Sachs disease, the course of the AB variant is slightly milder.

Although the molecular defects causing these rare inherited diseases are well understood, the clinical phenotypes of activator protein deficiencies vary considerably. The clinical manifestations depend on the residual activity of the defective metabolic step (Kolter and Sandhoff 1998). A relatively small residual activity which can still cope with the lipid influx into the lysosome and can be sufficient to avoid lipid storage and clinical manifestations. The GM2 AP is essential for the hydrolysis of ganglioside GM2 by HexA (Werth *et al.* 2001). Its deficiency leads to a complete block of ganglioside GM2 degradation and causes a storage disease with infantile onset. On the other hand, SAP-B and SAP-C stimulate the enzymatic hydrolysis of sulfatides and glucosylceramide, respectively. However, even in the absence of these activator proteins, the respective enzymes arylsulfatase A and β-glucosidase (Wilkening *et al.* 1998) exhibit a small residual activity against their membrane-bound substrates. Therefore, the inherited deficiency of either of these activator proteins results in a milder form of the storage disease with juvenile onset of the clinical symptomatology.

A mouse model for GM2 AP deficiency (GM2 AP $^{-/-}$; Liu *et al.* 1997) expresses an intermediate phenotype between Tay–Sachs mice (HexA$^{-/-}$) and Sandhoff mice (HexB $^{-/-}$; Sango *et al.* 1995; Phaneuf *et al.* 1996) (Chapter 11). They show an age-dependent onset of severe motor defects but have a normal lifespan. Storage of ganglioside GM2 and, to a lesser extent, glycolipid GA2 occurs in restricted regions of the brain which correspond to the affected regions in Tay–Sachs mice (Yamanaka *et al.* 1994; Cohen-Tannoudji *et al.* 1995; Taniike *et al.* 1995). A major difference is the additional storage of glycolipid GA2 in cerebellar neurones and glial cells of the GM2 AP knockout mice which correlates with impaired motor coordination. The low level of GA2 storage in the GM2 AP$^{-/-}$ mice supports the *in vitro* findings that the hexosaminidase-mediated degradation of GA2 can slowly proceed even in the absence of the GM2 AP, albeit at a reduced rate (Bierfreund *et al.* 1999).

Saposin B (or SAP-B)-deficient patients (Stevens *et al.* 1981; Schlote *et al.* 1991; Wrobe *et al.* 2000) show a severe storage of sulfatides (and slight storage of globotriaosylceramide) and have clinical manifestations related to MLD (Chapter 3). Late infantile MLD begins at about 1 year of age of the patients with psychomotoric retardation and growing dementia. Death occurs before the fifth year of age. The course of the juvenile form is similar but milder (death between 10 and 20 years), and the adult form shows variable phenotypes. The reported defects of SAP-B are due to homoallelic point mutations. Besides the functional inactivity, the half-life of the protein is strongly reduced. A first indication for the diagnosis are the lipid pattern and the SAP-B level in the urine (Li *et al.* 1985).

The deficiency of SAP-C results in the storage of glucosylceramide, the clinical picture corresponding to the juvenile form (visceromegalic and neuronopathic) of Gaucher disease (Christomanou *et al.* 1989). After growth retardation, ataxia, and a dementing process, death usually occurs in the second decade of life.

Currently, no human diseases are known that are caused by the isolated deficiency of SAP-A or -D. The two reports on patients with deficiency of the complete SAP precursor protein and, subsequently, all four saposins (Harzer *et al.* 1989, Hulkova *et al.* 2001) indicate that the clinical picture can be compared with Gaucher disease type II patients with extreme acute multiple motoric abnormalities and massive hepatosplenomegaly.

A mouse model for SAP precursor deficiency has been described (Fujita *et al.* 1996). The animals developed a clinical, pathological, and biochemical phenotype closely resembling that of the human disease. Recently, SAP-A($^{-/-}$) mice, created by the Cre/loxP system, were reported to develop slowly progressive hind leg paralysis with clinical onset at approximately 2.5 months and survival up to 5 months (Matsuda *et al.* 2001).

Pathophysiology of Niemann–Pick disease type C

Niemann–Pick disease was initially characterized by pathological changes including hepatosplenomegaly, sphingomyelin storage, and neurodegeneration. According to the clinical manifestations (see also Chapter 3), this heterogeneous neurovisceral disease has been classified into four subtypes: Niemann–Pick types A–D (NPA–NPD; Crocker and Farber 1958) and subsequently into types A–C (Crocker 1961), since type D seemed to be an ethnic allelic variant of type C, clinically indistinguishable from other forms of NPC (Greer *et al.* 1997). Types A and B are caused by a defect in lysosomal acid sphingomyelinase (Schuchman and Desnick 2001). Types C and D, on the other hand, have normal levels of sphingomyelinase activity but show defects in intracellular cholesterol transport (Patterson *et al.* 2001).

Niemann–Pick type C (see also Chapter 9) is an inherited autosomal recessive lipidosis. Defects in intracellular trafficking of exogenous cholesterol are associated with a complex endosomal–lysosomal storage of unesterified cholesterol, neutral and acidic glycolipids, especially gangliosides GM3 and GM2 (Zervas *et al.* 2001), sphingomyelin (less than in NPA or NPB), BMP, and phospholipids in liver and spleen (Patterson *et al.* 2001). The levels of individual lipids in this storage pattern are variable and no lipid is predominating. In the brain, there are elevated glycolipid levels but no increase of sphingomyelin and cholesterol, albeit some studies suggest that cholesterol transport in the brain is also defective.

The molecular bases of the disease are still unclear, but there is a direct link to mutations in the *NPC1* gene (Carstea *et al.* 1997), responsible for 95% of NPC (Millat *et al.* 1999). The minor disease locus for the remaining 5% has mutations in the *HE1* gene (Millat *et al.* 2001). *HE1* is the gene recently shown underlying the rare *NPC2* (Naureckiene *et al.* 2000), which was previously identified as a cholesterol-binding protein (maps to chromosome 14q24.3). HE1 is a soluble 16 kDa lysosomal glycoprotein which binds cholesterol with high affinity in a 1 : 1 stoichiometry (Okamura *et al.* 1999). Feeding of recombinant HE1 protein to NPC2 cells reduced the lysosomal accumulation of cholesterol derived from LDL. HE1 is ubiquitously expressed, with highest mRNA levels in testis, kidney, and liver (Naureckiene *et al.* 2000). It might function as a cholesterol carrier that regulates cholesterol transport from lipid bilayers, probably to transmembrane proteins, such as NPC1.

The NPC1 and NPC2 mutants show no differences in cholesterol or sphingolipid metabolism as well as in cellular and clinical phenotypes. The *NPC1* gene product is predicted to be an integral membrane protein with 13–16 transmembrane domains and a sterol-sensitive domain with homologies to HMG-CoA reductase. The NPC1 protein seems to be necessary for a post-plasma membrane cholesterol trafficking pathway which is involved in sorting processes (Cruz *et al.* 2000; Garver *et al.* 2002).

Our current understanding of the molecular bases of NPC is primarily derived from a strain of mutant BALB/*c* mice with neurovisceral lipidosis that has clear similarities to the human disease (Pentchev *et al.* 1984; Liu *et al.* 2000) (Chapter 11). In the mouse model, storage of unesterified cholesterol is observed and an impaired processing of exogenous cholesterol has been demonstrated.

Cultured cells from BALB/*c* mice are deficient in their ability to synthesize cholesterol esters and show the same elevated levels of unesterified cholesterol in intravesicular structures if they were fed LDL, but defects in internalization of LDL or in esterification can be excluded, since cell-free extracts of mutant cells show normal esterification activity (Pentchev *et al.* 1986). Therefore, it has been suggested that the defect underlying NPC has to be an impaired intracellular cholesterol trafficking.

The normal way of incorporating exogenous cholesterol is receptor-mediated endocytosis of LDL (Goldstein *et al.* 1985). The lipoprotein is targeted to early endosomes, rather than to late endosomes and lysosomes where cholesterol esters are hydrolysed to free cholesterol. This late endosomal compartment is both the end point of endocytosis and a sorting compartment (Gruenberg and Maxfield 1995). Cholesterol efflux from lysosomes is not well defined, but most of the cholesterol trafficks back, most probably by vesicular flow, to the plasma membrane (about two thirds) or to the ER where it can be esterified again (Neufeld *et al.* 1996). The cholesterol levels in the ER can regulate cellular cholesterol homoeostasis through sterol regulatory element-binding proteins (SREBPs). They work as transcription factors and have indirect influence on *de novo* synthesis and LDL uptake. Niemann–Pick disease type C cells show defects in the delivery of lysosomal cholesterol to the ER and the plasma membrane (Liscum and Faust 1989). As a downstream consequence, cholesterol-homoeostatic responses like *de novo* synthesis, LDL uptake, and cholesterol esterification are impaired.

In skin fibroblasts from NPC patients, the accumulating cholesterol is co-localized with BMP-rich late intraendosomal membrane structures (Kobayashi *et al.* 1999) which are suggested to function as a sorting machinery. The normal *NPC1* gene product is also found in this intraendosomal compartments, whereas the inactive mutated *NPC1* is distributed in the limiting membrane of the endosome (Watari *et al.* 1999). This suggests that cholesterol transport requires appropriate localization of *NPC1* in late endosomal structures.

Further studies by Davies *et al.* (2000) revealed that *NPC1* protein can act as a permease that transports fatty acids and other lipophilic molecules through membranes and therefore also out of the endosomal–lysosomal system. The protein, however, does not transport cholesterol or cholesterol esters. It remains unclear how a possible defect in fatty acid transport could result in cholesterol accumulation.

There are some hints that the cholesterol transport is affected through negatively charged lipids (especially BMP). Adding cations (Zn^{2+}) or BMP antibodies to cultured NPC patients' fibroblasts leads to an additional cholesterol accumulation.

Taken together, NPC1 eventually, together with NPC2 might act as a sensor for endocytosed cholesterol and facilitate delivery of excess free cholesterol to the ER for new esterification. For NPC1, it seems to be clear that the protein affects not only the sorting and trafficking of cholesterol (Ory 2000). Studies with [^{14}C]-sucrose revealed a more global retroendocytotic vesicular pathway defect (Neufeld *et al.* 1999). Other investigations give hints that the transport of ganglioside GM2 is also impaired (Watanabe *et al.* 1998; Zervas *et al.* 2001). Such more general theories could explain the multiple lipid storage in NPC.

Summary

Sphingolipid-activator proteins play an essential role in GSL catabolism. Glycosphingolipids are internalized from the plasma membrane and reach the acidic endosomal–lysosomal compartments of the cell via vesicular flow. According to our endocytosis model, the degradation occurs on intralysosomal vesicles by water-soluble exohydrolases. The activator proteins SAP-A to SAP-D and the GM2 AP are necessary *cofactors*.

In our current understanding, these activator proteins act by disturbing membrane phases, solubilizing glycolipids, and as in the case of SAP-C directly activating the degrading enzyme. They may also bind to their specific substrate to make it accessible for the degrading enzymes. The degradation is decisively influenced by vesicle diameter, the lateral pressure of the membranes, and their specific lipid composition with high amounts of BMP as a negatively charged phospholipid. *In vitro*, the presence of anionic lipids can be equally important to the presence of an activator. A defect in activator proteins leads to fatal GSL storage diseases.

In NPC, assumed to have a molecular defect in cholesterol trafficking, there is no enzyme defect known to date. The mostly affected protein is the product of the *NPC1* gene. It seems to be a regulatory protein for diverse intracellular transport processes from the endosomal–lysosomal compartment back to the plasma membrane and to the ER. Mutations in the genes *NPC1* and *NPC2* (HE1) can contribute to the disease which is characterized by a failure in cholesterol homoeostasis, which leads to cholesterol accumulation. NPC2/HE1 is a soluble lysosomal cholesterol-binding protein. The NPC1 protein, with multiple transmembrane domains and putative sterol-sensing domain, might act as a transfer protein for fatty acids through membranes. Until today, many aspects of the clinical phenotype of NPC remain unexplained.

References

Amidon, B., Brown, A., Waite, M. (1996). Transacylase and Phospholipases in the Synthesis of Bis(monoacylglycero)phosphate. *Biochemistry*, **35**, 13995–4002.

Berent, S. L. and Radin, N. S. (1981). Mechanism of activation of glucocerebrosidase by co-β-glucosidase (glucosidase activator protein). *Biochim Biophys Acta*, **664**, 572–82.

Bierfreund, U., Lemm, T., Hoffmann, A. *et al.* (1999). Recombinant GM2 activator protein stimulates *in-vivo* degradation of GA2 in GM2 gangliosidosis AB variant fibroblasts but exhibits no detectable binding of GA2 in an in vitro assay. *Neurochem Res*, **24**, 295–300.

Bradova, V., Smid, F., Ulrich-Bott, B., Roggendorf, W., Paton, B.C., Harzer, K. (1993). Prosaposin deficiency: further characterization of the sphingolipid activator protein-deficient sibs. Multiple glycolipid elevations (including lactosylceramidosis), partial enzyme deficiencies and ultrastructure of the skin in this generalized sphingolipid storage disease. *Hum Genet*, **92**, 143–52.

Brotherus, J. and Renkonen, O. (1977). Subcellular distributions of lipids in cultured BHK cells: evidence for the enrichment of lysobisphosphatidic acid and neutral lipids in lysosomes. *J Lipid Res*, **18**, 191–202.

Brown, D. A. and London, E. (2000). Structure and function of sphingolipid- and cholesterol-rich membrane rafts. *J Biol Chem*, **275**, 17221–4.

Burkhardt, J. K., Hüttler, S., Klein, A. *et al.* (1997). Accumulation of sphingolipids in SAP-precursor (prosaposin) deficient fibroblasts occurs within lysosomes and can be completely reversed by treatment with human SAP-precursor. *Eur J Cell Biol*, **73**, 10–18.

Carlsson, S. R., Roth, J., Piller, F., Fukuda, M. (1988). Isolation and characterization of human lysosomal membrane glycoproteins, h-LAMP-1 and h-LAMP-2. *J Biol Chem*, **263**, 18911–19.

Carstea, E. D., Morris, J. A., Coleman, K. G. *et al.* (1997). Niemann–Pick C1 disease gene: Homology to mediators of cholesterol homeostasis. *Science*, **277**, 228–31.

Ciaffoni, F., Salvioli, R., Tatti, M., Arancia, G., Crateri, P., Vaccaro, A. M. (2001). Saposin, D., solubilizes anionic phospholipid-containing membranes. *J Biol Chem*, **276**, 31583–9.

Chojnacki, T. and Dallner, G., (1988). The biological role of dolichol. *Biochem J*, **251**, 1–9.

Christomanou, H., Aignesberg, A., Linke, R. P. (1986). Immunochemical characterization of two activator proteins stimulating enzymic sphingomyelin degradation in vitro. Absence of one of them in a human Gaucher disease variant. *Biol Chem Hoppe-Seyler*, **367**, 879–90.

Christomanou, H., Chabás, A., Pampols, T., Guardiola, A. (1989). Activator protein deficient Gaucher disease. A second patient with the newly identified lipid storage disorder. *Klin Wochenschr*, **67**, 999–1003.

Cohen-Tannoudji, M., Marchand, P., Akli, S. *et al.* (1995). Disruption of murine Hexa gene leads to enzymatic deficiency and to neuronal lysosomal storage, similar to that observed in Tay–Sachs disease. *Mammalian Genome*, **6**, 844–9.

Conzelmann, E. and Sandhoff, K. (1978). AB variant of infantile GM2 gangliosidosis: Deficiency of a factor necessary for stimulation of hexosaminidase A-catalyzed degradation of ganglioside GM2 and glycolipid GA2. *Proc Natl Acad Sci USA*, **75**, 3979–83.

Conzelmann, E. and Sandhoff, K. (1979). Purification and characterization of an activator protein for the degradation of glycolipids GM2 and GA2 by hexosaminidase A. *Hoppe-Seyler Z Physiol Chem*, **360**, 1837–49.

Conzelmann, E., Burg, J., Stephan, G., Sandhoff, K. (1982). Complexing of glycolipids and their transfer between membranes by the activator protein for degradation of lysosomal ganglioside GM2. *Eur J Biochem*, **123**, 455–66.

Crocker, A. C. (1961). The cerebral defect in Tay–Sachs disease and Niemann–Pick disease. *J Neurochem*, **7**, 69–73.

Crocker, A. C. and Farber, S. (1958). Niemann–Pick disease: A review of eighteen patients. *Medicine (Baltimore)*, **37**, 1.

Cruz, J. C., Sugii, S., Yu, C., Chang, T. Y. (2000). Role of Niemann–Pick Type C1 Protein in Intracellular Trafficking of Low Density Lipoprotein-derived Cholesterol. *J Biol Chem*, **275**, 4013–21.

Davies, J. P., Chen, F. W., Ioannou, Y. A. (2000). Transmembrane molecular pump activity of Niemann–Pick C1 protein. *Science*, **290**, 2295–8.

Fabbro, D. and Grabowski, D. A. (1991). Human acid β-glucosidase. Use of inhibitory and activating monoclonal antibodies to investigate the enzyme's catalytic mechanism and saposin A and C binding sites. *J Biol Chem*, **266**, 15021–7.

Finn, L. S., Zhang, M., Chen, S. H., Scott, C. R. (2000). Severe type II Gaucher disease with ichthyosis, arthrogryposis and neuronal apoptosis: molecular and pathological analyses. *Am J Med Genet*, **91**, 222–6.

Fischer, G. and Jatzkewitz, H. (1975). The activator of cerebroside sulfatase. Purification from human liver and identification as a protein. *Hoppe-Seyler Z Physiol Chem*, **356**, 605–13.

Fürst, W., Machleidt, W., Sandhoff, K. (1988). The precursor of sulfatide activator protein is processed to three different proteins. *Biol Chem Hoppe-Seyler*, **369**, 317–28.

Fürst, W. and Sandhoff, K. (1992). Activator proteins and topology of lysosomal sphingolipid catabolism. *Biochim Biophys Acta*, **1126**, 1–16.

Fürst, W., Schubert, J., Machleidt. W., Meyer, E. H., Sandhoff, K. (1990). The complete amino-acid sequences of human ganglioside GM2 activator protein and cerebroside sulfate activator protein. *Eur J Biochem*, **192**, 709–14.

Fujita, N., Suzuki, K., Vanier, M. T. *et al.* (1996) Targeted disruption of the mouse sphingolipid activator protein gene: a complex phenotype, including severe leukodystrophy and wide-spread storage of multiple sphingolipids. *Hum Mol Genet*, **5**, 711–25.

Gärtner, S., Conzelmann, E., Sandhoff, K. (1983). Activator protein for the degradation of globotriaosylceramide by human α-galactosidase. *J Biol Chem*, **258**, 12378–85.

Garver, W. S., Krishnan, K., Gallagos, J. R., Michikawa, M., Francis, G. A., Heidenreich, R. A. (2002). Niemann–Pick C1 protein regulates cholesterol transport to the trans-Golgi network and plasma membrane caveolae. *J Lipid Res*, **43**, 579–89.

Giehl, A., Lemm, T., Bartelsen, O., Sandhoff, K., Blume, A. (1999). Interaction of the GM2 activator protein with phospholipid-ganglioside bilayer membranes and with monolayers at the air-water interface. *Eur J Biochem*, **261**, 650–8.

Goldstein, J. L., Brown, M. S., Anderson, R. G. W., Schneider. W. J. (1985). Receptor mediated endocytosis. *Annu Rev Cell Biol*, **1**, 1–40.

Greer, W. L., Riddell, D. C., Byers, D. M. *et al.* (1997). Linkage of Niemann–Pick disease type D to the same region of human chromosome 18 as Niemann–Pick disease type C. *Am J Hum Genet*, **61**, 139–42.

Gruenberg, J. and Maxfield, F. (1995). Membrane transport in the endocytic pathway. *Curr Opin Cell Biol*, **7**, 552–63.

Hannun, Y. A., Luberto, C., Argraves, K. M. (2001). Enzymes of sphingolipid metabolism: from modular to integrative signaling. *Biochemistry*, **40**, 4893–903.
Hannun, Y. A. and Obeid, L. M. (2002). The ceramide-centric universe of lipid-mediated cell regulation: Stress encounters of the lipid kind. *J Biol Chem*, **277**, 25847–50.
Harzer, K., Paton, B. C., Poulos, A. (1989). Sphingolipid activator protein (SAP) deficiency in a 16-week old atypical Gaucher disease patient and his fetal sibling; biochemical signs of combined sphingolipidosis. *Eur J Pediatr*, **149**, 31–9.
Henning, R. and Stoffel, W. (1973). Glycosphingolipids in lysosomal membranes. *Hoppe-Seyler's Z Physiol Chem*, **354**, 760–70.
Hepbildikler, S. T., Sandhoff, R., Kölzer, M., Proia, R. L., Sandhoff, K. (2002). Physiological substrates for human lysosomal β-Hexosaminidase S. *J Biol Chem*, **277**, 2562–72.
Hiesberger, T., Hüttler, S., Rohlmann, A., Schneider, W., Sandhoff, K., Herz, J. (1998). Cellular uptake of saposin (SAP) precursor and lysosomal delivery by the low density lipoprotein receptor-related protein (LRP). *EMBO J*, **17**, 4617–25.
Hineno, T., Sano, A., Kondoh, K., Ueno, S., Kakimoto, Y., Yoshida, K. (1991). Secretion of sphingolipid hydrolase activator precursor, prosaposin. *Biochem Biophys Res Commun*, **176**, 668–74.
Hiraiwa, M., Soeda, S., Kishimoto, Y., O'Brien, J. S. (1992). Binding and transport of gangliosides by prosaposin. *Proc Natl Acad Sci USA*, **89**, 11254–8.
Hiraiwa, M., Taylor, E. M., Campana, W. M., Darin, J. S., O'Brien, J. S. (1997). Cell death preventions, mitogen-activated protein kinase stimulation and increased sulfatide concentrations in Schwann cells and oligodendrocytes by prosaposin and prosaptide. *Proc Natl Acad Sci USA*, **94**, 4778–81.
Ho, M. W. and O'Brien, J. S. (1971). Gaucher's disease: deficiency of "acid" β-glucosidase and reconstruction of enzyme activity in vitro. *Proc Natl Acad Sci USA*, **68**, 2810–3.
Hulkova, H., Cervenkova, M., Ledvinova, J. *et al.* (2001). A novel mutation in the coding region of the prosaposin gene leads to a complete deficiency of prosaposin and saposins, and is associated with a complex sphingolipidosis dominated by lactosylceramide accumulation. *Hum Mol Genet*, **10**, 927–40.
Huwiler, A., Kolter, T., Pfeilschifter, J., Sandhoff, K. (2000). Physiology and pathophysiology of sphingolipid metabolism and signaling. *Biochim Biophys Acta*, **1485**, 63–99.
Im, D. S., Heise, C. E., Nguyen, T., O'Dowd, B. F., Lynch, K. R. (2001). Identification of a molecular target of psychosine and its role in globoid cell formation. *J Cell Biol*, **153**, 429–34.
Karlsson, K-A. (1989). Animal glycosphingolipids as membrane attachment sites for bacteria. *Annu Rev Biochem*, **58**, 309–50.
Kishimoto, Y., Hiraiwa, M., O'Brien, J. S. (1992). Saposins: structure, function, distribution and molecular genetics. *J Lipid Res*, **33**, 1255–67.
Klein, A., Henseler, M., Klein, C., Suzuki, K., Harzer, K., Sandhoff, K. (1994). Sphingolipid Activator Protein D (sap-D) Stimulates the Lysosomal Degradation of Ceramide in Vivo. *Biochem Biophys Res Commun*, **200**, 1440–8.
Klima, H., Tanaka, A., Schnabel, D. *et al.* (1991). Characterization of full-length cDNA and the gene coding for the human GM2 activator protein. *FEBS Lett*, **289**, 260–4.
Kobayashi, T., Beuchat, M.-H., Lindsay, M. *et al.* (1999). Late endosomal membranes rich in lysobisphosphatidic acid regulate cholesterol transport. *Nature Cell Biol*, **1**, 113–8.
Kobayashi, T., Strang, E., Fang, K., de Moerloose, P., Parton, R. G., Gruenberg, J. (1998). A lipid associated with the antiphospholipid syndrome regulates endosome structure and function. *Nature*, **392**, 193–7.
Kolter, T. and Sandhoff, K. (1998). Recent advances in the biochemistry of sphingolipidoses. *Brain Pathology*, **8**, 79–100.
Kolter, T. and Sandhoff, K. (1999). Sphingolipids–Their metabolic pathways and the pathobiochemistry of neurodegenerative diseases. *Angew Chem Int Ed*, **38**, 1532–68.
Kondoh, K., Hineno, T., Sano, A., Kakimoto, Y. (1991). Isolation and characterization of prosaposin from human milk. *Biochem Biophys Res Commun*, **181**, 286–92.
Kretz, K. A., Carson, G. S., Morimoto, S., Kishimoto, Y., Fluharty, A.L., O'Brien, J. S. (1990). Characterization of mutation in a family with saposin B deficiency: a glycosylation site defect. *Proc Natl Acad Sci USA*, **87**, 2541–4.

Kytzia, H.-J. and Sandhoff, K. (1985). Evidence for two different active sites on human hexosaminidase A– Interaction of GM2 activator protein with hexosaminidase A. *J Biol Chem*, **260**, 7568–72.

Li, S.C, Kihara, H., Serizawa, S. *et al.* (1985). Activator protein required for the enzymatic hydrolysis of cerebroside sulfate. Deficiency in urine of patients affected with cerebroside sulfatase activator deficiency and identity with activators for the enzymatic hydrolysis of GM1 ganglioside and globotriaosylceramide. *J Biol Chem*, **260**, 1867–71.

Liepinsh, E., Andersson, M., Ruysschaert, J. M., Otting, G. (1997). Saposin fold revealed by the NMR structure of NK-lysin. *Nature Struct Biol*, **10**, 793–5.

Linke, T., Wilkening, G., Lansmann, S. *et al.* (2001*a*). Stimulation of acid sphingomyelinase activity by lysosomal lipids and sphingolipid activator proteins. *Biol Chem*, **382**, 283–90.

Linke, T., Wilkening, G., Sadeghlar, F. *et al.* (2001*b*). Interfacial regulation of acid ceramidase activity. *J Biol Chem*, **276**, 5760–8.

Liscum, L. and Faust, J. R. (1989). Low density lipoprotein (LDL)-mediated suppression of cholesterol synthesis and LDL uptake is defective in Niemann–Pick type C fibroblasts. *J Biol Chem*, **262**, 17002–8.

Liu, Y., Hoffmann, A., Grinberg, A. *et al.* (1997). Mouse model of GM2 activator deficiency manifests cerebellar ganglioside storage and motor impairment. *Proc Natl Acad Sci USA*, **94**, 8138–43.

Liu, Y., Wu, Y.-P., Wada, R. *et al.* (2000). Alleviation of neuronal ganglioside storage does not improve the clinical course of the Niemann–Pick C disease mouse. *Hum Mol Genet*, **9**, 1087–92.

Mahuranm, D. J. (1998). The GM2 activator protein, its roles as a co-factor in GM2 hydrolysis and as a general glycolipid transport protein. *Biochim Biophys Acta*, **1393**, 1–18.

Marsh, D. (1996). Lateral pressures in membranes. *Biochim Biophys Acta*, **1286**, 183–223.

Matsuda, J., Vanier, M. T., Saito, Y., Tohyama, J., Suzuki, K. (2001). A mutation in the saposin A domain of the sphingolipid activator protein (prosaposin) gene results in a late-onset, chronic form of globoid cell leukodystrophy in the mouse. *Hum Mol Genet*, **10**, 1191–9.

Matsuzawa, Y. and Hostetler, K. Y. (1979). Degradation of bis(monoacylglycero)phosphate by an acid phosphodiesterase in rat liver lysosomes. *J Biol Chem*, **254**, 5997–6001.

Mehl, E. and Jatzkewitz, H. (1964). Eine Cerebrosidsulfatase aus Schweineniere. *Hoppe Seyler Z Physiol Chem*, **339**, 260–76.

Meier, E. M., Schwarzmann, G., Fürst, W., Sandhoff, K. (1991). The human GM2 activator protein: A substrate specific cofactor of hexosaminidase A. *J Biol Chem*, **266**, 1879–87.

Merrill, A. H., Jr and Sweely, C. C. (1996). In: Vance DE and Vance JE (eds) Biochemistry of lipids, lipoproteins and membranes, pp. 309–39, Elsevier, Amsterdam–New York.

Merrill, A. H., Jr (2002). De novo sphingolipid biosynthesis: A necessary, but dangerous, pathway. *J Biol Chem*, **277**, 25843–6.

Millat, G., Marcais, C., Rafi, M. A. *et al.* (1999). Niemann–Pick C1 disease: the I1061T substitution is a frequent mutant allele in patients of Western European descent and correlates with a classic juvenile phenotype. *Am J Hum Genet*, **65**, 1321–9.

Millat, G., Chikh, K., Naureckiene, S. *et al.* (2001). Niemann–Pick disease type C: spectrum of HE1 mutations and genotype/phenotype correlations in the NPC2 group. *Am J Hum Genet*, **69**, 1013–21.

Möbius, W., Herzog, V., Sandhoff, K., Schwarzmann, G. (1999). Intracellular distribution of a biotin-labeled ganglioside GM1 by immunoelectron microscopy after endocytosis in fibroblasts. *J Histochem Cytochem*, **47**, 1005–14.

Morimoto, S., Kishimoto, Y., Tomich, J. *et al.* (1990). Interaction of saposins, acidic lipids and glucosylceramidase. *J Biol Chem*, **265**, 1933–7.

Morimoto, S., Martin, B. M., Kishimoto, Y., O'Brien, J. S. (1988). Saposin D: A sphingomyelinase activator. *Biochem Biophys Res Commun*, **156**, 403–10.

Morimoto, S., Martin, B. M., Yamamoto, Y., Kretz, K. A., O'Brien, J. S. (1989). Saposin A: second cerebrosidase activator protein. *Proc Natl Acad Sci USA*, **86**, 3389–93.

Mundel, T. M., Heid, H. W., Mahuran, D. J., Kriz, W., Mundel, P. (1999). Ganglioside GM2 activator protein and vesicular transport in collecting duct intercalated cells. *J Am Soc Nephrol*, **10**, 435–43.

Munford, R. S., Sheppard, P.O., O'Hara, P. J. (1995). Saposin-like proteins (SAPLIP) carry out diverse functions on a common backbone structure. *J Lipid Res*, **36**,1653–63.

Nakamura, S.-I., Akisue, T., Jinnai, H. *et al.* (1998). Requirement of GM2 ganglioside activator for phospholipase D activation. *Proc Natl Acad Sci, USA*, **95**, 12249–53.

Nakano, T., Sandhoff, K., Stümper, J., Christomanou, H., Suzuki, K. (1989). Structure of full length cDNA coding for sulfatide activator, a co-β glucosidase and two other homologous proteins: two alternate forms of the sulfatide activator. *J Biochem*, **105**, 152–4.

Naureckiene, S., Sleat, D. E., Lackland, H. *et al.* (2000). Identification of HE1 as the second gene of Niemann–Pick C disease. *Science*, **290**, 2298–301.

Neufeld, E. B., Cooney, A. M., Pitha, J. *et al.* (1996). Intracellular Trafficking of Cholesterol Monitored with a Cyclodextrin. *J Biol Chem*, **271**, 21604–13.

Neufeld, E. B., Wastney, M., Patel, S. *et al.* (1999). The Niemann–Pick C1 Protein Resides in a Vesicular Compartment Linked to Retrograde Transport of Multiple Lysosomal Cargo. *J Biol Chem*, **274**, 9627–35.

O'Brien, J. S., Kretz, K. A., Dewji, N., Wenger, D. A., Esch, F., Fluharty, A. L. (1988). Coding of two sphingolipid activator proteins (SAP1 and SAP2) by same genetic locus. *Science*, **241**, 1098–101.

Okamura, N., Kiuchi, S., Tamba, M. *et al.* (1999). A porcine homolog of the major secretory protein of human epididymis, HE1, specifically binds cholesterol. *Biochim Biophys Acta*, **1438**, 377–87.

Ory, D. S. (2000). Niemann–Pick type C: A disorder of cellular cholesterol trafficking. *Biochim Biophys Acta*, **1529**, 331–9.

Patterson, M. C., Vanier, M. T., Suzuki, K. *et al.* (2001). Niemann–Pick disease type C: a lipid trafficking disorder. In : Scriver CR, Beaudet AL, Sly WS, and Valle D (eds) The metabolic and molecular bases of inherited disease, chapt 145, pp. 3611–33, Vol III, 8th edn, McGraw-Hill, New York.

Pentchev, P. G., Boothe, A. D., Kruth, H.S., Weintroub, H., Stivers, J., Brady, R. O. (1984). A genetic storage disorder in BALB/C mice with a metabolic block in esterification of exogenous cholesterol. *J Biol Chem*, **259**, 5784–91.

Pentchev, P. G., Comly, M. E., Kruth, H. S., Patel, S., Proestel, M., Weintroub, H. (1986). The cholesterol storage disorder of the mutant BALB/c mouse. *J Biol Chem*, **261**, 2772–7.

Peters, C. and von Figura, K. (1994). Biogenesis of lysosomal membranes. *FEBS Lett*, **346**, 108–14.

Phaneuf, D., Wakamatsu, N., Huang, J. Q. *et al.* (1996). Dramatically different phenotypes in mouse models of human Tay–Sachs and Sandhoff disease. *Hum Mol Genet*, **5**, 1–14.

Ponting, C. P. and Russell, R. B. (1995). Swaposins: circular permutations within genes encoding saposin homologues. *Trends Biochem Sci*, **20**, 179–80.

Pyne, S. and Pyne, N. (2000). Sphingosine 1-phosphate signalling via the endothelial differentiation gene family of G-protein-coupled receptors. *Pharmacol Ther*, **88**, 115–31.

Salvioli, R., Tatti, M., Ciaffoni. F., Vaccaro, A. M. (2000). Further studies on the reconstitution of glucosylceramidase activity by Sap C and anionic phospholipids. *FEBS Lett*, **472**, 17–21.

Sandhoff, K. (1977). The biochemistry of sphingolipid storage diseases. *Angew Chem Int Ed*, **16**, 273–85.

Sandhoff, K., Harzer, K., Wässle, W., Jatzkewitz, H. (1971). Enzyme alterations and lipid storage in three variants of Tay–Sachs disease. *J Neurochem*, **18**, 2469–89.

Sandhoff, K. and Kolter, T. (1996). Topology of glycosphingolipid degradation. *Trends Cell Biol*, **6**, 98–103.

Sandhoff, K., Kolter. T., Harzer, K. (2001). Sphingolipid activator proteins. In : Scriver CR, Beaudet AL, Sly WS, and Valle D (eds), The metabolic and molecular bases of inherited disease, chapt 134, pp. 3371–88, Vol III, 8th edn, McGraw-Hill, New York.

Sandhoff, R., Hepbildikler, S. T., Jennemann, R. *et al.* (2002). Kidney sulfatides in mouse models of inherited glycosphingolipid disorders. *J Biol Chem*, **277**, 20386–98.

Sango, K., Yamanaka, S., Hoffmann, A. *et al.* (1995). Mouse models of Tay–Sachs and Sandhoff diseases differ in neurologic phenotype and ganglioside metabolism. *Nature genetics*, **11**, 170–6.

Sarkar, S., Miwa, N., Kominami, H. *et al.* (2001). Regulation of mammalian phospholipase D2: interaction with and stimulation by GM2 activator. *Biochem J*, **359**, 559–604.

Sarmientos, F., Schwarzmann, G., Sandhoff, K. (1986). Specificity of human glucosylceramide beta-glucosidase towards synthetic glucosylsphingolipids inserted into liposomes. Kinetic studies in a detergent-free assay system. *Eur J Biochem*, **160**, 527–35.

Scheel, G., Acevedo, E., Conzelmann, E., Nehrkorn, H., Sandhoff, K. (1982). Model for the interaction of membrane-bound substrates and enzymes. Hydrolysis of ganglioside GD1a by sialidase of neuronal membranes isolated from calf brain. *Eur J Biochem*, **127**, 245–53.

Schepers, U., Glombitza, G. J., Lemm, T. *et al.* (1996). Molecular analysis of a GM2 activator deficiency in two patients with GM2 gangliosidosis AB-variant. *Am J Hum Genet*, **59**, 1048–56.

Schepers, U., Lemm, T., Herzog, V., Sandhoff, K. (2000). Characterization of Regulatory Elements in the 5'-Flanking Region of the GM2 Activator Gene. *Biol Chem*, **381**, 531–44.

Schlote, W., Harzer, K., Christomanou, H. *et al.* (1991). Sphingolipid activator protein 1 deficiency in metachromatic leukodystrophy with normal arylsulfatase A activity. A clinical, morphological, biochemical, and immunological study. *Eur J Pediatr*, **150**, 584–91.

Schnabel, D., Schröder, M., Fürst, W. *et al.* (1992). Simultaneous deficiency of sphingolipid activator proteins 1 and 2 is caused by a mutation in the initiation codon of their common gene. *J Biol Chem*, **267**, 3312–5.

Schnabel, D., Schröder, M., Sandhoff, K. (1991). Mutation in the sphingolipid activator protein 2 in a patient with a variant of Gaucher disease. *FEBS Lett*, **284**, 57–9.

Schröder, M., Schnabel, D., Hurwitz, R., Young, E., Suzuki, K., Sandhoff, K. (1993). Molecular genetics of GM2 gangliosidosis AB variant: A novel mutation and expression in BHK cells. *Human Genet*, **92**, 437–40.

Schröder, M., Schnabel, D., Suzuki, K., Sandhoff, K. (1991). A mutation in the gene of a glycolipid binding protein (GM2 activator) that causes GM2 gangliosidosis variant AB. *FEBS Lett*, **290**, 1–3.

Schuchman, E. H. and Desnick, R. J. (2001). Niemann–Pick disease types A and B: acid sphingomyelinase deficiencies. In: Scriver CR, Beaudet AL, Sly WS, and Valle D (eds). The metabolic and molecular bases of inherited disease, chapt 144, pp. 3589–610, Vol III, 8th edn, McGraw-Hill-New York.

Schütte, C.G., Lemm, T., Glombitza, G. J., Sandhoff, K. (1998). Complete localization of disulfide bonds in GM2 activator protein. *Protein Sci*, **7**, 1039–45.

Smiljanic-Georgijev, N., Rigat, B., Leung, A., Mahuran, D.J. (1997). Characterization of the affinity of the GM2 activator protein for glycolipids by a fluorescence dequenching assay. *Biochim Biophys Acta*, **1339**, 192–202.

Spiegel, S. and Milstien, S. (2002). Sphingosine 1-phosphate, a key cell signaling molecule. *J Biol Chem*, **277**, 25851–4.

Stevens, R. L., Fluharty, A. H., Kihara, H. *et al.* (1981). Cerebroside sulfatase activator deficiency induced metachromatic leukodystrophy. *Am J Hum Genet*, **33**, 900–6.

Suzuki, K. and Vanier, M. T. (1999). Lysosomal and Peroxisomal Diseases. In: Siegel GJ, Agranoff BW, Albers RW, Fisher SK, Uhler MD (eds), Basic Neurochemistry–Molecular, cellular and medical aspects, pp. 821–39, 6th edn, Lippincott-Raven, Philadelphia.

Swallow, D. M., Islam, I., Fox, M. F. *et al.* (1993). Regional localisation of the gene coding for the GM2 activator protein (GM2A) to chromosome 5q32–33 and confirmation of the assignment of GM2AP to chromosome 3. *Ann Hum Genet*, **57**, 187–93.

Taniike, M., Mohri, I., Eguchi, N. *et al.* (1999). An apoptotic depletion of oligodendrocytes in the twitcher, a murine model of globoid cell leukodystrophy. *J Neuropathol Exp Neurol*, **58**, 644–53.

Taniike, M., Yamanaka, S., Proia, R. L., Langaman, C., Bonc-Turentine, T., Suzuki, K. (1995). Neuropathology of mice with targeted disruption of Hexa gene, a model of Tay–Sachs disease. *Acta Neuropathol*, **89**, 296–304.

Tayama, M., Soeda, S., Kishimoto, Y. *et al.* (1993). Effects of saposins on acid sphingomyelinase. *Biochem J*, **290**, 401–4.

Vaccaro, A. M., Ciaffoni, F., Tatti, M. *et al.* (1995*a*). pH-dependent conformational properties of saposins and their interactions with phospholipid membranes. *J Biol Chem*, **270**, 30576–80.

Vaccaro, A. M., Salvioli, R., Barca. A. *et al.* (1995*b*). Structural analysis of saposin C and B. Complete localization of disulfide bridges. *J Biol Chem*, **270**, 9953–60.

Vaccaro, A. M., Salvioli, R., Tatti, M., Ciaffoni, F. (1999). Saposins and their interactions with lipids. *Neurochem Res*, **24**, 307–14.

Vaccaro, A.M., Tatti, M., Ciaffoni, F., Salvioli, R., Barca, A., Scerch, C. (1997). Effect of Saposins A and C on the Enzymatic Hydrolysis of Liposomal Glucosylceramide. *J Biol Chem*, **272**, 16862–7.

Varki, A. (1993). Biological roles of oligosaccharides: All of the theories are correct. *Glycobiol*, **3**, 97–130.

Vielhaber, G., Hurwitz, R., Sandhoff, K. (1997). Biosynthesis, processing, and targeting of sphingolipid activator protein (SAP-) precursor in cultured human fibroblasts. Mannose 6-phosphate receptor-independent endocytosis of SAP-precursor. *J Biol Chem*, **271**, 32438–46.

Vogel, A., Schwarzmann, G., Sandhoff, K. (1991). Glycosphingolipid specifity of the human sulfatide activator protein. *Eur J Biochem*, **200**, 591–7.

Watanabe, Y., Akaboshi, S., Ishida, G. *et al.* (1998). Increased levels of GM2 ganglioside in fibroblasts from a patient with juvenile Niemann–Pick disease type C. *Brain Developm*, **20**, 95–7.

Watari, H., Blanchette-Mackie, E. J., Dwyer, N. K. *et al.* (1999). Mutations in the leucine zipper motif and sterol-sensing domain inactivate the Niemann–Pick C1 glycoprotein. *J Biol Chem*, **274**, 21861–6.

Wenger, D. A., Sattler, M., Roth, S. (1982). A protein activator of galactosylceramide-β-galactosidase. *Biochim Biophys Acta*, **712**, 639–49.

Werth, N., Schuette, C. G., Wilkening, G., Lemm, T., Sandhoff, K. (2001). Degradation of membrane-bound ganglioside GM2 by β-hexosaminidase A. *J Biol Chem*, **276**, 12685–90.

Wilkening, G., Linke, T., Sandhoff, K. (1998). Lysosomal degradation on vesicular membrane surfaces. Enhanced glucosylceramide degradation by lysosomal anionic lipids and activators. *J Biol Chem*, **273**, 30271–8.

Wilkening, G., Linke, T., Uhlhorn-Dierks, G., Sandhoff, K. (2000). Degradation of membrane-bound Ganglioside GM1. *J Biol Chem*, **275**, 35814–9.

Wright, C., Li, S.-C, Rastinejad, F. (2000). Crystal structure of human GM2 activator protein with a novel β-cup topology. *J Mol Biol*, **304**, 411–22.

Wrobe, D., Henseler, M., Huettler, S., Pascual Pascual, S. I., Chabas, A., Sandhoff, K. (2000). A non-glycosylated and functionally deficient mutant (N215H) of the sphingolipid activator protein B (SAP-B) in a novel case of metachromatic leukodystrophy (MLD). *J Inherit Metab Dis*, **23**, 63–76.

Wu, Y. Y., Lockyer, J. M., Sugiyama, E., Pavlova, N. V., Li, Y.-T, Li, S.-C (1994). Expression and specifity of human GM2 activator protein. *J Biol Chem*, **269**, 16276–83.

Wu, Y. Y., Sonnino, S., Li, Y, Li, S (1996). Characterization of an alternatively spliced GM2 activator protein, GM2A protein. An activator protein which stimulates the enzymatic hydrolysis of N-acetylneuraminic acid, but not N-acetylgalactosamine, from GM2. *J Biol Chem*, **271**, 10611–5.

Xie, B., Kennedy, J. L., McInnes, B., Auger, D., Mahuran, D. (1992). Identification of a processed pseudogene related to the functional gene encoding the GM2 activator protein: localization of the pseudogene to human chromosome 3 and the functional gene to human chromosome 5. *Genomics*, **14**, 796–8.

Yamanaka, S., Johnson, M. D., Grinberg, A. *et al.* (1994). Targeted disruption of the Hexa gene results in mice with biochemical and pathologic features of Tay–Sachs disease. *Proc Natl Acad Sci USA*, **91**, 9975–9.

Zeller, C. B. and Marchase, R. B. (1992). Gangliosides as modulators of cell function. *Am J Physiol*, **262**, C 1341–55.

Zaltash, S. and Johansson, J. (1998). Secondary structure and limited proteolysis give experimental evidence that the precursor of pulmonary surfactant protein B contains three saposin-like domains. *FEBS Lett*, **423**, 1–4.

Zervas, M., Dobrenis, K., Walkley, S. U. (2001). Neurons in Niemann–Pick disease Type C accumulate gangliosides as well as unesterified cholesterol and undergo dendritic and axonal alterations. *J Neuropathol Exp Neurol*, **60**, 49–64.

Zschoche, A., Fürst, W., Schwarzmann, G., Sandhoff, K. (1994). Hydrolysis of lactosylceramide by human galactosylceramidase and GM1-β-galactosidase in a detergent-free system and its stimulation by sphingolipid activator proteins, *sap*-B and *sap*-C. *Eur J Biochem*, **222**, 83–90.

Chapter 9

Defects in transmembrane proteins

Yiannis A. Ioannou

Introduction

During the last 5 years, proteins found embedded within the membranes of the endosomal/lysosomal system have emerged as key regulators of many functions of this system. Their importance is exemplified by the occurrence of various disorders, each of which results from the deficiency of a single membrane protein. The severe phenotypes that are associated with these disorders, usually leading to neurodegeneration, emphasize their biological importance. A handful of these proteins has recently been identified and their initial characterization will be the focus of this chapter. However, before describing the characteristics of these endosomal/lysosomal membrane proteins, a brief discussion of our current understanding of this system is warranted.

Lysosomes are morphologically heterogeneous membrane-bound structures that were first isolated from rat liver in 1955 (de Duve *et al.* 1955). They were classified as a family of acid hydrolase-containing terminal compartments, found in all plant and animal cells, with the attributed function of intracellular or extracellular product degradation (de Duve and Wattiaux 1966). However, it gradually became clear that they were actually part of a complex system of vacuolar structures that were involved in such dynamic processes such as endocytosis, protein sorting, and membrane recycling (de Duve 1983) (Chapter 1). These structures could be distinguished by their morphology and assigned function: pre-lysosomes, or phagosomes, were storage vesicles that contained cytosolic materials but no enzymes; these fused with enzyme-containing vacuoles to form lysosomes, where digestion took place; post-lysosomes were the structures left when digestion was complete (de Duve and Wattiaux 1966). Eventually, pre-lysosomes were further characterized as early and late endosomes, to distinguish between two biochemically distinct vesicular populations. The complexity of this system revealed by these observations raised many questions regarding the role of these compartments within the cell as well as the mechanism of their regulation (see also Chapter 1), and although much progress has been made in understanding this system, a number of questions still remain.

The discovery of I-cell disease, or mucolipidosis type II (see Chapter 6), was instrumental in deciphering the pathway by which lysosomal acid hydrolases reached their final destination. I-Cell fibroblasts, which have dark cytoplasmic inclusions (Leroy and DeMars 1967), were found to contain reduced levels of acid hydrolases and to secrete high amounts of enzymes that could not be endocytosed by normal fibroblasts (Hickman and Neufeld 1972;

Sly *et al.* 1976). Eventually, it was demonstrated that I-cell fibroblasts are deficient in the phosphotransferase responsible for attaching *N*-acetylglucosamine (GlcNAc)-1-phosphate onto mannose residues of the oligosaccharide side chains of lysosomal enzymes in the endoplasmic reticulum (ER) (Reitman *et al.* 1981). This modification was shown to be the first step of a two-step reaction by which a mannose-6-phosphate (M6P) moiety is generated by first adding a GlcNAc-1-phosphate onto mannose residues of the oligosaccharide side chains of acid hydrolases (Willingham *et al.* 1981; Lobel *et al.* 1988; Oshima *et al.* 1988; Ma *et al.* 1991). In the second step, the GlcNAc moiety is clipped by a phosphodiesterase to produce an M6P residue (Waheed *et al.* 1981) that can bind to M6P receptors in the *trans*-Golgi network (TGN) (Lobel *et al.* 1988; Oshima *et al.* 1988; Ma *et al.* 1991), eventually leading to delivery of the enzymes to lysosomes (Chapter 6). In I-cell fibroblasts, the lack of available M6P moieties on enzymes precludes their binding to the receptor, leading to their secretion by default. Further investigation of this transport pathway revealed that the receptor and M6P ligand dissociate in the late endosomal compartment due to a radial drop in pH (Dahms *et al.* 1989). In addition, the receptor contains a cytoplasmic motif that prevents its entry into the lysosome where it could be degraded and instead allows it to recycle between the TGN, plasma membrane, and endosomes (Schweizer *et al.* 1997). Thus, a new definition emerged of the lysosome as an acid hydrolase-containing, M6P receptor-deficient compartment (Sahagian and Neufeld 1983).

The M6P pathway is not the only route for proteins to reach the lysosome (Barriocanal *et al.* 1986; Vega *et al.* 1991; Blagoveshchenskaya *et al.* 1998) (See also Chapter 6). Lysosomal integral membrane proteins contain signals in their cytoplasmic tails that target them from the TGN to the lysosome either directly or via the cell surface (Peters *et al.* 1990; Press *et al.* 1998). So far, two types of M6P-independent signals have been shown to be necessary and sufficient for the targeting of membrane proteins to the lysosome (Peters *et al.* 1990; Blagoveshchenskaya *et al.* 1998). The first, a tyrosine-based motif found in lysosome-associated membrane proteins (LAMPs) and lysosomal acid phosphatase (LAP), mediates sorting at the TGN, plasma membrane, and endosomes (Rohrer *et al.* 1996). Interestingly, it has been demonstrated that the spacing of the tyrosine-containing tail relative to the membrane is important, since altering this distance results in these proteins cycling between the plasma membrane and early endocytic compartments (Rohrer *et al.* 1996). The second M6P-independent motif is a di-leucine signal found in lysosome integral membrane protein II (LIMP II) and the insulin receptor (Vega *et al.* 1991; Sandoval *et al.* 1994; Haft *et al.* 1998). Recent evidence indicates that clathrin-coated vesicles recognize and sort proteins containing either the di-leucine or the tyrosine motifs to their proper compartment (Ohno *et al.* 1995; Liu *et al.* 1998).

Contrary to the original view of lysosomes as non-specific degradation centres, it is now known that under certain conditions proteins can be selectively targeted to the lysosome for degradation (for review see Dice 1990). A 73-kDa heat shock protein mediates this selective uptake and degradation under starvation conditions, indicating that lysosomes could play a role in the regulation of cellular protein concentrations under conditions of stress (see Danon disease below) (Cuervo *et al.* 1997).

The lysosome has been linked to other processes, which have only recently begun to be characterized. For example, in some cell types, a small proportion of lysosomes function as exocytic vesicles that are Ca^{2+} regulated and temperature- and ATP-dependent. These lysosomes can fuse with the plasma membrane and participate in regulated secretion (Rodriguez *et al.* 1997). The function of this process has been postulated to be membrane resealing in wounded cells, since a Ca^{2+} influx through damaged membranes could trigger lysosomal fusion with the plasma membrane (Miyake and McNeil 1995) and eventual repair of the plasma membrane (Reddy *et al.* 2001). Despite the progress made in elucidating the characteristics of the lysosome, information regarding the properties of the lysosomal membrane and the known or potential transmembrane transporters responsible for enabling metabolites and substrates to enter or exit the organelle is limited. In addition, virtually nothing is known about accessory proteins that may reside on the lysosomal membrane, either in an integral or in a peripheral fashion, on the cytosolic side of the membrane. Preliminary evidence suggests that such proteins might be involved in cell-cycle control, cell survival, and cell death (Garin *et al.* 2001).

Lysosomal storage diseases are classically known as a group of more than 40 different diseases that result from a deficiency of a particular lysosomal enzyme (for a recent review see Winchester *et al.* 2000) (Chapters 2–4). Because most lysosomal hydrolases work sequentially to remove terminal residues from their substrates, a deficiency of one enzyme can cause an accumulation of the constituents of an entire catabolic pathway, since the substrates for hydrolysis by downstream lysosomal enzymes in the pathway are no longer available. The undigested material remains trapped in lysosomes and is visible as deposits in grossly enlarged compartments. Disorders in this group are classified according to their accumulated substrates such as mucopolysaccharides, glycoproteins, glycogen, or sphingolipids (Chapter 2). The first characterization of a disorder of this type came in 1963 when Hers and colleagues determined that the lysosomal enzyme α-glucosidase was deficient in patients with glycogen storage disease type II or Pompe disease (Hers 1963) (see also the Foreword). Considerable progress has been made in the analysis of the genes and mutations causing these diseases (McKusick 1995; Scriver *et al.* 1995) (Chapter 4); however, their pathogenesis is less clear (Chapter 12). In some diseases, the stored material directly causes the symptoms of the disease. For example, in mucopolysaccharidosis type VI (Maroteaux–Lamy syndrome), failure to metabolize chondroitin sulfate and dermatan sulfate in the heart valve leads to cardiac problems (Chapter 3). In other disorders, the stored material appears to have effects on seemingly unrelated metabolic pathways, such as the accumulation of glycosphingolipids in several sphingolipidoses, which have been shown to inhibit the function of protein kinase C, causing secondary effects (Hannun and Bell 1987).

A new class of storage diseases has begun to emerge in which the defect is in a membrane protein that often, but not always, acts as a membrane transporter (Chapter 2). Inactivation of these proteins by mutation results in the accumulation of storage material in the endosomal/lysosomal system, leading to aberrant cell homoeostasis and disease. The nature of the accumulated substrate is not always clearly linked to the substrate(s) of a given transporter, leading to difficulties in elucidating the function of these proteins and the mechanisms of disease pathogenesis. For example, in Niemann–Pick C (NPC) disease, defects in the NPC1 protein are thought to result in cholesterol accumulation in the endosomal/lysosomal system (see below). However, recent studies suggest that in addition to cholesterol, other lipids such as gangliosides and sphingolipids and even some proteins accumulate in NPC disease. Furthermore, preliminary analysis of the substrate specificity of the NPC1 protein suggests that it does not transport cholesterol (see below) (Davies *et al.* 2000*a*).

The endosomal/lysosomal v-ATPase

Since most of the transport proteins that are discussed in this chapter utilize the proton gradient across the endosomal/lysosomal membranes to power transport, a brief description of how this electrochemical gradient is generated and maintained follows. In fact, since a multiprotein complex with a number of transmembrane subunits generates the electrochemical gradient, it is appropriate that it is discussed first, even though no diseases associated with a defect in v-ATPase activity are currently known.

The vacuolar ATPase (v-ATPase) is largely responsible for the acidification of cellular compartments, a process that has been shown to be essential for the formation of transport vesicles and the proper sorting of proteins through the endocytic as well as the secretory pathway (Yilla *et al.* 1993; Clague *et al.* 1994) (Chapter 1). v-ATPases are membrane-spanning multisubunit enzyme complexes that use the energy from ATP hydrolysis to generate a proton gradient. The v-ATPase is responsible for maintaining the acidic pH of all compartments along the endocytic pathway as well as in the Golgi and TGN (Moriyama and Nelson 1989; Wang and Gluck 1990). This control of pH homoeostasis has been shown to be required for proper processing and correct sorting of proteins to different cellular compartments (Oda *et al.* 1991; Arai *et al.* 1993; Palokangas *et al.* 1994; van Deurs *et al.* 1996). The importance of acidification in the targeting of lysosomal membrane proteins, however, is less clear. In yeast, inhibition of the pump by bafilomycin A1, a specific inhibitor of the v-type ATPase, results in the secretion of immature forms of soluble hydrolases but not of membrane proteins. However, strains in which the subunits of the v-ATPase are deleted exhibit sorting defects for both classes of proteins (Yamashiro *et al.* 1990; Morano and Klionsky 1994). It has been postulated that distinct mechanisms exist for the targeting of soluble and membrane vacuolar proteins, which respond differently when acidification is perturbed or abolished, but this is still a speculation (Morano and Klionsky, 1994).

Purification of the lysosomal v-ATPase (Arai *et al.* 1993) revealed a number of properties of this multiprotein pump. The complex is composed of a cytoplasmic V_1 domain and a transmembrane V_0 domain (Nelson 1992), arranged together to form a 'ball and stalk' structure (Stevens and Forgac 1997). The soluble V_1 domain is comprised of five to eight different subunits and is the site of ATP hydrolysis (Nelson 1992). V_1 domains that are dissociated with high pH buffers or chaotropic ions are capable of associating with the V_0 domain and also with each other (Zhang *et al.* 1994). The main components of this domain are three alternating A and B subunits that are clustered together to form a 'head', which is connected to the transmembrane domain by a stalk (Stevens and Forgac 1997). Both subunits contain several nucleotide-binding sites and ATP synthase motifs (Gogarten *et al.* 1989; Puopolo *et al.* 1991), and they are highly conserved through plants, yeast, and even archaebacteria (Denda *et al.* 1988; Nelson *et al.* 1989; Sudhof *et al.* 1989; Puopolo *et al.* 1992). It is thought that the A subunit, for which at least two isoforms have been found (Puopolo *et al.* 1991; van Hille *et al.* 1993), contains the actual catalytic site, since the B subunit lacks the consensus sequences that are important for ATP hydrolysis (Futai *et al.* 1994). Two isoforms of the B subunit have also been isolated. The B1 isoform is expressed at high levels in the kidney, with low-level expression in the placenta and lung, whereas the B2 isoform is found in all tissues but with highest expression in the brain and kidney (van Hille *et al.* 1994). The isoforms contain identical middle regions with highly variant amino- and carboxyl-terminal domains, but no functional differences have been detected (Gogarten and Starke 1992; Puopolo *et al.* 1992). The function of the B subunit remains unclear, although its similarity to the regulatory a subunit of the F_0F_1-ATPase has led to speculation that it could modify the catalytic properties of the enzyme (Futai *et al.* 1994; Liu *et al.* 1996). It has been shown that assembly of the B subunit on the membrane of the yeast vacuole requires the presence of both the A subunit and the 16K subunit of the V_0 domain (Umemoto *et al.* 1990).

The V_0 domain is a highly hydrophobic transmembrane complex, which forms the proton pore. Although the exact organization of the multiple subunits in this domain is unknown, a major component, the 16 kDa subunit, has a hexameric core that is extractable with organic solvents and is reactive to dicyclohexylcarbodiimide (DCCD), an inhibitor of proton translocation (Hanada *et al.* 1991). The 16K subunit appears to have evolved through gene duplication and modification of the proteolipid c subunit of the F_0 domain of the F_0F_1-ATPase (Mandel *et al.* 1988). Studies of this subunit have identified four transmembrane helices, including two amino acids that are identical in all species examined as well as in the c subunit of the F_0 domain (Hanada *et al.* 1991). One amino acid is found in the fourth transmembrane segment, the site of reaction with DCCD, and the other is found between the third and fourth helix, a region thought to be important for the interaction between the V_0 and V_1 domains (Hanada *et al.* 1991). The 16K subunit of the crustacean *Nephrops norvegicus* is able to complement yeast 16K mutants, further strengthening the idea that regions of interaction are highly conserved (Harrison *et al.* 1994). Isolation of gap junction-like structures in *Nephrops* revealed that this protein is the main component of these structures, which are responsible for cell–cell communication, lending further support for another role for this protein beyond proton translocation (Leitch and Finbow 1990).

The precise function of the V_0 domain is not clear. It is capable of restoring the ATPase activity of V_1 domains, but by itself lacks proton conductance ability when reconstituted into liposomes (Zhang *et al.* 1994). In addition, the 16K subunit is thought to contain the binding site for bafilomycin A1 that could work by inducing a conformational change of the catalytic site (Hanada *et al.* 1990, 1991; Yoshimori *et al.* 1991; Rautiala *et al.* 1993; Crider *et al.* 1994; Zhang *et al.* 1994). Yeast in which the 16K subunit is disrupted are unable to assemble their A and B subunits together and consequently have no functional enzyme complex or ATPase activity (Umemoto *et al.* 1990). Interestingly, storage of a partial proteolytic product of 16K has been found in the brains and kidneys of mouse models for Batten disease, a neuronal ceroid lipofuscinosis (Faust *et al.* 1994) (see below).

Studies into the function of the v-ATPase have revealed intriguing possibilities about the role of the lysosome in cell growth. Much insight comes from experiments of yeast vacuoles that contain this pump. Disruption of certain subunits of this pump complex abolishes ATPase activity in the vacuolar membrane, with subsequent disruption of vacuole acidification and defects in protein sorting (Nelson and Nelson 1990; Umemoto *et al.* 1990, 1991; Kane *et al.* 1992). These yeast cells have a conditional lethal phenotype, with an acidic pH optimum for growth and no growth at all in media above pH 6.5 (Nelson and Nelson 1990). The discovery of specific inhibitors of the ATPase has been extremely useful in elucidating the function of the lysosome and acidification in many cellular processes. Bafilomycin A1 is a macrolide antibiotic that specifically inhibits v-ATPases and also induces cells to undergo apoptosis (F.W. Chen and Y.A. Ioannou, unpublished observations) (Nishihara *et al.* 1995; Kinoshita *et al.* 1996; Okahashi *et al.* 1997; Long *et al.* 1998). The exact reason for this has not been determined; however, there are many potential consequences of disrupting the proton pump, including disruption of the proton motive force (PMF)—a requirement for the function of most, if not all, lysosomal membrane transporters (see below). Also, the v-ATPase complex contains many proteins, some of which transverse the lysosomal membrane as described above. One could hypothesize that disruption of any one of these proteins would result in a severe cellular phenotype given the function of this ATPase. The fact that no disorders have been attributed to defects in the v-ATPase pump suggests either that such disorders have not been characterized yet or that the resulting phenotype from such a deficit is too severe and is thus lethal.

Finally, the v-ATPase appears to play a role in cellular transformation. The association of the 16K subunit of the V_0 domain with the bovine or human papillomavirus type 1 E5 oncoprotein leads to cell transformation (Goldstein *et al.* 1991). Binding of the E5 protein to 16K causes tyrosine phosphorylation and thus activation of the epidermal growth factor and platelet-derived growth factor receptors (Martin *et al.* 1989; Sparkowski *et al.* 1995). These receptors can bind to the 16K subunit in the absence of the E5 protein (Goldstein *et al.* 1991). Currently, it is unclear whether the 16K subunit or the E5 oncoprotein is responsible for transformation. It has been shown that glutamic acid 143 in the fourth transmembrane domain of 16K is important for E5 binding (Andresson *et al.* 1995); this residue is highly conserved, and yeast mutants with this 16K mutant allele are not viable (Nelson and Nelson 1990). In mammalian cells, this mutant 16K protein acts as an oncoprotein in a dominant negative fashion (Goldstein *et al.* 1991). These results suggest that 16K is the first structural protein involved in tumorgenesis and emphasize the importance of the endosomal/lysosomal system in cell homoeostasis.

Niemann–Pick C disease

Niemann–Pick type C (NPC) is a rare autosomal recessive lipidosis characterized by the accumulation of unesterified cholesterol in lysosomes (Vanier *et al.* 1991; Pentchev *et al.* 1994) (Chapter 3). Patients exhibit progressive neurodegeneration and hepatosplenomegaly, which leads to death during early childhood (Patterson *et al.* 2001). The most prominent biochemical feature is the accumulation of LDL-derived unesterified cholesterol in the endosomal/lysosomal system (Vanier *et al.* 1991). In addition, cholesterol accumulates in the TGN and its relocation to and from the plasma membrane is delayed (Patterson *et al.* 2001). In fibroblasts, the defect in cholesterol exit from lysosomes is accompanied by attenuation in the downregulation of two key components of cholesterol homoeostasis—3-hydroxy-3-methylglutaryl coenzyme A reductase (HMG-Co A reductase) and the low-density lipoprotein receptor (Pentchev *et al.* 1986).

The gene mutated in most NPC patients, *NPC1*, maps to chromosome 18q11–12 (Carstea *et al.* 1997) and encodes an approximately 4.9 kb messenger RNA that is predicted to produce a 1278 amino acid protein. *NPC1* spans approximately 47 kb and contains 25 exons, ranging in size from 74 to 788 nucleotides, and introns ranging in size from 0.097 to 7 kb (Morris *et al.* 1999). More than 80 mutations have been described in *NPC1* patients (Carstea *et al.* 1997; Greer *et al.* 1998, 1999; Millat *et al.* 1999, 2001; Yamamoto *et al.* 1999; Sun *et al.* 2001), including nonsense and missense mutations as well as insertions, deletions, and duplications. These mutations are spread throughout the gene and do not suggest any functionally critical protein domains; however, there is a small cluster of mutations at the carboxyterminal third of the protein in a region containing cysteine residues that are conserved among the various *NPC1* orthologues (Greer *et al.* 1999).

In addition to NPC1, a small soluble protein originally identified as a major secreted protein from human epididymis (HE1) (Kirchhoff *et al.* 1996) was found to be mutated in the second complementation group of NPC disease, NPC2, which is responsible for about 5% of patients (Naureckiene *et al.* 2000) (Chapter 8). The protein receives the classical M6P modification for soluble lysosomal proteins and can reach the lysosome even when added exogenously onto cells in culture. Subcellular fractionation studies have confirmed that this small approximately 18 kDa soluble glycoprotein resides in the lysosome lumen (Naureckiene *et al.* 2000). Since, similar to NPC1, patients with NPC2 are characterized by an accumulation of free cholesterol in their endosomal/lysosomal system, NPC2 must play a role in the egress of cholesterol and other lipids from the endosomal/lysosomal membranes.

Analysis of the NPC1 sequence does not reveal any significant homologies to other proteins. However, transmembrane domains 3–7 (Fig. 9.1) show homology to the Patched (PTC) protein. Patched is a membrane-bound receptor for sonic hedgehog (Shh) (Marigo *et al.* 1996; Stone *et al.* 1996), a developmental signalling molecule that, in its active state, carries a covalently attached cholesterol moiety (Fietz *et al.* 1994; Lee *et al.* 1994). This sequence similarity is also shared by the sterol-sensing domains (SSDs) of HMG-R and sterol-regulated element cleavage-activating protein (SCAP). In HMG-R, the SSD plays a role in enzyme degradation when the cell 'senses' adequate levels of cholesterol, whereas in SCAP it may play a role in the activation of the sterol regulatory element-binding proteins (SREBPs), a family of transcription factors that regulates several critical enzymes in the salvage and *de novo* cholesterol pathways (Hua *et al.* 1996). Recently, a human gene homologous to *NPC1*, *Niemann–Pick C1-like 1* (*NPC1-L1*) (Davies *et al.* 2000*b*), was also found to contain an SSD domain, but its functional significance is not yet known.

NPC1 is a membrane glycoprotein that localizes to LAMP-positive organelles, presumably endosomes and lysosomes (Higgins *et al.* 1999; Neufeld *et al.* 1999; Patel *et al.* 1999). Further studies have demonstrated that NPC1 resides primarily in Rab7-positive late endosomes and only secondarily in lysosomes and the TGN (Higgins *et al.* 1999). This is an important distinction in view of data suggesting that cholesterol accumulation in *NPC1*$^{-/-}$ cells occurs primarily in late endosomes (Kobayashi *et al.* 1999), which are sorting sites for various cellular components. In addition, NPC1 cells seem to be defective in the efflux of endocytosed sucrose and in the sorting of the M6P receptor, suggesting that the retrograde movement of proteins and cargo from late endosomes to the TGN is perturbed (Kobayashi *et al.* 1999; Neufeld *et al.* 1999).

Further characterization of the effects of absent or mutated NPC1 protein suggests that *NPC1*$^{-/-}$ cells have a generalized block in lipid recycling from late endosomes to the Golgi and plasma membrane. A potential function for cholesterol in the modulation of lipid trafficking has been proposed (Puri *et al.* 1999). In those studies, BODIPY-labelled lactosyl ceramide (BLC; a glycosphingolipid) used to probe the distribution of the glycosphingolipid in normal and NPC1 cells following endocytosis from the plasma membrane is found to localize predominantly in the Golgi apparatus in normal cells (Puri *et al.* 1999). However, in cells from patients with sphingolipid storage disorders including NPC1, BLC is found in perinuclear vesicles characteristic of endosomes and lysosomes (Puri *et al.* 1999). When normal cells are grown in the presence of high levels of cholesterol (to induce cholesterol accumulation in the endosomal/lysosomal system), BLC is found in perinuclear vesicles similar to those seen in NPC1 cells, suggesting that cholesterol plays a role in modulating the movement of other lipids within the cell (Puri *et al.* 1999). Subsequent studies have implicated NPC1 in the regulation of lipid movement late in the endocytic pathway, presumably from late endosomes (Ko *et al.* 2001; Zhang *et al.* 2001*a*, *b*). Studies of NPC1 overexpression in CHO cells (Millard *et al.* 2000) indicate that ectopic expression of NPC1 (about 15-fold above endogenous levels) results in an increase in the transport of LDL cholesterol to the plasma membrane, lending further support to the idea that NPC1 is involved in subcellular lipid transport.

Analysis of its topological arrangement within membranes indicates that NPC1 contains 13 transmembrane domains (Fig. 9.1), three large lumenal hydrophilic loops and a cytoplasmic tail (Davies and Ioannou 2000). Within the cytoplasmic tail is a di-leucine motif that has been shown to direct the delivery of other membrane proteins to the endosomal/lysosomal system (Fukuda *et al.* 1988*a*). A number of glycosylation consensus sequences are scattered throughout the protein, most of which are apparently used *in vivo* (Davies and Ioannou 2000).

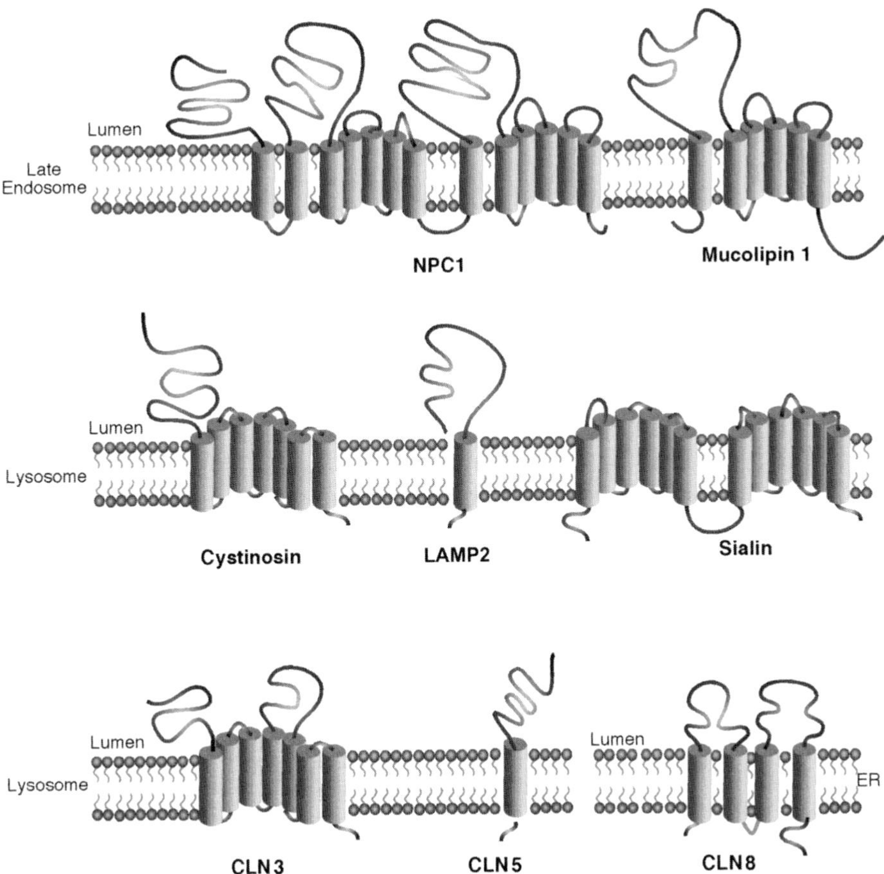

Fig. 9.1 The topologies of the various proteins discussed. The topology of NPC1 is known (Davies and Ioannou 2000) whereas the topologies of Cystinosin (Cherqui *et al.* 2001), Sialin (Verheijen *et al.* 1999) and LAMP2 (Fukuda 1991) are predicted based on preliminary experimental evidence. The topologies of the CLN proteins and mucolipin 1, however, are based on computer prediction and are not based on any experimental evidence. Thus, for the CLN proteins the location of the hydrophilic loops, whether lumenal or cytoplasmic, and the number of transmembrane domains will most likely change, as data on their structure and topology are reported.

Interestingly, a number of unique consensus sequences for a prokaryotic lipoprotein-attachment site, usually found in prokaryotic polytopic proteins, are found in prokaryotic permeases of the resistance–nodulation–division (RND) family. Further characterization of this relationship has revealed that NPC1 and members of the RND family share the same RND signature: six transmembrane domains separated by a large hydrophilic loop between transmembrane domains 1 and 2 (Davies *et al.* 2000*a*). This domain is repeated twice (Fig. 9.1).

Expression of human NPC1 in *E. coli* has demonstrated that NPC1 functions as a multidrug permease similar to its prokaryotic relatives (Tseng *et al.* 1999), positing NPC1 as the first mammalian member of this ancient family (Davies *et al.* 2000*a*). Transport studies in NPC1-expressing *E. coli* show that NPC1 can transport fatty acids very efficiently but not cholesterol or cholesterol esters. The lack of detectable NPC1 cholesterol transport activity in *E. coli* may be due to the lack of necessary accessory proteins or appropriate cholesterol acceptors in the prokaryotic membrane, or it may simply reflect the fact that NPC1 does not transport cholesterol. In fact, based on data from the Tangier disease transporter ABCA1, it seems reasonable that NPC1 may transport fatty acids or phospholipids as its primary substrates and only indirectly facilitate cholesterol movement (Wang *et al.* 2001). Alternatively, NPC1 may transport a group of lipids such as sphingolipids and gangliosides *en masse*.

Neuronal ceroid lipofuscinoses—Batten disease

The neuronal ceroid lipofuscinoses (CLN) are a class of neurodegenerative disorders characterized by the accumulation of autofluorescent ceroid lipopigment in the lysosome (Wisniewski *et al.* 2001). These diseases are characterized by progressive mental decline, motor dysfunction, epilepsy, and progressive blindness, leading to early death (Dawson and Cho 2000) (Chapter 3). The childhood forms of the disorder are inherited in an autosomal recessive manner and are caused by mutations in one of five genes: *CL1*, *CLN2*, *CLN3*, *CLN5*, and *CLN8*. Two additional genes, *CLN6* and *CLN7*, have recently been mapped to specific chromosomal locations, but their identity is still unknown. The genes responsible for the adult form of the disease, *CLN4*, are presently unknown. Although mutations in most of these genes, including 31 mutations for *CLN3*, four for *CLN5*, and one for *CLN8*, have recently been described (Mole *et al.* 2001), the precise functions of their encoded proteins are mostly unknown. The best-characterized protein is *CLN*1 which encodes palmitoyl : protein thioesterase and was the first to be identified (Vesa *et al.* 1995).

Of the lipofuscinoses, Batten disease, caused by a deficiency of *CLN3*, is one of the most common childhood neurodegenerative diseases and has received much attention recently (Luiro *et al.* 2001). Three of the five known genes, *CLN3* located on chromosome 16, *CLN5* located on chromosome 13, and *CLN8* located on 8p23, are predicted to encode proteins that contain potential transmembrane domains, suggesting that these proteins are embedded in a membrane (Fig. 9). Interestingly, *CLN3* and *CLN5* have been localized in the membranes of the endosomal/lysosomal system, as might be inferred from the lysosomal storage phenotype of the disease; *CLN8*, however, has been shown to reside in the ER (Lonka *et al.* 2000). Very little is currently known about the function of these proteins, due in part to their recent identification, although some data regarding *CLN3* are beginning to be reported.

As mentioned above, *CLN3* has been localized to the endosomal/lysosomal system, although there appears to be some confusion regarding its exact subcellular location (Pearce 2000). One report suggests that *CLN3* is a Golgi-resident protein (Kremmidiotis *et al.* 1999), whereas others assent that it resides in an endosomal/lysosomal compartment (Jarvela *et al.* 1998; Kida *et al.* 1999; Haskell *et al.* 2000). Interestingly, *CLN3* is not targeted to lysosomes in neuronal cells and has instead been found to associate with the synaptosomal fraction (Luiro *et al.* 2001). However, unlike *CLN1*, it is not found in synaptic vesicles, indicating that *CLN3* is localized to an as yet unknown membrane compartment in neurones (Luiro *et al.* 2001). These results emphasize the need for appropriate cell-culture systems to study proteins that cause tissue-specific phenotypes such as neural degeneration.

The causative role of the CLN proteins in the lipofuscinoses is still a mystery. How do these different proteins, some soluble and some membrane associated, result in the same disease phenotype when mutated? How does a protein that resides in the ER, *CLN8*, cause a lysosomal storage phenotype? The similarities between this disease and NPC (see above) cannot be ignored. In NPC disease, two seemingly unrelated proteins, *NPC1* (Carstea *et al.*

1997), a large transmembrane protein residing in late endosomal membranes, and *NPC2* (Naureckiene *et al.* 2000), a small soluble protein residing in lysosomes, cause similar phenotypes when mutated. However, although the phenotypes caused by these unrelated genes appear similar, upon careful inspection subtle differences between the phenotypes begin to emerge. It is possible that the phenotypes resulting from mutations in the various CLN proteins are similar but not identical and may require further characterization.

Alternatively, the various CLN proteins could interact with each other to form a multiprotein complex. Disruption of any one of these proteins would cause a disruption of the complex, yielding an identical phenotype no matter which protein was disrupted. However, no interaction between *CLN1*, *CLN2*, and *CLN3* has been detected by using a yeast two-hybrid system (Zhong *et al.* 2000). In addition, using a similar approach, no interaction could be detected between *CLN3* and a number of other proteins including the c subunit of the mitochondrial ATP synthase (Leung *et al.* 2001). An intriguing report suggests that *CLN3* might have a role in lysosome acidification as a regulator of lysosomal pH (Golabek *et al.* 2000). Even though the v-ATPase regulates the endosomal/lysosomal system pH (as described above), *CLN3* might interact with this multiprotein complex or may function in an accessory manner. It is also possible that *CLN3*, similar to *NPC1* and sialin (see below, Salla disease), might have a symport or antiport activity that involves the transport of protons across the endosomal/lysosomal membrane. In fact, it is very likely that *CLN3* utilizes a PMF for function, a property that seems to be shared by transmembrane transporters of the endosomal/lysosomal system.

Most of the questions raised must await further data to identify the exact function and properties of the membrane-associated CLN proteins. The availability of a mouse knockout model for *CLN3* (Katz and Johnson 2001) should provide further insights into the function of *CLN3* and disease pathogenesis.

Salla disease

Sialic acid released from the degradation of glycoproteins, glycolipids, and glycosaminoglycans in the lysosome must exit this organelle so that it can be reutilized. The lysosomal membrane transporter responsible for sialic acid and glucuronic acid transport was purified from rat liver (Havelaar *et al.* 1998). The 57 kDa protein correlates with transport activity of sialic and glucuronic acid and is inhibited by a number of aliphatic monocarboxylates. Interestingly, the transporter can recognize and transport a number of structurally different monosaccharides, including sialic, glucuronic, and iduronic acids (Havelaar *et al.* 1998).

Metabolic labelling of Salla disease fibroblasts with the tritiated ganglioside GM3 revealed that Salla fibroblasts are unable to incorporate this molecule in glycoproteins. In addition, the sphingolipids ceramide and lactosylceramide accumulate in the lysosomes of Salla fibroblasts, suggesting that accumulation of GM3 in the lysosome also affects enzymes involved in glycosphingolipid metabolism (Chigorno *et al.* 1996). Loading of Salla disease fibroblasts with GM1 ganglioside demonstrated that these cells accumulate GM2 and GM3 gangliosides and have a reduced turnover of breakdown products following desialosylation of various glycoconjugates (Pitto *et al.* 1996). These results suggest that accumulation of free sialic acid in lysosomes inhibits the action of lysosomal sialidase, reducing the breakdown of glycoconjugates and presumably contributing to the disease phenotype.

The locus for Salla disease was identified on 6q14-q15, and by using a positional cloning approach with a number of Finnish families, the causative gene has been identified (Verheijen *et al.* 1999). The predicted protein contains 495 amino acids, which correlates well with the 57 kDa molecular weight of the purified sialic acid transporter. It has been suggested that the transporter be called 'sialin' to reflect its major substrate, sialic acid. Homology searches have revealed that sialin is homologous to transporters belonging to the major facilitator superfamily (MFS), an ancient family of both eukaryotic and prokaryotic transporters (Verheijen *et al.* 1999). An interesting property of the MFS members is that energy for substrate transport is coupled to the symport of cations or anions. Similar to the properties of the *NPC1* protein described above, these transporters require a PMF for transport that is provided by the pH gradient across the lysosomal membrane. Thus, it appears that transmembrane transporters of the endosomal/lysosomal system take advantage of the electrochemical gradient across the membrane to power transport.

Danon disease

Danon disease is an X-linked disorder characterized by vacuolar cardiomyopathy and myopathy. The major pathological feature of Danon disease is the accumulation of intra-cytoplasmic vacuoles containing glycogen and other autophagic material in cardiac and skeletal muscle cells (Danon *et al.* 1981) (Chapter 3). The disease was first described in two unrelated 16-year-old boys who presented with mental retardation, cardiomegaly, and myopathy (Danon *et al.* 1981). Paradoxically, although muscle biopsies showed an accumulation of glycogen resembling acid maltase deficiency, acid maltase activity was normal. Thus, the disease was characterized as a general glycogenosis disorder of unknown aetiology. Eventually, the disease was characterized as 'lysosomal glycogen storage disease with normal acid maltase'.

The lysosomal membrane contains two major structural proteins of approximately 110–120 kDa, LAMP1 and LAMP2. The proteins were initially characterized in murine cells by using monoclonal antibodies raised against lysosomal membranes (Chen *et al.* 1985). Subsequent isolation and characterization of human LAMP1 and LAMP2 revealed that they were both sialoglycoproteins carrying polylactosaminoglycan (Carlsson *et al.* 1988). Further analysis showed that both proteins are synthesized as polypeptides of about 40–45 kDa and are extensively glycosylated (Mane *et al.* 1989). As might be expected, LAMP1 and LAMP2 contain 18 and 16 asparagine-linked oligosaccharides, respectively. However, some of these oligosaccharide chains are modified by poly-*N*-acetyl lactosamine, a unique modification that is not seen in other lysosomal proteins (Carlsson and Fukuda 1990). This extended polylactosamine modification contributes to the apparent high molecular weight exhibited by these proteins on SDS gels (approximately 120 kDa), since the predicted molecular weight of these proteins without oligosaccharides is approximately 40 kDa (Carlsson *et al.* 1988). In LAMP2, it has been found that an increase in polylactosamine glycosylation is associated with a slower transit of this protein through the Golgi complex during polarization of Madin–Darby canine kidney (MDCK) cells (Nabi and Rodriguez-Boulan 1993; Nabi and Dennis 1998).

Both LAMP1 and LAMP2 contain a single transmembrane domain and a short cytoplasmic tail (Fig. 9.1). Within this tail, a tyrosine-based sorting motif has been identified and shown to be ultimately responsible for targeting these proteins to the lysosome. Recent data suggest that sorting proteins, such as LAMP1 and LAMP2, containing a tyrosine-based targeting signal is distinct from the sorting of the M6P receptor, which occurs via clathrin-coated vesicles at the TGN (Karlsson and Carlsson 1998).

These related proteins appear to have evolved from the same ancestral gene, as evidenced by a comparison of their amino acid sequences following isolation of their cDNAs (Fukuda *et al.*

1988*b*). However, different genes on chromosomes 13q34 and Xq24-25 encode LAMP1 and LAMP2, respectively (Mattei *et al.* 1990). Isolation and characterization of the LAMP genes has revealed the existence of different isoforms of LAMP2. Avian LAMP2 was found to be encoded by at least three different transcripts, LAMP2a, LAMP2b, and LAMP2c, resulting in variant cytoplasmic and transmembrane domains (Hatem *et al.* 1995). It has been subsequently demonstrated that these different transcripts of avian LAMP2 arise from alternative splicing of a single gene (Gough *et al.* 1995). The function of these alternatively spliced mRNAs is beginning to be unravelled with the identification of an alternatively spliced LAMP2 transcript found to be highly expressed in human muscle (Konecki *et al.* 1995). This new transcript, h-LAMP2b, gives rise to a fully functional LAMP2 protein that retains the cytoplasmic tail Gly-Tyr-X-X motif and localizes to the lysosomal membrane (Konecki *et al.* 1995). Thus, it appears that different LAMP2 isoforms may be expressed in a tissue-specific manner. The functional significance of these observations is currently unknown.

Recently, the gene responsible for causing Danon disease was identified as LAMP2 (Nishino *et al.* 2000; Tanaka *et al.* 2000) by demonstrating mutations in 10 unrelated patients, including one of the original patients (Nishino *et al.* 2000). In addition, a mouse knockout model for LAMP2 exhibits an extensive accumulation of autophagic vacuoles with abnormal cardiac myocytes and heart contractility (Tanaka *et al.* 2000), lending further support for the role of LAMP2 in Danon disease. This marks the first example of a myopathy caused by a structural protein rather than a protein with enzymatic activity.

However, new evidence suggests that LAMP2 may have an additional non-structural function within the membranes of the endosomal/lysosomal system. For example, LAMP2a appears to function as a receptor for chaperone-mediated autophagy, a function that is not shared with other LAMP2 isoforms (Cuervo and Dice 2000). In rat liver, the LAMP2a isoform represents about 25% of total LAMP2 protein on the lysosomal membrane, and these levels correlate with the rate of chaperone-mediated autophagy (Cuervo and Dice 2000). Four positively charged amino acids at the cytoplasmic tail of LAMP2a are required for binding of substrate proteins. LAMP2a also responds to serum withdrawal in cultured fibroblasts and tends to multimerize (Cuervo and Dice 2000). LAMP2 has been purified from rat liver lysosomes in a soluble form lacking the transmembrane domain and cytoplasmic tail and was found to multimerize and form a tetrameric structure (Akasaki and Tsuji 1998).

It is currently not clear whether Danon disease is a result of a general loss of function of LAMP2 or whether loss of one of the isoforms such as LAMP2a or LAMP2b has a causative effect on disease pathogenesis. Based on mutation analysis of Danon alleles, however, it is suggested that the disease phenotype is most likely due to the absence of the LAMP2b isoform (Nishino *et al.* 2000). Of the 10 mutations identified, all but one are predicted to produce a protein that is truncated, without the transmembrane domain and cytoplasmic tail. In addition, LAMP2b is more abundantly expressed in heart, skeletal muscle, and brain, tissues affected in Danon disease, suggesting that the 2b isoform is responsible for the disease phenotype (Nishino *et al.* 2000).

Cystinosis

Cystinosis is an autosomal recessive condition caused by defects in the *CTNS* gene located on chromosome 17p13 (Town *et al.* 1998) (Chapter 3). This gene encodes a 367-amino acid protein called cystinosin that is predicted to contain seven transmembrane domains (Fig. 9.1) (Anikster *et al.* 1999). The major phenotype of this disease is cysteine accumulation in lysosomes, leading to the assumption that cystinosin is probably a cysteine transporter on the lysosomal membrane. Infantile nephropathic cystinosis is an early-onset form of the disease characterized by proximal tubular dysfunction, whereas a rarer late-onset form of the disease results in symptoms presenting at about 12–15 years of age (Attard *et al.* 1999). Mutation analysis of a number of cystinosis alleles suggests that the severe phenotype is caused by mutations that either cause a protein truncation or disrupt potential transmembrane domains, whereas the milder phenotype is caused by mutations that are predicted to have a minor effect on the protein (Attard *et al.* 1999).

Studies have shown that cystinosin is distinct from cysteine transporters found at the plasma membrane and that it exclusively transports cysteine. Recently, it has been shown that cystinosin is targeted to the lysosomal membrane via a GY-XX-Φ (Φ = hydrophobic amino acid) motif in the short cytoplasmic tail and a novel signal YF-PQA found in the third cytoplasmic loop (Cherqui *et al.* 2001). Additional data on the structure and function of cystinosin are not currently available, although a number of predictions can be inferred based on the discussion of other endosomal/lysosomal system membrane transporters. For example, the cystinosin transporter is most likely utilizing the lysosomal PMF for function, a hypothesis that can be easily tested using any one of the many agents that disrupt PMF gradients.

Mucolipidosis type IV

Mucolipidosis type IV (ML IV) was first described in 1974 as a lysosomal storage disorder due to the lysosomal accumulation of mucopolysaccharides and lipids. It has an autosomal recessive mode of inheritance and predominantly affects Ashkenazi Jews. Mucolipidosis type IV is characterized by severe progressive neurodegeneration, psychomotor retardation, and ophthalmological anomalies such as corneal opacity and retinal degeneration (Bach 2001) (Chapter 3).

The candidate locus for ML IV was identified on chromosome 19p13.2-13.3 using linkage analyses in 13 different families (Slaugenhaupt *et al.* 1999). Following the report of the ML IV chromosomal locus, three different groups independently reported identification of a gene located at 19p that is mutated in patients with ML IV (Bargal *et al.* 2000; Bassi *et al.* 2000; Sun *et al.* 2000). This gene encodes a protein with six predicted transmembrane domains (Fig. 9.1). Suggested names for the protein include 'mucolipin 1' (Sun *et al.* 2000) and 'mucolipidin' (Bassi *et al.* 2000); the 'mucolipin' designation appears to be the one most often used.

Mucolipin 1 is a new member of the transient receptor potential (TRP) cation channel family (Slaugenhaupt 2002). While the function of mucolipin 1 is still not known, studies in cultured ML IV cells have shown that the abnormal lysosomal storage seen in ML IV is due to a defect in late endosomal trafficking (Slaugenhaupt 2002). Further studies have indicated that the defect in ML IV lies in the endocytosis of various membrane components rather than their lysosomal degradation (Chen *et al.* 1998). In addition, ML IV cells appear to be unable to regulate their endosomal/lysosomal pH (Bach *et al.* 1999). Interestingly, mucolipin has been found on the plasma membrane when transiently expressed in COS7 cells (Bassi *et al.* 2000). Expression of a mucolipin green fluorescence protein (GFP) fusion in *Xenopus* oocytes has revealed that mucolipin colocalizes with lysosomal markers and can translocate to the plasma membrane upon treatment of the oocytes with the Ca^{2+} ionophore ionomycin (LaPlante *et al.* 2002). Recent data suggest that mucolipin1 is a Ca^{2+} channel that is also involved in late endosomal trafficking (LaPlante *et al.* 2002). This channel is permeable to Na^+ and K^+, whereas Ca^{2+} can modulate its activity.

Thus, ML IV, along with *NPC1*, belongs to a new group of disease-causing membrane proteins that are found on the membranes of the endosomal/lysosomal system and seem to transport molecules unrelated to the storage material found in these diseases. Both appear to regulate late endosome trafficking, but the mechanisms are as yet undetermined.

Summary

It is becoming increasingly evident that the lysosome is linked to many more cellular processes than it was first thought when described in the 1950s. Indeed, the integrity of this organelle and the proper functioning of the transporters found in its membranes are critical not only to the proper transport and degradation of various molecules, but also to more specialized functions. As the technologies of genomics and proteomics advance, the intricacies of the endosomal/lysosomal membranes will be elucidated. The question arises: Are there other, as yet undiscovered, transmembrane proteins that function in this system? It should be pointed out that other membrane proteins that have not been fully characterized, including the mouse transporter protein (MTP) (Cabrita *et al.* 1999), the STAR-related protein MLN64 (Alpy *et al.* 2001), and the ABC-type transporter ABCB9 (Zhang *et al.* 2000), have been localized to these compartments. The function of MTP in lysosomal membranes is currently unknown, but expression of this protein in yeast confers a drug-resistance phenotype, suggesting that MTP is a multidrug transporter (Hogue *et al.* 1999). MLN64 has been implicated in cholesterol egress from the late endosomal system (Alpy *et al.* 2001), whereas ABCB9 is a member of an expanding family of ABC transporters involved in lipid transport (Ioannou 2001). In addition, a recent proteomic analysis of the mammalian phagosome has identified other membrane proteins associated with the endosomal/lysosomal system (Garin *et al.* 2001), including two proteins known to associate with lipid rafts (Simons and Ikonen 1997)—flotillin-1 (Bickel *et al.* 1997) and stomatin (Snyers *et al.* 1999). Recently, a new protein with four transmembrane domains found on the membrane of late endosomes has been reported (Alpy *et al.* 2002). This new protein named MENTHO is related to MLN64 and its function is currently unknown.

The potential interaction of these membrane proteins with accessory proteins, either cytoplasmic or lumenal, has not been addressed due in part to the lack of data regarding such associations. A theme beginning to emerge from studies of these proteins is the apparent complexity of their regulation and function(s). Disease pathogenesis is not caused simply by abnormal accumulation of metabolites. A fact that is often overlooked is that these proteins exhibit a symport or antiport activity in order to power transport. The importance of this activity and the consequences of disrupting it have not been addressed. However, these activities almost certainly balance and regulate the activity of the v-ATPase to maintain the delicate electrochemical gradient across the endosomal/lysosomal membranes. As discussed above, the pH of the endosomal/lysosomal system is regulated to reflect the cellular stage of growth, so that actively proliferating cells maintain a more alkaline endosomal/lysosomal system than resting cells. It is also possible that transport of certain metabolites through the endosomal/lysosomal system signals downstream events such as DNA replication or preparation for cell division. Cells are known to monitor the availability of such raw materials as nucleotides prior to entering the cell cycle. However, virtually nothing is known about how cells sense the availability of other important materials such as lipids and other membrane components. This check could potentially be accomplished with the assistance of endosomal/lysosomal resident proteins.

In the case of disorders with brain dysfunction, we can hypothesize that if in fact the endosomal/lysosomal system is actively involved in the regulation of cell division, it could then potentially be abnormally stimulated in cells such as neurones, which do not have the ability to divide. The outcome of such abnormal stimulation would be apoptotic cell death, since the conflicting signals cannot be resolved (Chen and Ioannou 1999). It is of great interest that the brain pathology seen in most of the diseases described above involves the apoptotic death of neuronal cells. This common theme of neuropathology, coupled with the fact that communication of the endosomal/lysosomal system with the rest of the cell is disrupted, suggests that continued study of these proteins will provide intriguing insights into both the pathogenesis of these disorders and the interaction of intracellular signals with the endosomal/lysosomal system for maintaining cell homoeostasis.

Acknowledgements

These studies were supported in part by NIH grant R01 DK54736 and a grant from the March of Dimes Foundation and the Ara Parseghian Medical Research Foundation.

References

Akasaki, K. and Tsuji, H. (1998). Purification and characterization of a soluble form of lysosome-associated membrane glycoprotein-2 (LAMP-2) from rat liver lysosomal contents. *Biochem Mol Biol Int*, **46**, 197–206.

Alpy, F., Stoeckel, M. E., Dierich, A., Escola, J. M., Wendling, C., Chenard, M. P. *et al.* (2001). The steroidogenic acute regulatory protein homolog MLN64, a late endosomal cholesterol-binding protein. *J Biol Chem*, **276**, 4261–9.

Alpy, F., Wendling, C., Rio, M. C. and Tomasetto, C. (2002). MENTHO, a MLN64 homologue devoid of the START domain. *J Biol Chem*.

Andresson, T., Sparkowski, J., Goldstein, D. and Schlegel, R. (1995). Vacuolar H^+-ATPase mutants transform cells and define a binding site for the papillomavirus E5 oncoprotein. *J Biol Chem*, **270**, 6830–7.

Anikster, Y., Shotelersuk, V. and Gahl, W. A. (1999). CTNS mutations in patients with cystinosis. *Hum Mutat*, **14**, 454–8.

Arai, K., Shimaya, A., Hiratani, N. and Ohkuma, S. (1993). Purification and characterization of lysosomal H^+-ATPase. *J Biol Chem*, **268**, 5649–60.

Attard, M., Jean, G., Forestier, L., Cherqui, S., van't Hoff, W., Broyer, M. *et al.* (1999). Severity of phenotype in cystinosis varies with mutations in the CTNS gene: predicted effect on the model of cystinosin. *Hum Mol Genet*, **8**, 2507–14.

Bach, G. (2001). Mucolipidosis type IV. *Mol Genet Metab*, **73**, 197–203.

Bach, G., Chen, C. S. and Pagano, R. E. (1999). Elevated lysosomal pH in mucolipidosis type IV cells. *Clin Chim Acta*, **280**, 173–9.

Bargal, R., Avidan, N., Ben-Asher, E., Olender, Z., Zeigler, M., Frumkin, A. *et al.* (2000). Identification of the gene causing mucolipidosis type IV. *Nat Genet*, **26**, 118–23.

Barriocanal, J., Bonifacino, J., Yuan, L. and Sandoval, I. (1986). Biosynthesis, glycosylation, movement through the Golgi system, and transport to lysosomes by an N-linked carbohydrate-independent mechanism of three lysosomal integral membrane proteins. *J Biol Chem*, **261**, 16755–63.

Bassi, M. T., Manzoni, M., Monti, E., Pizzo, M. T., Ballabio, A. and Borsani, G. (2000). Cloning of the gene encoding a novel integral membrane protein, mucolipidin and identification of the two major founder mutations causing mucolipidosis type IV. *Am J Hum Genet*, **67**, 1110–20.

Bickel, P. E., Scherer, P. E., Schnitzer, J. E., Oh, P., Lisanti, M. P. and Lodish, H. F. (1997). Flotillin and epidermal surface antigen define a new family of caveolae-associated integral membrane proteins. *J Biol Chem*, **272**, 13793–802.

Blagoveshchenskaya, A., Norcott, J. and Cutler, D. (1998). Lysosomal targeting of P-selecting is mediated by a novel sequence within its cytoplasmic tail. *J Biol Chem*, **273**, 2729–37.

Cabrita, M. A., Hobman, T. C., Hogue, D. L., King, K. M. and Cass, C. E. (1999). Mouse transporter protein, a membrane protein that regulates cellular multidrug resistance, is localized to lysosomes. *Cancer Res*, **59**, 4890–7.

Carlsson, S. R. and Fukuda, M. (1990). The poly lactosaminoglycans of human lysosomal membrane glycoproteins LAMP-1 and LAMP-2. Localization on the peptide backbones. *J Biol Chem*, **265**, 20488–95.

Carlsson, S. R., Roth, J., Piller, F. and Fukuda, M. (1988). Isolation and characterization of human lysosomal membrane glycoproteins, h-LAMP-1 and h-LAMP-2. Major sialoglycoproteins carrying polylactosaminoglycan. *J Biol Chem*, **263**, 18911–9.

Carstea, E. D., Morris, J. A., Coleman, K. G., Loftus, S. K., Zhang, D., Cummings, C. *et al.* (1997). Niemann–Pick C1 disease gene: homology to mediators of cholesterol homeostasis. *Science*, **277**, 228–31.

Chen, F. W. and Ioannou, Y. A. (1999). Ribosomal proteins in cell proliferation and apoptosis. *Int Rev Immunol*, **18**, 429–48.

Chen, J. W., Murphy, T. L., Willingham, M. C., Pastan, I. and August, J. T. (1985). Identification of two lysosomal membrane glycoproteins. *J Cell Biol*, **101**, 85–95.

Chen, C. S., Bach, G. and Pagano, R. E. (1998). Abnormal transport along the lysosomal pathway in mucolipidosis, type IV disease. *Proc Natl Acad Sci USA*, **95**, 6373–8.

Cherqui, S., Kalatzis, V., Trugnan, G. and Antignac, C. (2001). The targeting of cystinosin to the lysosomal membrane requires a tyrosine-based signal and a novel sorting motif. *J Biol Chem*, **276**, 13314–21.

Chigorno, V., Tettamanti, G. and Sonnino, S. (1996). Metabolic processing of gangliosides by normal and Salla human fibroblasts in culture. A study performed by administering radioactive GM3 ganglioside. *J Biol Chem*, **271**, 21738–44.

Clague, M., Urbe, S., Aniento, F. and Gruenberg, J. (1994). Vacuolar ATPase activity is required for endosomal carrier vesicle formation. *J Biol Chem*, **269**, 21–4.

Crider, B., Xie, X. and Stone, D. (1994). Bafilomycin inhibits proton flow through the H^+ channel of vacuolar proton pumps. *J Biol Chem*, **269**, 17379–81.

Cuervo, A. M. and Dice, J. F. (2000). Unique properties of LAMP2a compared to other LAMP2 isoforms. *J Cell Sci*, **113** (Part 24), 4441–50.

Cuervo, A., Dice, J. F. and Knecht, E. (1997). A population of rat liver lysosomes responsible for the selective uptake and degradation of cytosolic proteins. *J Biol Chem*, **272**, 5606–15.

Dahms, N., Lobel, P. and Kornfeld, S. (1989). Mannose 6-phosphate receptors and lysosomal enzyme targeting. *J Biol Chem*, **264**, 12115–8.

Danon, M. J., Oh, S. J., DiMauro, S., Manaligod, J. R., Eastwood, A., Naidu, S. *et al.* (1981). Lysosomal glycogen storage disease with normal acid maltase. *Neurology*, **31**, 51–7.

Davies, J. P., Chen, F. W. and Ioannou, Y. A. (2000*a*). Transmembrane molecular pump activity of Niemann–Pick C1 protein. *Science*, **290**, 2295–8.

Davies, J. P., Levy, B. and Ioannou, Y. A. (2000*b*). Evidence for a Niemann–Pick C (NPC) gene family: identification and characterization of NPC1L1. *Genomics*, **65**, 137–45.

Davies, J. P. and Ioannou, Y. A. (2000). Topological analysis of NPC1 reveals that the orientation of the putative sterol-sensing domain is identical to that of HMG CoA and SCAP. *J Biol Chem*, **275**, 24367–74.

Dawson, G. and Cho, S. (2000). Batten's disease: clues to neuronal protein catabolism in lysosomes. *J Neurosci Res*, **60**, 133–40.

Denda, K., Konishi, J., Oshima, T., Date, T. and Yoshida, M. (1988). Molecular cloning of the beta-subunit of a possible non-F0F1 type ATP synthase from the acidothermophilic archaebacterium, *Sulfolobus acidocaldarius*. *J Biol Chem*, **263**, 17251–4.

van Deurs, B., Holm, P. and Sandvig, K. (1996). Inhibition of the vacuolar H^+-ATPase with bafilomycin reduces delivery of internalized molecules from mature multivesicular endosomes to lysosomes in HEp-2 cells. *Eur J Cell Biol*, **69**, 343–50.

Dice, J. F. (1990). Peptide sequences that target cytosolic proteins for lysosomal proteolysis. *TIBS*, **15**, 305–9.

de Duve, C. (1983). Lysosomes revisited. *Eur J Biochem*, **137**, 391–7.

de Duve, C. and Wattiaux, R. (1966). Functions of lysosomes. *Annu Rev Physiol*, **28**, 435–92.

de Duve, C., Pressman, B., Gianetto, R., Wattiaux, R. and Appelmans, F. (1955). Tissue fractionation studies: intracellular distribution patterns of enzymes in rat-liver tissue. *Biochem J*, **60**, 604–17.

Faust, J., Rodman, J., Daniel, P., Dice, J. and Bronson, R. (1994). Two related proteolipids and dolichol-linked oligosaccharides accumulate in motor neuron degeneration mice (mnd/mnd), a model for neuronal ceroid lipofuscinosis. *J Biol Chem*, **269**, 10150–5.

Fietz, M. J., Concordet, J.-P., Barbosa, R., Johnson, R., Krauss, S., McMahon, A. *et al.* (1994). The hedgehog gene family in *Drosophila* and vertebrate development. *Development*, 43–51.

Fukuda, M. (1991). Lysosomal membrane glycoproteins. Structure, biosynthesis, and intracellular trafficking. *J Biol Chem*, **266**, 21327–30.

Fukuda, M., Viitala, J., Matteson, J. and Carlsson, S. R. (1988*a*). Cloning of cDNAs encoding human lysosomal membrane glycoproteins, h-LAMP-1 and h-LAMP-2. *J Biol Chem*, **262**, 18920–8.

Fukuda, M., Viitala, J., Matteson, J. and Carlsson, S. R. (1988*b*). Cloning of cDNAs encoding human lysosomal membrane glycoproteins, h-LAMP-1 and h-LAMP-2. Comparison of their deduced amino acid sequences. *J Biol Chem*, **263**, 18920–8.

Futai, M., Park, M., Iwamoto, A., Omote, H. and Maeda, M. (1994). Catalysis and energy coupling of H^+-ATPase (ATP synthase): molecular biological approaches. *Biochim Biophys Acta*, **1187**, 165–70.

Garin, J., Diez, R., Kieffer, S., Dermine, J. F., Duclos, S., Gagnon, E. *et al.* (2001). The phagosome proteome: insight into phagosome functions. *J Cell Biol*, **152**, 165–80.

Gogarten, J. P. and Starke, T. (1992). Evolution and isoforms of V-ATPase subunits. *J Exp Biol*, **172**, 137–47.

Gogarten, J., Kibak, H., Dittrich, P., Taiz, L., Bowman, E., Bowman, B. *et al.* (1989). Evolution of the vacuolar H^+-ATPase: implications for the origin of eukaryotes. *Proc Natl Acad Sci USA*, **86**, 6661–5.

Golabek, A. A., Kida, E., Walus, M., Kaczmarski, W., Michalewski, M. and Wisniewski, K. E. (2000). CLN3 protein regulates lysosomal pH and alters intracellular processing of Alzheimer's amyloid-beta protein precursor and cathepsin D in human cells. *Mol Genet Metab*, **70**, 203–13.

Goldstein, D., Finbow, M., Andresson, T., McLean, P., Smith, K., Bubb, V. *et al.* (1991). Bovine papillomavirus E5 oncoprotein binds to the 16K component of vacuolar H^+-ATPases. *Nature*, **353**, 347–9.

Gough, N. R., Hatem, C. L. and Fambrough, D. M. (1995). The family of LAMP-2 proteins arises by alternative splicing from a single gene: characterization of the avian LAMP-2 gene and identification of mammalian homologs of LAMP-2b and LAMP-2c. *DNA Cell Biol*, **14**, 863–7.

Greer, W. L., Riddell, D. C., Gillan, T. L., Girouard, G. S., Sparrow, S. M., Byers, D. *et al.* (1998). The Nova Scotia (type D) form of Niemann–Pick disease is caused by a G3097(T transversion in NPC1. *Am J Hum Genet*, **63**, 52–4.

Greer, W. L., Dobson, M. J., Girouard, G. S., Byers, D. M., Riddell, D. C. and Neumann, P. E. (1999). Mutations in NPC1 highlight a conserved NPC1-specific cysteine-rich domain. *Am J Hum Genet*, **65**, 1252–60.

Haft, C., Sierra, M., Hamer, I., Carpentier, J.-L. and Taylor, S. (1998). Analysis of the juxtamembrane dileucine motif in the insulin receptor. *Endocrinology*, **139**, 1618–29.

Hanada, H., Moriyama, Y., Maeda, M. and Futai, M. (1990). Kinetic studies of chromaffin granule H^+-ATPase and effects of bafilomycin A1. *Biochem Biophys Res Commun*, **170**, 873–8.

Hanada, H., Hasebe, M., Moriyama, Y., Maeda, M. and Futai, M. (1991). Molecular cloning of cDNA encoding the 16 kDa subunit of vacuolar H^+-ATPase from mouse cerebellum. *Biochem Biophys Res Commun*, **176**, 1062–7.

Hannun, Y. and Bell, R. (1987). Lysosphingolipids inhibit protein kinase C: implications for the sphingolipidoses. *Science*, **235**, 670–4.

Harrison, M., Jones, P., Kim, Y., Finbow, M. and Findlay, J. (1994). Functional properties of a hybrid vacuolar H^+-ATPase in *Saccharomyces* cells expressing the *Nephrops* 16-kDa proteolipid. *Eur J Biochem*, **221**, 111–20.

Haskell, R. E., Carr, C. J., Pearce, D. A., Bennett, M. J. and Davidson, B. L. (2000). Batten disease: evaluation of CLN3 mutations on protein localization and function. *Hum Mol Genet*, **9**, 735–44.

Hatem, C. L., Gough, N. R. and Fambrough, D. M. (1995). Multiple mRNAs encode the avian lysosomal membrane protein LAMP-2, resulting in alternative transmembrane and cytoplasmic domains. *J Cell Sci*, **108**, 2093–100.

Havelaar, A. C., Mancini, G. M., Beerens, C. E., Souren, R. M. and Verheijen, F. W. (1998). Purification of the lysosomal sialic acid transporter. Functional characteristics of a monocarboxylate transporter. *J Biol Chem*, **273**, 34568–74.

Hers, H. (1963). Alpha-glucosidase deficiency in generalized glycogen-storage disease (Pompe disease). *Biochem J*, **86**, 11–6.

Hickman, S. and Neufeld, E. (1972). A hypothesis for I-cell disease: defective hydrolases that do not enter lysosomes. *Biochem Biophys Res Commun*, **49**, 992–9.

Higgins, M. E., Davies, J. P., Chen, F. W. and Ioannou, Y. A. (1999). Niemann–Pick C1 is a late endosome-resident protein that transiently associates with lysosomes and the trans-Golgi network. *Mol Genet Metab*, **68**, 1–13.

van Hille, B., Richener, H., Evans, D., Green, J. and Bilbe, G. (1993). Identification of two subunit A isoforms of the vacuolar H^+-ATPase in human osteoclastoma. *J Biol Chem*, **268**, 7075–80.

van Hille, B., Richener, H., Schmid, P., Puettner, I., Green, J. and Bilbe, G. (1994). Heterogeneity of vacuolar H^+-ATPase: differential expression of two human subunit B isoforms. *Biochem J*, **303**, 191–8.

Hogue, D. L., Kerby, L. and Ling, V. (1999). A mammalian lysosomal membrane protein confers multidrug resistance upon expression in *Saccharomyces cerevisiae*. *J Biol Chem*, **274**, 12877–82.

Hua, X., Sakai, J., Brown, M. S. and Goldstein, J. L. (1996). Regulated cleavage of sterol regulatory element binding proteins requires sequences on both sides of the endoplasmic reticulum membrane. *J Biol Chem*, **271**, 10379–84.

Ioannou, Y. A. (2001). Multidrug permeases and subcellular cholesterol transport. *Nat Rev Mol Cell Biol*, **2**, 657–68.

Jarvela, I., Sainio, M., Rantamaki, T., Olkkonen, V. M., Carpen, O., Peltonen, L. *et al.* (1998). Biosynthesis and intracellular targeting of the CLN3 protein defective in Batten disease. *Hum Mol Genet*, **7**, 85–90.

Kane, P., Kuehn, M., Howald-Stevenson, I. and Stevens, T. (1992). Assembly and targeting of peripheral and integral membrane subunits of the yeast vacuolar H^+-ATPase. *J Biol Chem*, **267**, 447–54.

Karlsson, K. and Carlsson, S. R. (1998). Sorting of lysosomal membrane glycoproteins LAMP-1 and LAMP-2 into vesicles distinct from mannose-6-phosphate receptor/g-adaptin vesicles at the trans-Golgi network. *J Biol Chem*, **273**, 18966–73.

Katz, M. L. and Johnson, G. S. (2001). Mouse gene knockout models for the CLN2 and CLN3 forms of ceroid lipofuscinosis. *Europ J Paediatr Neurol*, **5**, 109–14.

Kida, E., Kaczmarski, W., Golabek, A. A., Kaczmarski, A., Michalewski, M. and Wisniewski, K. E. (1999). Analysis of intracellular distribution and trafficking of the CLN3 protein in fusion with the green fluorescent protein in vitro. *Mol Genet Metab*, **66**, 265–71.

Kinoshita, K., Waritani, T., Noto, M., Takizawa, K., Minemoto, Y., Nishikawa, Y. *et al.* (1996). Bafilomycin A1 induces apoptosis in PC12 cells independently of intracellular pH. *FEBS Lett*, **398**, 61–6.

Kirchhoff, C., Osterhoff, C. and Young, L. (1996). Molecular cloning and characterization of HE1, a major secretory protein of the human epididymis. *Biol Reprod*, **54**, 847–56.

Ko, D. C., Gordon, M. D., Jin, J. Y. and Scott, M. P. (2001). Dynamic movements of organelles containing Niemann–Pick c1 protein: npc1 involvement in late endocytic events. *Mol Biol Cell*, **12**, 601–14.

Kobayashi, T., Beuchat, M.-H., Lindsay, M., Frias, S., Palmiter, R. D., Sakuraba, H. *et al.* (1999). Late endosomal membranes rich in lysobiphosphatidic acid regulate cholesterol transport. *Nat Cell Biol*, **1**, 113–8.

Konecki, D. S., Foetisch, K., Zimmer, K. P., Schlotter, M. and Lichter-Konecki, U. (1995). An alternatively spliced form of the human lysosome-associated membrane protein-2 gene is expressed in a tissue-specific manner. *Biochem Biophys Res Commun*, **215**, 757–67.

Kremmidiotis, G., Lensink, I. L., Bilton, R. L., Woollatt, E., Chataway, T. K., Sutherland, G. R. *et al.* (1999). The Batten disease gene product (CLN3p) is a Golgi integral membrane protein. *Hum Mol Genet*, **8**, 523–31.

LaPlante, J. M., Falardeau, J., Sun, M., Kanazirska, M., Brown, E. M., Slaugenhaupt, S. A. *et al.* (2002). Identification and characterization of the single channel function of human mucolipin-1 implicated in mucolipidosis type IV, a disorder affecting the lysosomal pathway. *FEBS Lett*, **532**, 183–7.

Lee, J. J., Ekker, S. C., von Kessler, D. P., Porter, J. A., Sun, B. I. and Beachy, P. A. (1994). Autoproteolysis in hedgehog protein biogenesis. *Science*, **266**, 1528–37.

Leitch, B. and Finbow, M. (1990). The gap junction-like form of a vacuolar proton channel component appears not to be an artifact of isolation: an immunocytochemical localization study. *Exp Cell Res*, **190**, 218–26.

Leroy, J. and DeMars, R. (1967). Mutant enzymatic and cytological phenotypes in cultured human fibroblasts. *Science*, **157**, 804–6.

Leung, K. Y., Greene, N. D., Munroe, P. B. and Mole, S. E. (2001). Analysis of CLN3-protein interactions using the yeast two-hybrid system. *Europ J Paediatr Neurol*, **5**, 89–93.

Liu, Q., Kane, P., Newman, P. and Forgac, M. (1996). Site-directed mutagenesis of the yeast V-ATPase B subunit (Vma2p). *J Biol Chem*, **271**, 2018–22.

Liu, S., Marks, M. and Brodsky, F. (1998). A dominant-negative clathrin mutant differentially affects trafficking of molecules with distinct sorting motifs in the class II major histocompatibility complex (MHC) pathway. *J Cell Biol*, **1998**, 1023–37.

Lobel, P., Dahms, N. and Kornfeld, S. (1988). Cloning and sequence analysis of the cation-independent mannose 6-phosphate receptor. *J Biol Chem*, **263**, 2563–70.

Long, X., Crow, M., Sollott, S., O'Neill, L., Menees, D., de Lourdes Hipolito, M. *et al.* (1998). Enhanced expression of p53 and apoptosis induced by blockade of the vacuolar proton ATPase in cardiomyocytes. *J Clin Invest*, **101**, 1453–61.

Lonka, L., Kyttala, A., Ranta, S., Jalanko, A. and Lehesjoki, A. E. (2000). The neuronal ceroid lipofuscinosis CLN8 membrane protein is a resident of the endoplasmic reticulum. *Hum Mol Genet*, **9**, 1691–7.

Luiro, K., Kopra, O., Lehtovirta, M. and Jalanko, A. (2001). CLN3 protein is targeted to neuronal synapses but excluded from synaptic vesicles: new clues to Batten disease. *Hum Mol Genet*, **10**, 2123–31.

Ma, Z., Grubb, J. and Sly, W. (1991). Cloning, sequencing, and functional characterization of the murine 46-kDa mannose 6-phosphate receptor. *J Biol Chem*, **266**, 10589–95.

McKusick, V. A. (1995). *Mendelian inheritance in man*. 11th edn. Baltimore, MD: Johns Hopkins University Press.

Mandel, M., Moriyama, Y., Julmes, J., Pan, Y., Nelson, H. and Nelson, N. (1988). cDNA sequence encoding the 16-kDA proteolipid of chromaffin granules implies gene duplication in the evolution of H^+-ATPases. *Proc Natl Acad Sci USA*, **85**, 5521–4.

Mane, S. M., Marzella, L., Bainton, D. F., Holt, V. K., Cha, Y., Hildreth, J. E. *et al.* (1989). Purification and characterization of human lysosomal membrane glycoproteins. *Arch Biochem Biophys*, **268**, 360–78.

Marigo, V., Davey, R. A., Zuo, Y., Cunningham, J. M. and Tabin, C. J. (1996). Biochemical evidence that patched is the hedgehog receptor. *Nature*, **384**, 176–9.

Martin, P., Vass, W., Schiller, J., Lowy, D. and Velu, T. (1989). The bovine papillomavirus E5 transforming protein can stimulate the transforming activity of EGF and CSF-1 receptors. *Cell*, **59**, 21–32.

Mattei, M. G., Matterson, J., Chen, J. W., Williams, M. A. and Fukuda, M. (1990). Two human lysosomal membrane glycoproteins, h-LAMP-1 and h-lamp-2, are encoded by genes localized to chromosome 13q34 and chromosome Xq24–25, respectively. *J Biol Chem*, **265**, 7548–51.

Millard, E. E., Srivastava, K., Traub, L. M., Schaffer, J. E. and Ory, D. S. (2000). Niemann–Pick type C1 (NPC1) overexpression alters cellular cholesterol homeostasis. *J Biol Chem*, **275**, 38445–51.

Millat, G., Marcais, C., Rafi, M. A., Yamamoto, T., Morris, J. A., Pentchev, P. G. *et al.* (1999). Niemann–Pick C1 disease: the I1061T substitution is a frequent mutant allele in patients of Western European descent and correlates with a classic juvenile phenotype. *Am J Hum Genet*, **65**, 1321–9.

Millat, G., Marcais, C., Tomasetto, C., Chikh, K., Fensom, A. H., Harzer, K. *et al.* (2001). Niemann–Pick C1 disease: correlations between NPC1 mutations, levels of NPC1 protein, and phenotypes emphasize the functional significance of the putative sterol-sensing domain and of the cysteine-rich luminal loop. *Am J Hum Genet*, **68**, 1373–85.

Miyake, K. and McNeil, P. (1995). Vesicle accumulation and exocytosis at sites of plasma membrane disruption. *J Cell Biol*, **131**, 1737–45.

Mole, S. E., Zhong, N. A., Sarpong, A., Logan, W. P., Hofmann, S., Yi, W. *et al.* (2001). New mutations in the neuronal ceroid lipofuscinosis genes. *Europ J Paediatr Neurol*, **5**, 7–10.

Morano, K. and Klionsky, D. (1994). Differential effects of compartment deacidification on the targeting of membrane and soluble proteins to the vacuole in yeast. *J Cell Sci*, **107**, 2813–24.

Moriyama, Y. and Nelson, N. (1989). H^+-Translocating ATPase in Golgi apparatus. *J Biol Chem*, **264**, 18445–50.

Morris, J. A., Zhang, D., Coleman, K. G., Nagle, J., Pentchev, P. G. and Carstea, E. D. (1999). The genomic organization and polymorphism analysis of the human Niemann–Pick C1 gene. *Biochem Biophys Res Commun*, **261**, 493–8.

Nabi, I. R. and Dennis, J. W. (1998). The extent of polylactosamine glycosylation of MDCK LAMP-2 is determined by its Golgi residence time. *Glycobiology*, **8**, 947–53.

Nabi, I. R. and Rodriguez-Boulan, E. (1993). Increased LAMP-2 polylactosamine glycosylation is associated with its slower Golgi transit during establishment of a polarized MDCK epithelial monolayer. *Mol Biol Cell*, **4**, 627–35.

Naureckiene, S., Sleat, D. E., Lackland, H., Fensom, A., Vanier, M. T., Wattiaux, R. *et al.* (2000). Identification of HE1 as the second gene of Niemann–Pick C disease. *Science*, **290**, 2298–301.

Nelson, N. (1992). The vacuolar H^+-ATPase—one of the most fundamental ion pumps in nature. *J Exp Biol*, **172**, 19–27.

Nelson, H. and Nelson, N. (1990). Disruption of genes encoding subunits of yeast vacuolar H^+-ATPase causes conditional lethality. *Proc Natl Acad Sci USA*, **87**, 3503–7.

Nelson, H., Mandiyan, S. and Nelson, N. (1989). A conserved gene encoding the 57-kDa subunit of the yeast vacuolar H^+-ATPase. *J Biol Chem*, **264**, 1775–8.

Neufeld, E. B., Wastney, M., Patel, S., Suresh, S., Cooney, A. M., Dwyer, N. K. *et al.* (1999). The Niemann–Pick C1 protein resides in a vesicular compartment linked to retrograde transport of multiple lysosomal cargo. *J Biol Chem*, **274**, 9627–35.

Nishihara, T., Akifusa, S., Koseki, T., Kato, S., Muro, M. and Hanada, N. (1995). Specific inhibitors of vacuolar type H^+-ATPases induce apoptotic cell death. *Biochem Biophys Res Commun*, **212**, 255–62.

Nishino, I., Fu, J., Tanji, K., Yamada, T., Shimojo, S., Koori, T. *et al.* (2000). Primary LAMP-2 deficiency causes X-linked vacuolar cardiomyopathy and myopathy (Danon disease). *Nature*, **406**, 906–10.

Oda, K., Nishimura, Y., Ikehara, Y. and Kato, K. (1991). Bafilomycin A1 inhibits the targeting of lysosomal acid hydrolases in cultured hepatocytes. *Biochem Biophys Res Commun*, **178**, 369–77.

Ohno, H., Stewart, J., Fournier, M., Bosshart, H., Rhee, I., Miyatake, S. *et al.* (1995). Interaction of tyrosine-based sorting signals with clathrin-associated proteins. *Science*, **269**, 1872–5.

Okahashi, N., Nakamura, I., Jimi, E., Koide, M., Suda, T. and Nishihara, T. (1997). Specific inhibitors of vacuolar H^+-ATPase trigger apoptotic cell death of osteoclasts. *J Bone Miner Res*, **12**, 1116–23.

Oshima, A., Nolan, C., Kyle, J., Grubb, J. and Sly, W. (1988). The human cation-independent mannose 6-phosphate receptor. *J Biol Chem*, **263**, 2553–62.

Palokangas, H., Metsikko, K. and Vaananen, K. (1994). Active vacuolar H^+-ATPase is required for both endocytic and exocytic processes during viral infection of BHK-21 cells. *J Biol Chem*, **269**, 17577–85.

Patel, S. C., Suresh, S., Kumar, U., Hu, C. Y., Cooney, A., Blanchette-Mackie, E. J. *et al.* (1999). Localization of Niemann–Pick C1 protein in astrocytes: implications for neuronal degeneration in Niemann–Pick type C disease. *Proc Natl Acad Sci USA*, **96**, 1657–62.

Patterson, M. C., Vanier, M. T., Suzuki, M. C., Morris, J. A., Carstea, E., Neufeld, E. B. *et al.* (2001). Niemann–Pick disease type C: A lipid trafficking disorder. In *The metabolic and molecular bases of inherited disease* (Scriver, C. R., Beadet, A. L., Valle, D. and Sly, W. S., ed.), pp. 3611–34. New York: McGraw-Hill.

Pearce, D. A. (2000). Localization and processing of CLN3, the protein associated to Batten disease: Where is it and what does it do? *J Neurosci Res*, **59**, 19–23.

Pentchev, P. G., Kruth, H. S., Comly, M. E., Butler, J. D., Vanier, M. T., Wenger, D. A. *et al.* (1986). Type C Niemann–Pick disease: a parallel loss of regulatory responses in both the uptake and esterification of low-density lipoprotein-derived cholesterol in cultured fibroblasts. *J Biol Chem*, **261**, 16775–80.

Pentchev, P. G., Brady, R. O., Blanchette-Mackie, E. J., Vanier, M. T., Carstea, E. D., Parker, C. C. *et al.* (1994). The Niemann–Pick C lesion and its relationship to the intracellular distribution and utilization of LDL cholesterol. *Biochim Biophys Acta*, **1225**, 235–43.

Peters, C., Braun, M., Weber, B., Wendland, M., Schmidt, B., Pohlmann, R. *et al.* (1990). Targeting of a lysosomal membrane protein: a tyrosine-containing endocytosis signal in the cytoplasmic tail of lysosomal acid phosphatase is necessary and sufficient for targeting to lysosomes. *EMBO J*, **9**, 3497–506.

Pitto, M., Chigorno, V., Renlund, M. and Tettamanti, G. (1996). Impairment of ganglioside metabolism in cultured fibroblasts from Salla patients. *Clin Chim Acta*, **247**, 143–57.

Press, B., Feng, Y., Hoflack, B. and Wandinger-Ness, A. (1998). Mutant Rab7 causes the accumulation of cathepsin D and cation-independent mannose 6-phosphate receptor in an early endocytic compartment. *J Cell Biol*, **140**, 1075–89.

Puopolo, K., Kumamoto, C., Adachi, I. and Forgac, M. (1991). A single gene encodes the catalytic 'A' subunit of the bovine vacuolar H^+-ATPase. *J Biol Chem*, **266**, 24564–72.

Puopolo, K., Kumamoto, C., Adachi, I., Magner, R. and Forgac, M. (1992). Differential expression of the 'B' subunit of the vacuolar H^+-ATPase in bovine tissues. *J Biol Chem*, **267**, 3696–706.

Puri, V., Watanabe, R., Dominguez, M., Sun, X., Wheatley, C. L., Marks, D. L. *et al.* (1999). Cholesterol modulates membrane traffic along the endocytic pathway in sphingolipid-storage diseases. *Nat Cell Biol*, **1**, 386–8.

Rautiala, T., Koskinen, A. and Vaananen, H. (1993). Purification of vacuolar ATPase with bafilomycin C1 affinity chromatography. *Biochem Biophys Res Commun*, **194**, 50–5.

Reddy, A., Caler, E. V. and Andrews, N. W. (2001). Plasma membrane repair is mediated by Ca(2+)-regulated exocytosis of lysosomes. *Cell*, **106**, 157–69.

Reitman, M., Varki, A. and Kornfeld, S. (1981). Fibroblasts from patients with I-cell disease and pseudo-Hurler polydystrophy are deficient in uridine 5′-diphosphate-*N*-acetylglucosamine : glycoprotein *N*-acetylglucosaminylphosphotransferase activity. *J Clin Invest*, **67**, 1574–9.

Rodriguez, A., Webster, P., Ortego, J. and Andrews, N. (1997). Lysosomes behave as Ca^{2+}-regulated exocytic vesicles in fibroblasts and epithelial cells. *J Cell Biol*, **137**, 93–104.

Rohrer, J., Schweizer, A., Russell, D. and Kornfeld, S. (1996). The targeting of LAMP1 to lysosomes is dependent on the spacing of its cytoplasmic tail tyrosine sorting motif relative to the membrane. *J Cell Biol*, **132**, 565–76.

Sahagian, G. and Neufeld, E. (1983). Biosynthesis and turnover of the mannose 6-phosphate receptor in cultured Chinese hamster ovary cells. *J Biol Chem*, **258**, 7121–8.

Sandoval, I., Arredondo, J., Alcalde, J., Noriega, A., Vandekerckhove, J., Jimenez, M. *et al.* (1994). The residues Leu(Ile)^{475}–Ile(Leu, Val, Ala)^{476}, contained in the extended carboxyl cytoplasmic tail, are critical for targeting of the resident lysosomal membrane protein LIMP II to lysosomes. *J Biol Chem*, **269**, 6622–31.

Schweizer, A., Kornfeld, S. and Rohrer, J. (1997). Proper sorting of the cation-dependent mannose 6-phosphate receptor in endosomes depends on a pair of aromatic amino acids in its cytoplasmic tail. *Proc Natl Acad Sci USA*, **94**, 14471–6.

Scriver, C. R., Beaudet, A., Sly, W. and Valle, D., ed. (1995). *The metabolic and molecular bases of inherited disease*, 7th edn. New York: McGraw-Hill.

Simons, K. and Ikonen, E. (1997). Functional rafts in cell membranes. *Nature*, **387**, 569–72.

Slaugenhaupt, S. A. (2002). The molecular basis of mucolipidosis type IV. *Curr Mol Med*, **2**, 445–50.

Slaugenhaupt, S. A., Acierno, J. S. Jr, Helbling, L. A., Bove, C., Goldin, E., Bach, G. *et al.* (1999). Mapping of the mucolipidosis type IV gene to chromosome 19p and definition of founder haplotypes. *Am J Hum Genet*, **65**, 773–8.

Sly, W., Lagwinska, E. and Schlesinger, S. (1976). Enveloped virus acquires membrane defect when passaged in fibroblasts from I-cell disease patients. *Proc Natl Acad Sci USA*, **73**, 2443–7.

Snyers, L., Umlauf, E. and Prohaska, R. (1999). Association of stomatin with lipid-protein complexes in the plasma membrane and the endocytic compartment. *Eur J Cell Biol*, **78**, 802–12.

Sparkowski, J., Anders, J. and Schlegel, R. (1995). E5 oncoprotein retained in the endoplasmic reticulum/*cis*-Golgi still induces PDGF receptor autophosphorylation but does not transform cells. *EMBO J*, **14**, 3055–63.

Stevens, T. and Forgac, M. (1997). Structure, function and regulation of the vacuolar (H^+)-ATPase. *Annu Rev Cell Dev Biol*, **13**, 779–808.

Stone, D. M., Hynes, M., Armanini, M., Swanson, T. A., Gu, Q., Johnson, R. L. *et al.* (1996). The tumour suppressor gene patched encodes a candidate receptor for sonic hedgehog. *Nature*, **384**, 129–33.

Sudhof, T., Fried, V., Stone, D., Johnston, P. and Xie, X. (1989). Human endomembrane H^+ pump strongly resembles the ATP-synthetase of Archaebacteria. *Proc Natl Acad Sci USA*, **86**, 6067–71.

Sun, M., Goldin, E., Stahl, S., Falardeau, J. L., Kennedy, J. C., Acierno, J. S. Jr *et al.* (2000). Mucolipidosis type IV is caused by mutations in a gene encoding a novel transient receptor potential channel. *Hum Mol Genet*, **9**, 2471–8.

Sun, X., Marks, D. L., Park, W. D., Wheatley, C. L., Puri, V., O'Brien, J. F. *et al.* (2001). Niemann–Pick C variant detection by altered sphingolipid trafficking and correlation with mutations within a specific domain of NPC1. *Am J Hum Genet*, **68**, 1361–72.

Tanaka, Y., Guhde, G., Suter, A., Eskelinen, E. L., Hartmann, D., Lullmann-Rauch, R. *et al.* (2000). Accumulation of autophagic vacuoles and cardiomyopathy in LAMP-2-deficient mice. *Nature*, **406**, 902–6.

Town, M., Jean, G., Cherqui, S., Attard, M., Forestier, L., Whitmore, S. A. *et al.* (1998). A novel gene encoding an integral membrane protein is mutated in nephropathic cystinosis. *Nat Genet*, **18**, 319–24.

Tseng, T.-T., Gratwick, K. S., Kollman, J., Park, D., Nies, D. H., Goffeau, A. *et al.* (1999). The RND permease superfamily: An ancient, ubiquitous and diverse family that includes human disease and development proteins. *J Mol Microbiol Biotechnol*, **1**, 107–25.

Umemoto, N., Ohya, Y. and Anraku, Y. (1991). VMA11, a novel gene that encodes a putative proteolipid, is indispensable for expression of yeast vacuolar membrane H^+-ATPase activity. *J Biol Chem*, **266**, 24526–32.

Umemoto, N., Yoshihisa, T., Hirata, R. and Anraku, Y. (1990). Roles of the VMA3 gene product, subunit c of the vacuolar membrane H^+-ATPase on vacuolar acidification and protein transport. *J Biol Chem*, **265**, 18447–53.

Vanier, M. T., Rodriguez-Lafrasse, C., Rousson, R., Gazzah, N., Juge, M.-C., Pentchev, P. G. *et al.* (1991). Type C Niemann–Pick disease: spectrum of phenotypic variation in disruption of intracellular LDL-derived cholesterol processing. *Biochim Biophys Acta*, **1096**, 328–37.

Vega, M., Rodriguez, F., Sequi, B., Cales, C., Alcade, J. and Sandoval, I. (1991). Targeting of lysosomal integral membrane protein LIMP II. *J Biol Chem*, **266**, 16269–72.

Verheijen, F. W., Verbeek, E., Aula, N., Beerens, C. E., Havelaar, A. C., Joosse, M. *et al.* (1999). A new gene, encoding an anion transporter, is mutated in sialic acid storage diseases. *Nat Genet*, **23**, 462–5.

Vesa, J., Hellsten, E., Verkruyse, L. A., Camp, L. A., Rapola, J., Santavuori, P. *et al.* (1995). Mutations in the palmitoyl protein thioesterase gene causing infantile neuronal ceroid lipofuscinosis. *Nature*, **376**, 584–7.

Waheed, A., Hasilik, A. and von Figura, K. (1981). Processing of the phosphorylated recognition marker in lysosomal enzymes. *J Biol Chem*, **256**, 5717–21.

Wang, Z. and Gluck, S. (1990). Isolation and properties of bovine kidney brush border vacuolar H^+-ATPase. *J Biol Chem*, **265**, 21957–65.

Wang, N., Silver, D. L., Thiele, C. and Tall, A. R. (2001). ABCA1 functions as a cholesterol efflux regulatory protein. *J Biol Chem*, **17**, 17.

Willingham, M., Pastan, I., Sahagian, G., Jourdian, G. and Neufeld, E. (1981). Morphologic study of the internalization of a lysosomal enzyme by the mannose 6-phosphate receptor in cultured Chinese hamster ovary cells. *Proc Natl Acad Sci USA*, **78**, 6967–71.

Winchester, B., Vellodi, A. and Young, E. (2000). The molecular basis of lysosomal storage diseases and their treatment. *Biochem Soc Trans*, **28**, 150–4.

Wisniewski, K. E., Kida, E., Golabek, A. A., Kaczmarski, W., Connell, F. and Zhong, N. (2001). Neuronal ceroid lipofuscinoses: classification and diagnosis. *Adv Genet*, **45**, 1–34.

Yamamoto, T., Nanba, E., Ninomiya, H., Higaki, K., Taniguchi, M., Zhang, H. *et al.* (1999). NPC1 gene mutations in Japanese patients with Niemann–Pick disease type C. *Hum Genet*, **105**, 10–6.

Yamashiro, C., Kane, P., Wolczyk, D., Preston, R. and Stevens, T. (1990). Role of vacuolar acidification in protein sorting and zymogen activation: a genetic analysis of the yeast vacuolar proton-translocating ATPase. *Mol Cell Biol*, **10**, 3737–49.

Yilla, M., Tan, A., Ito, K., Miwa, K. and Ploegh, H. (1993). Involvement of vacuolar H^+-ATPases in the secretory pathway of hepG2 cells. *J Biol Chem*, **268**, 19092–100.

Yoshimori, T., Yamamoto, A., Moriyama, Y., Futai, M. and Tashiro, Y. (1991). Bafilomycin A1, a specific inhibitor of vacuolar-type H^+-ATPase, inhibits acidification and protein degradation in lysosomes of cultured cells. *J Biol Chem*, **266**, 17707–12.

Zhang, J., Feng, Y. and Forgac, M. (1994). Proton conduction and bafilomycin binding by the V_0 domain of the coated vesicle A-ATPase. *J Biol Chem*, **269**, 23518–23.

Zhang, F., Zhang, W., Liu, L., Fisher, C. L., Hui, D., Childs, S. *et al.* (2000). Characterization of ABCB9, an ATP binding cassette protein associated with lysosomes. *J Biol Chem*, **275**, 23287–94.

Zhang, M., Dwyer, N. K., Love, D. C., Cooney, A., Comly, M., Neufeld, E. *et al.* (2001*a*). Cessation of rapid late endosomal tubulovesicular trafficking in Niemann–Pick type C1 disease. *Proc Natl Acad Sci USA*, **98**, 4466–71.

Zhang, M., Dwyer, N. K., Neufeld, E. B., Love, D. C., Cooney, A., Comly, M. *et al.* (2001*b*). Sterol-modulated glycolipid sorting occurs in Niemann–Pick C1 late endosomes. *J Biol Chem*, **276**, 3417–25.

Zhong, N. A., Moroziewicz, D. N., Ju, W., Wisniewski, K. E., Jurkiewicz, A. and Brown, W. T. (2000). CLN-encoded proteins do not interact with each other. *Neurogenetics*, **3**, 41–4.

Section III

Model systems and pathophysiological mechanisms

Chapter 10

Simple non-mammalian systems

David A. Pearce

Introduction

Animal models for disease have always been important in researching the pathogenesis of disease and for the testing of potential therapeutic interventions (see also Chapter 11). Mice in particular have been widely used as the development of molecular genetic approaches has facilitated an easier and more rapid manipulation of expressed genes. There are in fact several engineered mouse models used for the study of neurodegenerative and indeed lysosomal storage diseases (Chapter 11). With the advent of genome sequencing, homologous or orthologous genes and proteins to those associated with human disease can now be accessed in the yeast *Saccharomyces cerevisiae* and *Schizosaccharomyces pombe,* the nematode worm *Caenorhabditis elegans,* and the fruitfly *Drosophila melanogaster,* and hopefully in the near future in zebrafish *Danio rerio.* The contribution to date towards understanding the function of proteins associated with human disease in these model systems can be related to the complexity of the model organism, and also to when the sequence of the model organism was completed. It is no coincidence that sequencing of the entire genome for *S. cerevisiae,* worm, and fruit fly which was completed in 1996, 1998, and 2000, respectively, reflects their respective genome sizes of 12 Mb, 97 Mb, and 120 Mb, respectively . Therefore, as will be reflected in this chapter the simplest of model systems, *S. cerevisiae,* has the most published reports on functional studies of orthologues to human disease not only due to the fact that it is the simplest to manipulate, but also because its genome was the first to be completed. Completion of the *C. elegans* and *Drosophila* genomes was more recent with an increasing number of papers using *C. elegans* as a disease model appearing in press, and I am sure that there will be an increasing number utilizing *Drosophila* as a disease model. For the first time, a researcher can choose to work on a gene or protein without knowing what the contribution of that protein is to the biology of that organism, or the effect the mutation of that protein will have on that organism. The primary motivation for working on that protein in that organism would be to model a protein function, or in most cases loss of protein function on how it causes disease.

The use of yeast such as *S. cerevisiae* and *S. pombe* as simple eukaryotic models for disease is attractive because of the ease with which they can be cultured and the wealth of tools available for genetic manipulation. Although a single-celled organism, it is well established that many biological pathways have been conserved from yeast to man, and this review will hopefully establish that the primordial proteins involved in lysosome function and trafficking to the lysosome exist in yeast. The use of invertebrate systems such as *C. elegans* and *Drosophila* is attractive for the study of a given biological paradigm such as disease, because genetic interactions can be used to define cellular cascades that mediate for example, lysosomal storage. Although there are obvious differences between humans and invertebrates, particularly at the anatomic level, there is clear conservation between basic biological processes. The effect of a cellular defect can be monitored on an organismal level. Both *C. elegans* and *Drosophila* have a relatively rapid generation time, a good understanding of their genetics, and well-developed transgenic technology for selection of mutations, genetic interactions, and for the expression of human genes of interest. With regard to researching the central nervous system (CNS), both *C. elegans* and *Drosophila* can be utilized for different reasons. For example in *C. elegans* each neurone can be identified, and in *Drosophila* sophisticated behaviours can be monitored. Finally, the utility of using *D. rerio* as a model is fast becoming recognized. A complete genome sequence should become available within the next couple of years, which along with the ongoing development of genetic tools will elevate the use of this model system for disease study. *D. rerio* has proven to be an excellent model for developmental biologists, which will prove valuable in understanding and recognizing any early contribution of a genetic defect in a metabolic pathway to the overall pathophysiology of the disease such as those that occur in many lysosomal storage diseases.

Proteins associated with lysosomal storage diseases and their orthologues in model organisms

Table 10.1 lists lysosomal storage diseases along with the gene/protein that has been shown to be defective in each disease. Where possible, the name of an orthologous protein from *S. cerevisiae*, *S. pombe*, *C. elegans*, *D. melanogaster*, and *D. rerio* based on the searching of public databases and sequence alignments with the percent homology is shown. As will be evident, many of the designations represent assignations from sequencing projects, rather than gene names, as these gene products remain essentially unstudied in these organisms. As these orthologues are ultimately studied, gene/protein names will surely be assigned; however, this author suggests that perhaps an assumption of the name designated for the human protein would be most appropriate and best serve researchers of lysosomal storage diseases. It is important at this point to recognize that many of the orthologues listed in Table 10.1 are based on sequence alignment. Functional data on many of these proteins/sequences are still required to confirm whether these are truly homologous proteins to those associated with the disease. Furthermore, per cent homologies for *D. rerio* are not listed as related sequences are ESTs, and the whole protein sequence is not available.

Studies of orthologous proteins associated with lysosomal storage diseases

This section reviews those proteins that are associated with lysosomal storage diseases and what has been reported on their function in model systems.

Table 10.1 List of lysosomal storage diseases along with the gene/protein that has been shown to be defective in each disease

Lysosomal disorder/ gene name/ protein description or function	Organism	Homologous protein or sequence ID	Percent identity
Pompe disease	*Drosophila melanogaster*	GH04962	29
GAA		CG11909	22
Acid α-glucosidase	*Caenorhabditis elegans*	D2096.3	36
		R05F9.12	35
	Saccharomyces cerevisiae	Rot2p	29
	Schizosaccharomyces pombe	Agl1p	35
GM1 gangliosidosis	*D. melanogaster*	CG3132	43
GLB		CG9092	40
β-Galactosidase	*C. elegans*	T19B10.3	40
		H22K11.2	33
Tay–Sachs disease	*D.melanogaster*	CG1318	34
HEXA		CG8824	31
β-Hexosaminidase A	*C. elegans*	T14F9.3	38
Sandhoff disease	*D. melanogaster*	CG1318	35
HEXB		CG8824	34
β-Hexosaminidase B	*C. elegans*	T14F9.3	44
Fabry disease	*D. melanogaster*	CG5731	47
GLA		CG7997	47
α-Galactosidase	*C. elegans*	R07B7.11	44
	S. cerevisiae	Mel6p	33
		Mel5p	33
		Mel2p	33
	S. pombe	Spac869.07cp	36
Gaucher disease	*D. melanogaster*	CG10299	32
GBA	*C. elegans*	F11E6.1	42
Glucocerebrosidase		F11E6.1A	42
Metachromatic	*D. melanogaster*	CG7402	29
Leukodystrophy		CG5584	30
ARSA		CG8646	28
Arylsulfatase A	*C. elegans*	R1014.1	37
		C54D2.4	36
		K09C4.8	25
	S. pombe	Spbpb1od8.02cp	25
Krabbe disease	*C. elegans*	C29E4.10	29
GALC			
Galactosylceramidase			
Niemann–Pick types A and B	*D. melanogaster*	CG3376	43
SMPD1		CG15534	33
Acid sphingomyelinase		CG15533	33
	C. elegans	ASM-1	34
		ASM-2	32

Table 10.1 *(continued)*

Lysosomal disorder/ gene name/ protein description or function	Organism	Homologous protein or sequence ID	Percent identity
		W03G1.7	31
	S. cerevisiae	Phm5p	25
	S. pombe	Spbc713.07cp	26
Niemann–Pick type C	*Danio rerio*	AI722583	NA
NPC1	*D. melanogaster*	NPC1	44
Unknown		CG12092	39
		CG11212	23
	C. elegans	NPC-1	28
		PTR-19	23
		NPC-2	24
	S. cerevisiae	Ncr1p	33
Niemann–Pick type C(2)	*D. melanogaster*	CG7291	37
HE1/NPC2		CG3153	27
Unknown		CG11315	27
	C. elegans	R148.6	25
Farber disease	*C. elegans*	K11D2.2	39
ASAH		F27E5.1	37
Acid ceramidase			
Wolman disease	*D. melanogaster*	LIP3	39
LIPA		CG6113	38
Acid lipase		CG8093	39
	C. elegans	YE7E12B.B	42
		F54F3.3	44
		ZK6.7	46
	S. cerevisiae	Tgl1p	33
		Yil012p	28
		Ylr020p	26
	S. pombe	Spbc16a3.12cp	31
		Spcc1672.09p	33
Hurler/Scheie syndrome (MPSI)	*D. melanogaster*	CG6201	31
IDUA			
α-L-Iduronidase			
Hunter syndrome (MPS II)	*D. melanogaster*	CG12014	45
IDS		CG14291	25
Iduronate sulfatase		CG7402	24
	C. elegans	D1014.1	27
	S. cerevisiae	Mcd4p	26
	S. pombe	Spbpb10d8.02cp	23
Sanfilippo A (MPS IIIA)	*D. melanogaster*	CG14291	55
SGSH		CG6725	25
Heparan *N*-Sulfatase		CG8646	26

	C. elegans	D1014.1	29
	S. pombe	Spbpb10d8.02cp	22
Sanfilippo B (MPS IIIB) NAGLU α-*N*-Acetylglucosaminidase	*D. melanogaster*	CG13397	43
	C. elegans	K09E4.4	36
Morquio A (MPS IVA) GALNS Galactosamine-6 sulfatase	*D. melanogaster*	CG7402	29
		CG8646	27
		CG5584	29
	C. elegans	D1014.1	27
		C54D2.4	22
	S. pombe	Spbpb10d8.02cp	27
		Spcc1672.09p	33
Maroteaux-Lamy (MPS VI) ARSB Arylsulfatase B	*D.melanogaster*	CG7402	37
		CG8646	35
		CG5584	41
	C. elegans	D1014.1	29
		C54D2.4	26
		K09C4.8	22
	S. pombe	Spbpb10d8.02cp	26
Sly syndrome (MPS VII) GUSB β-Glucuronidase	*D. melanogaster*	CG15117	46
		CG2135	43
	C. elegans	Y105E8B.N	29
		Y105E8A.VV	29
α-Mannosidosis MANB α-Mannosidase	*D. melanogaster*	GH02419	46
		CG5322	43
	C. elegans	F55D10.1	37
		F58H1.1	26
β-Mannosidosis MANBA β-Mannosidase	*D. melanogaster*	CG12583	36
		CG12582	34
	C. elegans	F33G3.4	34
Fucosidosis FUCA1 α-L-Fucosidase	*D. rerio*	AW184653	NA
	D. melanogaster	CG6128	46
	C. elegans	W03G11.3	46
Aspartylglucosaminuria AGA *N*-Aspartyl-β-Glucosaminidase	*D. rerio*	AI436940	NA
	D. melanogaster	CG1827	56
		CG10474	50
		CG4372	37
	C. elegans	R04B3.2	47
	S. pombe	Spac823.09cp	25
Galactosialidosis PPGB Unknown	*D. melanogaster*	CG4572	27
		DS00365.3	22
	C. elegans	F41C3.5	39
		F13D12.6	40
	S. cerevisiae	Ybr139p	31
		Prc1p	31
		Kex1p	27
	S. pombe	Cpy1p	31
		Spbc16g5.09p	30

Table 10.1 *(continued)*

Lysosomal disorder/ gene name/ protein description or function	Organism	Homologous protein or sequence ID	Percent identity
Schindler disease	*D. melanogaster*	CG5731	52
NAGA		CG7997	46
α-*N*-Acetyl-	*C. elegans*	R07B7.11	45
galactosaminidase	*S. cerevisiae*	Mel5p	35
		Mel6p	35
		Mel2p	30
	S. pombe	Spac869.07cp	33
Salla disease	*D. melanogaster*	CG4288	42
SLC17A5		CG4330	39
Sialic acid transporter		PICOT	41
	C. elegans	C38C10.2	41
		EAT-4	36
		K10G9.1	38
	S. cerevisiae	Dal5p	23
		Tna1p	22
	S. pombe	Liz1p	24
		Spbc1683.12p	22
Mucolipidosis IV	*D. melanogaster*	CG8743	44
ML4/MCOLN1		CG6504	23
Mucolipin-1	*C. elegans*	CUP-5	39
Infantile neuronal ceroid	*D. melanogaster*	CG12108	55
lipofuscinosis		CG4851	29
PPT1			
Protein thiolesterase	*C. elegans*	F44C4.5	54
	S. pombe	SPBC530.12c	31
Juvenile neuronal ceroid	*D. melanogaster*	CG5582	40
lipofuscinosis	*C. elegans*	CLN-3.1	41
CLN3		CLN-3.2	42
Unknown		CLN-3.3	40
	S. cerevisiae	Btn1p	39
	S. pombe	Spac607.09cp	37
Prosaposin	*D. melanogaster*	SAP-R	25
PSAP	*C. elegans*	T08A9.7	29
Saposins A-D		C28C12.6	24
Cystinosis	*D. melanogaster*	CG17119	50
CTNS	*C. elegans*	C41C4.7	36
Cystinosin	*S. cerevisiae*	Ers1p	31

Source: This table correlates data found on public databases at www.proteome.com, www.ncbi.nlm.nih.gov, genome-www.stanford.edu, www3.ncbi.nlm.nih.gov/Omim, and mcrcr2.med.nyu.edu/murphp01/lysosome/dischart.htm and through blasting of sequences at www.ncbi.nlm.nih.gov/BLAST.

There were no identifiable homologues to the proteins associated with the following diseases: Sanfilippo C (MPS IIIC), *N*-acetylglucosaminide acetyltransferase; Sanfilippo D (MPS IIID), *N*-acetylglucosamine-6-sulfatase; Morquio B (MPS IVB), β-galactosidase; sialidosis, α-neuraminidase; mucolipidosis II (I-cell disease) and mucolipidosis III (pseudo-Hurler polydystrophy), *N*-acetylglucosamine-1-phosphotransferase; late infantile neuronal ceroid lipofuscinosis (CLN2), TPP-1 protease; variant late infantile neuronal ceroid lipofuscinosis (CLN5), protein of unknown function. NA, per cent homologies for *D. rerio* are not listed as related sequences are ESTs, and the whole protein sequence is not available.

Pompe disease

The *ROT2* gene of *S. cerevisiae* is non-essential and encodes Rot2p, the α-subunit of glucosidase II, and has 29% homology to the acid α-glucosidase (GAA) which is associated with Pompe disease. Acid α-glucosidase is a lysosomal enzyme, while Rot2p associates with the endoplasmic reticulum (ER). However, it is possible that Rot2p and its processing activity represent the primordial function of this protein. Essentially, Rot2p is involved in the second step of N-glycan processing in the ER. α-glucosidase I encoded by *CWH41* cleaves the terminal α1,2-linked glucose and the α-glucosidase II removes the two α1,3-linked glucose residues from the Glc3Man9GlcNAc2 oligosaccharide precursor while the α1,2-mannosidase encoded by *MNS1* removes one specific mannose to form a single isomer of Man8GlcNAc2. Trimming by these glycosidases is not essential for the formation of N-glycan outer chains, and mutants lacking these enzymes indicate that α-glucosidases I and II may play an indirect role in cell wall β1,6-glucan formation and that the α1,2-mannosidase is involved in ER quality control (Herscovics 1999). A lack of Rot2p has also been shown to result in a decrease in the degradation of misfolded proteins by the ER degradation system (Jakob *et al.* 1998). Studies of Rot2p are yet to correlate to pheno-genotypic characteristics of Pompe disease, most likely due to the differing sub-cellular localization. However, close analysis of conserved regions between GAA and Rot2p suggests that catalytic function may be similar between the two proteins. Therefore, further understanding of the biochemical activity of Rot2p may aid in the complete characterization of the GAA protein. Further detail on the classification of this group of enzyme activities can be found in Henrissat and Davies (2000) and Bourne and Henrissat (2001). The agl protein from *S. pombe* has been shown to have 35% homology to GAA, and to have a characteristic α-glucosidase activity (Okuyama *et al.* 2001). However, further functional studies on the agl protein have not been reported. The primary defect associated with Pompe disease is lysosomal storage or accumulation of glycogen as a result of a lack of activity of the α-glucosidase or acid maltase.

Fabry disease and Schindler disease

MEL2, MEL5, and *MEL6* are non-essential polymorphic genes of *S. cerevisiae* which encode the α-galactosidase, GLA (melibiase) proteins Mel2p, Mel5p, and Mel6p, which share 33% homology to GLA, which is associated with Fabry disease, and 35% homology to α-*N*-acetyl-galactosaminidase (NAGA), which is associated with Schindler disease. Yeast GLA catalyses the conversion of melibiose into galactose and glucose. Despite numerous publications on the expression of these gene products, most studies have focused on understanding the redundancy of these proteins, which will not be addressed in this review. However, one interesting study indicated that cerulenin which inhibits lipid formation on growing yeasts, but does not affect protein synthesis and selective permeability does result in partial inhibition of the secretion of GLA. Furthermore, there is a parallel accumulation of GLA in membranous structures, particularly at the plasma membrane (Martinez *et al.* 1982). Both Fabry and Schindler disease are associated with metabolic deficiencies of the GLA and NAGA enzymes, respectively.

Niemann–Pick disease

PHM5 is a non-essential gene of *S. cerevisiae* that encodes a vacuolar polyphosphatase sharing 25% homology to acid sphingomyelinase (SMPD1), which is associated with Niemann–Pick types A and B. Although a gene/protein name has been designated, unfortunately no functional studies have been reported for this protein. It would appear that Phm5p would not be a functional homologue of SMPD1, but as these enzymes share similarity, there may be relevance with regard to activation or regulation of their subsequent activities. Two acid sphingomyelinases have been identified in *C. elegans* and termed asm-1 and asm-2 based on 34 and 32% homology, respectively, to SMPD (Lin *et al.* 1998). However, functional information on these proteins in this model system is still unavailable. The *NCR1* gene of *S. cerevisiae* is non-essential and Ncr1p shares 33% identity with NPC1, which is associated with Niemann–Pick type C. Like its human counterpart, Ncr1p is a transmembrane protein that is believed to be involved, to some degree, in the regulation of sphingolipid and cholesterol content and distribution in the cell. Two NPC1 homologues have been identified in *C. elegans*, npc-1 and npc-2, which are 28% and 24% homologous to human NPC1, respectively (see Chapter 9). In addition, the *C. elegans* ptr-1 gene product shows 19% homology. The ptr-1 gene product, like its counterpart in *D. melanogaster*, is a member of the patched family of proteins that bear a conserved sterol-sensing domain. This sterol-sensing domain is also present in all NPC1 proteins, and has led to the suggestion that NPC1 may be a regulatory protein for the trafficking of sterols within the cell (Chapter 9).

Wolman disease

TGL1 is a non-essential gene of *S. cerevisiae* that encodes a triglyceride lipase that shares 33% homology to the acid lipase (LIPA) that is associated with Wolman disease (Chapter 3). Tgl1p has been shown to associate with lipid particles, and strains lacking this protein accumulate ergosteryl esters (Athenstaedt *et al.* 1999). This is of relevance as the primary sterol in yeast is ergosterol, as opposed to cholesterol. Therefore, mutation of Tgl1p leading to the accumulation of ergosteryl esters is analogous to the accumulation of cholesteryl esters in Wolman disease. It is likely that much information can be attained from the study of Tgl1p in determining the molecular effects of lacking a functional LIPA. Interestingly, two uncharacterized gene products identified from the sequencing of the yeast genome, *YIL012w* and *YLR020c* share 28 and 26% homology with LIPA. Deletion studies have shown that both *YIL012w* and *YLR020c* are non-essential, and while there are no functional studies on these proteins, it is significant that *Ylr020p* shows a degree of similarity to triacylglycerol lipase. *D. melanogaster* has been shown to possess three lipase homologues, LIP1, LIP2, and LIP3 each with approximately 39% homology to LIPA. Close examination of the sequence of these three proteins reveals that LIP3 is most like the lysosomal acid lipase and that this homologue is expressed only during larval development (Pistillo *et al.* 1998), which might suggest that any metabolic consequence of lacking this protein would be imprinted developmentally.

Hunter syndrome (MPS II)

The *MCD4* gene of *S. cerevisiae* shares 26% homology to iduronate sulfatase (IDS) which is associated with MPS II (Chapter 3). Although the Mcd4p does not appear to be an IDS enzyme, the homology is nonetheless significant to report on the function of this yeast protein, which may be pertinent in understanding how the conserved regions contribute to the regulation of the enzyme. Deletion of *MCD4* (*mcd4-Δ*) is lethal, indicating that the function of this protein is essential to yeast. *Mcd4p* is a multimembrane-spanning protein that localizes to the ER and contains a large NH2-terminal ER lumenal domain (Gaynor *et al.*

1999), although some reports indicate that the protein also traffics to the vacuole (Packeiser *et al.* 1999). *Mcd4p* lumenal domain contains three conserved motifs found in mammalian phosphodiesterases and nucleotide pyrophosphatases. Mutations in *MCD4* that are not lethal result in defective ER-to-Golgi transport of GPI-anchored proteins, and strains bearing these mutations exhibit marked morphological defects, most notably the accumulation of distorted, ER- and vesicle-like membranes (Gaynor *et al.* 1999).

Galactosialidosis

The PPGB protein associated with galactosialidosis has significant homology to the uncharacterized gene product *YBR138p* (31%), *Prc1p* (31%), and *Kex1p* (27%) in *S. cerevisiae*. Deletion of any of these proteins from yeast does not result in lethality; however, there have been several studies on the function of, and the effect of deleting either *Prc1p* (*prc1-Δ*) or *Kex1p* (*kex1-Δ*). Both *Prc1p* and *Kex1p* are carboxypeptidases that localize to the vacuole and Golgi, respectively (Bryant and Boyd 1993). *Prc1p* is believed to be responsible for the proteolysis of certain vacuolar proteins. *Kex1p* has been shown to be involved in the C-terminal processing of precursors to secrete mature proteins (Cooper and Bussey 1992). Many questions remain in elucidating the molecular basis of galactosialidosis (Chapter 7). Deducing how the altered function of PPGB, which if it has a role in proteolytic processing of enzymes, will be important in understanding why this defect results in lysosomal storage. The yeast models *prc1-Δ*, *kex1-Δ*, and *ybr138-Δ* will certainly be valuable tools in such studies. A homologue showing 31% similarity to PPGB in *S. pombe*, *Cpy1p*, has also been shown to be a vacuolar carboxypeptidase (Tabuchi *et al.* 1997), which presumably is also involved in the processing or degradation of protein substrates.

Salla disease

The sialic acid transport protein (SLC17A5) has been shown to be mutated in Salla disease. Eukaryotes have many proteins that are considered either small molecule transporters or permeases, and yeast is no exception. However, *S. cerevisiae* bears two proteins with significant homology to SLC17A5, notably Dal5p and Tna1p, which are 23 and 22% homologous to SLC17A5, respectively. Dal5p has been characterized as an allantoate and ureidosuccinate permease (Turoscy and Cooper 1987; Rai *et al.* 1988) and is a member of the allantoate permease family of major facilitator superfamily (MFS). Deletion of *Dal5p* (*dal5-Δ*) is not lethal but does result in an inability to take up allantoate or ureidosuccinate from growth media (Chisholm *et al.* 1987; Turoscy and Cooper 1987). *Tna1p*, is also a member of the MFS, and has been shown to be a nicotinic acid permease (Llorente and Dujon 2000). Deletion of *Tna1p* (*tna1-Δ*) is not lethal but does result in a near complete inability to take up nicotinic acid (Llorente and Dujon 2000). Further study of these yeast homologues, particularly by way of manipulation of these proteins will no doubt yield valuable data, as researchers look for ways to compensate for transport defects associated with Salla disease. In *S. pombe*, *Liz1p* is predicted to be a small molecule transporter and is 24% homologous to SLC17A5. Functional studies on the effect of deleting *Liz1p* have suggested that the protein may in fact be involved in the transportation across membranes of uracil precursors (Moynihan and Enoch, 1999). The eat-4 protein of *C. elegans* is 36% homologous to SLC17A5. Studies on eat-4 in *C. elegans* highlight the utility of this organism for understanding neuronal function and the neurologic effect of lacking a particular protein. It has been shown that eat-4 functions presynaptically and is necessary for glutamatergic neurotransmission (Bellocchio *et al.* 1998; Lee *et al.* 1999; Rankin and Wicks 2000). Mutations in eat-4 result in a number of sensory deficits in response to, or avoidance of external stimuli (Berger *et al.* 1998; Lee *et al.* 1999; Zheng *et al.* 1999).

Mucolipidosis IV

CUP-5 of *C. elegans* is 39% homologous to mucolipin-1, which is associated with mucolipidosis IV. It was recently reported that mutation of the CUP-5 protein resulted in an enhanced rate of uptake of fluid-phase markers, a decrease in the rate of degradation of endocytosed protein and an accumulation of large vacuoles (Fares and Greenwald 2001). Interestingly, the same study revealed that by overexpressing CUP-5, the opposite to these phenotypes occurs, suggesting that CUP-5 is involved in the regulation of endocytosis (Fares and Greenwald 2001). Mucolipidosis IV has an associated alteration in the endocytosis of lipids that accumulate in large vesicles, and it would appear that further study of this *C. elegans* model for mucolipidosis IV will yield valuable information on the function of mucolipin-1 and the course of the disease.

Batten disease

The *BTN1* gene of *S. cerevisiae* encodes a protein that shares 39% identity to CLN3, which is, associated with juvenile neuronal ceroid lipofuscinoses (Batten disease) (Chapters 3 and 9). Deletion of *BTN1* (*btn1*-Δ) in yeast results in an elevated ability to acidify the growth medium due to an elevated activity of plasma membrane H^+-ATPase, resulting from an abnormally acidic vacuole of pH 5.8 rather than the normal 6.1 (Pearce and Sherman 1998; Pearce *et al.* 1999). However, these phenomena are only seen in the early phases of growth in *btn1*-Δ. As *btn1*-Δ strains grow, altered vacuolar pH, which is presumed to be the primary defect, becomes normalized. Our most recent studies have shown that through this normalization of vacuolar pH, a depletion in the levels of the basic amino acids arginine and lysine occurs (Chattopadhyay and Pearce 2002). Interestingly, the *BTN2* gene product that is upregulated in *btn1*-Δ strains (Pearce *et al.* 1999) has been shown to been involved in the localizing of *Rsg1p* which has a role in regulating the uptake of arginine and lysine from the external environment (Urano *et al.* 2000; Chattopadhyay and Pearce 2002). *Btn1p* localizes to the vacuolar compartment (Croopnick *et al.* 1998; Pearce *et al.* 1999), and *btn1*-Δ strains show genetic interactions with mutations in proteins involved in trafficking to the vacuole (Pearce, unpublished observation). Therefore, *btn1*-Δ results in a disturbance in trafficking and vacuolar content of yeast. *C. elegans* has three orthologues to human CLN3, cln3.1, cln3.2, and cln3.3. Although studies of these gene products are in an early stage, it is apparent that their expression may be regulated developmentally (Hill *et al.* 2000; Jiang *et al.* 2001). Although there are currently no reported studies on the *Drosophila* CLN3 orthologue, it is significant to mention that yeast Btn2p (which is upregulated in *btn1*-Δ) shows 38% similarity over 104 amino acids to the human HOOK1 protein. *Drosophila* HOOK1 functions in the endocytosis of transmembrane ligands and apparently acts as a negative regulator of the fusion of mature multivesicular bodies (MVBs) to the late endosome and lysosome (Sunio *et al.* 1999). HOOK1 will be covered in a later section on the use of *Drosophila* in dissecting out pathways involved in endosome/lysosome trafficking. However, despite the fact that Btn2p and HOOK1 do not appear to be true orthologues, there appears to be similarity in the proteins that interact *in vivo* with Btn2p and HOOK1 in yeast and human, respectively (Chattopadhyay and Pearce, in preparation). This may indicate an evolutionary divergence at a particular point in this HOOK1/Btn2p trafficking pathway (Pearce, 2000).

Biogenesis and trafficking to the lysosome

To gain a complete understanding of an organelle such as the lysosome, it will be important to identify not only how the proteins that form it reach the lysosome, but also how the lysosome is formed. A defect in the delivery of a certain protein to the lysosome will leave a lysosome lacking that particular protein and have four possible negative effects on lysosomal function. First, an absence of a protein that is required for a specific function will create a lesion in a biochemical pathway such that this pathway is no longer completed. This would result in an inability to complete a biochemical process that is presumably necessary. Second, an incomplete biochemical pathway could lead to the accumulation of the enzyme's substrate, which could subsequently interfere with the lysosomal environment so as to disturb the activity of other lysosomal proteins. Third, a loss of a protein may not directly lead to an accumulation of this enzyme substrate but could lead to the accumulation of other proteins through an alteration in the lysosomal environment precipitated by the loss of this protein. Fourth, if the protein in question is involved in a pathway where it has multiple substrates, such as processing or protein modification for example, then the activity or function of several other proteins may not be controlled due to their not being activated or deactivated. Any of the three other consequences described could also affect a protein involved in processing of protein modification and result in this last case. The use of model systems to dissect out the intricacies of what contribution a protein has to lysosomal function or trafficking has been personified by studies on vacuolar/lysosomal biogenesis in the yeast *S. cerevisiae*, and studies on the causation of eye colour mutations in *D. melanogaster*. Very recently, a few studies on *C. elegans* have shown the potential for this organism in contributing to our understanding of lysosomal biogenesis. The following overviews on studies in yeast, worm, and fly are brief and applicable to biogenesis of the vacuole/lysosome; however, more detail can be obtained from the cited review articles that specifically address in more detail this ever expanding area of biology.

Yeast

How proteins may end up at the vacuole in yeast can be categorized into six pathways, carboxypeptidase Y pathway, alkaline phosphatase pathway (ALP), endocytosis, cytoplasm to vacuole pathway, autophagy, and inheritance, although strictly speaking, inheritance is not a distinct pathway. However, within these categories, there is significant overlap. A schematic representation of the six pathways that deliver materials to the vacuole and some of the proteins that have been characterized to be involved in these processes is presented in Fig. 10.1. This is a modified version of a figure from Mullins and Bonifacino (2001).

Many proteins that ultimately reside in the vacuole, for example subunits of the vacuolar ATPase, are sorted through the carboxypeptidase Y, or CPY pathway. CPY is a soluble vacuolar hydrolase, and isolation of mutants in the CPY pathway was often achieved by looking for defects in the intracellular distribution of this protein. Proteins trafficked by the CPY pathway move from the Golgi apparatus to the pre-vacuolar compartment (PVC) and on the

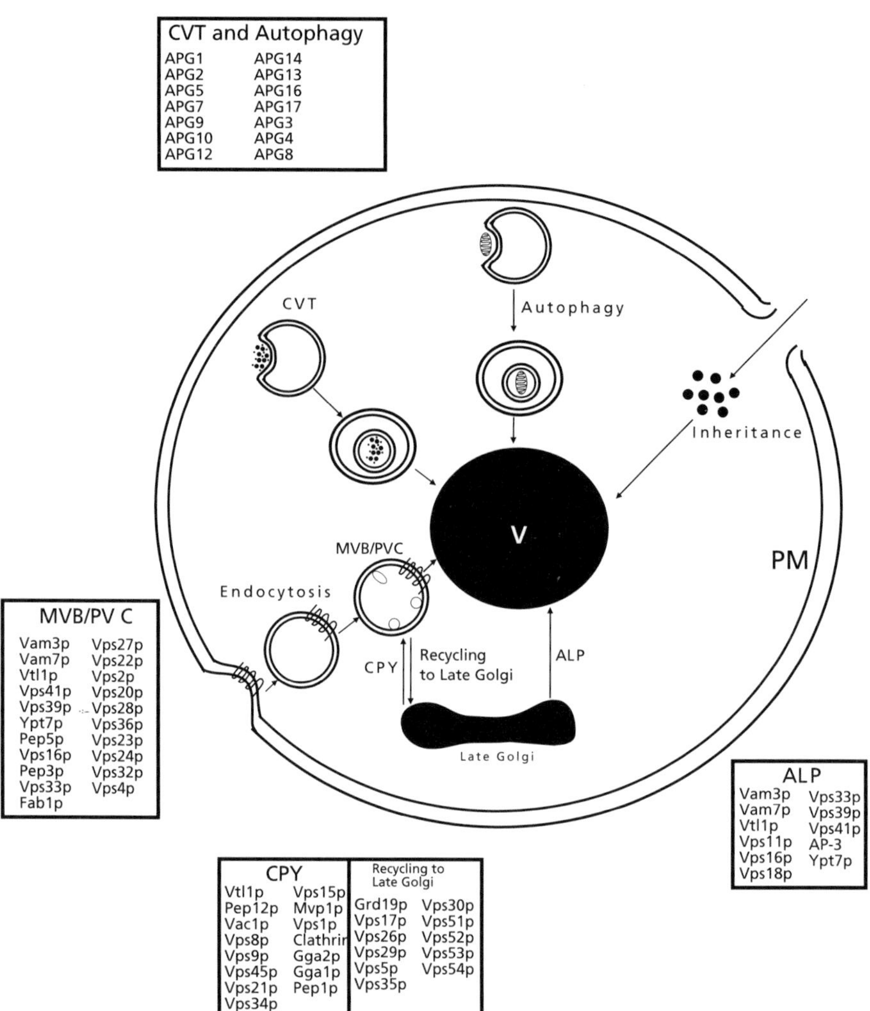

Fig. 10.1 Six modes by which materials can be delivered to the yeast vacuole, and some of the proteins that have been characterized to be involved in these processes.

1. Endocytosis from the plasma membrane to multivesicular bodies MVB/prevacuolar compartment (PVC). Here endocytosed material is internalized into luminal vesicles or recycled. Mature MVB's may fuse with the vacuolar membrane for turnover of their content in the vacuole.
2. Cytoplasm to Vacuole (CVT) pathway. Cytoplasmic proteins are internalized in a double membrane CVT vesicle, which fuses to the vacuolar membrane.
3. Autophagy. This is similar to the CVT-pathway, but is apparently active under conditions of nutrient starvation. Cytoplasmic proteins are internalized into a double membrane autophagosome, which fuses to the vacuolar membrane for turnover of their content in the vacuole.
4. Inheritance. Vesicles travel from mother to daughter and merge to form the vacuole.
5. Carboxypeptidase Y (CPY) pathway. Sorting of synthesized proteins from late Golgi to MVB/PVC, where delivery to the vacuole as described above occurs.
6. Alkaline Phosphatase pathway (ALP). A direct sorting of certain proteins to the vacuole from the late Golgi.

vacuole (Fig. 10.1). At least 50 proteins, many designated as vacuolar protein sorting (VPS) proteins have been shown to have a function in the CPY pathway. These proteins were often identified by a defect in the sorting of CPY itself, or due to altered vacuolar morphology. In brief, the Pep1p (Vps10p), transmembrane protein binds or cross-links to CPY at the Golgi apparatus. At the PVC, Pep1p disassociates from CPY and returns or recycles to the Golgi, requiring a complex composed of Vps29p, Vps26p, Vps35p, Vps5p, and Vps17p (Kohrer and Emr 1993; Seaman *et al.* 1997, 1998). Disruption of this complex leads to Pep1p being mislocalized to the vacuole.

Similarly, mutations in Vps52p, Vps53p, or Vps54p, which associate with the Golgi apparatus, result in Pep1p being mis-sorted to the vacuole (Conibear and Stevens 2000). The sorting to the PVC requires proteins involved in vesicle formation, clathrin and Vps1p (Payne *et al.* 1988; Vater *et al.* 1992; Dell'Angelica *et al.* 2000; Hirst *et al.* 2000). Vps21p, Vps9p, Vac1p, Vps19, Vps45p, Pep12p, Vti1p, and Sec18p are involved in targeting and fusion with the PVC (Graham and Emr 1991; Horazdovsky *et al.* 1994; Piper *et al.* 1994; Becherer *et al.* 1996; Burd *et al.* 1997; von Mollard *et al.* 1997; Hama *et al.* 1999). Phosphorylation of specific lipids involved in these processes is brought about by the Vps15p and Vps34p kinases (Stack *et al.* 1993, 1995). Mutations in Vps27p and Vps28p result in the accumulation of enlarged PVCs (Piper *et al.* 1995; Reider *et al.* 1996), suggesting a function at the PVC membrane. Similarly, mutations in Vps4p alter the PVC, and as Vps4p has been shown to bind to the PVC in an ATP-dependent fashion, it has been proposed that Vps4p could be central to regulating interactions with other proteins to the PVC (Babst *et al.* 1998). The final step of fusion of the PVC to the vacuole itself requires the GTPase, Ypt7p, the v-SNARE and t-SNARE, Vti1p and Vam3p, respectively, Vam7p, a docking complex composed of Vps16p, Vps33p, Pep3p, and Pep5p (the class C Vps-complex) and perhaps two other proteins, and another complex composed of Vps39p and Vps41p (Darsow *et al.* 1997; Nakamura *et al.* 1997; Radisky *et al.* 1997; Rieder and Emr 1997; Wada *et al.* 1997; Sato *et al.* 1998; Wurmser *et al.* 2000; Cheever *et al.* 2001). Most recently the class C Vps-complex has been implicated in membrane docking and fusion at the Golgi to PVC and PVC to vacuole stages (Peterson and Emr 2001). There is overlap of the latter steps of the CPY pathway with the ALP pathway (Stepp *et al.* 1997), which will be described next. A specific review on phosphoinositide signalling and its importance in the regulation of membrane trafficking, and particularly the biogenesis of the vacuole by Odorizzi *et al.* (2000) covers many aspects not covered in this overview.

The (ALP)pathway involves trafficking directly from the Golgi apparatus to the vacuole, with no involvement of the PVC (Fig.10.1). This sorting pathway is mediated by the yeast equivalent to the AP-3 adaptor complex, Apl5p, Apl6p, Apm3p, and Aps3p (Dell'Angelica *et al.* 1997; Panek *et al.* 1997; Simpson *et al.* 1997), and by Vps41p and Vam2p (Cowles *et al.* 1997; Stepp *et al.* 1997). Vps41p has been shown to associate with AP-3 and Vps39p, and as mutations in either Vps39p or Vps41p result in processing defects of ALP, it is thought that these proteins are required for AP-3 vesicle formation (Nakamura *et al.* 1997; Rehling *et al.* 1999; Darsow *et al.* 2001). As alluded to above, overlap with the CPY pathway exists with mis-sorting of vacuolar hydrolases (Raymond *et al.* 1992; Nakamura *et al.* 1997). A thorough review of sorting between the Golgi and vacuole can be found in Conibear and Stevens (2000) and an overview on yeast vacuole biogenesis in Bryant and Stevens (1998).

Endocytosis can be summarized as the uptake of extracellular material and plasma membrane components into the cell (Fig. 10.1). Early studies on yeast endocytosis focused on using the pheromone α-factor, and the receptors that it bound, which became internalized as a complex and degraded in the vacuole (Davis *et al.* 1993; Schandel and Jenness 1994). Furthermore, these early studies showed that the receptor–ligand complex passed through two internal membrane compartments, termed early and late endosomes before being degraded in the vacuole (Singer and Reizman 1990; Singer-Kruger *et al.* 1993). More recently, the use of the fluorescent compound FM4-64 which travels from the plasma membrane to the vacuole *via* punctate endocytic intermediates in a time-, temperature-, and energy-dependent way has been utilized (Vida and Emr 1995). Consequently, mutations in the aptly named *END*-genes that create defects at points from plasma membrane to vacuole could be isolated on the basis of cell sorting and the fluorescence in the cell. In fact, *End3p* and *End4p* which are important in the early stages of the endocytic pathway were identified by mutations in the genes that encode them by this type of screen (Raths *et al.* 1993). After internalization, marker proteins of endocytosis intersect with proteins targeted for delivery to the vacuole at late endosomes or the PVC. As with the other pathways discussed in this section, considerable overlap of function and phenotype exists. A recent report indicated that mutations in Vps4p, whose function in the CPY pathway was described earlier, produced an internalization defect, suggesting that Vps4p probably has an important role at multiple steps in the endocytic and trafficking pathways (Zhan *et al.* 2001). The trafficking of proteins through the endocytic pathway is tightly linked to the function of many proteins known to associate with the cytoskeleton. The powerful techniques afforded to the yeast molecular biologist are fast distinguishing the contribution of many proteins that have a role in endocytosis at the actin cytoskeleton, with clathrin coats, and the formation and movement of vesicles. For example, proteins such as the epsins have four family members in yeast, Ent1p, Ent2p, Ent3p, and Ent4p, and may act at multiple points in the endocytic pathway (Wendland *et al.* 1999). Several reviews go into considerable detail on endocytosis, namely, Bryant and Stevens (1998), Munn (2000, 2001), Baggett and Wendland (2001).

Autophagy is the transport of proteins to the vacuole in response to nutrient deprivation, such that cells can facilitate degradation of large amounts of intracellular protein, (Fig. 10.1). Autophagy itself can be described as two types, depending on the type and size of the cargo that is being autophagocytosed. Microautophagy is the invagination of the vacuolar membrane, which results in the formation of a membrane-bound intravacuole vesicle containing small portions of the cytosol. The contents of this intravacuole vesicle can then be degraded by vacuolar hydrolases. Macroautophagy involves the formation of an autophagosome, which is a double membrane structure, around either bulk cytosol or organelles (Takeshige *et al.* 1992; Baba *et al.* 1994). The autophagosome fuses to the vacuole to release a single membrane autophagic body into the vacuole lumen (Takeshige *et al.* 1992). Autophagy in yeast can be seen under nutrient-limited conditions in vacuolar protease-deficient yeast strains by the accumulation of autophagic vesicles, the contents of which can be distinguished from the cytosol, inside the vacuole (Simeon *et al.* 1992; Takeshige *et al.* 1992). A number of *apg/aut* mutants have been identified through their inability to survive during nutrient starvation (Tsukada and Ohsumi 1993; Thumm *et al.* 1994), and several of the proteins identified from subsequent characterization of these mutants are listed in Fig. 10.1. It is pertinent to point out that much overlap occurs between the function of proteins in Fig. 10.1, and this is particularly evident with the cvt and autophagy pathways (Baba *et al.* 1997; Klionsky and Ohsumi 1999). An excellent and more detailed review of the processes and proteins involved in autophagy and cytoplasm-to-vacuole pathways has been published by Klionsky and Ohsumi (1999).

Inheritance of vacuoles from mother to daughter cells is coordinated by the cell cycle. After cytokinesis, vesicles are transported and deposited in the growing bud, or daughter cell, and by homotypic fusion form one or a few large vacuoles (Conradt *et al.* 1992). Many mutants defective in vacuolar inheritance have been reported and designated *vac* mutants, and several proteins associated with these mutations have been characterized (Wang *et al.* 1996, 1998, 2001; Bonangelino *et al.* 1997). Again, there is significant overlap with the proteins with alternative vacuolar biogenesis pathways; in particular many Vps proteins have a role in vacuolar inheritance. A more detailed review of vacuolar inheritance, including the functional overlap of proteins involved in vacuolar inheritance can be found by Bryant and Stevens (1998). It is interesting to note that while the inheritance of different organelles is controlled independently from that of the vacuole, some of the processes involved, such as a requirement for cytoskeletal involvement show overlap in mechanism (Warren and Wickner 1996; Catlett and Weisman 2000).

Worm

C. elegans is contributing to our understanding of lysosomal biogenesis. An initial report utilized a green fluorescent protein (GFP) reporter fused to vitellogenin and expressed in oocytes (Grant and Hirsh 1999). In combination with RNA interference, this system was used to show that defects in the endocytosis of the vitellogenin–GFP fusion could be produced and that mechanisms of endocytosis in *C. elegans* were conserved from higher organisms. Furthermore, this study was used to isolate mutations in receptor-mediated endocytosis, the so-called 'rme' mutants, or proteins (Grant and Hirsh 1999). The rme-2 protein was subsequently shown to be a low-density lipoprotein receptor (Grant and Hirsh 1999). A study on the transport of cholesterol using the fluorescent analogue, dehydroergosterol, identified many mutants that have defects, including rme-2, which failed to accumulate dehydroergosterol in oocytes and embryos (Matyash *et al.* 2001). The rme-8 protein has been shown to be required for receptor-mediated endocytosis, and in certain cell types localizes to the membrane of large endosomes (Zhang *et al.* 2001). The rme-1 protein associates with the endocytic recycling compartment, and mutations in the protein result in endocytic recycling defects, with the suggestion that the defect may be in the exit of membrane proteins from recycling endosomes (Grant *et al.* 2001; Lin *et al.* 2001). So far, it would appear that rme mutants result in developmental defects. An arrest in development was shown to occur when expression of auxillin, which is required for clathrin-mediated endocytosis, is decreased (Greener *et al.* 2001).

Fly

Although yeast as a tool for elucidating the machinery of lysosomal biogenesis is very valuable, due to the considerable conservation, a complete understanding of lysosomal biogenesis needs to be gained from a multicellular organism, as some proteins shown to be involved in these processes do not exist in yeast. *Drosophila* eye colour mutations are a relatively well-studied phenomenon, and as many as 80 mutations have been characterized that result in an altered eye colour phenotype. Many of these mutations have been shown to be in proteins involved in the synthesis of the pigments that give colour; however, many of the proteins are involved in the trafficking of proteins to either pigment granules or the lysosome (Lloyd *et al.* 1998). Mutations in *Drosophila* that result in the eye colour phenotypes of *light, carnation,* and *deep-orange* are in homologues to Vps41p, Vps33p, and Pep3p, respectively (Rieder and Emr 1997; Lloyd *et al.* 1998; Sevrioukov *et al.* 1999). Each of these proteins functions at different points in different vacuolar sorting pathways in yeast, as described in the previous section. Interestingly, Vps41p may associate with AP-3, and mutations in the δ-subunit of AP-3 in *Drosophila* result in defective pigment granule biogenesis and the *garnet* eye colour phenotype (Ooi *et al.* 1997; Simpson *et al.* 1997). Furthermore, defects in AP-3 σ-, μ-, and β- subunits have been associated with a decrease in pigment granules responsible for the *orange, carmine,* and *ruby* eye colour mutants (Mullins *et al.* 1999; Mullins *et al.* 2000; Kretzschmar *et al.* 2000). These are of extreme pertinence to diseases of lysosome-like organelles or storage granules, such as Hermansky–Pulak disease, which are covered in more detail later in this chapter.

Not all proteins found to be involved in trafficking to the lysosome are conserved throughout all model systems. The HOOK1 protein from *Drosophila* was originally isolated due to the *hook* mutation showing a bristle phenotype, and HOOK1 is a novel protein involved in the endocytosis of transmembrane ligands (Kramer and Phistry 1996, 1999). *Drosophila* HOOK1 apparently acts as a negative regulator of the fusion of mature MVBs to the late endosome and lysosome (Sunio *et al.* 1999). In a study on the *Drosophila* larval neuromuscular junction, HOOK1 and deep-orange protein (Pep3p) were found to be highly enriched at the synapse (Narayanan *et al.* 2000). In the same study, it is noted that mutations in *hook* (HOOK1) and *deep-orange* (Pep3p) result in an increase and a decrease in the synapse size, respectively. The fact that HOOK1 and deep-orange protein can be generally stated to have a negative and positive regulatory role on endocytic trafficking, respectively, led to the suggestion that these protein may have a role in regulating the composition of the synaptic plasma membrane (Narayanan *et al.* 2000). Therefore, the studies on HOOK1 emphasize the fact that components of the lysosomal biogenesis pathway in higher eukaoryotes may not always be present in yeast. Furthermore, the same can be said when we compare various model systems to mammals. Several of the disorders listed in Table 10.1 do not have a model system counterpart, and a report from the group of Kramer, establishes that an HOOK1-like protein, namely HOOK3, associates with the Golgi apparatus (Walenta *et al.* 2001). This leads to the intriguing possibility that a family of HOOK proteins has evolved and diverged through invertebrates to vertebrates such that different members are present at more than one organelle or membrane, and are involved as a family in more than one type of vesicular trafficking.

Proteins associated with disease and with lysosome biogenesis and their orthologues in model organisms

Table 10.2 lists diseases that have defects affecting the transport machinery for lysosomes or lysosome-related organelles such as melanosomes, platelet storage granules, and cytolytic granules. Where possible, the name of an orthologous protein from *S. cerevisiae, S. pombe, C. elegans,* and *D. melanogaster* based on the searching of public databases and sequence alignments along with the per cent homology is shown. Unfortunately, homologues in *D. rerio* do not appear in the databases yet, but are likely to be identified through sequencing of this organism genome. As with the lysosomal storage diseases, many of the designations represent assignations from sequencing projects, rather than gene names, as these gene products remain essentially unstudied in these organisms.

Table 10.2 Diseases that have defects affecting the transport machinery for lysosomes or lysosome-related organelles

Disorder/gene name	Organism	Homologous protein or sequence ID	Percent identity
Hermansky–Pudlak syndrome type 1	*Drosophila melanogaster*	CG12855	25
HPS1			
Hermansky–Pudlak syndrome type 2	*D. melanogaster*	RB	50
AP3B1		BAP	30
		BETACOP	20
	Caenorhabditis elegans	R11A5.1	39
		Y71H2B.10	29
	Saccharomyces cerevisiae	Apl6p	28
		Apl2p	25
		Apl1p	25
	Schizosaccharomyces pombe	Apl6p	31
		Apl2p	28
		Apl1p	25
Chediak–Higashi syndrome	*D. melanogaster*	CG11814	25
CHS1		CG1332	41
		CG6734	29
	C. elegans	VT23B5.2	33

Table 10.2 *(continued)*

Disorder/gene name	Organism	Homologous protein or sequence ID	Percent identity
		F10F2.1	26
	S. cerevisiae	Bph1p	28
	S. pombe	Spbc3h7.16p	29
Griscelli disease with haemophagic	*D. melanogaster*	80H7.4:EG	62
syndrome		Rab3	44
Rab27		Rab10	40
	C. elegans	Y87G2A.4	66
		Rab-3	44
		T23H2.5	41
	S. cerevisiae	Sec4p	44
		Ypt31p	37
		Ypt1p	36
	S. pombe	Ypt2p	47
		Ypt1p	39
		Ypt3p	34

Source: This table correlates data found on public databases at www.proteome.com, www.ncbi.nlm.nih.gov, genome-www.stanford.edu and www3.ncbi.nlm.nih.gov/Omim. LAMP2, which is associated with Danon disease, has no apparent homologues in model organisms.

Studies of orthologous proteins implicated in diseases that are involved in lysosome biogenesis

This section will review those proteins that are associated with diseases associated with defects in biogenesis of lysosome-like organelles and what has been reported on their function in model systems.

Hermansky–Pulak disease Type 2

The Apl6p, Apl2p and Apl1p of *S. cerevisiae* are all large subunits or β-adaptin of the clathrin-associated (AP) complex, and show 28, 25, and 25% homology to AP3B1, respectively, which is associated with Hermansky–Pulak syndrome. Collectively, these proteins have been shown to be involved in clathrin-dependent Golgi functions, including the sorting to, or biogenesis of, the vacuolar organelles (Rad *et al.* 1995; Stepp *et al.* 1997). Mutation of these genes results in deficiencies in the transport of certain proteins to the vacuole. As adaptor complexes are associated to the formation of vesicles and the incorporation of cargo into vesicular membranes, it has been a logical speculation that the lysosome-like organelle defects associated with Hermansky–Pulak disease types 1 and 2 are a result of a defect in the transport machinery to these organelles.

Chediak–Higashi syndrome

The Bph1p of *S. cerevisiae* is 28% homologous to CHS1, which has been associated with Chediak–Higashi syndrome. Although deletion of *BPH1* (*bph1*-Δ) does not result in any obvious phenotype (Shea *et al.* 1994), a failure to grow on glucose media at low pH in the presence of acetic acid has led to the suggestion of a function in transporting small organic molecules (Oliver 1996). Correlation to a transport function is still required to establish whether Bph1 serves as a viable model for Chediak–Higashi syndrome. Despite weak overall homology to proteins involved in vacuolar trafficking, motifs associated with this function suggest a potential role in vesicular trafficking, which may be much more in line with the potential function of this protein as determined by defects associated with the disease.

Griscelli disease with haemophagic syndrome

The Rab27 protein that is associated with Griscelli disease with haemophagic syndrome is 44, 37, and 36% homologous to Sec4p, Ypt31p, and Ypt1p of *S. cerevisiae*, respectively. There have been many studies on these proteins that reveal that they are GTP-binding proteins required for vesicular trafficking between the Golgi and plasma membrane (Sec4p), formation of trans-Golgi vesicles (Ypt31p), and transport between ER and Golgi (Ypt1p) (Benli *et al.* 1996; Jedd *et al.* 1997; Lazar *et al.* 1997 GarciaRanea and Valencia 1998;). Studies on Ypt2p, Ypt1p, and Ypt3p of *S. pombe*, which are 47, 39, and 34% homologous to Rab27, respectively, also indicate that mutation of these proteins result in defects in vesicular trafficking (Craighead *et al.* 1993; Tang *et al.* 2000). Interestingly, mutations in the *C. elegans* homologue, rab-3, which is 44% similar to Rab27, have been shown to result in a depletion of certain vesicles and have a direct effect on synaptic transmission presumably due to this effect on vesicles (Nonet *et al.* 1997; Iwasaki and Toyonaga 2000). Similarly, rab-3 of *D. melanogaster*, which is 44% homologous to rab27, has been shown to associate with synaptic vesicles and be involved in neurotransmission (Diantonio *et al.* 1993). Collectively, these studies correlate to the presumed role of rab-27 in the exocytosis of cytolyic granules from T cells, which is uncontrolled in Griscelli disease with haemophagic syndrome.

Summary

It is apparent that virtually all diseases that are classed as lysosomal storage diseases have some sort of neurodegenerative aspect to their course. It is often assumed that the unique nature of cell types such as neurones within the brain, makes them particularly susceptible to the effects of lysosomal storage. In fact, there could be many biological explanations as to why neurones are in fact susceptible to dysfunction in the presence of lysosomal storage. There is a need to understand the biology of the lysosome, and to not only deduce the function of each protein component of the lysosome, but how the function of each of these proteins affects other proteins. Furthermore, studies on the biogenesis of the lysosome are revealing that altered function, and perhaps storage of material at the lysosome may not result from a direct dysfunction at the lysosome, but rather as a result of a defect in a protein that is involved in the trafficking of proteins to the lysosome. Trafficking of proteins to and from acidic compartments that emanate from, or associate with, the lysosome, such as the early or late endosomes is of extreme importance to the function of neurones. Many orthologues of proteins involved in the trafficking of proteins in yeast are involved in the trafficking of vesicles in neurones, particularly those at the synapse. Many studies utilizing *C. elegans* and *Drosophila* are focused on understanding neural development and neuronal function, and many proteins whose primordial function in yeast is in trafficking have a clear function in neurones. A disturbance in synaptic transmission could result from a defect in the machinery involved in transporting proteins to the synapse, or a defect in the acidic environment of the endosome/lysosome, from which many of these proteins may at some point reside. Alterations in synapse function through an alteration in the trafficking of proteins to the synapse may contribute to or even result directly in neuronal dysfunction and degeneration.

Acknowledgements

I wish to thank Yasser Elshatory for preparing Fig. 10.1 and careful editing, Brandeis Knibbs for helping with the references and Dr. Paul Roberts for useful comments during the preparation of this chapter. Some of the unpublished research published herein was supported by NIH R01 NS36610.

References

Athenstaedt, K., Zweytick, D., Jandrositz, A., Kohlwein, S. D. and Daum, G. (1999). Identification and characterization of major lipid particle proteins of the yeast *Saccharomyces cerevisiae*. *J Bacteriol*, **181**, 6441–8.

Baba, M., Takeshige, K., Baba, N. and Ohsumi, Y. (1994). Ultrastructural analysis of the autophagic process in yeast: detection of autophagosomes and their characterization. *J Cell Biol*, **124**, 903–913.

Baba, M., Osumi, M., Scott, S. V., Klionsky, D. J. and Ohsumi, Y. (1997). Two distinct pathways for targeting proteins from the cytoplasm to the vacuole/lysosome. *J Cell Biol*, **139**, 1687–95.

Babst, M., Wendland, B., Estepa, E. J. and Emr, S. D. (1998). The vps4p AAA ATPase regulates membrane association of a Vps protein complex required for normal endosome function. *EMBO J*, **17**, 2982–93.

Baggett, J. J. and Wendland, B. (2001). Clathrin function in yeast endocytosis. *Traffic*, **2**, 297–302.

Becherer, K. A., Rieder, S. E., Emr, S. D. and Jones, E. W. (1996). Novel syntaxin homologue, Pep12p, required for the sorting of lumenal hydrolases to the lysosome-like vacuole in yeast. *Mol Biol Cell*, **7**, 579–94.

Bellocchio, E. E., Hu, H., Pohorille A, Chan, J., Pickel, V. M. and Edwards, R. H. (1998). The localization of the brain-specific inorganic phosphate transporter suggests a specific presynaptic role in glutamatergic transmission. *J Neurosci*, **18**, 8648–59.

Benli, M., Doring, F., Robinson, D. G., Yang, X. and Gallwitz, D. (1996). Two GTPase isoforms, Ypt31p and Ypt32p, are essential for Golgi functions in yeast. *EMBO J*, **15**, 6460–75.

Berger, A. J., Hart, A. C. and Kaplan, J. M. (1998). G alpha-induced neurodegeneration in *Caenorhabditis elegans*. *J Neurosci*, **18**, 2871–80.

Bonangelino, C. J., Catlett, N. L. and Weisman, L. S. (1997). Vac7p, a novel vacuolar protein, is required for normal vacuole inheritance and morphology. *Mol Cell Biol*, **17**, 6847–58.

Bourne, Y. and Henrissat, B. (2001). Glycoside hydolases and glycosyltransferases: families and functional modules. *Curr Opin Struct Biol*, 593–600.

Bryant, N. J. and Boyd, A. (1993). Immunnoisolation of Kex2p-containing organelles from yeast demonstrates colocalisation of three processing proteinases to a single Golgi compartment. *J Cell Sci*, **106**, 815–22.

Bryant, N. J. and Stevens, T. H. (1998). Vacuole biogenesis in *Saccharomyces cerevisiae*: protein transport pathways to the yeast vacuole. *Microbiol Mol Biol Rev*, **62**, 230–47.

Burd, C. G., Peterson, M., Cowles, C. R. and Emr, S. D. (1997). A novel Sec18p/NSF-dependent complex required for Golgi-to-endosome transport in yeast. *Mol Biol Cell*, **8**, 1089–104.

Catlett, N. L. and Weisman, L. S. (2000). Divide and multiply: organelle partitioning in yeast. *Curr Opin Cell Biol*, **12**, 509–16.

Chattopadhyay, S. and Pearce, D. A. (2002). Btn2p-mediated changes in arginine and lysine uptake: altered arginine and lysine content in the vacuole of batten disease yeast (in press).

Cheever, M. L., Sato, T. K., de Beer, T., Kutateladze, T. G., Emr, S. D. and Overduin, M. (2001). Phox domain interaction with PtdIns(3)P targets the Vam7 t-SNARE to vacuole membranes. *Nat Cell Biol*, **3**, 613–8.

Chisholm, V. T., Lea, H. Z., Rai, R. and Cooper, T. G. (1987). Regulation of allantoate transport in wild-type and mutant strains of *Saccharomyces cerevisiae*. *J Bacteriol*, 169, 1684–90.

Conibear, E. and Stevens, T. H. (2000). Vps52p, Vps53p, and Vps54p form a novel multisubunit complex required for protein sorting at the yeast late Golgi. *Mol Biol Cell*, **11**, 305–23.

Conradt, B., Shaw, J., Vida, T., Emr, S. and Wickner, W. (1992). In vitro reactions of vacuole inheritance in *Saccharomyces cerevisiae*. *J Cell Biol*, **119**, 1469–79.

Cooper, A. and Bussey, H. (1992). Yeast Kex1p is a Golgi-associated membrane protein: deletions in a cytoplasmic targeting domain result in mislocalization to the vacuolar membrane. *J Cell Biol*, **119**, 1459–68.

Cowles, C. R., Odorizzi, G., Payne, G. S. and Emr, S. D. (1997). The AP-3 adaptor complex is essential for cargo-selective transport to the yeast vacuole. *Cell*, **91**, 109–18.

Craighead, M. W., Bowden, S., Watson, R. and Armstrong, J. (1993). Function of the ypt2 gene in the exocytic pathway of *Schizosaccharomyces pombe*. *Mol Biol Cell*, **4**, 1069–76.

Croopnick, J. B., Choi, H. C. and Mueller, D. M. (1998). The subcellular location of the yeast *Saccharomyces cerevisiae* homologue of the protein defective in the juvenile form of Batten disease. *Biochem Biophys Res Commun*, **250**, 335–41.

Darsow, T., Rieder, S. E. and Emr, S. D. (1997). A multispecificity syntaxin homologue, Vam3p, essential for autophagic and biosynthetic protein transport to the vacuole. *J Cell Biol*, **138**, 517–29.

Darsow, T., Katzmann, D. J., Cowles, C. R. and Emr, S. D. (2001). Vps41p function in the alkaline phosphatase pathway requires homo-oligomerization and interaction with AP-3 through two distinct domains. *Mol Biol Cell*, **12**, 37–51.

Davis, N. G., Horecka, J. L. and Sprague, G. F. Jr (1993). Cis- and trans-acting functions required for endocytosis of the yeast pheromone receptors. *J Cell Biol*, **122**, 53–65.

Dell'Angelica, E. C., Ooi, C. E. and Bonifacino, J. S. (1997). Beta3A-adaptin, a subunit of the adaptor-like complex AP-3. *J Biol Chem*, **272**, 15078–84.

Dell'Angelica, E. C., Puertollano, R., Mullins, C. *et al.* (2000). GGAs: a family of ADP ribosylation factor-binding proteins related to adaptors and associated with the Golgi complex. *J Cell Biol*, **149**, 81–94.

Diantonio, A., Burgess, R. W., Chin, A. C., Deitcher, D. L., Scheller, R. H. and Schwarz, T. L. (1993). Identification and characterization of *Drosophila* genes for synaptic vesicle proteins. *J Neurosci*, **13**, 4924–35.

Fares, H. and Greenwald, I. (2001). Regulation of endocytosis by CUP-5, the *Caenorhabditis elegans* mucolipin-1 homolog. *Nat Genet*, **28**, 64–8.

GarciaRanea, J. A. and Valencia, A. (1998). Distribution and functional diversification of the ras superfamily in *Saccharomyces cerevisiae*. *FEBS Lett*, **434**, 219–25.

Gaynor, E. C., Mondesert, G., Grimme, S. J., Reed, S. I., Orlean, P. and Emr, S. D. (1999). MCD4 encodes a conserved endoplasmic reticulum membrane protein essential for glycosylphosphatidylinositol anchor synthesis in yeast. *Mol Biol Cell*, **10**, 627–48.

Graham, T. R. and Emr, S. D. (1991). Compartmental organization of Golgi-specific protein modification and vacuolar protein sorting events defined in a yeast sec18 (NSF) mutant. *J Cell Biol*, **114**, 207–18.

Grant, B. and Hirsh, D. (1999). Receptor-mediated endocytosis in the *Caenorhabditis elegans* oocyte. *Mol Biol Cell*, **10**, 4311–26.

Grant, B., Zhang, Y., Paupard, M. C., Lin, S. X., Hall, D. H. and Hirsh, D. (2001). Evidence that RME-1, a conserved *C. elegans* EH-domain protein, functions in endocytic recycling. *Nat Cell Biol*, **3**, 573–9.

Greener, T., Grant, B., Zhang, Y. *et al.* (2001). *Caenorhabditis elegans* auxilin: a J-domain protein essential for clathrin-mediated endocytosis in vivo. *Nat Cell Biol*, **3**, 215–19.

Hama, H., Tall, G. G. and Horazdovsky, B. F. (1999). Vps9p is a guanine nucleotide exchange factor involved in vesicle-mediated vacuolar protein transport. *J Biol Chem*, **274**, 15284–91.

Henrissat, B. and Davies, G. J. (2000). Glycoside hydrolases and glycosyltransferases. Families, modules, and implications for genomics. *Plant Physiol*, **124**, 1515–9.

Herscovics, A. (1999). Processing glycosidases of *Saccharomyces cerevisiae*. *Biochim Biophys Acta*, **1426**, 275–85.

Hill, A. A., Hunter, C. P., Tsung, B. T., Tucker-Kellogg, G. and Brown, E. L. (2000). Genomic analysis of gene expression in *C. elegans*. *Science*, **290**, 809–12.

Hirst, J., Lui, W. W., Bright, N. A., Totty, N., Seaman, M. N. and Robinson, M. S. (2000). A family of proteins with gamma-adaptin and VHS domains that facilitate trafficking between the trans-Golgi network and the vacuole/lysosome. *J Cell Biol*, **149**, 67–80.

Horazdovsky, B. F., Busch, G. R. and Emr, S. D. (1994). VPS21 encodes a rab5-like GTP binding protein that is required for the sorting of yeast vacuolar proteins. *EMBO J*, **13**, 1297–309.

Iwasaki, K. and Toyonaga, R. (2000). The Rab3 GDP/GTP exchange factor homolog AEX-3 has a dual function in synaptic transmission. *EMBO J*, **19**, 4806–16.

Jakob, C. A., Burda, P., Roth, J. and Aebi, M. (1998). Degradation of misfolded endoplasmic reticulum glycoproteins in *Saccharomyces cerevisiae* is determined by a specific oligosaccharide structure. *J Cell Biol*, **142**, 1223–33.

Jedd, G., Mulholland, J. and Segev, N. (1997). Two new Ypt GTPases are required for exit from the yeast trans-Golgi compartment. *J Cell Biol*, **137**, 563–80.

Jiang, M., Ryu, J., Kiraly, M., Duke, K., Reinke, V. and Kim, S. K. (2001). Genome-wide analysis of developmental and sex-regulated gene expression profiles in *Caenorhabditis elegans*. *Proc Natl Acad Sci USA*, **98**, 218–23.

Klionsky, D. J. and Ohsumi, Y. (1999). Vacuolar import of proteins and organelles from the cytoplasm. *Annu Rev Cell Dev Biol*, **15**, 1–32.

Kohrer, K. and Emr, S. D. (1993). The yeast VPS17 gene encodes a membrane-associated protein required for the sorting of soluble vacuolar hydrolases. *J Biol Chem*, **268**, 559–69.

Kramer, H. and Phistry, M. (1996). Mutations in the *Drosophila* hook gene inhibit endocytosis of the boss transmembrane ligand into multivesicular bodies. *J Cell Biol*, **133**, 1205–15.

Kramer, H. and Phistry, M. (1999). Genetic analysis of hook, a gene required for endocytic trafficking in *Drosophila*. *Genetics*, **151**, 675–84.

Kretzschmar, D., Poeck, B., Roth, H. *et al.* (2000). Defective pigment granule biogenesis and aberrant behavior caused by mutations in the *Drosophila* AP-3 beta adaptin gene ruby. *Genetics*, **155**, 213–23.

Lazar, T., Gotte, M. and Gallwitz, D. (1997). Vesicular transport: how many Ypt/Rab-GTPases make a eukaryotic cell? *Trends Biochem Sci*, **22**, 468–72.

Lee, R. Y., Sawin, E. R., Chalfie, M., Horvitz, H. R. and Avery, L. (1999). EAT-4, a homolog of a mammalian sodium-dependent inorganic phosphate cotransporter, is necessary for glutamatergic neurotramsmission in *Caenorhabditis elegans*. *J Neurosci*, **19**, 159–67.

Lin, X., Hengartner, M. O. and Kolesnick, R. (1998). *Caenorhabditis elegans* contains two distinct acid sphingomyelinases. *J Biol Chem*, **273**, 14374–79.

Lin, S. X., Grant, B., Hirsh, D. and Maxfield, F. R. (2001). Rme-1 regulates the distribution and function of the endocytic recycling compartment in mammalian cells. *Nat Cell Biol*, **3**, 567–72.

Llorente, B. and Dujon, B. (2000). Transcriptional regulation of the *Saccharomyces cerevisiae* DAL5 gene family and identification of the high affinity nicotinic acid permease TNA1 (YGR260w). *FEBS Lett*, **475**, 237–41.

Lloyd, V., Ramaswami, M. and Kramer, H. (1998). Not just pretty eyes: *Drosophila* eye-colour mutations and lysosomal delivery. *Trends Cell Biol*, **8**, 257–9.

Martinez, J. P., Elorza, M. V., Gozalbo, D. and Sentandreu, R. (1982). Regulation of alpha-galactosidase synthesis in *Saccharomyces cerevisiae* and effect of cerulenin on the secretion of this enzyme. *Biochim Biophys Acta*, **716**, 158–68.

Matyash, V., Geier, C., Henske *et al.* (2001). Distribution and transport of cholesterol in *Caenorhabditis elegans*. *Mol Biol Cell*, **12**, 1725–36.

von Mollard, G. F., Nothwehr, S. F. and Stevens, T. H. (1997). The yeast v-SNARE Vtilp mediates two vesicle transport pathways through interactions with the t-SNAREs Sed5p and Pep12p. *J Cell Biol*, **137**, 1511–24.

Moynihan, E. B. and Enoch, T. (1999). Lizlp, a novel fission yeast membrane protein, is required for normal cell division when ribonucleotide reductase is inhibited. *Mol Biol Cell*, **10**, 245–57.

Mullins, C. and Bonifacino, J. S. (2001). The molecular machinery for lysosome biogenesis. *Bioessays*, **23**, 333–43.

Mullins, C., Hartnell, L. M., Wassarman, D. A. and Bonifacino, J. S. (1999). Defective expression of the mu3 subunit of the AP-3 adaptor complex in the *Drosophila* pigmentation mutant carmine. *Molecular General Genetics*, **262**, 401–412.

Mullins, C., Hartnell, L. M. and Bonifacino, J. S. (2000). Distinct requirements for the AP-3 adaptor complex in pigment granule and synaptic vesicle biogenesis in *Drosophila melanogaster*. *Mol Gen Genet*, **263**, 1003–14.

Munn, A. L. (2000). The yeast endocytic membrane transport System. *Microsc Res Technol*, **51**, 547–562.

Munn, A. L. (2001). Molecular requirements for the internalisation step of endocyto: insights from yeast. *Biochim Biophys Acta*, **1535**, 236–57.

Nakamura, N., Hirata, A., Ohsumi, Y. and Wada, Y. (1997). Vam2/vps41p and Vam6/Vps39p are components of a protein complex on the vacuolar membranes and involved in the yeast *Saccharomyces cerevisiae*. *J Biol Chem*, **272**, 11344–9.

Narayanan, R., Kramer, H. and Ramaswami, M. (2000). *Drosophila* endosomal proteins hook and deep orange regulate synapse size but not synaptic vesicle recycling. *J Neurobiol*, **45**, 105–19.

Nonet, M. L., Staunton, J. E., Kilgard, M. P. *et al.* (1997). *Caenorhabditis elegans* rab-3 mutant synapses exhibit impaired function and are partially depleted of vesicles. *J Neurosci*, **17**, 8061–73.

Odorizzi, G., Babst, M. and Emr, S. D. (2000). Phosphoinositide signaling and the regulation of membrane trafficking in yeast. *Trends Biochem Sci*, **25**, 229–35.

Okuyama, M., Okuno, A., Shimizu, N., Mori, H., Kimura, A. and Chiba, S. (2001). Carboxyl group of residue Asp647 as possible proton donor in catalytic reaction of alpha-glucosidase from *Schizosaccharomyces pombe*. *Eur J Biochem*, **268**, 2270–80.

Oliver, S. G. (1996). From DNA sequence to biological function. *Nature*, **379**, 597–600.

Ooi C. E., Moreira, J. E., Dell'Angelica, E. C., Poy, G., Wassarman, D. A. and Bonifacino, J. S. (1997). Altered expression of a novel adaptin leads to defective pigment granule biogenesis in the *Drosophila* eye color mutant garnet. *EMBO J*, **16**, 4508–18.

Packeiser, A. N., Urakov, V. N., Polyakova, Y. A. *et al.* (1999). A novel vacuolar protein encoded by SSU21/MCD4 is involved in cell wall integrity in yeast. *Yeast*, **15**, 1485–501.

Panek, H. R., Stepp, J. D., Engle, H. M. *et al.* (1997). Suppressors of YCK-encoded yeast casein kinase 1 deficiency define the four subunits of a novel clathrin AP-like complex. *EMBO J*, **16**, 4194–204.

Payne, G. S., Baker, D., van Tuinen, E. and Schekman, R. (1988). Protein transport to the vacuole and receptor-mediated endocytosis by clathrin heavy chain-deficient yeast. *J Cell Biol*, **106**, 1453–61.

Pearce, D. A. (2000). Localization and processing of CLN3, the protein associated to Batten disease: where is it and what does it do? *J Neurosci Res*, **59**, 19–23.

Pearce, D. A. and Sherman, F. (1998). A yeast model for the study of Batten disease. *Proc Natl Acad Sci USA*, **95**, 6915–8.

Pearce, D. A., Ferea, T., Nosel, S. A., Das, B. and Sherman, F. (1999). Action of BTN1, the yeast orthologue of the gene mutated in Batten disease. *Nat Genet*, **22**, 55–8.

Peterson, M. R. and Emr, S. D. (2001). The class c vps complex functions at multiple stages of the vacuolar transport pathway. *Traffic*, **2**, 476–86.

Piper, R. C., Whitters, E. A. and Stevens, T. H. (1994). Yeast Vps45p is a Sec1p-like protein required for the consumption of vacuole-targeted, post-Golgi transport vesicles. *Eur J Cell Biol*, **65**, 305–18.

Piper, R. C., Cooper, A. A., Yang, H. and Stevens, T. H. (1995). VPS27 controls vacuolar and endocytic traffic through a prevacuolar compartment in *Saccharomyces cerevisiae*. *J Cell Biol*, **131**, 603–17.

Pistillo, D., Manzi, A., Tinow, A., Boyl, P. P., Graziani, F. and Malva, C. (1998). The *Drosophila* melanogaster lipase homologs: a gene family with tissue and developmental specific expression. *J Mol Biol*, **276**, 877–85.

Rad, M. R., Phan, H. L., Kirchrath, L. *et al.* (1995). *Saccharomyces cerevisiae* Ap12p, a homologue of the mammalian clathrin AP beta subunit, plays a role in clathrin-dependent Golgi functions. *J Cell Sci*, **108**, 1605–15.

Radisky, D. C., Snyder, W. B., Emr, S. D. and Kaplan, J. (1997). Characterization of VPS41, a gene required for vacuolar trafficking and high-affinity iron transport in yeast. *Proc Natl Acad Sci USA*, **94**, 5662–6.

Rai, R., Genbauffe, F. S. and Cooper, T. G. (1988). Structure and transcription of the allantoate permease gene (DAL5) from *Saccharomyces cerevisiae*. *J Bacteriol*, **170**, 266–71.

Rankin, C. H. and Wicks, S. R. (2000). Mutations of the *Caenorhabditis elegans* brain specific inorganic phosphate transporter eat-4 affect habituation of the tap-withdrawal response without affecting the response itself. *J Neurosci*, **20**, 4337–44.

Raths, S., Rohrer, J., Crausaz, F. and Riezman, H. (1993). end3 and end4: two mutants defective in receptor-mediated and fluid-phase endocytosis in *Saccharomyces cerevisiae*. *J Cell Biol*, **120**, 55–65.

Raymond, C. K., Howald-Stevenson, I., Vater, C. A. and Stevens, T. H. (1992). Morphological classification of the yeast vacuolar protein sorting mutants: evidence for a prevacuolar compartment in class E vps mutants. *Mol Biol Cell*, **3**, 1389–402.

Rehling, P., Darsow, T., Katzmann, D. J. and Emr, S. D. (1999). Formation of AP-3 transport intermediates requires Vps41 function. *Nat Cell Biol*, **1**, 346–53.

Reider, S. E., Banta, L. M., Kohrer, K., McCaffery, J. M. and Emr, S. D. (1996). Multilamellar endosome-like compartment accumulates in the yeast vps28 vacuolar protein sorting mutant. *Mol Biol Cell*, **7**, 985–99.

Rieder, S. E. and Emr, S. D. (1997). A novel RING finger protein complex essential for a late step in protein transport to the yeast vacuole. *Mol Biol Cell*, **8**, 2307–27.

Sato, T. K., Darsow, T. and Emr, S. D. (1998). Vam7p, a SNAP-25-like molecule, and Vam3p, a syntaxin homolog, function together in yeast vacuolar protein trafficking. *Mol Cell Biol*, **18**, 5308–19.

Schandel, K. A. and Jenness, D. D. (1994). Direct evidence for ligand-induced internalization of the yeast alpha-factor pheromone receptor. *Mol Cell Biol*, **14**, 7245–55.

Seaman, M. N., Marcusson, E. G., Cereghino, J. L. and Emr, S. D. (1997). Endosome to Golgi retrieval of the vacuolar potein sorting receptor, Vps10p, requires the function of the VPS29, VPS30, and VPS35 gene products. *J Cell Biol*, **137**, 79–92.

Seaman, M. N., McCaffery, J. M. and Emr, S. D. (1998). A membrane coat complex essential for endosome-to-Golgi retrograde transport in yeast. *J Cell Biol*, **142**, 665–81.

Sevrioukov, E. A., He, J. P., Moghrabi, N., Sunio, A. and Kramer, H. (1999). A role for the deep orange and carnation eye color genes in lysosomal delivery in *Drosophila*. *Mol Cell*, **4**, 479–86.

Shea, J. E., Toyn, J. H. and Johnston, L. H. (1994). The budding yeast U5 snRNP Prp8 is a highly conserved protein which links RNA splicing with cell cycle progression. *Nucleic Acids Res*, **22**, 5555–64.

Simeon, A., van der Klei, I. J., Veenhuis, M. and Wolf, D. H. (1992). Ubiquitin, a central component of selective cytoplasmic proteolysis, is linked to proteins residing at the locus of non-selective proteolysis, the vacuole. *FEBS Lett*, **301**, 231–5.

Simpson, F., Peden, A. A., Christopoulou, L. and Robinson, M. S. (1997). Characterization of the adaptor-related protein complex, AP-3. *J Cell Biol*, **137**, 835–45.

Singer, B. and Riezman, H. (1990). Detection of an intermediate compartment involved in transport of alpha-factor from the plasma membrane to the vacuole in yeast. *J Cell Biol*, **110**, 1911–22.

Singer-Kruger, B., Frank, R., Crausaz, F. and Riezman, H. (1993). Partial purification and characterization of early and late endosomes from yeast. Identification of four novel proteins. *J Biol Chem*, **268**, 14376–86.

Stack, J. H., DeWald, D. B., Takegawa, K. and Emr, S. D. (1995). Vesicle-mediated protein transport: regulatory interactions between the Vps15 protein kinase and the Vps34 PtdIns 3-kinase essential for protein sorting to the vacuole in yeast. *J Cell Biol*, **129**, 321–34.

Stack, J. H., Herman, P. K., Schu, P. V. and Emr, S. D. (1993). A membrane-associated complex containing the Vps15 protein kinase and the Vps34 PI 3-kinase is essential for protein sorting to the yeast lysosome-like vacuole. *EMBO J*, **12**, 2195–204.

Stepp, J. D., Huang, K. and Lemmon, S. K. (1997). The yeast adaptor protein complex, AP-3, is essential for the efficient delivery of alkaline phosphatase by the alternate pathway to the vacuole. *J Cell Biol*, **139**, 1761–74.

Sunio, A., Metcalf, A. B. and Kramer, H. (1999). Genetic dissection of endocytic trafficking in *Drosophila* using a horseradish peroxidase-bride of sevenless chimera: hook is required for normal maturation of multivesicular endosomes. *Mol Biol Cell*, **10**, 847–59.

Tabuchi, M., Iwaihara, O., Ohtani, Y. *et al.* (1997). Vacuolar protein sorting in fission yeast: cloning, biosynthesis, transport, and processing of carboxypeptidase Y from *Schizosaccharomyces pombe*. *J Bacteriol*, **179**, 4179–89.

Takeshige, K., Baba, M., Tsuboi, S., Noda, T. and Ohsumi, Y. (1992). Autophagy in yeast demonstrated with proteinase-deficient mutants and conditions for its induction. *J Cell Biol*, **119**, 301–11.

Tang, Z., Kuo, T., Shen, J. and Lin, R. J. (2000). Biochemical and genetic conservation of fission yeast Dsk1 and human SR protein-specific kinase1. *Mol Cell Biol*, **20**, 816–24.

Thumm, M., Egner, R., Koch, B. *et al.* (1994). Isolation of autophagocytosis mutants of *Saccharomyces cerevisiae*. *FEBS Lett*, **349**, 257–80.

Tsukada, M. and Ohsumi, Y. (1993). Isolation and characterization of autophagy-defective mutants of *Saccharomyces cerevisiae*. *FEBS Lett*, **333**, 169–74.

Turoscy, V. and Cooper, T. G. (1987). Ureidosuccinate is transported by the allantoate transport system in *Saccharomyces cerevisiae*. *J Bacteriol*, **169**, 2598–600.

Urano, J., Tabancay, A. P., Yang, W. and Tamanoi, F. (2000). The *Saccharomyces cerevisiae* Rheb G-protein is involved in regulating canavanine resistance and arginine uptake. *J Biol Chem*, **275**, 11198–206.

Vater, C. A., Raymond, C. K., Ekena, K., Howald-Stevenson, I. and Stevens, T. H. (1992). The VPS1 protein, a homolog of dynamin required for vacuolar protein sorting in *Saccharomyces cerevisiae*, is a GTPase with two functionally separable domains. *J Cell Biol*, **119**, 773–86.

Vida, T. A. and Emr, S. D. (1995). A new vital stain for visualizing vacuolar membrane dynamics and endocytosis in yeast. *J Cell Biol*, **128**, 779–92.

Wada, Y., Nakamura, N., Ohsumi, Y. and Hirata, A. (1997). Vam3p, a new member of syntaxin related protein, is required for vacuolar assembly in the yeast *Saccharomyces cerevisiae*. *J Cell Sci*, **110**, 1299–306.

Walenta, J. H., Didier, A. J., Liu, X. and Kramer, H. (2001). The Golgi-associated hook3 protein is a member of a novel family of microtubule-binding proteins. *J Cell Biol*, **152**, 923–34.

Wang, Y. X., Zhao, H., Harding, T. M. *et al.* (1996). Multiple classes of yeast mutants are defective in vacuole partitioning yet target vacuole proteins correctly. *Mol Biol Cell*, **7**, 1375–89.

Wang, Y. X., Catlett, N. L. and Weisman, L. S. (1998). Vac8p, a vacuolar protein with armadillo repeats, functions in both vacuole inheritance and protein targeting from the cytoplasm to vacuole. *J Cell Biol*, **140**, 1063–74.

Wang, Y. X., Kauffman, E. J., Duex, J. E. and Weisman, L. S. (2001). Fusion of docked membranes requires the armadillo repeat protein Vac8p. *J Biol Chem* (epub ahead of print).

Warren, G. and Wickner, W. (1996). Organelle inheritance. *Cell*, **84**, 395–400.

Wendland, B., Steece, K. E. and Emr, S. D. (1999). Yeast epsins contain an essential N-terminal ENTH domain, blind clathrin and are required for endocytosis. *EMBO J*, **18**, 4383–93.

Wurmser, A. E., Sato, T. K. and E. M. R. S. D. (2000). New component of the vacuolar class C-Vps complex couples nucleotide exchange on the Ypt7 GTPase to SNARE-dependent docking and fusion. *J Cell Biol*, **151**, 551–62.

Zhan, R., Stevenson, B. J., Schroder-Kohne, S., Zanolari, B., Riezman, H. and Munn, A. L. (2001). End13p/Vps4p is required for efficient transport from early to late endosomes in *Saccharomyces cerevisiae. J Cell Sci*, **114**, 1935–47.

Zhang, Y., Grant, B. and Hirsh, D. (2001). RME-8, a conserved J-domain protein, is required for endocytosis in *Caenorhabditis elegans. Mol Biol Cell*, **12**, 2011–21.

Zheng, Y., Brockie, P. J., Mellem, J. E., Madsen, D. M. and Maricq, A. V. (1999). Neuronal control of locomotion in *C. elegans* is modified by a dominant mutation in the GLR-1 ionotropic glutamate receptor. *Neuron*, **24**, 347–61.

Chapter 11

Spontaneous and engineered mammalian storage disease models

John J. Hopwood, Allison C. Crawley and Rosanne M. Taylor

Lysosomal storage disorders are inherited disorders of lysosomal organelle dysfunction. The relative rarity of storage diseases, their broad heterogeneous clinical presentation, and varied genetic background, together with ethical restrictions, make studies to understand their pathophysiology or to evaluate the efficacy of therapies difficult in humans. Animals with lysosomal disorders have long been of considerable importance in the development of therapy and in understanding the pathophysiology of these disorders in patients. Authentic animal models complement patients with their availability, genetic homogeneity, and their convenience and flexibility to enable the design of relatively simple experiments. Over the past 20 years, a large number of animal models have been identified and studied. Over the past 5 years in particular, results have encouraged the extension of these studies to natural history studies and clinical trials of therapies in patients.

This chapter summarizes the spontaneous and induced mammalian animal models and discusses their characteristics relative to their human disease equivalent. The advantages and limitations of each model relative to the human disorder are also discussed.

A number of lysosomal storage diseases are grouped according to the nature of the material or undigested substrate that is stored in lysosomes. The major storage disease groups include the sphingolipidoses, mucopolysaccharidoses, glycoproteinoses, glycogen storage disorders, mucolipidoses, and the neuronal ceroid lipofuscinoses.

A word of caution: while the advantages of specific animal models are obvious, species differences in development and metabolic pathways must be appreciated if the goal of these studies is to improve the quality of life of humans affected by lysosomal storage diseases. The creation of mouse models of human disease by gene targeting has enabled the evaluation of the pathophysiology of many of these disorders. Although many of these models provide reasonably accurate copies of the human disease, many do not precisely match their human equivalent.

Sphingolipidoses

There are a number of sphingolipids. These are made from a common core of ceramide (sphingosine fatty acid esters) esterified to sialated oligosaccharides to form gangliosides, to neutral oligosaccharides to form globosides, or to phosphocholine to form sphingomyelin. Inherited defects in the degradation of sphingolipids represent a major group of storage diseases known as the sphingolipidoses (see Chapter 2). Animal models for all of the sphingolipidoses have been identified, and their details are described and listed in Table 11.1.

Table 11.1 Sphingolipidoses

1. SAP precursor deficiency	Prosaposin (contains saposins A, B, C, and D); substrates include multiple glycolipids.
Murine	Targeted disruption of the prosaposin gene, at exon 3 with the neomycin-resistance gene, produced a model that resembles the biochemical and clinical phenotype of patients, except affected mice do not have organomegaly. Mice survive birth to develop a rapidly progressive neurological disease before death at about 5 weeks. Demyelination and storage of periodic acid–Schiff (PAS)-positive material throughout the nervous system and abnormal cells in liver and spleen were observed. Most prominent materials stored in brain, liver, and kidney are ceramide, glucosylceramide, galactosylceramide, sulfatide, and globotriosylceramide. The ultrastructural features of inclusions in these mice appear to be different from those of other known sphingolipidoses (Fujita *et al.* 1996; Oya *et al.* 1998).
Murine	Introduction of the amino acid substitution C106F into the saposin A domain of prosaposin eliminated one of three conserved disulfide bonds (Matsuda *et al.* 2001). Saposin A-deficient mice slowly developed progressive hind leg paralysis with onset at 2–3 months and survival up to 5 months. Tremors and shaking only became obvious at the terminal stage. Tissue and chemical pathology of this model were quantitatively identical, but clinically milder, to that seen in infantile globoid cell leukodystrophy (Krabbe). Thus, it was proposed that saposin A is required for the lysosomal turnover of galactosylceramide.
2. Niemann–Pick disease types A/B	Lysosomal sphingomyelinase; substrates include sphingomyelin
Murine	Targeted disruption, using two different methods, gave essentially the same phenotype—normal at birth and up to 3 months, ataxia at 5 months, and death between 6 and 8 months (Horinouchi *et al.* 1995; Otterbach and Stoffel 1995). Knockout mice have considerably higher numbers of enlarged and often multinucleated macrophages in their pulmonary airspaces at a few weeks of age. These mice also have elevated levels of sphingomyelin in their airways at 10 weeks of age. Histology of alveolar walls of the affected mice shows increased cellularity (Dhami *et al.* 2001). The central nervous system (CNS) has lipid storage vacuoles in neurones and an almost complete absence of Purkinje cells in 3-month-old affected animals (Sarna *et al.* 2001). This model mimics type A Niemann–Pick patients who often present with hepatosplenomegaly and nervous system involvement in early infancy and die in the first 10 years of life as a result of neurodegeneration.
Murine	A transgenic knockout strategy was used to create a mouse able to stably express low levels of lysosomal sphingomyelinase in the complete absence of secretory sphingomyelinase. These mice exhibit approximately 15% of wild-type enzyme activity in their brain. Other organs had 1–14% of wild-type activity. Mice develop without severe neurologic disease and have normal lifespans. Low expression of lysosomal sphingomyelinase in brain is able to preserve CNS function (Marathe *et al.* 2000). This mouse, without CNS involvement, provides a model for Niemann–Pick type B where patients present as older children or adults with hepatosplenomegaly without signs of CNS dysfunction.

Feline	Several reports have appeared on the occurrence of lysosomal sphingomyelinase deficiency in cats including Siamese (Wenger *et al.* 1980), Balinese (Baker *et al.* 1984) and Black Oriental Shorthair (Cuddon *et al.* 1989) breeds. Neurological disease was prominent in each.
Canine	One report on lysosomal sphingomyelinase deficiency has been reported in dogs (miniature Poodle) (Bundza *et al.* 1979). The affected animal exhibited some neurological disease.
3. Niemann–Pick disease type C	Lysosomal membrane cholesterol trafficking; two genes: *NPC1*, a polytropicmembrane-bound protein with putative sterol-sensing domain; *NPC2*, epididymal secretory glycoprotein 1.
Murine	Initially, Pentchev *et al* (1980) described this disease in a strain of BALB/c mice with loss of coordination, weight loss, and premature death. Miyawaki *et al* (1982) described C57BL/6JS mice with similar clinical findings. These two independently derived colonies played a pivotal role in delineating the biochemical basis of this disorder. One, a BALB/c mouse presented with clinical and biochemical features of this disorder (Pentchev *et al.* 1984); the other, a C57BL/KS mouse was originally characterized as a sphingomyelinosis because of attenuated sphingomyelinase activity and excess sphingomyelin accumulation (Miyawaki *et al.* 1986; Kitagawa 1987). Retarded myelination and cerebellar degeneration have been described (Weintraub *et al.* 1985; Higashi *et al.* 1993). Myelination of regenerating axons was retarded in affected mice following sciatic nerve crush (Goodrum and Pentchev 1997). The functional disturbance in *NPC1* appears to disrupt vesicular transport of cholesterol, glycolipids, and other components necessary for the maintenance of neurones (Liu *et al.* 2000; Ong *et al.* 2001). Brains of affected mice had signs of extensive damage throughout, including neurofibrillary tangles and intracellular storage of various compounds. Loss of cerebellar Purkinje cells was the most specific damage (Yadid *et al.* 1998).
Murine	The mutation in the *NPC1* gene is an insertion of an 824 bp sequence along with a 703 bp deletion of genomic sequence consisting of 44 bp of exon sequence. The resulting transcript results in a truncated protein that is one-third the size of the wild-type protein and excludes 11 of 13 transmembrane domains (Loftus *et al.* 1997).
Feline	A domestic short-hair 9-week-old kitten presented with progressive neurological dysfunction and histopathological lesions consistent with a lysosomal storage disorder. Large numbers of foamy macrophages were seen in the liver, spleen, lymph nodes, and lung (Lowenthal *et al.* 1990; Brown *et al.* 1994; March *et al.* 1997). Affected cats displayed a subtle intention tremor noticed initially at 8–12 weeks of age. The disease was rapidly progressive, with the tremor becoming more pronounced and developing severe dysmetria and ataxia. Cats died or were euthanized between 12 and 43 weeks of age. Pathological findings included accumulation of substrate within neurones throughout the CNS and axonal spheroid formation. The clinical and pathological findings in these cats are comparable to those in the human form of the disease (Munana *et al.* 1994). Cell complementation studies confirmed the involvement of *NPC1* gene in the pathology (Somers *et al.* 1999).

Table 11.1 *(continued)*

4. Wolman disease	Acid lipase; substrates include cholesterol esters and triglycerides.
Murine	Targeted disruption of the mouse lysosomal lipase gene was used to create a knockout model of cholesterol ester storage disease with massive accumulation of triglycerides and cholesteryl esters in several organs. Affected mice are fertile and can be bred to produce progeny. The histopathology of the model is reported to mimic the human disease (Du *et al.* 1998; 2001).
5. Gaucher	Glucocerebrosidase; substrate, glucosylceramide.
Murine	Targeted disruption was used to develop Gaucher mice. Homozygous mice die *in utero* or within 34 h of birth, with extensive lysosomal storage of glucosyl ceramide (Tybulewicz *et al.* 1992). This model is similar to acute infantile type (collodion baby).
Murine	A knock-in process was used to produce mice homologous for L444P, RecNcil, or D456P. L444P homozygotes have more glucosylceramidase activity and less storage than RecNcil homozygotes—both variants died within 48 h of birth (Liu *et al.* 1998). Studies of the nature of storage of glucosylceramide species in the RecNcil homozygous mouse show that omega-hydroxylated glucosylceramides, which are protein-bound to the epidermal cornified cell envelope of the transgenic mouse, accumulate up to 35-fold, whereas levels of related protein-bound ceramides and fatty acids were decreased to normal control levels (Doering *et al.* 1999).
Ovine	Gaucher has been identified in newborn lambs (Hopwood, unpublished observations).
Canine	Gaucher disease was identified in Sydney silky terriers in Sydney. Dogs had very low glucosylceramidase activity in peripheral blood leucocytes, diagnostic of Gaucher. They developed tremors and ataxia from 3 months of age and progressed to severe neurological disease by 6 months (Farrow *et al.* 1982).
6. Krabbe	Galactocerebrosidase; substrates include galactocerebroside and galactosylshingosine.
Murine	'Twitcher' is a naturally occurring model that has abundant and characteristic inclusions in lymph nodes and kidney (Takahashi *et al.* 1983, 1984). Mice exhibit stunted growth, tremor, and abnormal postural reactions that begin at 20 days and progress to severe tremor, ataxia, hind limb weakness, and paralysis, and despite intensive care, die before 3 months of age. The affected mouse is an authentic model for Krabbe, a genetic demyelinating disorder (Komiyama and Suzuki 1994). The nonsense mutation is in codon 339 (TGG to TGA) (Sakai *et al.* 1996). Affected mice develop clinical signs at the onset of myelin remodelling from day 15 (Taniike and Suzuki 1994) and, if untreated, die by day 35. The pathology is very similar to that seen in human disease, with the accumulation of toxic psychosine as the primary cause of the pathogenesis (Suzuki and Suzuki 1995). Immune and inflammatory responses to myelin degradation play a central role in the rapid progress of the disease (Suzuki and Ohno 1995). Major histocompatibility complex (MHC) class II expression worsens the severity of disease (Matsushima *et al.* 1994), while interleukin-6

	(IL-6) upregulation during twitcher disease reduces the disruption of the blood—brain barrier and gliosis (Pedchenko and Levine 1999). Oliogodendrocytes are lost through apoptosis (Taniike *et al.* 1999).
Murine	Doubly deficient mice (deficient in galactosylceramide synthase-galactocerebrosidase synthesis and Twitcher deficient in galactocerebroside catabolism) developed later, mild signs (Ezoe *et al.* 2000).
Murine	Homologous recombination was used to produce the H168C mutation in the mouse galactocerebrosidase gene. These mice developed symptoms that were delayed by about 2 weeks compared to the natural 'Twitcher' mouse. The H168C mice accumulate psychosine and show pathological changes in the CNS and peripheral nervous systems at a slower rate and live about 2 weeks longer than the 'Twitcher' mice (Luzi *et al.* 2001).
Canine	West Highland white and cairn terriers have been reported with progressive accumulation of psychosine in the brain and inclusions in kidney. This model has the characteristic pathological findings in the nervous system seen in Krabbe patients (Igisu and Suzuki 1984; Cozzi *et al.* 1998; Wenger *et al.* 1999). Y158S was shown to be the mutation causing the Krabbe phenotype (Victoria *et al.* 1996).
Canine	Affected Irish setters with a 78 bp insertion in their galactocerebrosidase gene have been identified (Wenger *et al.* 2001).
Canine	Kelpie dogs with severe galactocerebrosidase deficiency have been identified. Dogs developed hind limb ataxia, paresis, and mild tremor at 4 months and progressed to paralysis by 6 months of age. The pathological findings resembled those in cairn and West Highland white terriers (Taylor, unpublished observations).
Monkey	Baskin *et al.* (1989) first described a monkey with a Krabbe phenotype. A 2 bp deletion was shown to cause the reduced galactocerebrosidase activity (Luzi *et al.* 1997). Two affected monkeys were identified in a colony. Both were unaffected at birth. One rapidly lost weight and developed volitional tremors, whereas the other developed tremors at day 92 and had severely decreased nerve conduction and was euthanized at day 158 (Baskin *et al.* 1998).
Feline	A domestic long-haired kitten was identified with clinical signs that included hypotonia, mental regression, and death by 2 years of age. Loss of oligodendrocytes, myelin loss, gliosis, and the perivascular accumulation of large mononuclear cells with fine cytoplasmic vacuoles in the peripheral nervous system and CNS were observed (Sigurdson *et al.* 2002).
The clinical and pathological characteristics of this group of models are similar to those observed in human disease.	
7. Krabbe	Saposin A deficiency; substrates include galactocerebroside and galactosylsphingosine.
Murine	Homologous recombination was used to produce the C106F mutation in the mouse prosaposin gene to cause a dysfunction of saposin A. Homozygous mice slowly developed progressive hind leg paralysis with clinical onset at about 2.5 months and survival up to 5 months of age. Tremors and shaking are not prominent until the terminal stage. Affected mice develop a late-onset, **Table** chronic form of globoid cell leukodystrophy, clearly indicating that saposin A is indispensable for the degradation of galactosylceramide (Matsuda *et al.* 2001).

Table 11.1 *(continued)*

8. Metachromatic leukodystrophy (MLD)	Arylsulfatase A; galactose-3-sulfatase; substrates, non-reducing end 3-sulfate ester on galactosyl residues of sulfated galactosylceramide(sulfatide), lactosylceramide, seminolipid, and lysosulfatide.
MLD as a spontaneously occuring disease has only been described in humans but a knockout model was generated. Compared to the classical MLD phenotype in humans, the most striking difference in the MLD mouse is the lack of demyelination of the CNS.	
Murine	Targeted disruption of exon 4 with a neomycin-resistance gene was used to produce a mouse with lysosomal storage of sulfatide in neuronal tissues predominantly in white matter with less storage in grey matter. Homozygous affected mice have an extremely mild phenotype, with many mice living beyond 20 months. Affected mice show various neurologic and behavioural pathologies. Gait patterns are affected. In their second year, affected mice develop a head tremor (Hess *et al.* 1996). Hyperactivity, neuromotor defects, and impaired learning and memory were studied in this model (D'Hooge *et al.* 2001). Six-month-old affected mice displayed only slight impairment in special learning and memory tests, whereas 12-month-old mice are obviously impaired in these tests. The mice were hyperactive, motor incoordinate, and slow in these tests. These results may relate to the decline of motor and cognitive functions in these affected mice. Brainstem auditory-evoked potentials were shown to coincide with loss of spiral ganglion cells in affected mice, assessed by histological examination and morphometric analysis. A significant delay in the wave pattern in the 6-month-old mice was completely absent in 9- and 12-month-old affected mice (D'Hooge *et al.* 1999*a*). Two-year-old affected mice showed altered walking characterized by shorter pace, later evolving into severe ataxia with tremor. Cerebellar histology in these mice showed that they had lost most of the calbindin immunoreactivity from their Purkinje cell dendrites, which also show simplified dendrite architecture. A considerable loss of Purkinje cells was also observed (D'Hooge *et al.* 1999*b*).
9. GM1 Gangliosidosis	Lysosomal β-galactosidase; substrates include non-reducing end β-galactosyl residues on keratan sulfate fragments, glycolipids, and glycopeptides. All animal models of GM1 gangliosidosis show CNS manifestations. Skeletal dysplasia is present in most GM1 gangliosidosis patients and animal models but not in affected mice. This difference may reflect the very low levels of keratan sulfate in mice or the time needed for these dysplasias to form.
Murine	Targeted disruption of exon 6 in the β-galactosidase gene with a neomycin-resistance gene led to mice that were normal at birth but develop progressive spastic diplegia within a few months after birth, show no overt clinical phenotype up to 4–5 months, and die of emaciation at 7–10 months of age. Vacuolated neurones appear in the spinal cord 3 days after birth. Vacuolation extended to neurones in the brainstem, cerebral cortex, hippocampus, and thalamus, and ballooning neurones became prominent with age. Tremor, ataxia, and abnormal gait become apparent in older mice (Hahn *et al.* 1997; Matsuda *et al.* 1997*a*,*b*; Itoh *et al.* 2001).
Feline	The first report of GM1 gangliosidosis in cats was in the Siamese breed by Baker and colleagues (Baker *et al.* 1971). A more slowly progressive disease was reported in the Korat breed. These Korat cats presented at 7 months with a slowly progressive neurological disease. At 21 months, the brain contained diffuse vacuolations and enlarged neurones. The clinical progression, survival time,

	biochemistry, and histology of this cat appeared somewhat different than the Siamese models of GM1 gangliosidosis and was believed similar to the human juvenile form of the disorder. (Demaria *et al.* 1998). GM1 gangliosidosis was also diagnosed in three cats that presented with clinical signs of cerebellar dysfunction, including ataxia, intention tremors, truncal sway, and generalized muscular tremors. GM1 ganglioside accumulated in brain and liver (Dial *et al.* 1994). The disease in these cats is different to that in the Korat cat. Cox *et al.* (1998, 1999) reported alterations in the growth hormone/insulin-like growth factor I pathways and thymocyte development in this model.
Canine	GM1 gangliosidosis has been reported in Beagle crossbreed dogs (Read *et al.* 1976), English Springer Spaniels (Alroy *et al.* 1985), Portuguese Water dogs and other breeds (Saunder *et al.* 1988). Pathology in Portuguese Water dogs was caused by an R60H change in the β-galactosidase gene (Wang *et al.* 2000). Progressive skeletal dysplasia was observed, with lesions observed at 2 months of age, characterized by retarded endochondral ossification and osteoporosis. These lesions were similar to those in a child with this disorder (Alroy *et al.* 1995). A 6-month-old Shiba dog with a 1-month history of progressive motor dysfunction presented with ataxia, intention tremor of the head, and dysmetria. These clinical signs were suggestive of a cerebellar disorder. Distended neurones packed with membranous cytoplasmic bodies were identified throughout the CNS (Yamato *et al.* 2000). Retarded endochondral ossification and osteoporosis were present, causing progressive skeletal dysplasia (Alroy *et al.* 1995). Alaskan huskies exhibited proportional dwarfism and progressive neurological impairment with signs of cerebellar dysfunction at 5–7 months of age (Muller *et al.* 2001). Importantly, retarded endochondral ossification, osteoporosis, and chondrocytic hypertrophy were observed in 2-month-old affected dogs. These changes are similar to those in a GM1 gangliosidosis child (Alroy *et al.* 1995).
Ovine	Lambs at 1 month presented with neurological signs and died early with ballooned neurones showing characteristic whorled membranes consistent with a gangliosidosis. Affected lambs had deficient β-galactosidase and normal *N*-acetylneuraminidase activities (Skelly *et al.* 1995). Three adult Romney ewes were identified with distended neurones containing granular eosinophilic storage material during a large neuropathological study of clinically normal sheep. The affected neurones were confined to the striatum. Phenotype suggested that these sheep are similar to human type 3 disease (Ryder and Simmons 2001).
Bovine	Friesian calves were reported with an accumulation of GM1 gangliosides in neurones with minimal morphologic hepatic changes. Vision was impaired at the late stage of the disease (Sheahan *et al.* 1974).
10. (A) GM2 Gangliosidosis type 1 (Tay–Sachs disease)	β-Hexosaminidase A, α-subunit; substrates include GM2 and higher brain gangliosides, glycoproteins, and glycosaminoglycans with β-*N*-acetylhexosaminyl residues.
Murine	Three different targeted disruptions (exon 8 or 11) of the α-subunit gene were used to produce a near total deficiency of β-hexosaminidase A and normal β-hexosaminidase B activities (Yamanaka *et al.* 1994; Cohen-Tannoudji *et al.* 1995; Taniike *et al.* 1995; Phaneuf *et al.* 1996). These mice, in contrast to classical Tay–Sachs patients, show no clinical phenotype or behavioural activities till at least 1 year. Restrictive regions of the brain, particularly in neurones in the cerebral cortex and others, are seen to progressively

Table 11.1 *(continued)*

	store GM2 gangliosides, with little relative storage in cerebellum and brainstem. No storage in the visceral organs was reported. Late-onset disease in these mice was observed in females after repeated breeding (Jeyakumar *et al.* 2002).
Deer	Two juvenile sibling male Muntjak deer with depression, ataxia, and visual deficits were shown to be deficient in β-hexosaminidase A activity. Brain and retina had characteristic inclusion bodies with massive accumulation of GM2 ganglioside in the cerebral cortex of both animals (Fox *et al.* 1999).
(B) GM2 gangliosidosis type 2 (Sandhoff disease)	β-Hexosaminidases A and B, β-subunit; substrate of the B form include glycoproteins, oligosaccharides, glycosaminoglycans, and glycolipids with β-*N*-acetylhexosaminyl residues.
Murine	Two different targeted disruptions (exon 2 or 13) of the β-subunit gene were used to produce mice deficient in both β-hexosaminidase A and β-hexosaminidase B activities but with small amounts of β-hexosaminidase S activity (Sango *et al.* 1995; Phaneuf *et al.* 1996). At 3 months, these mice underwent a progressive and severe neurological change in motor function, reflected in balance and coordination that lead to a complete loss of limb movement at 4 months with muscle wasting and hind limb rigidity. Death occurs at about 4–5 months. Lysosomal storage of GM2 ganglioside is extensive throughout neurones of cerebellum, brainstem, spinal cord, and others. Apoptotic death of neurones was seen in the Sandhoff, but not the Tay–Sachs, model with two to four times more GM2 ganglioside in the Sandhoff, compared to the Tay–Sachs mice. There is extensive intracytoplasmic storage of GM2 ganglioside in the dorsal root ganglion (Sango *et al.* 2002).
Feline	Sandhoff disease has been reported several times in cats beginning with a report by Cork and colleagues (1977). Affected cats show MR evidence of delayed myelination consistent with decreased myelin in the subcortical and internal capsule region (Kroll *et al.* 1995). A deletion of a single base in the β-subunit gene of Korat cats leads to a frameshift and a premature stop codon to produce β-hexosaminidase B deficiency and pathology in brain and liver typical of Sandhoff (Muldoon *et al.* 1994).
Canine	German short pointers have been described wih Sandhoff disease (Singer and Cork 1989). A golden retriever with a deficiency in both β-hexosaminidase A and β-hexosaminidase B activities and elevated GM2 ganglioside in CSF has also been reported (Yamato *et al.* 2002).
Porcine	Pigs with GM2 gangliosidosis have been reported (Pierce *et al.* 1976; Kosanke *et al.* 1978)
Double mutant murine	Crossbreeding of mice homozygous-disrupted for α-subunit and β-subunit genes produced mice with a total deficiency of β-hexosaminidase A, B, and S activities (Sango *et al.* 1995; Suzuki *et al.* 1998). Humans with these deficiencies have not been described. These mice, besides exhibiting gangliosidosis features, displayed dysmorphic features, dysostosis multiplex, and secretion of glycosaminoglycans characteristics of the mucopolysaccharidoses (Suzuki *et al.* 1997).

Activator deficiency	GM2 Activator; substrates include GM2 ganglioside.
Murine	Targeted disruption of exons 3 and 4 of the mouse GM2 activator gene produces a model that presents with intermediate phenotype between Tay–Sachs and Sandhoff diseases. They have an age-dependent onset of severe motor defects with a normal life expectancy. Lysosomal storage of GM2 ganglioside, and to a lesser extent GA2 glycolipid, in restricted areas of the brain (e.g. large middle layer pyramidal neurones with little storage in spinal cord or visceral organs) is seen in this model. It is claimed that the major difference between this model and Tay–Sachs mice is the additional storage of GA2 glycolipid in middle layer neurones, suggesting that the GM2 activator is also needed to degrade GA2 glycolipid in mice (Liu *et al.* 1997).
Canine	GM2 gangliosidosis in Japanese Spaniels has been reported to be due to a deficiency of the GM2 activator protein (Ishikawa *et al.* 1987).
11. Fabry	α-Galactosidase A; substrates include globotriaosylceramide, galabiosylceramide, and blood group substances with α-galactosyl residues.
Murine	Targeted disruption of the α-galactosidase A gene created mice by homologous recombination using a replacement-type vector containing both the neomycin-resistance gene, for positive selection, and the thymidine kinase, which completely lack α-galactosidase A activity. Affected mice appeared clinically normal at 10 weeks of age. Concentric lamellar inclusions were identified in kidney by ultra-structural analysis. Marked accumulation of ceramidetrihexoside was identified in kidney and liver of affected mice (Ohshima *et al.* 1997).
12. Schindler	α-Galactosidase B; substrates include sialated and asialoglycopeptides, glycosphingolipids, and oligosaccharides with non-reducing end α-*N*-acetygalactosaminyl residues.
Murine	Gene targeting techniques were used to create a mouse model. Lysosomal storage, consisting of flocculent particular material with concentric lamellar figures and multivesicular bodies, is observed in the CNS, kidney, and other organs. Neuronal storage is varied in distribution and intensity, and is seen in interstitial or mesenchymal cells in the brain, dorsal root ganglia, kidney, and other tissues. Storage is greatest in the sub-mucosal and myentric plexus of the gastrointestinal tract, with least storage in the CNS. The widespread storage in these mice appears to mimic the unique pathology of Schindler patients, particularly to that seen in type II or late-onset patients (Wang *et al.* 1993).
13. Farber lipogranulomatosis	Lysosomal ceramidase; substrate includes ceramide.
No animal models have been identified.	
14. Multiple sulfatase deficiency	Enzyme factor required for the post-translational modification of an active-site cysteine to α-formylglycine.
No animal models have been identified.	

All of the sphingolipidoses animal models have abundant neuronal storage. Significant visceral storage has been noted only in the feline model and GM2 gangliosidosis patients. The GM2 gangliosidosis mouse models have different clinical courses and phenotypes to Tay–Sachs, Sandhoff, and GM2 activator-deficient patients. In humans, GM2 ganglioside is degraded exclusively by β-hexosaminidase A activity in combination with an activator. Therefore, in these three human syndromes that result from a deficiency of α-subunit, β-subunit, or activator activity, a total block of GM2 ganglioside turnover occurs with massive storage within neurones, leading to their degeneration. However, in mice, two pathways can degrade GM2 ganglioside. One is identical to the human pathway. The other appears unique to mouse with sialidase able to degrade GM2 ganglioside to an intermediate that can be degraded by either β-hexosaminidase A or hexosaminidase B activities. Thus, the β-hexosaminidase A-deficient mouse does not have a Tay–Sachs phenotype: storage of ganglioside is reduced or prevented because ganglioside turnover through the alternate pathway via the mouse sialidase and the action of β-hexosaminidase B; a deficiency of β-hexosaminidase A and B activities in mice will lead to a Sandhoff phenotype. In the GM2 activator-deficient mouse, GM2 ganglioside turnover is blocked in both pathways leading to a phenotype similar to Tay–Sachs (Kolter and Sandhoff 1998; Gravel *et al.* 2001).

Mucopolysaccharidoses

There are a number of mucopolysaccharides, also known as glycosaminoglycans, such as dermatan sulfate, heparan sulfate, keratan sulfate, and chondroitin sulfate. These glycosaminoglycans are made from up to 20–30 sulfated repeating disaccharide structures. A stepwise process involving a number of endo- and exohydrolase and *N*-acetyltransferase activities degrades these complex carbohydrate structures. These enzymes, located in the lysosome, are mostly sulfatases and glycosidases that display extremely tight substrate specificities. Animal models are available for most mucopolysaccharidoses (MPSs) types except MPS IIIC (Table 11.2). Some mouse MPS models arose spontaneously as part of a process of natural selection, such as those that exist for MPS IIIA and MPS VII. However, most of the mouse MPS models have been produced by the application of homologous recombination. This technique has provided an opportunity to generate animal models where naturally occurring models are yet to be found. Although mouse models have provided convenient laboratory models to evaluate therapies and to study the pathophysiology of each MPS type, care should be taken in accepting these models as copies the human disease. There are obvious differences between humans and mice, particularly with skeletal dysplasias being considerably reduced in mice.

Glycoproteinoses

The glycoproteinoses represent a group of storage diseases caused by deficiencies of hydrolases required for the lysosomal degradation of the complex glyco moiety of glycoproteins (Table 11.3). This group has provided important lessons in understanding the pathogenesis of lysosomal storage in general. Heterozygote testing in large herds of α-mannosidosis-susceptible cattle and planned breeding strategies have made considerable economic gains in this industry.

Glycogen lysosomal storage disorders

This group represents a storage disease that involves the turnover of glycogen (Table 11.4).

Table 11.2 Mucopolysaccharidoses

1. MPS I (Hurler and Scheie syndromes)	α-L-Iduronidase; α-iduronosyl residues on non-reducing end heparan and dermatan sulfate fragments.
Murine	Targeted disruption of exon 6 was used to produce a mouse model with normal appearance at birth that develops a flattened facial profile and thickened digits by 3 weeks, flared ribs, and thickening of facial bones by a few weeks. However, there was no obvious growth deficiency or mortality seen within the first 20 weeks. Widespread lysosomal storage in hepatocytes, neurones, and renal tubular cells were noted at 8 weeks of age. The central nervous system (CNS) of affected mice showed progressive neuronal loss within the cerebellum. In addition, brain showed increased levels of GM2 and GM3 gangliosides (Clarke *et al.* 1997).
Feline	An α-L-iduronidase-deficient cat has been described (Haskins *et al.* 1979). A 3 bp deletion in the feline iduronidase was linked to the enzyme deficiency (He *et al.* 1999). The affected cat had progressive lameness, a broad face with depressed nasal bridge, small ears, corneal clouding, and multiple bone dysplasia.
Canine	An α-L-iduronidase-deficient dog has been described as the result of an IVI + IG > A mutation in the canine α-L-iduronidase gene (Menon *et al.* 1992). Affected dogs are stunted, have enlarged hearts, and have normal liver and spleen. Dogs have facial dysmorphia, corneal clouding, cardiac valvular insufficiencies, bone disease resulting in gait abnormalities, and storage vacuoles in CNS (Shull *et al.* 1982).
2. MPS II (Hunter syndrome)	Iduronate-2-sulfatase; substrates include iduronosyl-2-sulfate esters on non-reducing-end heparan and dermatan sulfate fragments.
Murine	Targeted disruption of exons 4 and part of 5 was used to produce 2-sulfatase-deficient mice. Affected mice had skeletal abnormalities and distorted faces by 10 weeks of age. MPS II mice weighed less than wild-type and secreted elevated amounts of glycosaminoglycans, and clearly elevated in liver, kidney, lung, and heart valves. Lymph nodes and synoviocytes were vacuolated at 4 weeks of age. Vacuolation was widespread, including heart valves and cerebellar neurones, with neuronal necrosis of the brainstem and spinal cord obvious in 60-week-old affected mice (Lamsa *et al.* 2002; Muenzer *et al.* 2002).
Canine	The causative mutation in the affected dog is not known. Phenotype in a Labrador retriever is of coarse facial features, macrodactyly, unilateral corneal dystrophy, generalized osteopenia, and progressive neurologic deterioration (Wilkerson *et al.* 1998).

Table 11.2 (*continued*)

3. MPS IIIA (Sanfilippo syndrome)	Sulfamidase; substrates includes non-reducing end glucosaminyl-*N*-sulfate esters on heparan sulfate fragments.
Murine	Naturally occurring model with a D31N change in the mouse sulfamidase gene (Bhattacharyya *et al.* 2001). Affected mice had storage vacuoles in neurones containing membranous and floccular materials, with some having classical zebra body morphology. Lysosomal storage was also seen in cells of other tissues. Affected mice died at 7–10 months of age (Bhaumik *et al.* 1999).
Canine	A 3 bp 737–739delCCA resulting in the loss of threonine at position 246 was identified in the sulfamidase gene of wire-haired dachshunds leading to progressive neurologic disease without apparent somatic involvement (Aronovich *et al.* 2000). A pelvic limb ataxia was observed at 3 years of age, which gradually progressed within 1–2 years to severe generalized spinocerebellar ataxia. Mild cerebral cortical atrophy and dilations in the lateral ventricles are grossly evident. Cerebellar Purkinje cells, neurones of the brainstem nuclei, and dorsal ganglia were distended with brightly autofluorescent material. Mentation remained normal throughout the course of the disease. Clinical and pathologic features of the model were reported to mimic human MPS III (Fischer *et al.* 1998).
Canine	A 708–709insC mutation has been shown to cause MPS IIIA pathology in Huntaway dogs (Yogalingam *et al.* 2002). The mutation causes severe CNS degeneration. The index case developed symptoms at 1.5 years of age. Disease progressed rapidly over 1 month. Progressive ataxia and hypermetria caused difficulty with jumping. The animal exhibited loss of learned behaviour, such as defecating in kennel (Jolly *et al.* 2000).
4. MPS IIIB (Sanfilippo syndrome)	α-*N*-Acetyl glucosaminidase; substrates include non-reducing end α-*N*-acetyglucosaminyl residues on heparan sulfate fragments.
Murine	Targeted disruption of exon 6 in the α-*N*-acetylglucosaminidase gene produced mice that were healthy and fertile while young, could survive for 8–12 months, are totally deficient in α-*N*-acetylglucosaminidase, have massive accumulation of heparan sulfate in liver and kidney, and have elevation of gangliosides GM2 and GM3 in brain. Vacuolation is seen in many cells, including macrophages, epithelial cells, and neurones, and becoming more prominent with age. Although most vacuoles contained finely granular material characteristic of glycosaminoglycan accumulation, large pleiomorphic inclusions were seen in some neurones and pericytes in the brain. At 4.5 months, abnormal hypoactive behaviour was observed in an open field test (Li *et al.* 1999). Attenuated plasticity in neurones and astrocytes was reported in the affected mice (Li *et al.* 2002).

Canine	A naturally occurring mutation in schipperke dogs led to dysmetria, hind limb ataxia, and wide-based stance with truncal swaying. Neurological examination identified signs consistent with cerebellar disease (Ellinwood *et al.* 2001).
Bovine	(Hopwood, unpublished observations)
5. MPS IIIC (Sanfilippo syndrome)	AcetylCoA : glucosamine-*N*-acetyl transferase.
No animal models have been identified.	
6. MPS IIID (Sanfilippo syndrome)	Glucosamine-6-sulfatase; substrates include non-reducing end residues of glucosamine-6-sulfate esters on heparan and keratan sulfate fragments.
Caprine	Identified post mortem in a goat (Thompson *et al.* 1992) and mutation R102X identified (Cavanagh *et al.* 1995). The goat model has similar clinical and histological properties to humans with MPS III. Goats develop systemic and CNS heparan sulfate glycosaminoglycan (HS-GAG) accumulation, secondary storage of lipids, and severe, progressive dementia (Downs-Kelly *et al.* 2000).
7. MPS IVA (Morquio syndrome)	*N*-Acetylgalactosamine-6-sulfatase; substrates include, non-reducing end 6-sulfated esters on *N*-acetygalactosaminyl and galactosyl residues on chondroitin sulfate and keratan sulfate fragments, respectively.
Murine	Targeted disruption of exon 2 in the mouse *N*-acetylgalactosamine-6-sulfatase gene produced a model corresponding to a mild form of Morquio syndrome. Growth or mortality is not reduced in mice that are seen to accumulate glycosaminoglycans in liver, kidney, and spleen at 8 weeks of age. Storage did not increase dramatically with age. Radiological examination revealed only minimal changes in skeleton (Tomatsu *et al.* 2002*a*).
8. MPS VI (Maroteaux–Lamy syndrome)	Arylsulfatase B; *N*-acetylgalactosamine-4-sulfatase; substrates include non-reducing end 4-sulfated esters on *N*-acetylgalactosaminyl residues on dermatan and chondroitin sulfate fragments.
Murine	Targeted disruption with the neomycin-resistance gene of exon 5 in arylsulfatase B gene produced mice with an MPS VI phenotype. Mice developed progressive symptoms, at 4 weeks, facial dysmorphism became obvious, long bones were shortened, and pelvic and costal abnormalities were observed. Major alterations in bone formation with perturbed cartilaginous tissues in newborns and widened, perturbed, and persisting growth plates in adult animals were seen. All major parenchymal organs show storage of glycosaminoglycans preferentially in interstitial cells and macrophages. Affected mice are fertile, and mortality is not elevated after 15 months (Evers *et al.* 1996).

Table 11.2 *(continued)*

Rat	A spontaneous 507–508insC mutation (Kunieda *et al.* 1995) in the Ishibashi hairless strain was found in rats exhibiting facial dysmorphia and growth retardation, with disease features closely resembling the human disease. Skeletal abnormalities became evident in affected animals from 3 weeks of age. Histologically, accumulation of glycosaminoglycans was observed in reticuloendothelial cells, cartilage, and other connective tissues, and bone growth plates were widened and irregular (Yoshida *et al.* 1993).
Feline	Originally described in Siamese cats, disease characteristics closely parallel disease in humans clinically and histologically, with lysosomal storage in many cell types including chondrocytes, smooth muscle cells, and corneal keratocytes. Skeletal dysplasia, shortened body length, reduced body weight, spinal cord compression, and hind limb paresis have been observed (Jezyk *et al.* 1977; Crawley *et al.* 1998). Animals exhibiting the classical severe phenotype are homozygous for an L476P mutation (Yogalingam *et al.* 1996).
Feline	A mild clinical phenotype with joint degeneration but normal skeletal growth has been described in cats heterozygous for L476P and D520N mutations (Crawley *et al.* 1998; Yogalingam *et al.* 1998).
Canine	A miniature pinscher exhibited growth retardation, corneal clouding, facial dysmorphia, and skeletal abnormalities. Widespread vacuolation of connective tissues including macrophages, chondrocytes, and smooth muscle cells was observed. Long bone and vertebral morphology were severely affected (Neer *et al.* 1995).
9. MPS VII (Sly syndrome)	β-Glucoronidase; substrates include, non-reducing end β-glucuronosyl residues on dermatan and heparan and chondroitin sulfate fragments.
Murine	Affected mice have shortened lifespan, dysmorphic features, skeletal dysplasia, and widespread lysosomal storage of glycosaminoglycans (Birkenmeier *et al.* 1989). Mutation identified as 1470delC (Sands and Birkenmeier 1993).
Murine	Spontaneously formed in a C3H/HeOuJ strain from the insertion of an intracisternal A particle element into intron 8 of the glucuronidase gene. Although the phenotype of these mice is similar to 1470delC homozygous mice, except lysosomal distension is less prominent, with the brain showing striking meganeurite formation that is seen only occasionally in the 1470delC mice (Vogler *et al.* 2001). These meganeurites have been described in both human and animal storage diseases and are thought to interfere with cell function by altering electrical properties of neurones (Purpura and Suzuki 1976).

Murine	Using targeted mutagenesis, Tomatsu *et al.* (2002*b*) generated E536A and E536Q, corresponding to active-site nucleophile replacements E540A and E540Q in human β-glucuronidase, and L175F, corresponding to the most common human mutation, L176F. The E536A mouse had no detectable β-glucuronidase activity in all tissues tested and displayed a severe phenotype like that of the originally described MPS VII mice carrying the 1470delC. E536Q and L175F mice had low levels of residual activity and milder phenotypes. All three mutant MPS models showed progressive lysosomal storage in many tissues but had different rates of accumulation. The amount of urinary glycosaminoglycan excretion paralleled the clinical severity, with urinary glycosaminoglycans remarkably higher in E536A mice than in E536Q or L175F mice. Molecular analysis showed that the β-glucuronidase mRNA levels were quantitatively similar in the three mutant mouse strains and normal mice. These models mimic different clinical phenotypes of human MPS VII and should be useful in studying pathogenesis and the efficacy of therapies.
Feline	Walking difficulties and an enlarged abdomen have been reported for affected cats. Facial dysmorphia, large paws, corneal clouding, granulation of neutrophils, and vacuolated lymphocytes have been described (Gitzelmann *et al.* 1994). E351K was identified as the disease-causing mutation (Fyfe *et al.* 1999).
Feline	An affected cat had skeletal dysmorphism, flattened facial profile, β-glucoronidase deficiency and urinary glycosaminoglycans (Taylor, unpublished observations).
Canine	Dogs with MPS VII have facial and skeletal dysmorphism and corneal opacity. They have large heads and short maxilla and develop progressive hind limb weakness after weaning, which progresses. The joints are lax and joint capsules are swollen, and there is extensive skeletal disease with bilateral femoral head luxation, epiphyseal lesions, and vertebral dysplasia. Dogs have hepatomegaly with vacuolated cytoplasm in hepatocytes, keratocytes, fibroblasts, and chondrocytes, and in cells of the synovial membrane, retinal pigment epithelium, neurones, and cardiac valves. Neurones had cytoplasmic vacuoles (Haskins *et al.* 1984, 1991). R166H identified in the dog β-glucuronidase gene was shown to cause the pathology (Ray *et al.* 1998*a*,*b*, 1999). The corneal endothelium was severely vacuolated but still functioned to maintain corneal hydration. Clouding was due to storage in stromal keratinocytes (Mollard *et al.* 1996). Affected dogs had mitral valve insufficiency, thickened aortic valves, and dilated aorta with thickened walls with extensive vacuolation (Sammarco *et al.* 2000).

Table 11.3 Glycoproteinoses

1. α-Fucosidosis	Lysosomal α-fucosidase; substrates include non-reducing end α-fucosyl residues on glycolipid and glycopeptide fragments.
Canine	A 14 bp deletion in an English springer spaniel introduces a premature stop codon (Occhiodoro and Anson 1996) Progressive ataxia, dysphagia, and wasting results from the accumulation of fucose-containing oligosaccharides in the central nervous system (CNS) and peripheral nervous system (Kelly *et al.* 1983). Affected dogs lose learned behaviour and develop hypermetria and mild ataxia by 12–18 months of age. They progress to severe ataxia with proprioceptive deficits, nystagmus, disorientation, and severe incoordination by 3 years (Taylor *et al.* 1987). Enlarged peripheral nerves can be palpated and are a prominent finding in the brachial, lumbosacral plexi, and vagus nerve at post mortem. Extensive cytoplasmic vacuolation is found throughout most visceral organs (liver, spleen, lymph node, salivary gland, pancreas, intestine, thyroid, and skin), peripheral nerves (in Schwann cells and macrophages), and the CNS (neurones and glia). Large perivascular cuffs of vacuolated phagocytes are found in the meninges, brain, and endoneurium (Taylor and Farrow 1988). Affected dogs are infertile (sperm defects) with severe epididymal lesions of vacuolation. Biochemical studies showed that canine alpha-L-fucosidase acts preferentially on the alpha-(1–3)-linked fucose at the non-reducing end and that removal of alpha-(1–6)-linked asparagine-linked *N*-acetylglucosamine is rate-limiting in the lysosomal catabolism of fucosylated N-linked glycans (Barker *et al.* 1988).
2. β-Mannosidosis	β-Mannosidase; substrates include non-reducing end β-mannosyl residues on *N*-acetylglucosaminylaspartartyl residues.
Caprine	Affected Nubian goats were affected at birth and unable to rise or walk. All had facial dysmorphia, dome-shaped skulls, carpal contractures, nystagmus, marked intention tremor, and deafness. There was widespread cytoplasmic vacuolation correlated with accumulation of oligosaccharides in the brain and kidney, with paucity of myelin in the cerebrum and cerebellum, ventricular dilation, extensive cytoplasmic vacuolation, axonal spheroids, and myelin paucity (Jones and Dawson 1981; Jones *et al.* 1983). A single base deletion resulted in a reading frameshift and premature termination to produce a shortened polypeptide (Leipprandt *et al.* 1996). This lysosomal storage disorder has a relatively milder phenotype in humans.
Cattle	Severe pathology occurs during fetal development in Salers and involves demyelination and dysmyelination. Affected neonatal calves were unable to rise and had intention tremors. Post-mortem findings included variable dilatation of the lateral cerebral ventricles and paucity of white matter of the cerebrum and cerebellum, and mild-to-marked bilateral kidney enlargement (Abbitt *et al.* 1991). β-Mannosidosis was also reported in a Nebraska cowherd (Baker and Sears 1998). A transition mutation was identified that caused a stop codon 22 amino acids short of the normal C-terminal (Leipprandt *et al.* 1999; Chen *et al.* 1995).
3. α-Mannosidosis	Acid α-mannosidase; substrates include non-reducing end α-mannosyl residues on complex oligosaccharides N-linked to polypeptides.
Murine	Disruption of exon 2 within the lysosomal α-mannosidase gene with a neomycin-resistance gene was used to produce affected mice. Homologous mutant mice have deficient α-mannosidase activity and elevated urinary secretion of mannose–oligosaccharides,

	consistent with mannosidosis. Mannose–oligosaccharides are elevated in liver, kidney, spleen, and brain. The morphological lesions and their topographical distribution are similar to those seen in the human syndrome (Stinchi *et al.* 1999).
Guinea pig	An R227W mutation (Berg and Hopwood 2002) in the acid α-mannosidase gene results in guinea pigs with stunted growth, progressive mental dullness, behavioural abnormalities, and abnormal posture and gait. Affected animals showed a deficiency of acidic α-mannosidase activity in leucocytes, plasma, fibroblasts, and whole-liver extracts. Widespread neuronal vacuolation is observed throughout the CNS, including the cerebral cortex, hippocampus, thalamus, cerebellum, midbrain, pons, medulla, and the dorsal and ventral horns of the spinal cord of affected guinea pigs. Lysosomal vacuolation also occurs in many other visceral tissues and is particularly severe in pancreas, thyroid, epididymis, and peripheral ganglion. Axonal spheroids are observed in some brain regions, but gliosis and demyelination are not observed. Ultrastructurally, most vacuoles in both the CNS and the visceral tissues are lucent or contain fine fibrillar or flocculent material. Rare large neurones in the cerebral cortex contained fine membranous structures. Skeletal abnormalities are very mild (Crawley *et al.* 1999).
Feline	The first of several reports of α-mannosidosis in cats was in the Persian breed in 1982 (Vandevelde *et al.* 1982; Cummings *et al.* 1988). A 583–586del in the cat acid α-mannosidase gene (Berg *et al.* 1997) was found to cause progressive neurological signs with tremors, loss of balance, nystagmus, and myelin loss throughout the cerebrum and cerebellum of affected cats. Inada *et al.* (1996) reported that cerebellar dysfunction in affected cats from the age of 7–8 weeks onwards became progressively worse. Magnetic resonance imaging indicated that the cerebellum size of the diseased cats was markedly reduced. Extensive destruction of Purkinje cells was observed microscopically. The disease in cats shows clinical, morphologic, and biochemical features closely resembling the human disease (Vite *et al.* 2001). Affected cats showed progressively worsening neurological signs that included tremors, loss of balance, nystagmus, slow motor nerve conduction velocity, and increased F-wave latency. Single-nerve fibre teasing revealed significant demyelination/remyelination in affected cats. Magnetic resonance imaging of the CNS revealed diffuse white matter signal abnormalities throughout the brain of affected cats. Histology confirmed myelin loss throughout the cerebrum and cerebellum (Vite *et al.* 2001).
Cattle	Different mutations F321L and R221H have been identified in Angus and Galloway cattle, respectively (Tollersrud *et al.* 1997). Affected animals have progressive ataxia, incoordination, tremor, aggressive behaviour, and early death (Hocking *et al.* 1972; Dorling 1984; Jolly and Walkley 1997). There is foamy cytoplasmic vacuolation in neurones in the cerebral cortex, thalamus, brainstem, and cerebellum, with axonal spheroids. Visceral organs with vacuolation are liver (Kupffer's cells), lymph nodes (macrophage), and the pancreas. Considerable phenotypic variation occurs in cattle, depending on the breed, as Galloway breed calves were stillborn or died neonatally, while Angus calves survived 1–7 months (Healy *et al.* 1990).
4. Aspartylglucosaminuria	Aspartylglucosaminidase; substrate includes mostly *N*-acetylglucosaminylaspartaryl.
Murine	Targeted disruption of exon 3 in the mouse aspartylglucosaminidase gene produces affected animals that completely lack aspartylglucosaminidase activity, and that gradually deteriorate clinically. At the age of 5–10 months, a massive accumulation of aspartylglucosamine is detected in affected mice along with lysosomal vacuolation, axonal swelling in the gracile nucleus, and

Table 11.3 *(continued)*

	impaired neuromotor coordination. A significant number of older male mice have massively swollen bladders, which is not caused by obstruction, but is most likely related to the impaired function of the nervous system. A widespread atrophy in the CNS was detected. The oldest animals (20 months old) display neuronal loss and gliosis, particularly in the regions where the most severe neuronal vacuolation is found. The severe ataxic gait of the older mice was probably due to the dramatic loss of Purkinje cells, intensive astrogliosis, and vacuolation of neurones in the deep cerebellar nuclei, and the severe vacuolation of the cells in vestibular and cochlear nuclei. The impaired bladder function and subsequent hydronephrosis are secondary to involvement of the CNS (Kaartinen *et al.* 1996).
Murine	Exon 8 in the mouse aspartylglucosaminidase gene is disrupted with the neomycin-resistance gene to produce affected mice (Jalanko *et al.* 1998). This model was generated to mimic a human genotype. Affected mice showed storage in brain, liver, kidney, and skin. Lysosomal storage was present in 19-day-old fetuses. Affected mice are fertile, and up to 11 months of age had normal movement and behavioural characteristics. However, affected mice had slowly worsening performance in learning and special ability tests. The model mimics the disease in humans who show characteristic slowly progressing mental retardation and relatively mild skeletal abnormalities.
5. Galactosialidosis	Protective protein/cathepsin A; substrates include α2–3- and α2–6-linked siayloligosaccharide structures on glycopeptides and glycolipids.
Murine	Targeted disruption of the protective protein gene produced a mouse model that correlates with the most severe form in humans. Affected mice present with signs soon after birth and have a shorter lifespan. There is a regional distribution of cells showing vacuolation of specific cells such as neurones and glial cells (Zhou *et al.* 1995).
Ovine	These sheep had mild neurologic signs at 4–6 months, with rapid progression over 2–8 weeks to severe ataxia and coma. Marked vacuolation of neurones with clinical severity mainly associated with the extent of neuronal storage (Ahern-Rindell *et al.* 1988).
6. Sialidosis	Lysosomal neuraminidase; substrates include non-reducing end neuraminyl residues on glycopeptides and glycolipids.
Murine	The mutation in SM/J mice was identified as L209I and believed to cause a partial deficiency of lysosomal neuraminidase. Reduced activity is caused by an altered affinity by the enzyme for its substrate (Rottier *et al.* 1998). The residual neuraminidase activity in these mice is too high to provoke a sialidosis phenotype.
Murine	Targeted disruption of the mouse neuraminidase gene produced a model that is completely deficient in enzyme activity. These null mice have progressive nephropathy, severe ataxia, progressive deformity of the spine, age-related extramedullary haematopoiesis, lack of early degeneration of cerebellar Purkinje cells, and shortened lifespan. Affected mice develop similar clinical abnormalities to patients with early-onset sialidosis, including severe nephropathy, progressive oedema, splenomegaly, kyphosis, and excretion of sialylated oligosaccharides (de Geest *et al.* 2002).

Table 11.4 Glycogen Storage

1. Pompe	Acid α-glucosidase; substrates include lysosomal glycogen fragments.
Murine	Knockout by targeted disruption of exon 13 in murine acid α-glucosidase in embryonic stem cells was used to produce affected mice. Glycogen-containing lysosomes are seen, affecting liver, heart, and skeletal muscles at birth. Glycogen storage becomes more severe with time, leading to muscle wasting by 10 months of age, with limb girdle weakness and kyphosis following. Heart is typically enlarged and electrocardiogram is abnormal. Lysosomal storage is evident in Schwann cells of peripheral nerves and in a subset of neurones in the central nervous system (CNS). Affected mice show impaired performance of skeletal muscle, with loss of developed torque found to be disproportionate to loss in muscle mass. The model parallels the pathological criteria of the human infantile form of Pompe. Despite the serious tissue pathology, these mice do not have a markedly shortened lifespan. Affected mice are fertile and can be crossed (Bijvoet *et al.* 1998, 1999; Hesselink *et al.* 2002). Although less than seen in infantile patients, affected mice have markedly increased left ventricular weight and wall thickness that reflect cardiac abnormalities (Kamphoven *et al.* 2001). The disease phenotype in knockout mice depends upon the genetic background. A severe phenotype with progressive cardiomyopathy and profound muscle wasting, with a phenotype similar to that in patients with infantile Pompe, is observed in knockout 129/C57Bl/6 mice, whereas mice with a background of 129/C57Bl/6 crossed with FVB gave a phenotype with a later age of onset (Raben *et al.* 2000; 2001). A mouse model with a deletion of exon 6 has unimpaired strength and mobility up to 6 months of age despite indistinguishable biochemical and pathological changes (Raben *et al.* 1998).
Bovine	Two mutations have been identified in Brahmans and one in shorthorns (Palmer *et al.* 1994). All three mutations (more common 1057ΔTA and less common 1783T and 1351T) cause premature termination of translation (Dennis *et al.* 2000, 2002; Dennis and Healy 2001). Affected Brahman calves show signs at 6 months of age of ill-thrift and weakness. Increased amounts of high-molecular weight oligosaccharides were found in urine. Fine cytoplasmic vacuolation of neurones was present in the brain and spinal cord, skeletal muscle, myocardium, and Purkinje fibres. Periodic acid–Schiff-stained material was found in lymphocytes (Reichmann *et al.* 1993; Healy *et al.* 1995).
Canine	Affected Lapland dogs produce near normal amounts of α-glucosidase protein but without enzyme activity (Walvoort *et al.* 1982). Except for the presence of oesophageal dilation, this model closely parallels the infantile form of Pompe in humans. Glycogen storage is generalized but particularly affected skeletal, cardiac, oesophageal, and smooth muscle (Walvoort *et al.* 1985).
Feline	CNS glycogen storage has been reported in the cat (Reuser 1993).
2. Danon	LAMP2 deficiency.
Murine	Vacuolar cardioskeletal myopathy, as well as pancreatic, hepatocytic, endothelial, and leucocyte vacuolation (Saftig *et al.* 2001).

Mucolipidoses

The mucolipidoses reflect the complex nature of the biogenesis pathway for lysosomal proteins involving a mannose phosphate receptor-mediated pathway required for the translocation of mannose-6-phosphorylated lysosomal enzyme from the Golgi, via endosomal compartments to the lysosome (Table 11.5).

Table 11.5 Mucolipidoses

Mucolipidoses	A deficiency of *N*-acetylglucosamine-1-phosphotransferase results in multiple lysosomal protein substrates failing to be phosphorylated, leading to a generalized deficiency of many lysosomal hydrolases in the lysosome. Although these hydrolases are still active towards their natural substrate, they are not found in the lysosome and appear in elevated amounts in peripheral circulation.
Feline	Short-hair cat presented at 7 months with retarded growth, abnormal facial features, retinal changes, stiffness of skin and progressive hind limb paresis. Radiography revealed a severely deformed spinal column, bilateral hip luxation with hip dysplasia, an abnormally shaped skull, and generalized decreased bone opacity (Hubler *et al.* 1996; Bosshard *et al.* 1996).

Neuronal ceroid lipofuscinoses

Neuronal ceroid lipofuscinoses (NCLs) are now recognized as the most common neurodegenerative diseases in children and young adults (Table 11.6). There are possibly eight distinct genes involved in this group of disorders. Animal models have played an important part in elucidating the genes involved and the nature of the pathology causing NCL (Jolly *et al.* 1992; Jolly and Walkley 1999). As with other lysosomal storage diseases, animal models will prove invaluable in studies to develop effective therapies.

The past decade has seen significant advances in our understanding of the molecular genetic basis of the NCL, a clinically and genetically heterogeneous group of childhood neurodegenerative storage disorders. Recent research has been able to identify genes, improve diagnostics, and evaluate treatment by using a number of animal models that have been identified with these disorders.

Table 11.6 Neuronal ceroid lipofuscinoses

1. CLN1 (Batten)	Palmitoyl protein thioesterase.
Murine	Targeted disruption of *PPT1* or *PPT2* genes coding for lysosomal thioesterase leads to neurological disease consistent with infantile Batten disease in humans (Gupta *et al.* 2001).
2. CLN2 (Batten)	Tripeptidyl peptidase I.
Murine	Neurodegenerative symptoms (Sleat and Lobel, unpublished).
Canine	Tibetan terrier dogs (Riis *et al.* 1992; Sohar *et al.* 1999).
3. CLN3 (Vogt–Spielmeyer)	Multiple membrane-spanning protein, function not known.
Murine	Targeted disruption of the *CLN3* gene was achieved by deletion of most of exon 1 and all of exons 2–6 by insertion of the neomycin-resistance gene. Batten-like neuronal storage and widespread and progressive intracellular accumulation of autofluorescent material with multilaminar rectilinear/fingerprint appearance under electron microscope. Mice also displayed neuropathological abnormalities with certain cortical interneurones and hypertrophy of many interneuronal populations in the hippocampus (Katz *et al.* 1999; Mitchison *et al.* 1999) and retinal pathology affecting function (Seigel *et al.* 2002).
Murine	Created by disruption of exons 1–6 in the *CLN3* gene. Affected mice are clinically normal at 5 months of age, with intracellular accumulation of autofluorescent material similar to that seen in juvenile patients (Greene *et al.* 1999).
Murine	Deletion of exons 7 and 8 from the *CLN3* gene was produced to match a common mutation identified in the juvenile-onset form in humans (Cotman *et al.* 2002). These knock-in mice, with the common 1 kb CLN3 deletion seen in humans, at the murine Cln3 locus deletion produced alternately spliced mRNAs and protein similar to the human equivalents. The affected mice although exhibiting accrual of membrane deposits from before birth that were high in liver and select neuronal populations, CNS was normal. The affected mice had degenerative changes in retina, cerebral cortex, and cerebellum, as well as had neurological deficits and premature death (Cotman *et al.* 2002).
Canine	Border collies developed mental, motor, and visual signs between 15 and 22 months of age, with rapid progression to severe neurological disease (Taylor and Farrow 1992). Dogs had gait and visual deficits and became progressively demented. Tissues contained granular, sudan black positive, autofluorescent material in neurones and some viscera. Widespread inclusions in the retina did not disrupt its architecture (Taylor and Farrow 1992). English setters have also been reported as a model for juvenile ceroid lipofuscinosis (Koppang 1992; Lingaas *et al.* 1998).

Table 11.6 (*continued*)

Ferret	Affected ferrets had progressive hind limb ataxia with a swaying gait, preservation of retinal structure, ventricular dilation, neurone loss, and autofluorescent inclusions (France and Taylor, unpublished).
4. CLN6 (Batten, late infantile)	311-Amino acid protein with seven predicted transmembrane domains, function not known.
Murine	A 1 bp insertion in the *CLN6* gene has been identified (Wheeler *et al.* 2002).
Ovine	Severe and progressive neurodegeneration of the cerebral cortex of South Hampshire sheep (Palmer *et al.* 1992; Jolly and Walkley 1999). This model represents a mutation in a gene orthologous to that mutated in the human late infantile variant of CLN6 (Broom *et al.* 1998, 1999).
Ovine	Cook *et al.* (2002) reported behavioural changes and visual impairment initially at 7–12 of months of age in Merino sheep. The disease progressed, with associated motor disturbances and, at later stages, seizures, to premature death by 27 months of age. At necropsy, there was severe cerebrocortical atrophy associated with neuronal loss. Storage bodies isolated from fresh brain, liver, and pancreas formed electron-dense aggregates that consisted mainly of the hydrophobic protein, subunit c of mitochondrial ATP synthase. Clinically and pathologically, the disease in the Merino was reported to be similar to CLN6 in South Hampshire sheep. Cook *et al.* (2002) proposed that the disease in both breeds represents mutation at the same gene locus in chromosomal region OAR7q13–15.
5. CLN8 (Northern Epilepsy)	Protein function not known.
Murine	A 267–268insC in codon 90 to give a frameshift and a truncated protein was identified (Ranta *et al.* 1999). This naturally occurring model has behavioural deficits that become prominent at 4–5 months of age, with onset of gross motor symptoms at 6 months (Bolivar *et al.* 2002).

Summary

Forty years ago, Hers (1963) developed the concept of lysosomal storage as an explanation for Pompe disease (see Foreword). In the time since, an outstanding breadth of knowledge has been revealed about the cell biology, genetics, and pathophysiology of these rare diseases. Most of this knowledge of the normal process of lysosomal function and biogenesis has come from studies of lysosomal storage diseases themselves. The abundance of animal models for these disorders has been of considerable benefit to this process. At present, there are more than 45 different lysosomal storage diseases. They are all genetic disorders with a group incidence of 1:5000 births that generally have devastating outcomes leading to early death. For the moment, there is promise of development of effective therapies for patients who have lysosomal diseases that, in general, do not involve the CNS. The selection of appropriate animal models to develop and evaluate therapies to prevent particular pathologies will continue to be of considerable importance.

Recently, a number of therapies have reached clinical trials assisted by studies in animal models to optimize their clinical effect. Particular examples include a study demonstrating improved efficacy following bone marrow transplantation in fucosidosis dogs before the onset of clinical CNS symptoms (Taylor *et al.* 1992) the ability of enzyme replacement to prevent muscle pathology in knockout Pompe mice (Bijvoet *et al.* 1998) and the efficacy of enzyme replacement therapy in mucopolysaccharidosis type VI cats to prevent skeletal pathology, all of which is, dependent on dose and early treatment (Crawley *et al.* 1997).

At present, there is a need to develop safe and effective therapies to prevent CNS pathology that is common amongst the lysosomal storage diseases. The availability of many appropriate animal models for these disorders provides an important resource to speed the development of therapies to the clinic.

Editors' note

While this chapter has focused on mammalian models of lysosomal diseases as requested of its authors, there too are a least two reports of inherited lysosomal diseases in another major vertebrate group, namely birds. A lysosomal storage disease resembling MPS involving brain, spinal cord, liver, and spleen has been described in a 6-month-old male emu (*Dromaius novaehollandiae*) (Kim and Taylor, 1996). Subsequent genetic, enzymatic and pathologic studies revealed this to be MPS IIIB disease (Aronovich *et al.* 2001).

Japanese quail (*Coturnix coturnix japonica*) with a storage disease characteristic of glycogenosis type II (Pompe disease) found in man have been documented. Affected animals exhibited a lack of α-glucosidase (acid maltase) and were incapable of wing movement. Histologically they demonstrated glycogen deposits in skeletal, cardiac and smooth muscle, as well as nerve cells of the brain and spinal cord (Matsui *et al.* 1983). These animals have been the subject of both enzyme replacement (Kikuchi *et al.* 1998) and gene therapy (Lin *et al.* 2002) studies with success in the former study being revealed by the treated birds' ability to fly.

References

Abbitt, B., Jones, M. Z., Kasari, T. R. *et al.* (1991). β-Mannosidosis in twelve Salers calves. *J Am Vet Med Assoc*, **198**, 109–13.

Ahern-Rindell, A. J., Prieur, D. J., Murnane, R. D. *et al.* (1988). Inherited lysosomal storage disease associated with deficiencies of beta-galactosidase and alpha-neuraminidase in sheep. *Am J Med Genet*, **31**, 39–56.

Ahern-Rindell, A. J., Kretz, K. A. and O'Brien, J. S. (1996). Comparison of the canine and human acid β-galactosidase gene. *Am J Med Genet*, **63**, 340–5.

Alroy, J., Orgad, U., Ucci, A. A. *et al.* (1985). Neurovisceral and Skeletal GM1-Gangliosidosis in Dogs with β-Galactosidase Deficiency. *Science*, **229**, 470–2.

Alroy, J., Knowles, K., Schelling, S. H., Kaye, E. M. and Rosenburg, A. E. (1995). Retarted bone formation in G(M1)-gangliosidosis—a study of he infantile form and comparison with two canine models. *Virchows Arch*, **426**, 141–8.

Aronovich, E. L., Carmichael, K. P., Morizono, H. et al. (2000). Canine heparan sulfate sulfamidase and the molecular pathology underlying Sanfilippo syndrome type A in Dachsunds. *Genomics*, **68**, 80–4.

Aronovich, E. L., Johnston, J.M., Wang, P., Giger, U., Whitley, C.B. (2001). Molecular basis of mucopolysaccharidosis type IIIB in emu (*Dromaius novaehollandiae*): an avian model of Sanfilippo syndrome type B. *Genomics*, **74**, 299–305

Baker, W. C. and Sears, G. L. (1998). β-Mannosidosis in a Nebraska cow herd. *Compendium Cotin Educ Pract Vet*, **20** (Suppl. S), S138ff.

Baker, H. J., Lindsay, J. R., McKhann, G. M. and Farrell, D. F. (1971). Neuronal GM1 Gangliosidosis in a Siamese Cat with β-Galactosidase Deficiency. *Science*, **174**, 838–9.

Baker, H. J., Wood, P. A., Wenger, D. A. et al. (1987). Sphingomyelin Lipidosis in a Cat. *Vet Pathol*, **24**, 386–91.

Barker, C., Dell, A., Rogers, M., Alhadeff, J. A. and Winchester, B. (1988). Canine alpha-L-fucosidase in relation to the enzymic defect and storage products in canine fucosidosis. *Biochem J*, **254**, 861–8.

Baskin, G., Alroy, J., Li, Y.-T. *et al.* (1989). Galactosylceramide lipidosis in Rhesus monkeys. *Lab Invest*, **60**, 7A.

Baskin, G. B., Ratterree, M., Davison, B. B. *et al.* (1998). Genetic galactocerebrosidase deficiency (globoid cell leukodystrophy, Krabbe disease) in Rhesus monkeys (*Macaca mulatta*). *Lab Anim Sci*, **48**, 476–82.

Berg, T. and Hopwood, J. J. (2002). α-Mannosidosis in the guinea pig: cloning of the lysosomal α-mannosidase cDNA and identification of a missense mutation causing α-mannosidosis. *Biochim Biophys Acta*, **1586**, 169–76.

Berg, T., Tollersrud, O. K., Walkley, S. U., Siegel, D. and Nilssen, O. (1997). Purification of feline lysosomal α-mannosidase, determination of its cDNA sequence and identification of a mutation causing α-mannosidosis in Persian cats. *Biochem J*, **328**, 863–70.

Bhattacharyya, R., Gliddon, B., Beccari, T., Hopwood, J. J. and Stanley, P. (2001). A novel missense mutation in lysosomal sulfamidase is the basis of MPS IIIA in a spontaneous mouse mutant. *Glycobiology*, **11**, 99–103.

Bhaumik, M., Muller, V. J., Rozaklis *et al.* (1999). A mouse model for mucopolysaccharidosis type IIIA (Sanfilippo syndrome). *Glycobiology*, **9**, 1389–96.

Bijvoet, A. G., van de Kamp, E. H., Kroos, M. A. *et al.* (1998). Generalized glycogen storage and cardiomegaly in a knockout mouse model of Pompe disease. *Hum Mol Genet*, **7**, 53–62.

Bijvoet, A. G. A., van Hirtum, H., Vermey, M. *et al.* (1999). Pathological features of glycogen storage disease type II highlighted in the knockout mouse model. *J Pathol*, **189**, 416–24.

Birkenmeier, E. H., Davisson, M. T., Beamer, W. G. *et al.* (1989). Murine mucopolysaccharidosis type VII. Characterization of a mouse with β-glucuronidase deficiency. *J Clin Invest*, **83**, 1258–66.

Bolivar, V. J., Ganus, J. S. and Messer, A. (2002). The development of behavioral abnormalities in the motor neuron degeneration (mnd) mouse. *Brain Res*, **937**, 74–82.

Bosshard, N. U., Hubler, M., Arnold, S., Briner, J. *et al.* (1996). Spontaneous mucolipidosis in a cat—an animal model of human I-cell disease. *Veterinary Pathology*, **33**, 1–13.

Broom, M. F., Zhou, C. M., Broom, J. E. *et al.* (1998). Ovine neuronal ceroid lipofuscinosis—a large animal model syntenic with the human neuronal ceroid lipofuscinosis variant CLN6. *J Med Genet*, **35**, 717–21.

Broom, M. F., Zhou, C. M. and Hill, D. F. (1999). Progress toward positional cloning of ovine neuronal ceroid lipofuscinosis, a model of the human late-infantile variant CLN6. *Mol Genet Metab*, **66**, 373–5.

Brown, D. E., Thrall, M. A., Walkley, S. U. *et al.* (1994). Feline Niemann–Pick disease type C. *Am J Pathol*, **144**, 1412–5.

Bundza, A., Lowden, J. A. and Charlton, K.M. (1979). Niemann–Pick Disease in a Poodle Dog. *Vet Pathol*, **16**, 530–8.

Cavanagh, K. T., Leipprandt, J. R., Jones, M. Z. and Friderici, K. (1995). Molecular defect of caprine *N*-acetylglucosamine-6-sulfatase deficiency. A single base substitution creates a stop codon in the 5'-region of the coding sequence. *J Inherit Metab Dis*, **18**, 96–101.

Chen, H., Leipprandt, J. R., Traviss, C. E. *et al.* (1995). Molecular cloning and characterization of bovine β-mannosidase. *J Biol Chem*, **270**, 3841–8.

Clarke, L. A., Russell, C. S., Pownall *et al.* (1997). Murine mucopolysaccharidosis type I: targeted disruption of the murine α-L-iduronidase gene. *Hum Mol Genet*, **6**, 503–11.

Cohen-Tannoudi, M., Marchand, P., Akli, S. *et al.* (1995). Disruption of murine Hexa gene leads to enzymatic deficiency and to neuronal lysosomal storage, similar to that observed in Tay–Sachs disease. *Mamm Genome*, **6**, 844–9.

Cook, R. W., Jolly, R. D., Palmer, D. N., Tammen, I., Broom, M. F. and McKinnon, R. (2002). Neuronal ceroid lipofuscinosis in Merino sheep. *Aust Vet J*, **80**, 292–7.

Cork, L. C., Munnell, J. F., Lorenz, M. D., Murphy, J. V., Baker, H. J. and Rattazzi, M. C. (1977). GM2 Gangliosidosis Lysosomal Storage Disease in Cats with β-Hexosaminidase Deficiency. *Science*, **196**, 1014–7.

Cotman, S. L., Vrbanac, V., Lebel, L. A. *et al.* (2002). Cln3 (Deltaex7/8) knock-in mice with the common JNCL mutation exhibit progressive neurologic disease that begins before birth. *Hum Mol Genet*, **11**, 2709–21.

Cox, N. R., Ewald, S. J., Morrison, N. E. *et al.* (1998). Thymic alterations in feline GM1 gangliosidosis. *Vet Immunol Immunopathol*, **63**, 335–53.

Cox, N. R., Morrison, N. E., Sartin, J. L. *et al.* (1999). Alterations in the growth hormone/insulin-like growth factor 1 pathways in feline GM1 gangliosidosis. *Endocrinology*, **140**, 5698–704.

Cozzi, F., Vite, C. H., Wenger, D. A., Victoria, T. and Haskins, M. E. (1998). MRI and electrophysiological abnormalities in a case of canine globoid cell leucodystrophy. *J Small Anim Pract*, **39**, 401–5.

Crawley, A. C., Niedzielski, K. H., Issac, E. L., Davey, R. C., Byers, S., Hopwood, J. J. (1997). Enzyme replacement therapy from birth in a feline model of mucopolysaccharidosis type VI. *J Clin Invest*, **99**, 651–62.

Crawley, A. C., Yogalingam, G., Muller, V. J. and Hopwood, J. J. (1998). Two mutations within a feline mucopolysaccharidosis type VI colony cause three different clinical phenotypes. *J Clin Invest*, **101**, 109–19.

Crawley, A. C., Jones, M. Z., Bonning, L. E., Finnie, J. W. and Hopwood, J. J. (1999). Alpha-mannosidosis in the guinea pig: a new animal model for lysosomal storage disorders. *Pediatr Res*, **46**, 501–9.

Cuddon, P. A., Higgin, R. J., Duncan, I. D., Miller, S. P. F., Parent, J. M. and Moser, A. B. (1989). Polyneuropathy in Feline Niemann–Pick Disease. *Brain*, **112**, 1429–43.

Cummings, J.F., Wood, P.A., de Lahunta, A., Walkley, S.U. and LeBoeuf, L. (1988). The Clinical and Pathologic Heterogeneity of Feline Alpha-Mannosidosis. *J Vet Int Med*, **2**, 163–70.

D'Hooge, R., Coenen, R., Gieselmann, V., Lullmann-Rauch, R. and de Deyn, P. P. (1999*a*). Decline in brain-stem auditory-evoked potentials coincides with loss of spiral ganglion cells in arylsulfatase A-deficient mice. *Brain Res*, **847**, 352–6.

D'Hooge, R., Hartmann, D., Manil, J. *et al.* (1999*b*). Neuromotor alterations and cerebellar deficits in aged arylsulfatase A-deficient transgenic mice. *Neurosci Lett*, **273**, 93–6.

D'Hooge, R., van Dam, D., Franck, F., Gieselmann, V. and de Deyn, P. P. (2001). Hyperactivity, neuromotor defects, and impaired learning and memory in a mouse model for metachromatic leukodystrophy. *Brain Res*, **907**, 35–43.

Demaria, R., Divari, S., Bo, S. *et al.* (1998). β-Galactosidase deficiency in a Korat cat—a new form of feline G(M1)-gangliosidosis. *Acta Neuropathol*, **96**, 307–14.

Dennis, J. A. and Healy, P. J. (2001). Genotyping Shorthorn cattle for generalised glycogenosis. *Aust Vet J*, **79**, 773–5.

Dennis, J. A., Moran, C. and Healy, P. J. (2000). The bovine α-glucosidase gene: coding region, genomic structure, and mutations that cause bovine generalised glycogenosis. *Mamm Genome*, **11**, 206–12.

Dennis, J. A., Healy, P. J. and Reichmann, K. G. (2002). Genotyping Brahman cattle for generalised glycogenosis. *Aust Vet J*, **80**, 286–91.

Dhami, R., He, X. X., Gordon, R. E. and Schuchman, E. H. (2001). Analysis of the lung pathology and alveolar macrophage function in the acid sphingomyelinase-deficient mouse model of Niemann–Pick disease. *Lab Invest*, **81**, 987–99.

Dial, S. M., Mitchell, T. W., Lecouteur, R. A. *et al.* (1994). GM1 gangliosidosis (type-II) in 3 cats. *J Am Anim Hosp Assoc*, **30**, 355–9.

Doering, T., Proia, R. L. and Sandhoff, K. (1999). Accumulation of protein-bound epidermal glucosylceramides in β-glucocerebrosidase deficient type 2 Gaucher mice. *FEBS Lett*, **447**, 167–70.

Dorling, P. R. (1984). Lysosomal storage diseases in animals. In *Lysosomes in biology and medicine* (Dingle, J. T. and Dean, R. T., ed.), pp. 347–79. Amsterdam: Elsevier.

Downs-Kelly, E., Jones, M. Z., Alroy, J. *et al.* (2000). Caprine mucopolysaccharidosis IIID: a preliminary trial of enzyme replacement therapy. *J Mol Neurosci*, **15**, 251–62.

Du, H., Duanmu, M., Witte, and Grabowski, G. A. (1998). Targeted disruption of the mouse lysosomal acid lipase gene: long-term survival with massive cholesteryl ester and triglyceride storage. *Hum Mol Genet*, **7**, 1347–54.

Du, H., Schiavi, S., Levine, M., Mishra, J., Heur, M. and Grabowski, G. A. (2001). Enzyme therapy for lysosomal acid lipase deficiency in the mouse. *Hum Mol Genet*, **10**, 1639–48.

Ellinwood, N. M., Wang, P., Skeen, T. *et al.* (2001). Canine Mucopolysaccharidosis type IIIB: Sanfilippo type B syndrome identified in Schipperke dogs, 16th Annual MPS Conference, June 21–24, UCLA Sunset Village, USA.

Evers, M., Saftig, P., Schmidt, P. *et al.* (1996). Targeted disruption of the arylsulfatase B gene results in mice resembling the phenotype of mucopolysaccharidosis VI. *Proc Natl Acad Sci USA*, **93**, 8214–9.

Ezoe, T., Vanier, M. T., Oya, Y. *et al.* (2000). Twitcher mice with only a single active galactosylceramide synthase gene exhibit clearly detectable but therapeutically minor phenotypic improvements. *J Neurosci Res*, **59**, 179–87.

Farrow, B. R. H., Hartley, W. J., Pollard, A. C. *et al.* (1982). Gaucher disease in the dog. *Prog Clin Biol Res*, **95**, 645–53.

Fischer, A., Carmichael, K. P., Munnell, J. F. *et al.* (1998). Sulfamidase deficiency in a family of Dachshunds: a canine model of mucopolysaccharidosis IIIA (Sanfilippo A). *Pediatr Res*, **44**, 74–82.

Fox, J., Li, Y. T., Dawson, G. *et al.* (1999). Naturally occurring G(M2) gangliosidosis in two Muntjak deer with pathological and biochemical features of human classical Tay–Sachs disease (type B G(M2) gangliosidosis). *Acta Neuropathol*, **97**, 57–62.

Fujita, N., Suzuki, K., Vanier, M. T. *et al.* (1996). Targeted disruption of the mouse sphingolipid activator protein gene—a complex phenotype, including severe leukodystrophy and wide-spread storage of multiple sphingolipids. *Hum Mol Genet*, **5**, 711–25.

Fyfe, J. C., Kurzhals, R. L., Lassaline, M. E. *et al.* (1999). Molecular basis of feline β-glucuronidase deficiency: an animal model of mucopolysaccharidosis VII. *Genomics*, **58**, 121–8.

de Geest, N., Bonten, E., Mann, L. *et al.* (2002). Systemic and neurologic abnormalities distinguish the lysosomal disorders sialidosis and galactosialidosis in mice. *Hum Mol Genet*, **11**, 1455–64.

Gitzelmann, R., Bosshard, N. U., Supertifurga, A. *et al.* (1994). Feline mucopolysaccharidosis VII due to β-glucuronidase deficiency. *Vet Pathol*, **31**, 435–43.

Goodrum, J. F. and Pentchev, P. G. (1997). Cholesterol, reutilization during myelination of regenerating PNS axons is impaired in Niemann–Pick disease type C mice. *J Neurosci Res*, **49**, 389–92.

Gravel, R. A., Kaback, M. M., Proia, R. L. *et al.* (2001). The GM2 gangliosidosis. In *The metabolic and molecular bases of inherited disease* (Scriver, C. R., Beaudet, A. L., Sly, W. S. and Valle, D. ed.), pp. 3827–76, 8th edn. New York: McGraw-Hill.

Greene, N. D. E., Bernard, D. L., Taschner, P. E. M. *et al.* (1999). A murine model for juvenile NCL: Gene targeting of mouse Cln3. *Mol Genet Metab*, **66**, 309–13.

Gupta, P., Soyombo, A. A., Atashband, A., Wisniewski, K. E. *et al.* (2001). Disruption of *PPT1* or *PPT2* causes neuronal ceroid lipofuscinosis in knockout mice. *PNAS*, **98**, 13566–71.

Hahn, C. N., Martin, M. D., Schroder, M. *et al.* (1997). Generalized CNS disease and massive G(M1)-ganglioside accumulation in mice defective in lysosomal acid β-galactosidase. *Hum Mol Genet*, **6**, 205–11.

Haskins, M. E., Jezyk, P. F., Desnick, R. J. *et al.* (1979). α-L-Iduronidase deficiency in a cat: a model of mucopolysaccharidosis I. *Pediatr Res*, **13**, 1294–7.

Haskins, M. E., Desnick, R. J., Di Ferrante, N. *et al.* (1984). β-Glucuronidase deficiency in a dog: a model of human mucopolysaccharidosis type VII. *Pediatr Res*, **18**, 980–4.

Haskins, M. E., Aguirre, G. D., Jezyk, P. F. *et al.* (1991). Animal model of human disease, mucopolysaccharidosis type VII. *Am J Pathol*, **138**, 1553–5.

He, X. X., Li, C. M., Simonaro, C. M. *et al.* (1999). Identification and characterization of the molecular lesion causing mucopolysaccharidosis type I in cats. *Mol Genet Metab*, **67**, 106–12.

Healy, P. J., Harper, P. A. and Dennis, J. A. (1990). Phenotypic variation in bovine alpha-mannosidosis. *Res Vet Sci*, **49**, 82–4.

Healy, P. J., Nicholls, P. J., Martiniuk, F., Tzall, S., Hirschhorn, R. and Howell, J. M. (1995). Evidence of molecular heterogeneity for generalised glycogenosis between and within breeds of cattle. *Aust Vet J*, **72**, 309–11.

Hess, B., Saftig, P., Hartmann, D. *et al.* (1996). Phenotype of arylsulfatase A-deficient mice—relationship to human metachromatic leukodystrophy. *Proc Natl Acad Sci USA*, **93**, 14821–6.

Hesselink, R. P., Gorselink, M., Schaart, G. *et al.* (2002). Impaired performance of skeletal muscle in α-glucosidase knockout mice. *Muscle Nerve*, **25**, 873–83.

Higashi, Y., Murayama, S., Pentchev, P. G. and Suzuki, K. (1993). Cerebellar degeneration in the Niemann–Pick type C mouse. *Acta Neuropathol (Berl)*, **85**, 175–84.

Hocking, J. D., Jolly, R. D. and Batt, R. D. (1972). Deficiency of α-mannosidase in Angus cattle. *Biochem J*, **128**, 69–78.

Horinouchi, K., Erlich, S., Perl, D. P. *et al.* (1995). Acid sphingomyelinase deficient mice: a model of types A and B Niemann–Pick disease. *Nat Genet*, **10**, 288–93.

Hubler, M., Haskins, M. E., Arnold, S. *et al.* (1996). Mucolipidosis type II in a domestic Shorthair cat. *J Small Anim Pract*, **37**, 435–41.

Igisu, H. and Suzuki, K. (1984). Progressive accumulation of toxic metabolite in a genetic leukodystrophy. *Science*, **284**, 753–5.

Inada, S., Mochizuki, M., Izumo, S. *et al.* (1996). Study of hereditary cerebellar degeneration in cats. *Am J Vet Res*, **57**, 296–301.

Ishikawa, Y., Li, S.-C., Wood, P. A. and Li, Y.-T. (1987). Biochemical Basis of Type ABG M2 Gangliosidosis in a Japanese Spaniel. *J Neurochem*, **48**, 860–4.

Itoh, M., Matsuda, J., Suzuki, O. *et al.* (2001). Development of lysosomal storage in mice with targeted disruption of the β-galactosidase gene: a model of human G(M1)-gangliosidosis. *Brain Dev*, **23**, 379–84.

Jalanko, A., Kenhunen, K., McKinney, C. E. *et al.* (1998). Mice with an aspartylglucosaminuria mutation similar to humans replicate the pathophysiology in patients. *Hum Mol Genet*, **7**, 265–72.

Jeyakumar, M., Smith, D., Eliott-Smith, E. *et al.* (2002). An inducible mouse model of late onset Tay–Sachs disease. *Neurobiol Dis*, **10**, 201–10.

Jezyk, P. F., Haskins, M. E., Patterson, D. F. *et al.* (1977). Mucopolysaccharidosis in a cat with arylsulfatase B deficiency: a model for Maroteaux–Lamy syndrome. *Science*, **198**, 834–6.

Jolly, R. D. and Walkley, S. U. (1997). Lysosomal storage diseases of animals: an essay in comparative Pathology. *Vet Pathol*, **34**, 527–48.

Jolly, R. D. and Walkley, S. U. (1999). Ovine ceroid lipofuscinosis: postulated mechanism of neurodegeneration. *Mol Genet Metab*, **66**, 376–80.

Jolly, R. D., Martinus, R. D. and Palmer, D. N. (1992). Sheep and other animals with ceroid-lipofuscinoses: their relevance to Batten disease. *Am J Med Genet*, **42**, 609–14.

Jolly, R. D., Allan, F. J., Collett, M. G. *et al.* (2000). Mucopolysaccharidosis IIIA (Sanfilippo syndrome) in a New Zealand Huntaway dog with ataxia. *N Z Vet J*, **48**, 144–8.

Jones, M. Z. and Dawson, G. (1981). Caprine β-mannosidosis. *J Biol Chem*, **266**, 5185–8.

Jones, M. Z., Cunningham, J. G., Dade, A. W. *et al.* (1983). Caprine β-mannosidosis: clinical and pathological features. *J Neuropathol Exp Neurol*, **42**, 268–85.

Kaartinen, V., Mononen, I., Voncken, J. W. *et al.* (1996). A mouse model for the human lysosomal disease aspartylglycosaminuria. *Nat Med*, **2**, 1375–8.

Kamphoven, J. H. J., Stubenitsky, R., Reuser, A. J. J. *et al.* (2001). Cardiac remodeling and contractile function in acid α-glucosidase knockout mice. *Physiol Genomics*, **5**, 171–9.

Katz, M. L., Shibuya, H., Liu, P. C. *et al.* (1999). A mouse gene knockout model for juvenile ceroid-lipofuscinosis (Batten disease). *J Neurosci Res*, **57**, 551–6.

Kelly, W. R., Clague, A. E., Barns, R. J. *et al.* (1983). Canine α-L-fucosidosis: a storage disease of Springer Spaniels. *Acta Neuropathol (Berl)*, **60**, 9–13.

Kikuchi, T., Yang, H.W., Pennybacker, M., Ichihara, N., Mizutani, M., Van Hove, J.L., Chen, Y.T. (1998). Clinical and metabolic correction of pompe disease by enzyme therapy in acid maltase-deficient quail. *J Clin Invest*, **101**, 827–33.

Kim, D. Y., Cho, D. Y., Taylor, H.W. (1996). Lysosomal storage disease in an emu (*Dromaius novaehollandiae*). *Vet Pathol*, **33**, 365–6.

Kitagawa, T. (1987). An animal model of human acid sphingomyelinase deficiency (Niemann–Pick disease) and the study of its enzyme replacement. *Jinrui Idengaku Zasshi*, **32**, 55–69.

Kolter, T. and Sandhoff, K. (1998). Glycosphingolipid degradation and animal models of GM2 gangliosidoses. *J Inherit Metab Dis*, **21**, 548–63.

Komiyama, A. and Suzuki, K. (1994). Progressive dysfunction of Twitcher Schwann cells is evaluated better *in vitro* than *in vivo*. *Brain Res*, **637**, 106–13.

Koppang, N. (1992). English Setter model and juvenile ceroid-lipofuscinosis in man. *Am J Med Genet*, **42**, 599–604.

Kosanke, S.D., Pierce, K. R. and Bay, W. W. (1978). Clinical and biochemical abnormalities in porcine GM2 gangliosidosis. *Veterinary Pathology*, **15**, 685–99.

Kroll, R. A., Pagel, M. A., Roman-Goldstein, S. *et al.* (1995). White matter changes associated with feline G(M2) gangliosidosis (Sandhoff disease)—correlation of MR findings with pathologic and ultrastructural abnormalities. *Am J Neuroradiol*, **16**, 1219–26.

Kunieda, T., Simonaro, C. M., Yoshida, M. *et al.* (1995). Mucopolysaccharidosis type VI in rats: isolation of cDNAs encoding arylsulfatase B, chromosomal localization of the gene, and identification of the mutation. *Genomics*, **29**, 582–7.

Lamsa, J. C., Garcia, A., Dacosta, J. *et al.* (2002). *7th International Symposium on MPS and Related Diseases, June, Paris.* p. 61.

Leipprandt, J. R., Kraemer, S. A., Haithcock, B. E. *et al.* (1996). Caprine β-mannosidase: sequencing and characterization of the cDNA and identification of the molecular defect of caprine β-mannosidosis. *Genomics*, **37**, 51–6.

Leipprandt, J. R., Chen, H., Horvath, J. E., Qiao, X. T., Jones, M. Z. and Friderici, K. H. (1999). Identification of a bovine β-mannosidosis mutation and detection of two β-mannosidase pseudogenes. *Mamm Genome*, **10**, 1137–41.

Li, H. H., Yu, W. H., Rozengurt, N. *et al.* (1999). Mouse model of Sanfilippo syndrome type B produced by targeted disruption of the gene encoding alpha-*N*-acetylglucosaminidase. *Proc Natl Acad Sci USA*, **96**, 14505–10.

Li, H. H., Zhao, H. Z., Neufeld, E. F., Cai, Y. and Gomez-Pinilla, F. (2002). Attenuated plasticity in neurons and astrocytes in the mouse model of Sanfilippo syndrome type B. *J Neurosci Res*, **69**, 30–8.

Lin, C. Y., Ho, C. H., Hsieh, Y.H., Kikuchi, T. (2002) Adeno-associated virus-mediated transfer of human acid maltase gene results in a transient reduction of glycogen accumulation in muscle of Japanese quail with acid maltase deficiency. *Gene Ther*, **9**, 554–63.

Lingaas, F., Aarskaug, T., Sletten, M. *et al.* (1998). Genetic markers linked to neuronal ceroid lipofuscinosis in English Setter dogs. *Anim Genet*, **29**, 371–6.

Liu, Y. J., Hoffmann, A., Grinberg, A. *et al.* (1997). Mouse model of G(M2) activator deficiency manifests cerebellar pathology and motor impairment. *Proc Natl Acad Sci USA*, **94**, 8138–43.

Liu, Y. J., Suzuki, K., Reed, J. D. *et al.* (1998). Mice with type 2 and 3 Gaucher disease point mutations generated by a single insertion mutagenesis procedure. *Proc Natl Acad Sci USA*, **95**, 2503–8.

Liu, Y. J., Wu, Y. P., Wada, R. *et al.* (2000). Alleviation of neuronal ganglioside storage does not improve the clinical course of the Niemann–Pick C disease mouse. *Hum Mol Genet*, **9**, 1087–92.

Loftus, S. K., Morris, J. A., Carstea, E. D. *et al.* (1997). Murine model of Niemann–Pick C disease: mutation in a cholesterol homeostasis gene. *Science*, **277**, 232–5.

Lowenthal, A. C., Cummings, J. F., Wenger, D. A. *et al.* (1990). Feline sphingolipidosis resembling Niemann–Pick type C disease. *Acta Neuropathol (Berl)*, **81**, 189–97.

Luzi, P., Rafi, M. A., Victoria, T., Baskin, G. B. and Wenger, D. A. (1997). Characterization of the rhesus monkey galactocerebrosidase (GALC) cDNA and gene and identification of the mutation causing globoid cell leukodystrophy (Krabbe disease) in this primate. *Genomics*, **42**, 319–24.

Luzi, P., Rafi, M. A., Zaka, M. *et al.* (2001). Generation of a mouse with low galactocerebrosidase activity by gene targeting: a new model of globoid cell leukodystrophy (Krabbe disease). *Mol Genet Metab*, **73**, 211–23.

Marathe, S., Miranda, S. R. P., Devlin, C. *et al.* (2000). Creation of a mouse model for non-neurological (type B) Niemann–Pick disease by stable, low level expression of lysosomal sphingomyelinase in the absence of secretory sphingomyelinase: relationship between brain intra-lysosomal enzyme activity and central nervous system function. *Hum Mol Genet*, **9**, 1967–76.

March, P. A., Thrall, M. A., Brown, D. E. *et al.* (1997). GABAergic neuroaxonal dystrophy and other cytopathological alterations in feline Niemann–Pick disease type C. *Acta Neuropathol*, **94**, 164–72.

Matsuda, J., Suzuki, O., Oshima, A. *et al.* (1997*a*). β-Galactosidase-deficient mouse as an animal model for G(M1)-gangliosidosis. *Glycoconj J*, **14**, 729–36.

Matsuda, J., Suzuki, O., Oshima, A. *et al.* (1997*b*). Neurological manifestations of knockout mice with β-galactosidase deficiency. *Brain Dev*, **19**, 19–20.

Matsuda, J., Vanier, M. T., Saito, Y. *et al.* (2001). A mutation in the saposin A domain of the sphingolipid activator protein (prosaposin) gene results in a late-onset, chronic form of globoid cell leukodystrophy in the mouse. *Hum Mol Genet*, **10**, 1191–9.

Matsui, T., Kuroda, S., Mizutani, M., Kiuchi, Y., Suzuki, K., Ono, T. (1983). Generalized glycogen storage disease in Japanese quail (*Coturnix coturnix japonica*). *Vet Pathol*, **20**, 312–21

Matsushima, G. K., Taniike, M., Glimcher, L. H. *et al.* (1994). Absence of MHC class II molecules reduces CNS demyelination, microglial/macrophage infiltration, and twitching in murine globoid cell leukodystrophy. *Cell*, **78**, 645–56.

Menon, K. P., Tieu, P. T. and Neufeld, E. F. (1992). Architecture of the canine IDUA gene and mutation underlying canine mucopolysaccharidosis I. *Genomics*, **14**, 763–8.

Mitchison, H. M., Bernard, D. J., Greene, N. D. E. *et al.* (1999). Targeted disruption of the Cln3 gene provides a mouse model for Batten disease. *Neurobiol Dis*, **6**, 321–34.

Miyawaki, S., Mitsuoka, S., Sakiyama, T. and Kitagaura, T. (1982). Sphingomyelinosis, a new mutation in a mouse. *J Hered*, **73**, 257–63.

Miyawaki, S., Yoshida, H., Mitsuoka, S., Enomoto, H. and Ikehara, S. (1986). A mouse model for Niemann–Pick disease. Influence of genetic background on disease expression in spm/spm mice. *J Hered*, **77**, 379–84.

Mollard, R. J., Telegan, P., Haskins, M. and Aguirre, G. (1996). Corneal endothelium in mucopolysaccharide storage disorders. Morphologic studies in animal models. *Cornea*, **15**, 25–34.

Muenzer, J., Lamsa, J. C., Garcia, A., Dacosta, J., Garcia, J. and Treco, D. A. (2002). Enzyme replacement therapy in mucopolysaccharidosis type II (Hunter syndrome): a preliminary report. *Acta Paediatr Suppl*, **91**, 98–9.

Muldoon, L. L., Neuwelt, E. A., Page, M. A. and Weiss, D. L. (1994). Characterization of the molecular defect in a feline model for type II G(M2)-gangliosidosis (Sandhoff disease). *Am J Pathol*, **144**, 1109–18.

Muller, G., Alldinger, S., Moritz, A. *et al.* (2001). GM1 Gangliosidosis in Alaskan Huskies: clinical and pathologic findings. *Vet Pathol*, **38**, 281–90.

Munana, K. R., Luttgen, P. J., Thrall, M. A., Mitchell, T. W. and Wenger, D. A. (1994). Neurological manifestations of Niemann–Pick disease type C in cats. *J Vet Intern Med*, **8**, 117–21.

Neer, T. M., Dial, S. M., Pechman, R. *et al.* (1995). Clinical vignette. Mucopolysaccharidosis type VI in miniature pinscher. *J Vet Intern Med*, **9**, 429–33.

Occhiodoro, T. and Anson, D. S. (1996). Isolation of the canine alpha-L-fucosidase cDNA and definition of the fucosidosis mutation in English springer spaniels. *Mamm Genome*, **7**, 271–4.

Ohshima, T., Murray, G. J., Swaim, W. D. *et al.* (1997). α-Galactosidase A deficient mice—a model of Fabry disease. *Proc Natl Acad Sci USA*, **94**, 2540–4.

Ong, W. Y., Kumar, U., Switzer, R. C. *et al.* (2001). Neurodegeneration in Niemann–Pick type C disease mice. *Exp Brain Res*, **14**, 218–31.

Otterbach, B. and Stoffel, W. (1995). Acid sphingomyelinase-deficient mice mimic the neurovisceral form of human lysosomal storage disease (Niemann–Pick disease). *Cell*, **81**, 1053–61.

Oya, Y., Nakayasu, H., Fujita, N., Suzuki, K. and Suzuki, K. (1998). Pathological study of mice with total deficiency of sphingolipid activator proteins (SAP knockout mice). *Acta Neuropathol*, **96**, 29–40.

Palmer, D. N., Fearnley, I. M., Walker, J. E. *et al.* (1992). Mitochondrial ATP synthase subunit c storage in the ceroid-lipofuscinoses (Batten disease). *Am J Med Genet*, **42**, 561–7.

Palmer, D. G., Dorling, P. R. and Howell, J. M. (1994). Bovine glycogenosis type II: the molecular defect in Shorthorn cattle. *Neuromuscul Disord*, **4**, 39–48.

Pedchenko, T. V. and LeVine, S. M. (1999). IL-6 deficiency causes enhanced pathology in Twitcher (globoid cell leukodystrophy) mice. *Exp Neurol*, **158**, 459–68.

Pentchev, P. G., Gal, A. E., Booth, A. D. *et al.* (1980). A lysosomal storage disorder in mice characterized by a dual deficiency of sphingomyelinase and glucocerebrosidase. *Biochim Biophys Acta*, **619**, 669–79.

Pentchev, P. G., Boothe, A. D., Kruth, H. S. *et al.* (1984). A genetic storage disorder in BALB/*c* mice with a metabolic block in esterification of exogenous cholesterol. *J Biol Chem*, **259**, 5784–91.

Phaneuf, D., Wakamatsu, N., Huang, J.-Q. *et al.* (1996). Dramatically different phenotypes in mouse models of human Tay–Sachs and Sandhoff diseases. *Hum Mol Genet*, **5**, 1–14.

Pierce, K. R., Kosanke, S.D., Bay, W. W. and Bridges, C. H. (1976). Porcine cerebrospinal lipodystrophy (GM2 gangliosidosis). *American J Pathology*, **83**, 419–22.

Purpura, D. P. and Suzuki, K. (1976). Distortion of neuronal geometry and formation of aberrant synapses in neuronal storage disease. *Brain Res*, **116**, 1–21.

Raben, N., Nagaraju, K., Lee, E. *et al.* (1998). Targeted disruption of the acid α-glucosidase gene in mice causes an illness with critical features of both infantile and adult human glycogen storage disease type II. *J Biol Chem*, **273**, 19086–92.

Raben, N., Nagaraju, K., Lee, E. and Plotz, P. (2000). Modulation of disease severity in mice with targeted disruption of the acid α-glucosidase gene. *Neuromuscul Disord*, **10**, 283–91.

Raben, N., Lu, N., Nagaraju, K. *et al.* (2001). Conditional tissue-specific expression of the acid α-glucosidase (GAA) gene in the GAA knockout mice: implications for therapy. *Hum Mol Genet*, **10**, 2039–47.

Ranta, S., Zhang, Y. H., Ross, B. *et al.* (1999). The neuronal ceroid lipofuscinoses in human EPMR and mnd mutant mice are associated with mutations in CLN8. *Nat Genet*, **23**, 233–6.

Ray, J., Bouvet, A., Desanto, C. *et al.* (1998*a*). Cloning of the canine β-glucuronidase cDNA, mutation identification in canine MPS VII, and retroviral vector-mediated correction of MPS VII cells. *Genomics*, **48**, 248–53.

Ray, J., Haskins, M. E. and Ray, K. (1998*b*). Molecular diagnostic tests for ascertainment of genotype at the mucopolysaccharidosis type VII locus in dogs. *Am J Vet Res*, **59**, 1092–5.

Ray, J., Scarpino, V., Laing, C. and Haskins, M. E. (1999). Biochemical basis of the β-glucuronidase gene defect causing canine mucopolysaccharidosis VII. *J Hered*, **90**, 119–23.

Read, D. H., Harrington, D. D., Keenan, T. W. and Hinsman, E. J. (1976). Neuronal-Visceral GM1 Gangliosidosis in a Dog with β-Galactosidase Deficiency. *Science*, **194**, 442–5.

Reichmann, K. G., Twist, J. O. and Thistlethwaite, E. J. (1993). Clinical, diagnostic and biochemical features of generalised glycogenosis type II in Brahman cattle. *Aust Vet J*, **70**, 405–8.

Reuser, A.J. J. (1993). Molecular Biology, Therapeutic Trials and Animal Models of Lysosomal Storage Diseases—Type II Glycogenosis as an Example. *Annales de Biologie Clinique*, **51**, 218–19.

Riis, R. C., Cummings, J. F., Loew, E. R. and de Lahunta, A. (1992). Tibetan Terrier model of canine ceroid lipofuscinosis. *Am J Med Genet*, **42**, 615–21.

Rottier, R. J., Bonten, E. and d'Azzo, A. (1998). A point mutation in the neu-1 locus causes the neuraminidase defect in the SM/J mouse. *Hum Mol Genet*, **7**, 313–21.

Ryder, S. J. and Simmons, M. M. (2001). A lysosomal storage disease of Romney sheep that resembles human type 3 G(M1) gangliosidosis. *Acta Neuropathol*, **101**, 225–8.

Saftig, P., Tanaka, Y., Lullmann-Rauch, R. and von Figura, K. (2001). Disease model: LAMP-2 enlightens Danon disease [Review]. *Trends Mol Med*, **7**, 37–9.

Sakai, N., Inui, K., Tatsumi, N. *et al.* (1996). Molecular cloning and expression of cDNA for murine galactocerebrosidase and mutation analysis of the twitcher mouse, a model of Krabbe's disease. *J Neurochem*, **66**, 1118–24.

Sammarco, C., Weil, M., Just, C. *et al.* (2000). Effects of bone marrow transplantation on the cardiovascular abnormalities in canine mucopolysaccharidosis VII. *Bone Marrow Transplant*, **25**, 1289–97.

Sands, M. S. and Birkenmeier, E. H. (1993). A single-base-pair deletion in the β-glucuronidase gene accounts for the phenotype of murine mucopolysaccharidosis type VII. *Proc Natl Acad Sci USA*, **90**, 6567–71.

Sango, K., Yamanaka, S., Hoffmann, A. *et al.* (1995). Mouse models of Tay–Sachs and Sandhoff diseases differ in neurologic phenotype and ganglioside metabolism. *Nat Genet*, **11**, 170–6.

Sango, K., Yamanaka, S., Ajiki, K., Tokashiki, A. and Watabe, K. (2002). Lysosomal storage results in impaired survival but normal neurite outgrowth in dorsal root ganglion neurones from a mouse model of Sandhoff disease. *Neuropathol Appl Neurobiol*, **28**, 23–34.

Sarna, J., Miranda, S. R. P., Schuchman, E. H. and Hawkes, R. (2001). Patterned cerebellar Purkinje cell death in a transgenic mouse model of Niemann Pick type A/B disease. *Eur J Neurosci*, **13**, 1873–80.

Saunders, G. K., Wood, P. A., Myers, R. K., Shell, L. G. and Carithers, R. (1988). GM1Gangliosidosis in Portuguese Water Dogs: Pathologic and Biochemical Findings. *Vet Pathol*, **25**, 265–9.

Seigel, G. M., Lotery, A., Kummer, A. *et al.* (2002). Retinal pathology and function in a Cln3 knockout mouse model of juvenile neuronal ceroid lipofuscinosis (Batten disease). *Mol Cell Neurosci*, **19**, 515–27.

Sheahan, R. J. and Donnelly, W. J. C. (1974). Enzyme histochemical alterations in the brain of Friesian calves with GM1 gangliosidosis. *Acta Neuropathol (Berl)*, **30**, 73–4.

Shull, R. M., Munger, R. J., Spellacy, E. *et al.* (1982). Canine alpha-L-iduronidase deficiency. A model of mucopolysaccharidosis I. *Am J Pathol*, **109**, 244–8.

Sigurdson, C. J., Basaraba, R. J., Mazzaferro Ema and Gould, D. H. (2002). Globoid cell-like leukodystrophy in a domestic Longhaired cat. *Vet Pathol*, **39**, 494–6.

Singer, H. S. and Cork, L. C. (1989). Canine GM2 Gangliosidosis: Morphological and Biochemical Analysis. *Vet Pathol*, **26**, 114–20.

Skelly, B. J., Jeffrey, M., Franklin, R. J. M. and Winchester, B. G. (1995). A new form of ovine GM1 gangliosidosis. *Acta Neuropathol*, **89**, 374–9.

Sohar, J., Sleat, D. E., Jadot, M. and Lobel, P. (1999). Biochemical characterization of a lysosomal protease deficient in classical late infantile neuronal ceroid lipofuscinosis (LINCL) and development of an enzyme-based assay for diagnosis and exclusion of LINCL in human specimens and animal models. *J Neurochem*, **73**, 700–11.

Somers, K. L., Wenger, D. A., Royals, M. A. *et al.* (1999). Complementation studies in human and feline Niemann–Pick type C disease. *Mol Genet Metab*, **66**, 117–21.

Stinchi, S., Lullmann-Rauch, R., Hartmann, D. *et al.* (1999). Targeted disruption of the lysosomal alpha-mannosidase gene results in mice resembling a mild form of human alpha-mannosidosis. *Hum Mol Genet*, **8**, 1365–72.

Suzuki, K. and Ohno, M. (1995). Expression of immune-related molecules in a murine genetic demyelinating disease. *Prog Brain Res*, **105**, 289–94.

Suzuki, K. and Suzuki, K. (1995). The Twitcher mouse – a model for Krabbe disease and for experimental therapies. *Brain Pathol*, **5**, 249–58.

Suzuki, K., Sango, K., Proia, R. L. and Langaman, C. (1997). Mice deficient in all forms of lysosomal β-hexosaminidase show mucopolysaccharidosis-like pathology. *J Neuropathol Exp Neurol*, **56**, 693–703.

Suzuki, K., Vanier, M. T. and Suzuki, K. (1998). Induced mouse models of abnormal sphingolipid metabolism [Review]. *J Biochem*, **124**, 8–19.

Takahashi, H., Igisu, H., Suzuki, K. and Suzuki, K. (1983). Murine globoid cell leukodystrophy (the twitcher mouse). The presence of characteristic inclusions in the kidney and lymph nodes. *Am J Pathol*, **112**, 147–54.

Takahashi, H., Igisu, H., Suzuki, K. and Suzuki, K. (1984). Murine globoid cell leukodystrophy: the twitcher mouse. An ultrastructural study of the kidney. *Lab Invest*, **50**, 42–50.

Taniike, M. and Suzuki, K. (1994). Spacio-temporal progression of demyelination in twitcher mouse: with clinico-pathological correlation. *Acta Neuropathol*, **88**, 228–36.

Taniike, M., Yamanaka, S., Proia, R. L. *et al.* (1995). Neuropathology of mice with targeted disruption of Hexa gene, a model of Tay–Sachs disease. *Acta Neuropathol (Berl)*, **89**, 296–304.

Taniike, M., Mohri, I., Eguchi, N. *et al.* (1999). An apoptotic depletion of oligodendrocytes in the twitcher, a murine model of globoid cell leukodystrophy. *J Neuropathol Exp Neurol*, **58**, 644–53.

Taylor, R. M. and Farrow, B. R. H. (1988). Animal model series. Fucosidosis. *Comp Pathol Bull*, **20**, 2–5.

Taylor, R. M. and Farrow, B. R. H. (1992). Ceroid lipofuscinosis in the Border Collie dog: retinal lesions in an animal model of juvenile Batten disease. *Am J Med Genet*, **42**, 622–7.

Taylor, R. M., Farrow, B. R. H. and Healy, P. J. (1987). Canine Fucosidosis: clinical findings. *J Small Anim Pract*, **28**, 291–300.

Taylor, R. M., Farrow, B. R. H. and Stewart, G. J. (1992). Amelioration of clinical disease following bone marrow transplantation in fucosidase-deficient dogs. *Am J Med Genet*, **42**, 628–32.

Thompson, J. N., Jones, M. Z., Dawson, G. and Huffman, P. S. (1992). *N*-Acetylglucosamine 6-sulfatase deficiency in a Nubian goat: a model of Sanfilippo syndrome type D (mucopolysaccharidosis IIID). *J Inherit Metab Dis*, **15**, 760–8.

Tollersrud, O. K., Berg, T., Healy, P., Evjen, G., Ramachandran, U. and Nilssen, O. (1997). Purification of bovine lysosomal alpha-mannosidase, characterization of its gene and determination of two mutations that cause α-mannosidosis. *Eur J Biochem*, **246**, 410–9.

Tomatsu, S., Orii, K. O., Vogler, C. *et al.* (2002*a*). Mouse model of Morquio syndrome produced by targeted mutagenesis. *7th International Symposium on MPS and Related Diseases, June, Paris.* p. 37.

Tomatsu, S., Orii, K. O., Vogler, C. *et al.* (2002*b*). Missense models [Gustm(E536A)Sly, Gustm(E536Q)Sly, and Gustm(L175F)Sly] of murine mucopolysaccharidosis type VII produced by targeted mutagenesis. *Proc Natl Acad Sci USA*, **99**, 14982–7.

Tybulewicz, V. L., Tremblay, M. L., LaMarca, M. E. *et al.* (1992). Animal model of Gaucher's disease from targeted disruption of the mouse glucocerebrosidase gene. *Nature*, **357**, 407–10.

Vandevelde, M., Fankhauser, R., Bichsel, P., Wiesmann, U. and Herschkowitz (1982). Hereditary Neurovisceral Mannosidosis Associated with -Mannosidase Deficiency in a Family of Persian Cats. *Acta Neurpathol*, **58**, 64–8.

Victoria, T., Rafi, M. A. and Wenger, D. A. (1996). Cloning of the canine GALC cDNA and identification of the mutation causing globoid cell leukodystrophy in West Highland White and Cairn Terriers. *Genomics*, **33**, 457–62.

Vite, C. H., McGowan, J. C., Braund, K. G. *et al.* (2001). Histopathology, electrodiagnostic testing, and magnetic resonance imaging show significant peripheral and central nervous system myelin abnormalities in the cat model of α-mannosidosis. *J Neuropathol Exp Neurol*, **60**, 817–28.

Vogler, C., Levy, B., Galvin, N. *et al.* (2001). A novel model of murine mucopolysaccharidosis type VII due to an intracisternal A particle element transposition into the β-glucuronidase gene: clinical and pathologic findings. *Pediatr Res*, **49**, 342–8.

Walvoort, H. C., Slee, R. G. and Koster, J. F. (1982). Canine glycogen storage disease type II. A biochemical study of an acid α-glucosidase-deficient Lapland dog. *Biochim Biophys Acta*, **715**, 63–9.

Walvoort, H. C., Dormans, J. A. and van den Ingh, T. S. (1985). Comparative pathology of the canine model of glycogen storage disease type II (Pompe's disease). *J Inherit Metab Dis*, **8**, 38–46.

Wang, A. M., Stewart, C. L. and Desnick, R. J. (1993). α-*N*-Acetylgalactosaminidase: Characterization of the murine cDNA and genomic sequences and generation of mice by targeted gene disruption. *Am J Hum Genet*, **53**, 99.

Wang, Z. H., Zeng, B., Shibuya, H. *et al.* (2000). Isolation and characterization of the normal canine β-galactosidase gene and its mutation in a dog model of GM1 gangliosidosis. *J Inherit Metab Dis*, **23**, 593–606.

Weintraub, H., Abramovici, A., Sandbank, U. *et al.* (1985). Neurological mutation characterized by dysmyelination in NCTR-BALB/*c* mouse with lysosomal lipid storage disease. *J Neurochem*, **45**, 665–72.

Wenger, D. A., Sattler, M., Kudoh, T., Snyder, S. P. and Kingston, R. S. (1980). Niemann–Pick Disease: A Genetic Model in Siamese Cats. *Science*, **208**, 1471–3.

Wenger, D. A., Victoria, T., Rafi, M. A. *et al.* (1999). Globoid cell leukodystrophy in Cairn and West Highland White Terriers. *J Hered*, **90**, 138–42.

Wenger, D. A., Suzuki, K., Suzuki, Y. and Suzuki, K. (2001) Galactosylceramide lipidosis: globoid cell leukodystrophy. In *The metabolic and molecular bases of inherited disease* (Scriver, C. R., Beaudet, A. L., Sly, W. S. and Valle, D. ed.), pp. 3669–94, 8th edn. New York: McGraw-Hill.

Wheeler, R. B., Sharp, J. D., Schultz, R. A. *et al.* (2002). The General mutated in variant late infantile neuronal ceroid lipofuscinosis (CLN6) and in nclf mutant mice encodes a novel predicted transmembrane protein. *Am J Hum Genet*, **70**, 537–42.

Wilkerson, M. J., Lewis, D. C., Marks, S. L. and Prieur, D. J. (1998). Clinical and morphologic features of mucopolysaccharidosis type II in a dog: naturally occurring model of Hunter syndrome. *Vet Pathol*, **35**, 230–3.

Yadid, G., Sotnikbarkai, I., Tornatore, C. *et al.* (1998). Neurochemical alterations in the cerebellum of a murine model of Niemann–Pick type C disease. *Brain Res*, **799**, 250–6.

Yamanaka, S., Johnson, M. D., Grinberg, A. *et al.* (1994). Targeted disruption of the hexa gene results in mice with biochemical and pathologic features of Tay–Sachs disease. *Proc Natl Acad Sci USA*, **91**, 9975–9.

Yamato, O., Ochiai, K., Masuoka, Y. *et al.* (2000). GM1 gangliosidosis in Shiba dogs. *Vet Rec*, **146**, 493–6.

Yamato, O., Matsuki, N., Satoh, H. *et al.* (2002). A Golden Retriever dog is described with total hexosaminidase deficiency and raised GM2 ganglioside in CSF. The animal represents a model for human Sandhoff disease. *J Inherit Metab Dis*, **25**, 319–20.

Yogalingam, G., Litjens, T., Bielicki, J. *et al.* (1996). Feline mucopolysaccharidosis type VI. Characterization of recombinant *N*-acetylgalactosamine 4-sulfatase and identification of a mutation causing the disease. *J Biol Chem*, **271**, 27259–65.

Yogalingam, G., Hopwood, J. J., Crawley, A. and Anson, D. S. (1998). Mild feline mucopolysaccharidosis type VI. Identification of an *N*-acetylgalactosamine-4-sulfatase mutation causing instability and increased specific activity. *J Clin Biochem*, **273**, 13421–9.

Yogalingam, G., Pollard, T., Gliddon, B., Jolly, R. D. and Hopwood, J. J. (2002). Identification of a mutation causing mucopolysaccharidosis type IIIA in New Zealand Huntaway dogs. *Genomics*, **79**, 150–3.

Yoshida, M., Noguchi, J., Ikadai, H., Takahashi, M. and Nagase, S. (1993). Arylsulfatase B-deficient mucopolysaccharidosis in rats. *J Clin Invest*, **91**, 1099–104.

Zhou, X. Y., Morreay, H., Rottier, R. *et al.* (1995). Mouse model for the lysosomal disorder galactosialidosis and correction of the phenotype with over-expressing erythroid precursor cells. *Genes Dev*, **9**, 2623–34.

Chapter 12

Pathogenic cascades and brain dysfunction

Steven U. Walkley

Introduction

Lysosomal storage diseases that affect the brain are most commonly characterized by insidious onset and slow, but relentless, progression. Children with storage diseases often exhibit little or no evidence of disease at birth, but the final clinical outcome, which may be years in the making, manifests as severe neurological dysfunction that reduces both the length and the quality of life. The severity of end-stage disease thus stands in sharp contrast to the apparent normalcy of early life in most affected individuals. This distinctive feature of many lysosomal diseases indicates that the primary gene defects do not, in themselves, necessarily impede an orderly and normal development of many organ systems, including brain. Rather, what is suggested is that recruitment of a host of downstream or cascade events, which take time to accrue, is the ultimate cause of cell and organ dysfunction. Importantly, this finding offers a glimmer of hope that if corrective measures could be taken to intervene early in the disease process, significant neurological dysfunction might be prevented. Whether this treatment is directed at the gene itself or at some subsequent point in the cascade, the more that is understood about events set in motion by the original metabolic defect the more likely the possibility for full interdiction of the disease process. Detailed knowledge of disease cascades, for example, would reveal which accrued deficits are reversible and specific time windows critical for successful intervention. Finally, as readily illustrated in earlier chapters in this book, it is important to recognize that molecular and cellular analyses of pathogenic cascades in storage diseases provide unique windows for understanding the intricacies of *normal* cell function (Garrod 1928). This could be viewed as a silver lining to otherwise tragic conditions.

A clinical maelstrom

Lysosomal disorders, as reviewed in Chapter 3, variously affect many tissues and organ systems including bone and cartilage, the liver, kidneys and other visceral organs, the immune system, and the brain and related neural tissues. For brain, early developmental milestones, including acquisition of walking and language, may occur with minimal or no delay, but are subsequently followed by stasis, and later, by loss of acquired skills. This progressive spiral of neurological decline in storage diseases differs from that seen in disorders like cerebral palsy and phenylketonuria in which a pathogenic insult during a key period of early brain development leads to specific deficits and a more static clinical condition in later life. Clinical symptoms in storage diseases typically begin after birth during infantile, late infantile, juvenile, or adult periods and, generally speaking, the earlier the onset, the more severe the course and the shorter the lifespan. Essentially, all aspects of brain function are susceptible to compromise in the full range of lysosomal diseases with neurological involvement. Motor dysfunction is common and may include dysarthria, dysphagia, myoclonus, hypo- and hypertonia, choreoathetosis, dystonia, tremors, ataxia, and spastic tetraparesis. Sensory disturbances range from visual impairment to hearing loss; exaggerated startle responses (hyperacusis) may also be observed. Seizures are prominent in some types of storage diseases and may be refractory to pharmacological therapies [e.g. in the neuronal ceroid lipofuscinoses (NCLs)] (Hofmann and Peltonen 2001); other storage diseases either lack seizures or exhibit this feature only in late disease [e.g. many of the mucopolysaccharidoses (MPSs)] (Neufeld and Muenzer 2001). Autonomic disturbances and sleep disorders are often-cited clinical features of many storage diseases. Behavioural abnormalities including mental disturbances and psychosis may occur and in some cases have been reported to exacerbate with onset of puberty. Not surprisingly, cognitive deficits are a common occurrence and include mild-to-severe mental retardation, and in older patients, dementia. Not only do clinical neurological deficits cover a wide and diverse spectrum depending on the disease type, but presenting signs of individual diseases also show substantial variation. In aspartyglucosaminuria, for example, speech delay typically occurs first and is followed only later by motor dysfunction, behavioural abnormalities, and mental decline (Aula *et al.* 2001). In Niemann–Pick type C (NPC) disease, non-specific behavioural problems, for example in school, have been reported to precede other clinical features including vertical supranuclear gaze palsy, a well known hallmark of this disorder (Patterson *et al.* 2001). In the NCL disorders, children with the infantile form (CLN1) typically first exhibit seizures, whereas in the juvenile form (CLN3), visual impairment is the presenting sign. However, both of these disease types subsequently progress to include significant psychomotor retardation, with the juvenile form also demonstrating seizures and the infantile form, blindness (Hofmann and Peltonen 2001).

The wide spectrum of clinical neurological dysfunction that characterizes storage disorders reveals an extensive impact of genetically induced disturbances of the endosomal–lysosomal system on the cellular elements of brain and their coordinate functions. As outlined below, the cellular/molecular generators of this dysfunction at the level of the neurone and its support cells, with few exceptions, have yet to be determined.

The pathogenic cascade in brain

To a significant degree, an explanation of disease cascades responsible for cell dysfunction and organ failure in lysosomal disorders must address not just cell-intrinsic events that occur directly or indirectly as a result of the primary genetic defect, but also the effects of disordered function of one cell type on the operations of others. For an organ like brain, countless examples exist, including both neuronal–glial and neuronal–neuronal interactions. In addition to brain-intrinsic events, the effect of compromise of other organs (e.g. liver) on brain must also be determined. The latter theme emerges with some importance with the development of new therapies (see Chapter 13) that may substantially benefit peripheral tissues like liver but leave neurones behind the blood-brain barrier largely untouched by the corrective agent. Thus, understanding the pathogenesis of lysosomal disease is necessarily a multi-tiered process requiring the assessment of molecular-cellular issues in both organ and organ-system operations.

Diseases of the endosomal–lysosomal system, like many genetic diseases, are characterized by a *divergence* of cascading events such that a functional defect in one protein ultimately gives rise to an array of complex clinical manifestations (Herschkowitz and Schulte 1984; Walkley 1988). Thus, a single defective catabolic enzyme may lead to the accumulation of one or more substrates characterized by cleavage sites uniquely dependent on that enzyme for degradation (Chapter 4). This event affecting lysosomes is followed by a host of seemingly unrelated events that impact all parts of the neurone. For example, as described in detail below, both ectopic dendritogenesis affecting many excitatory neurones and neuroaxonal dystrophy affecting inhibitory (GABAergic) neurones are characteristic features of Tay–Sachs disease (Walkley 1998). Both occur downstream to the absence of β-hexosaminidase, though exact causative mechanisms remain unclear. Interestingly, these two cellular defects are also prominent features of a host of other storage diseases with radically different molecular derangements. This latter finding indicates that, in addition to a divergence of events in the pathologic cascade, there is also a second important principle of *convergence*. That is, storage diseases with widely differing primary genetic errors may nonetheless develop the very same or dramatically similar cell-pathological features. Identifying such commonalities between metabolically distinct storage disorders can offer important clues as to those factors responsible for generating individual pathological effects, as will be illustrated below.

The why, where, and what of storage

The original concept of lysosomal disorders posited that a metabolic block in intracellular digestion in the lysosome secondary to an inherited defect in a degradative enzyme led to intralysosomal accumulation of all of the complex molecules that required the missing enzyme for their degradation (see Foreword; Hers 1965). This insightful view was successful in setting the stage for understanding an entire family of brain diseases (Hers and Van Hoof 1973). However, explanations for the 'why' of substrate accumulation in storage diseases now extends well beyond the lack of activity of a single lysosomal hydrolase resulting from a mutation in the gene encoding that enzyme (Chapters 2 and 4). Thus, we also recognize the loss of degradative capacity in cells secondary to defects in lysosomal enzyme processing (Chapter 5), in targeting of enzymes to the lysosome (Chapter 6), in protection/stabilization of enzymes within the lysosome (Chapter 7), and even in non-enzyme lysosomal and other organellar proteins (Chapters 8 and 9).

Just as the 'why' of storage has become more complex than originally conceived, so too has the 'where'. If storage is simply lysosomal and the lysosome only an end-organelle (as originally conceived), this would argue that cell dysfunction would occur principally only as a result of substrate accumulation exceeding manageable cell volume. Thus, according to this 'cytotoxicity hypothesis' (Desnick *et al.* 1976), there is limited storage capacity for tertiary lysosomes and at some point mechanical disruption of the cytoplasm is deleterious to affected cells. Increasingly, however, lysosomes are not simply viewed as end-organelles but rather as part of a continuum consisting of the entire endosomal–lysosomal system (Chapter 3). This is an important advance in the consideration of pathogenic cascades of storage disorders, since endosomes are known to be intimately involved in a variety of

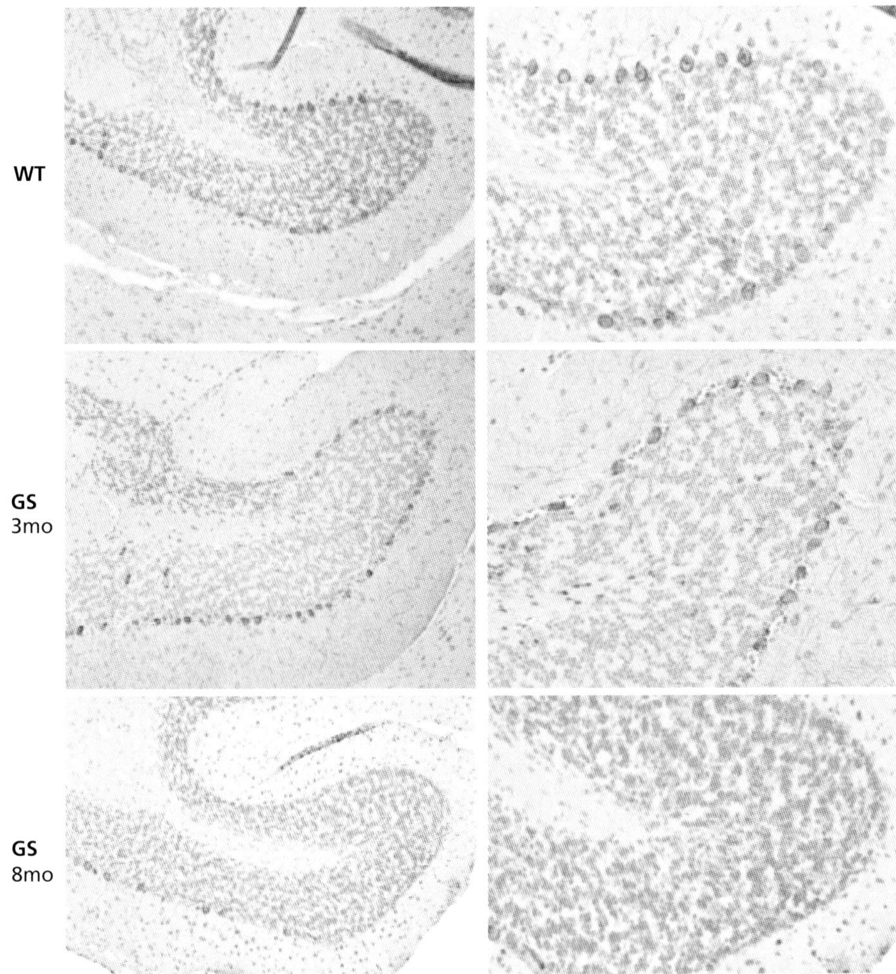

Plate 7 Wild-type (WT), 3-month-old PPCA$^{-/-}$ (GS, 3 months) and 8-month-old PPCA$^{-/-}$ mice were perfused with 4% paraformaldehyde and the brains were fixed in 10% neutral-buffered formalin, processed, and embedded in paraffin. 10 μm sections were stained with an anti-PEP19 antibody, recognizing preferentially Purkinje cells, and counterstained with haematoxylin. The anterior lobes of the cerebellum are shown.

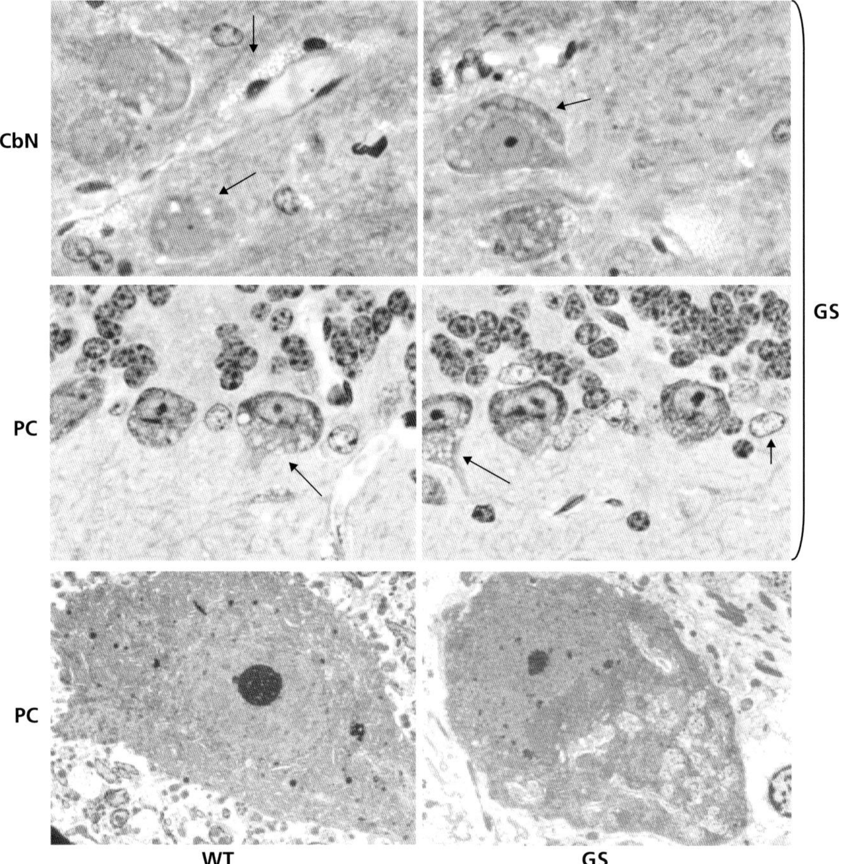

Plate 8 *Upper panels*: The brain of a GS mouse aged 8 months was fixed and embedded in plastic. Sections of 1 μm thickness were stained in toluidine blue. *Top row* (GS): deep cerebellar nucleus (CbN). *Bottom row* (GS): Purkinje cells (PC). *Lower panels*: The brains of two mice, PPCA$^{-/-}$ and wild type of 7 months of age, were fixed in 4% buffered glutaraldehyde, postfixed in OsO_4, dehydrated, and embedded in Spurr. The ultrathin sections (80 nm) were stained with uranyl acetate and lead citrate.

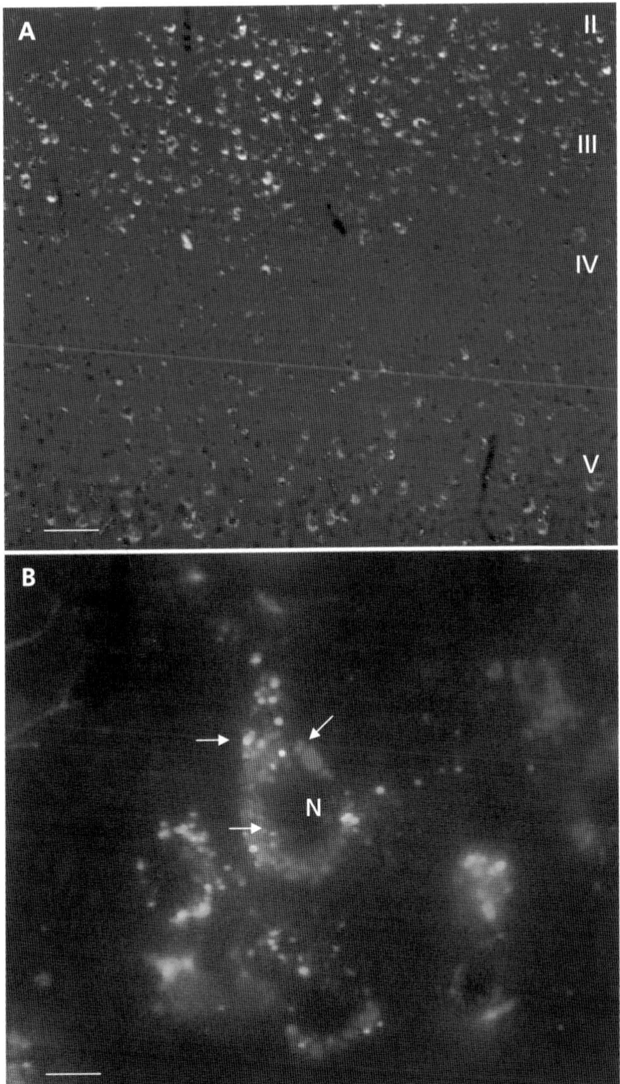

Plate 9 Multiple substrate accumulation in neurons of the cerebral cortex in a murine model of MPS III B disease (tissues kindly provided by Dr. E. Neufeld). (A) Low magnification view of cerebral cortex showing significant accumulation of GM2 (green fluorescence), GM3 (red fluorescence) and free cholesterol (filipin labeling seen as blue fluorescence). Note that GM2 is more conspicuous in upper cortical layers (II,III) while GM3 predominates in lower layers (V). (B) Higher magnification view of a layer III pyramidal neuron exhibiting GM2 (see upper left arrow), GM3 (upper right arrow) and filipin (lower left arrow) labeling. Note the lack of significant co-localization between GM2 and GM3 gangliosides. GM3 and cholesterol appear co-localized more commonly than GM2 and cholesterol. Calibration bar in (A) equals 100 mm and in (B) 10 mm.

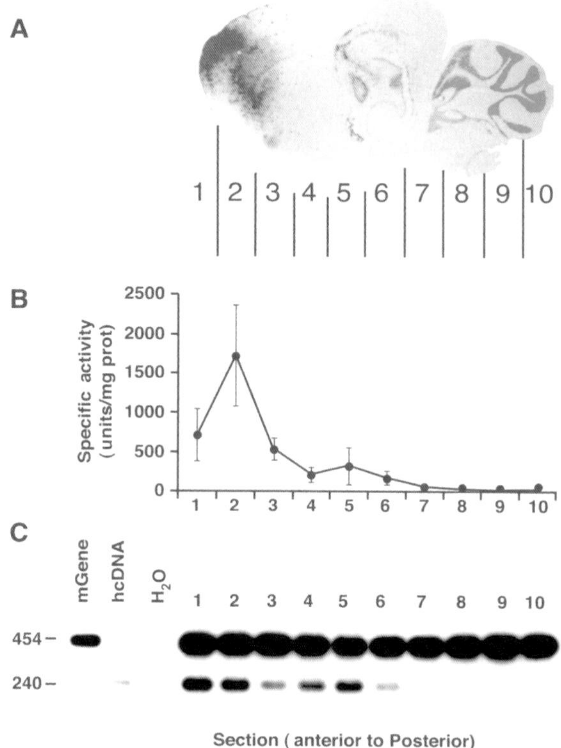

Plate 10 β-Glucuronidase (GUSB) activity and the recombinant adeno-associated virus (AAV) genome are concentrated near the injection sites in mucopolysaccharidosis VII (MPS VII) mice that received intracranial injections of AAV at birth. Histochemical staining demonstrates a concentration of GUSB activity (red) near the injection sites in the anterior cortex and hippocampus (A). Quantitative biochemical assays performed on homogenates from 1 mm coronal sections show that increased GUSB-specific activities are observed in the cortex and hippocampus (B). The data represent the mean and one standard deviation from assays performed on sections from three AAV-injected mice. Relatively more polymerase chain reaction (PCR) product from the AAV-encoded human GUSB cDNA (240, hcDNA) is observed in sections from the anterior cortex and hippocampus when compared to other regions of the brain (C). The PCR product (454, mGene) from the murine GUSB gene served as an internal control. The numbers (1–10) in each panel correspond to the specific 1 mm section from the injected brains.

cellular events, including signal transduction (Parton and Dotti 1993; Bevan *et al.* 1996; Ceresa and Schmid 2000). Lysosomal enzymes are known to be present in endosomes as well as lysosomes, with a pH gradient existing along this continuum (Chapter 1). Furthermore, compounds that could be degraded to their simplest components in lysosomes do not necessarily reach this stage before being recycled to other parts of the cell. For example, after GM2 ganglioside enters the endosomal–lysosomal system (or is generated there by degradation of higher order gangliosides) it will be degraded by β-hexosamindase (in conjunction with the GM2-activator protein) to GM3. Alternatively, it may leave the endosomal–lysosomal system intact and be recycled directly to the Golgi, where it is utilized in the synthesis of higher order gangliosides (Sonderfeld *et al.* 1985; Trinchera and Ghidoni 1990; Trinchera *et al.* 1990). This transit from late endosome to Golgi may be mediated by a protein known as NPC1 (Zervas *et al.* 2001*a*), a deficiency of which leads to a complex cholesterol–glycosphingolipid storage disease known as NPC disease (Chapter 9). The 'where' of storage therefore must address not only the nature of the organelles with abnormal sequestration of materials, but also the consequences of this involvement on the broader functions of the endosomal–lysosomal system. Likewise, alternate pathways and shunting of materials that cannot be degraded, and the consequences of their appearance elsewhere in cells, must also be considered.

Interestingly, the 'what' of storage has similarly emerged as a more complex issue in recent years. Initially, it was understood that the primary storage material could be easily predicted on the basis of, for example, the catalytic features of a defective lysosomal hydrolase (Hers and Van Hoof 1973). Primary storage compounds were found to consist of glycosphingolipids (GSLs) (particularly gangliosides), glycoproteins and oligosaccharides, glycosaminoglycans (GAGs), cholesterol, and glycogen, with diseases classified accordingly as glycosphingolipidoses, glycoproteinoses, MPSs, and so forth (Chapter 2). In addition to the major, primary storage material, less abundant accumulation of other substrates were sometimes found and explained on the basis that their degradation was dependent on the same missing enzyme. For example, the storage of oligosaccharides with β-glycosidically linked *N*-acetylglucosaminyl residues accompanies GM2 ganglioside accumulation secondary to a deficiency of β-hexosaminidase in Sandhoff disease. More recently, it has become apparent that materials unrelated to the primary degradative defect can also accumulate in storage diseases. Examples of this are in the MPS disorders and in some glycoproteinoses (α-mannosidosis), where there is substantial intraneuronal accumulation of GM2 and GM3 gangliosides even though there is no evidence that these gangliosides require the missing enzymes for degradation (Siegel and Walkley 1994; Walkley 1995). Furthermore, in many such cases significant levels of cholesterol storage accompany this increase in glycolipids, again without evidence of primary degradative errors (McGlynn *et al.* 2003). Finally, in some storage diseases, the nature of the primary versus secondary storage materials remains ill defined. The best examples of this can be found in the NCL disorders. Originally viewed as diseases in which 'ceroid' and lipofuscin were stored (hence the original disease name), they are now believed to be characterized principally by the accumulation of subunit c of mitochondrial ATP synthase (Hofmann and Peltonen 2001). However, apart from the late infantile form (CLN2) in which subunit c may be a substrate for the missing peptidase (Ezaki *et al.* 2002), no explanation for why this particular protein accumulates in the other NCL disorders is presently available.

A final consideration that goes beyond the why, where, and what of storage is a determination of the overall consequences of the storage process on cell function. Numerous scenarios are plausible: (1) Sequestration within the endosomal–lysosomal system may cause the function of a compound to be lost or compromised. For example, numerous proteoglycans with heparan sulfate side chains are believed to have critical roles in brain development ranging from pattern formation to axon guidance and synaptogenesis (Bandtlow and Zimmermann 2000). Failure to degrade specific GAG moieties, for example in Sanfilippo disease, could conceivably impede the normal function of the parent proteoglycan molecules. (2) Sequestration may deprive the cell of vital molecules that require the stored material or its derivatives for their synthesis. For example, the massive accumulation of gangliosides in lysosomes in the GM1 and GM2 gangliosidoses conceivably could deprive neurones of precursor materials for normal GSL synthesis (Schwarzmann and Sandhoff, 1990). Neurones may respond to this deficit by increasing GSL synthesis concomitantly with ganglioside storage, further enhancing storage. (3) Sequestration may exaggerate or prolong the function of a stored compound that normally would be eliminated. This may explain the correlation between the accumulation of GM2 ganglioside and a recapitulation of dendritogenesis in mature neurones in storage diseases (Walkley *et al.* 1995b). (4) Chronic sequestration may secondarily disrupt the normal functioning of the endosomal–lysosomal system and lead to a multiplicity of defects including abnormalities in trafficking, degradation, or endosome-mediated signal transduction. This may explain why, in many storage diseases, numerous materials unrelated to the primary degradative enzyme are sequestered within cells (Marks and Pagano 2002, McGlynn *et al.* 2003). (5) Sequestered compounds may be directly or indirectly toxic to cells, an idea that has been proposed for accumulating psychosine in Krabbe disease (Miyatake and Suzuki 1972) and for subunit c of mitochondrial ATP synthase in NCL disorders (Walkley *et al.* 1996; McGeoch and Palmer 1999).

Glycosphingolipids

A variety of GSLs are believed to depend on the lysosome for degradation (Chapter 8). Sequential removal of the terminal moieties of the hydrophilic chains down to the ceramide backbone is followed by its degradation to sphingosine and fatty acids. Sialic acid-containing glycolipids known as gangliosides are one of the most prominent groups of GSLs degraded within the lysosome. Although most abundant in neurones, gangliosides are found in most types of cells. They are reported to be synthesized in the Golgi (Yusuf *et al.* 1984; Sandhoff and Echten 1994; Yu 1994) and possibly elsewhere (Stern and Tiemeyer 2001) and to be chiefly localized to the outer leaflet of the plasmalemma. From here, they enter the endosomal system for subsequent degradation and recycling (Sandhoff and Kolter 1996). The function of gangliosides is poorly understood but they have been implicated in a variety of biological processes ranging from cell adhesion to neuritogenesis (Ledeen 1985; Yates 1986). Much of the interest in their potential function has centred on their structure: they have variable polar carbohydrate head groups that extend from the plasmalemma but are anchored in the membrane by hydrophobic tails. As such, gangliosides are poised to selectively interact with other membrane constituents. There is evidence that gangliosides are transported to the plasmalemma in exocytic vesicles (Sandhoff and Schwarzmann 1989) and that these vesicles contain glycosylphosphatidylinositol (GPI)-anchored proteins, since inhibitors of GSL synthesis alter transport of such proteins (Futerman 1995). A variety of studies indicate that gangliosides can interact with and have modulatory effects on specific membrane proteins (e.g. growth factor receptors) (Weis and Davis 1990; Bremer 1994; Mutoh *et al.* 1995; Rabin and Mocchetti 1995; Yates *et al.* 1995). In the last few years evidence has mounted that gangliosides and other GSLs at the cell surface are co-localized with cholesterol in specialized patches of membrane rather than being dispersed randomly (Brown and London 1998; Hakomori 2000; Kasahara and Sanai 2000). These specialized microdomains have been variously referred to as 'rafts', DIGS (detergent-insoluble glycolipid-enriched complexes), GEMs (glycosphingolipid-enriched microdomains), and GSDs (glycosphingolipid-signalling domains). In addition to gangliosides, a variety of proteins have been found to be associated with rafts. These include GPI-anchored proteins, protein receptors (including receptor tyrosine kinases), and several signal transduction elements (e.g. Rho GTPases). The concept that has emerged is that rafts are signalling platforms that link receptor–ligand interactions at the cell surface with signal-transduction events inside the cell (Hakomori 2000). There is also evidence that rafts may be associated with actin, thus providing a connection to the cytoskeleton (Brdickova *et al.* 2001). Studies have suggested the presence of rafts within endosomes (Kobayashi and Hirabayashi 2000) consistent with signal-transduction events occurring in this compartment (Ceresa and Schmid 2000).

The glycosphingolipidoses comprise one of the larger categories of lysosomal disorders (Chapters 2 and 3). Disorders include those with storage of GM1 and GM2 gangliosides (e.g. Tay–Sachs, Sandhoff, etc.), sphingomyelin (e.g. Niemann–Pick disease type A), glucosylceramide (e.g. Gaucher), galactosylceramide (e.g. Krabbe), sulfatide [e.g. metachromatic leukodystrophy (MLD)], and ceramide (e.g. Farber). Interestingly, the accumulation of GSLs is not limited to diseases with primary catabolic defects involving this class of compounds. For example, lactosylceramide and glucosylceramide, as well as GM2 and GM3 gangliosides, are known to accumulate in NPC disease, which has been widely regarded as a primary cholesterol storage disorder (but see discussion below). Elevations of GM2 and GM3 gangliosides have also been documented in neurones in MPS diseases (Fig. 12.1) as well as in α-mannosidosis, a glycoproteinosis (Goodman *et al.* 1991; Walkley 1998). The reason(s) for storage of gangliosides in these disorders is not well understood, although for MPS secondary inhibition of key lysosomal hydrolases responsible for ganglioside degradation by accumulating GAGs has been proposed (Kint *et al.* 1973; Avila and Convit 1975; Baumkotter and Cantz 1983). This explanation has recently been re-examined, however, with the discovery that storage of GM2 and GM3 gangliosides occurs in part in organelles distinct from those with GAG storage as well as from each other (Fig. 12.1) (McGlynn *et al.* 2003). That these same two gangliosides are consistently elevated in diverse types of storage diseases (and are essentially undetectable in normal neurones) suggests the possibility of a common defect involving disordered trafficking and/or metabolism.

A key question in the analysis of storage disease pathogenic cascades, as described earlier, is whether accumulation of a particular substrate in any way alters its function—either positively or negatively. In the case of gangliosides, so little is currently understood as to their function that it is difficult to make this assessment. One potential pathogenic mechanism, however, is that the massive storage of GM1 or GM2 ganglioside in the respective disorders may lead to a relative *deficiency* of precursor molecules for ganglioside synthesis (Schwarzmann and Sandhoff 1990). If correct, a possible outcome would be an alteration in the relative activities of enzymes within the ganglioside synthetic pathway. Control of this synthetic pathway is not well understood, though most enzymes have been characterized (Sandhoff and Echten 1994; Yu 1994), and relative changes in activity are reported to occur during early brain development (Yu *et al.* 1988). As detailed in the next section, GM2 ganglioside is expressed at significant levels in post-migratory neurones of the cerebral cortex, coincident with dendritic sprouting and differentiation, but is essentially undetectable in most mature neurones (Walkley *et al.* 2000). Heightened

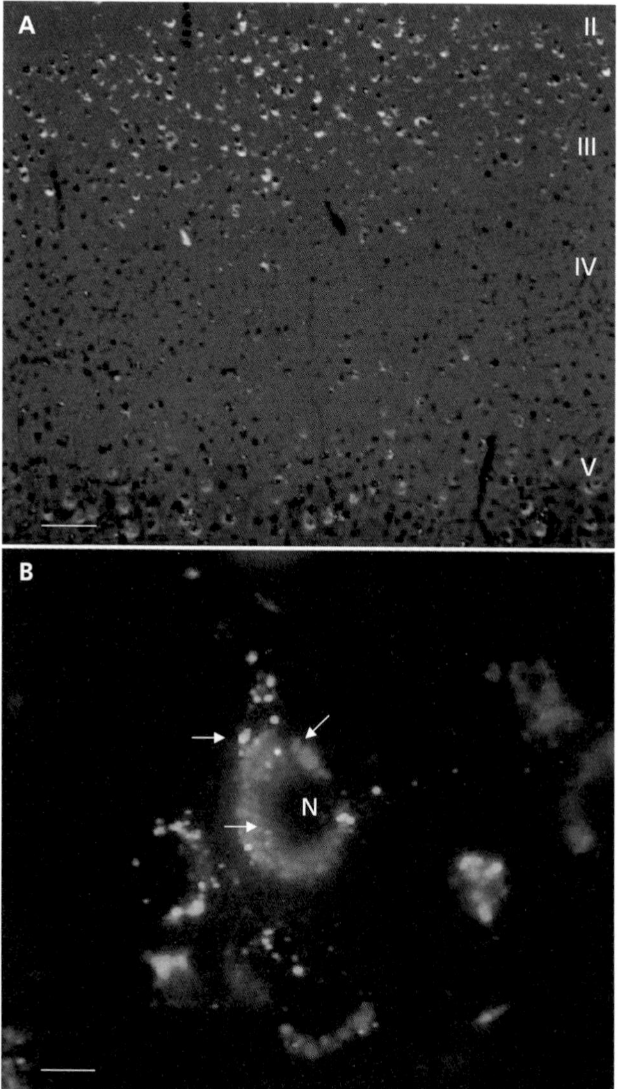

Fig.12.1 Multiple substrate accumulation in neurons of the cerebral cortex in a murine model of MPS III B disease (tissues kindly provided by Dr. E. Neufeld). (A) Low magnification view of cerebral cortex showing significant accumulation of GM2 (green fluorescence), GM3 (red fluorescence) and free cholesterol (filipin labeling seen as blue fluorescence). Note that GM2 is more conspicuous in upper cortical layers (II,III) while GM3 predominates in lower layers (V). (B) Higher magnification view of a layer III pyramidal neuron exhibiting GM2 (see upper left arrow), GM3 (upper right arrow) and filipin (lower left arrow) labeling. Note the lack of significant co-localization between GM2 and GM3 gangliosides. GM3 and cholesterol appear co-localized more commonly than GM2 and cholesterol. Calibration bar in (A) equals 100 μm and in (B) 10 μm. **See Plate 9**.

expression of this ganglioside in human fetal brain and certain tumours led to its identification as an oncofetal antigen in earlier studies (Tai *et al.* 1983). In normal mature brain, GM2 synthesis in neurones is reduced relative to the production of other, more complex gangliosides (e.g. GM1). As discussed in detail below, increases in GM2 ganglioside that occur in storage diseases are accompanied by the growth of ectopic dendrites in a variety of storage diseases, most notably Tay–Sachs. This phenomenon may represent an example of renewal or prolongation of function of a particular storage substrate in the absence of its normal degradation.

While there is little to suggest that gangliosides are toxic, there is evidence that the ganglioside precursor molecule, ceramide, has the ability to induce apoptosis (Hannun and Luberto 2000), and a storage disease characterized by ceramide accumulation (Farber disease) exhibits increased cell death in a variety of tissues (Li *et al.* 2002). Likewise, in Krabbe disease, production of the abnormal GSL metabolite, psychosine, has been hypothesized to play a role in the destruction of oligodendroglia (Wenger *et al.* 2001).

Glycosaminoglycans

Proteoglycans are glycoproteins in which the carbohydrate moieties consist of polysaccharides containing amino sugars, i.e. GAGs (e.g. heparan-, chondroitin-, and dermatan sulfates). Like the GSLs described above, many types of proteoglycans are found in brain where they reside in the outer leaflet of the plasmalemma and in other membranes from which they are ultimately trafficked to the endosomal–lysosomal system for degradation. The degradation of these complex molecules requires several lysosomal enzymes including proteases, glycosidases, and sulfatases. One group of proteoglycans is represented by the syndecans, which are transmembrane proteins with heparan sulfate side chains that are widely expressed in neurones (Ethell *et al.* 2000). Another group, the glypicans, also contains heparan sulfate side chains but are attached to membranes by GPI anchors. Heparan sulfate-containing proteoglycans at the cell surface bind to a large variety of heparan sulfate-binding proteins including growth factors, ligands of the extracellular matrix, and other cell-surface molecules (Bandtlow and Zimmermann 2000). In this way, they are believed to have functions involving numerous developmental processes from neurogenesis to axon and dendrite maturation, although details of precise mechanisms in most cases are still lacking (Rapraeger 2001; Yamaguchi 2001). Other classes of proteoglycans possess chondroitin sulfate side chains (brevicans, lecticans, versicans, aggrecans, etc.) and are reported to be the most abundant types of proteoglycan in the nervous system (Bovolenta and Fernaud-Espinosa 2000). Possible functions are again diverse and include effects on cell–cell interactions to axon growth and targeting. For most proteoglycans, gene knockout studies in mice are not yet available. However, mutation of GPC3, the gene for glypican-3, has recently been shown to be the cause of Simpson–Golabi–Behmel syndrome, a severe developmental disorder characterized by dysmorphisms related to prenatal and postnatal overgrowth (Cano-Gauci *et al.* 1999).

As for the glycosphingolipidoses, a key question in the pathogenesis of MPS disorders is whether an error in proteoglycan degradation in itself leads to a defect in the normal function of the parent molecules. Given the noted involvement of many proteoglycans in developmental events, as evidenced by the GPC3 mutation described above, and the apparent normal brain development that occurs in most MPS disorders, it presently appears that faulty degradation of GAGs in brain may not in itself significantly disturb the function of parent proteoglycans. Whether this speculation might hold true for other tissues or organ systems, some of which (e.g. cartilage) exhibit severe abnormalities in MPS disease, remains to be determined.

Glycoproteins and oligosaccharides

As for GSLs and proteoglycans describe above, numerous glycoproteins also reside at the plasmalemma, as well as elsewhere in cells, and eventually move to the endosomal–lysosomal system for degradation and/or recycling. There is increasing awareness of the critical role of protein modification through covalent attachment of carbohydrates in signal-transduction pathways (Dwek 1996; Schachter 2001). This diverse array of glycoproteins eventually enters the endosomal–lysosomal system and comes into contact with numerous hydrolases responsible for their degradation, including α- and β-mannosidases, β-hexosaminidase, β-galactosidase, α-*N*-acetylgalactosaminidase, sialidase, aspartylglucosamidase, and α-fucosidase. Proteases and peptidases also reside here to degrade the protein backbones of individual glycoprotein molecules. Disorders lacking activity of the enzymes responsible for degrading the glycan portion of the glycoprotein result in accumulation of specific oligosaccharides (Chapter 4). Since many of the same oligosaccharide linkages found in glycoproteins are also found in glycolipids and in proteoglycans, a deficiency of one of these enzymes can lead to storage of multiple types of oligosaccharide-containing molecules. This is borne out clinically by the presence of MPS-like features in children with many of the glycoproteinoses (Thomas 2001).

A key question in the pathogenesis of the glycoproteinoses again is whether there are secondary storage-induced defects in glycoprotein synthesis, trafficking, or function that occur as a result of the catabolic defect and that contribute to brain dysfunction. If not, pathogenesis would be restricted to the direct and indirect consequences of accumulation of the various oligosaccharides and secondary storage products. One approach that may eventually yield insight into this issue is the comparison of pathogenic cascades in the glycoproteinoses with genetic disorders known to directly involve defects in the synthesis of glycoproteins. A large and expanding group of diseases caused by defects in *N*-glycosylation of proteins are now being recognized. Indeed, storage diseases known as mucolipidoses and caused by defects in lysosomal enzyme targeting via the mannose-6-phosphate epitope (Chapter 6) are appropriately classified as this type of disorder. Disorders of glycoprotein synthesis are known as congenital disorders of glycosylation (CDG, previously referred to as carbohydrate-deficient glycoprotein syndromes) (Jaeken and Matthijs 2001; Schachter 2001) and typically exhibit dramatic clinical consequences involving multiple organs, often including severe brain disease.

Cholesterol

As an integral component of membranes in all cells, elaborate homoeostatic pathways exist to regulate the synthesis, trafficking, and degradation of cholesterol. Lysosomal storage of cholesterol occurs as accumulation of cholesterol esters (and triglycerides) secondary to acid lipase deficiency in Wolman disease and in cholesterol ester storage disease (Assmann and Seedorf 2001). Wolman disease is a severe lipidosis, generally leading to death by 1 year of age, whereas cholesterol ester disease is, more benign. In the CNS, storage within neurones has been described in one study of Wolman disease (Kahana *et al.* 1968), but most reports suggest that accumulation of cholesterol esters is limited to oligodendroglia, microglia, and other non-neuronal cells (Byrd and Powers 1979). Neurones in peripheral ganglia, however, have been documented to accumulate significant amounts of sudanophilic lipids (Kamoshita and Landing 1968) which were believed to represent cholesterol esters. The lack of CNS neuronal accumulation of cholesterol ester was recently reconfirmed in a mouse knockout for acid lipase (Du *et al.* 2001), a finding that suggests either that cholesterol esters are not being generated in normal neurones, or that alternative pathways for cholesterol ester processing are present.

A second neuronal storage disorder in which cholesterol accumulation has received a great deal of attention is NPC disease. As reviewed elsewhere (Chapter 9), this disorder is caused by a defect in a transmembrane protein known as NPC1 or, less frequently, in a soluble lysosomal protein known as NPC2 (Chapter 8). The cholesterol connection in this disorder derives from the discovery that loading NPC fibroblasts with LDL-cholesterol elicited significant increases in intracellular levels of free cholesterol as revealed by filipin staining (Pentchev *et al.* 1985). Other studies have also documented dramatic increases in cholesterol synthesis in organs like liver. Cholesterol storage in brain was first believed absent, but more recent studies have unequivocally revealed significant increases in free cholesterol in neurones (Zervas *et al.* 2001*b*). The metabolic defect in NPC disease is complicated by the finding that GSL storage (e.g. GM2 and GM3 gangliosides, as well as lactosylceramide and glucosylceramide) also occurs, particularly in brain (Zervas *et al.* 2001*a*). A key question in terms of NPC1 function is whether its primary role involves shuttling of cholesterol or GSLs, or both (Chapter 9). Studies evaluating mice deficient in both NPC1 and in the enzyme responsible for synthesis of GM2 and higher order gangliosides [β1,4-*N*-acetylgalactosaminyltransferase (GalNAcT)] have shown that cholesterol accumulation in these double mutants is reduced and occurs in neurones that store GM3 ganglioside (Gondré-Lewis *et al.* 2003). These findings are consistent with the view that in NPC1-deficient neurones, cholesterol accumulation occurs principally in parallel with, or secondary to, the metabolism and/or trafficking of gangliosides, rather than vice versa. The suggestion is therefore that NPC1 function in neurones may involve the shuttling and/or recycling of simple gangliosides, possibly as a control for ganglioside homoeostasis (Zervas *et al.* 2001*b*). This view is supported by recent studies showing that the treatment of NPC disease-affected animals with an inhibitor of GSL synthesis delayed clinical onset and prolonged life (Zervas *et al.* 2001*a*) (Chapter 15), whereas drugs affecting cholesterol synthesis have shown little or no benefit (reviewed in Patterson *et al.* 2001).

Accumulation of free cholesterol accompanies ganglioside storage in a variety of glycosphingolipidoses (e.g. see Pagano *et al.* 2000; Marks and Pagano, 2002). This in fact has long been known as a feature of Tay–Sachs disease in which the cholesterol was believed to autoassemble with GM2 ganglioside within lysosomes to form so-called membranous cytoplasmic bodies (MCBs) (Samuels *et al.* 1963). That is, non-degraded ganglioside would passively combine with cholesterol in the lysosome and form membranes. A more recent, provocative speculation is that the GSL storage diseases actually represent 'log jams' of GSL–cholesterol rafts within the endosomal–lysosomal system (Puri *et al.* 1999; Simons and Gruenberg 2000; Lusa, *et al.* 2001). This attractive hypothesis suggests the possibility of substantial interference with a variety of signal-transduction events involving endosomes. Both the passive ganglioside–cholesterol autoassembly hypothesis, and the concept of the so-called raft log-jam predict that the sequestered gangliosides and cholesterol would be co-localized to common vesicles in affected neurones. However, studies localizing cholesterol and GM2 ganglioside in both Sandhoff and NPC diseases (in mouse models) have indicated that the two substrates often occur in separate cell compartments (Zervas *et al.* 2001*a*). Cholesterol accumulation has also recently been found to accompany ganglioside storage in MPS disorders which are believed to lack primary involvement of GSL degradation (McGlynn *et al.* 2003). Once again, a significant portion of the identified free cholesterol appeared to be sequestered independently of GM2 and GM3 gangliosides (Fig. 12.1).

Glycogen

While there are many types of glycogen storage diseases (Chen, 2001), the vast majority are not lysosomal in nature. Glycogen storage secondary to lysosomal α-glucosidase (acid maltase) deficiency, also known as Pompe disease, was the prototype disease in the initial characterization of lysosomal disorders (Hers 1965; Forward). Glycogen is believed to enter the lysosome by autophagocytosis, with glucose being the final breakdown product. In most cells, it has been viewed as unlikely that this event contributes significantly to energy metabolism (Hirshhorn and Reuser 2001). Since the accumulation of glycogen does not significantly deprive cells of glucose, and since no toxic secondary products have been recognized, it has been presumed that the pathogenic cascade in cases of Pompe disease derives solely from the constipation of the lysosomal system (Winchester 1996). Clinical disease in individuals with α-glucosidase deficiency principally involves hepatomegaly, cardiomegaly, and hypotonia. Clinical neurological disease is not reported, though some degree of lysosomal glycogen storage in CNS neurones and glia has been documented (Martin *et al.* 1973). Glycogen storage in neurones is also reported in a rare disorder, Danon disease, in which activity of α-glucosidase is normal (Danon *et al.* 1981). This disorder has recently been reported to be caused by a defect in lysosomal associated membrane protein-2 (LAMP-2) (Nishino *et al.* 2000; Tanaka *et al.* 2000). In this case, the storage of glycogen is believed to be accompanied by defects in autophagocytosis, and most cases are associated with mental retardation as well as skeletal myopathy and cardiomyopathy.

Ceroid lipofuscin

The term 'neuronal ceroid lipofuscinosis' (NCL) was coined on the basis of an electron microscopic study as applied to so-called juvenile amaurotic idiocy (Batten–Spielmeyer–Vogt disease), also known as Batten disease (Zeman and Donahue 1963; Zemen and Dyken 1969). The goal to distinguish this disorder from Tay–Sachs and related glycosphingolipidoses and MPSs was successful in that the ultrastructural features of inclusion bodies in Batten disease-affected cells were dramatically different than other storage diseases. The NCL term gained wide acceptance but in several respects is misleading in that storage occurs in both neural and non-neural cells, and the accumulating autofluorescent lipopigment may be neither 'ceroid' nor 'lipofuscin'. The NCL or Batten disorders were largely left behind during the rapid advancements of the 1970s and 1980s that saw storage substrate and lysosomal enzyme deficiencies clearly defined, and then genes cloned, for most other types of storage disorders. Recent advances, however, have been dramatic and have led to the discovery of many of the genes responsible for NCL disease (CLN1-8) (Peltonen *et al.* 2000). Two of the identified genes code for proteins believed to be lysosomal proteases (CLN1 and CLN2), although questions have arisen as to whether one of them, palmitoyl protein thioesterase (CLN1p), exhibits a lysosomal location in neurones (Lehtovirta *et al.* 2001). Other identified proteins (those of CLN3, CLN5, CLN6, and CLN8) are transmembrane proteins of unknown function (Gao *et al.* 2002; Hofmann and Peltonen 2001), although some may have a lysosomal location (Isosomppi *et al.* 2002; Vesa *et al.* 2002). The latter study also reports that the CLN5 protein may directly interact with CLN2 and CLN3 proteins, providing a possible common mechanism for disease production. The nature of the material accumulating in the NCL disorders has also seen significant advances and is now believed to be primarily a single protein, subunit c of mitochondrial ATP synthase, consistent with classification as lysosomal proteinoses (Palmer *et al.* 1992). Storage of subunit c has now been documented in all forms of NCL disease, including CLN1 (Elleder *et al.* 1997), although the latter also exhibits substantial accumulation of saposins A and D, proteins critical for GSL degradation (Hofmann and Peltonen 2001). Recently, mice in which the gene for the lysosomal protease, cathepsin D, has been ablated also have been found to exhibit features of NCL disease, including the storage of subunit c (Koike *et al.* 2000). It is not known exactly why subunit c accumulates in cells in NCL disease, nor has the significance of its storage been established. Interestingly, this same protein has also been reported to accumulate to some degree in MPS disease, the gangliosidoses, and other storage diseases (Lake and Hall 1993; Elleder *et al.* 1997), even though these disorders otherwise bear little resemblance to NCL diseases.

The cellular consequences of storage

In the original studies on the pathology of Tay–Sachs disease, it was recognized that neurones contained abnormal amounts of granular material that distorted neuronal cell bodies and proximal processes (Sachs 1887, 1903; Sachs and Strauss 1910). Subsequent reports established this 'storage' as the pathologic hallmark of a large group of paediatric brain diseases (Suzuki, 1976). With the advent of electron microscopy it became evident that it was often possible to categorize a given disease by the ultrastructural features of the sequestered material, with Tay–Sachs disease exhibiting MCBs (Terry and Weiss 1963), the MPSs 'zebra bodies' (Loeb *et al.* 1968), the NCL disorders 'fingerprint bodies' and 'curvilinear bodies' (Zeman and Donahue 1963; Zemen 1976) and so forth. As detailed above, closer inspection of the storage process revealed substantial heterogeneity within a given disease category and within different cells of any one disease. While it might be assumed that the ensuing disease cascades in storage diseases would be as numerous as the many types of polymeric molecules known to accumulate, current evidence suggests otherwise. Indeed, at the cellular level, as few as five broad and somewhat overlapping disease paths can currently be identified. One involves a renewal of dendritic sprouting ('ectopic dendritogenesis'), complete with new synapse formation, and occurs specifically on a limited set of excitatory neurones. A second involves axons and is seen as formation of enlargements or 'spheroids' (neuroaxonal dystophy), occurring predominately in inhibitory (GABAergic) neurones. These two disease cascades have been identified principally in the glycosphingolipidoses and in some other storage disorders with secondary storage of gangliosides. A third and prominent disease cascade is seen as massive, early death of neurones as documented in the NCL disorders. This loss of neurones typically is regionally selective and often involves the cerebral cortex. A fourth disease cascade involves abnormalities predominating in glia and is accompanied by severe loss of myelin, often with grey matter remaining intact. This cascade principally characterizes the leukodystrophies (MLD and Krabbe disease). Demyelination may also be observed in the poliodystrophies described above, though there are notable exceptions, and myelin loss may be caused by different mechanisms. Finally, a fifth disease cascade involves microglial activation and its consequences and may impact many types of storage diseases. Details are provided below.

Neuronal perikarya and dendrites

The lysosomal system of neurones is believed to be localized chiefly within the perikaryal space, whereas endosomal vacuoles are considerably more widespread in dendrites and axons (Chapter 1). Early studies on storage diseases revealed that the accumulating materials in neurones are principally within perikarya and in disorders like the NCLs, the characteristic storage bodies are often corralled in the lower perikaryal space between the nucleus and axon hillock. In disorders with ganglioside storage, ganglioside-laden vesicles are again most abundant in perikarya but may also be found in dendrites, particularly along the cytoplasmic side of the plasmalemma of apical dendrites of cortical pyramidal neurones. In Purkinje cells of the cerebellum, the presence of so-called 'megadendrites' has been documented, i.e. very prominent enlargements within main stem dendrites that closely resemble storage in perikarya (Goldman *et al.* 1981). Typically, most types of neurones exhibit accumulation of storage vacuoles principally within perikarya. Volume increases may cause cell swelling and rounding of perikaryal contours, but more commonly in most types of neurones it is the axon hillock which preferentially swells to accommodate the volume increase. The resulting enlargement is identifiable by both silver (Bielschowsky 1932) and Golgi staining (Purpura and Suzuki 1976) (Fig. 12.2A), and has been referred to as a meganeurite by Purpura and colleagues. Importantly, from a functional view, meganeurites force the initial segment of the axon—the sodium channel-rich 'trigger zone' for action potential generation—to be displaced distally away from the perikaryon, probably with negative consequences for orderly synaptic integration over the soma-dendritic domain (Purpura and Suzuki 1976; Walkley and Pierok 1986). These studies also establish an important distinction between meganeurites, which occur proximal to the axonal initial segment and axonal spheroids (discussed below) which occur distal to this region.

While the so-called meganeurite can be an impressive component of cellular pathology in storage diseases, an even more remarkable abnormality occurring at the axon hillock is ectopic dendritogenesis (Fig. 12.2B–D). This phenomenon was originally discovered in the AB variant form of GM2 gangliosidosis and later in Tay–Sachs disease (Purpura and Suzuki 1976; Purpura 1978). Morphologically, mature pyramidal neurones in cerebral cortex of children with these diseases exhibited an unusual sprouting of new primary dendrites from the axon hillock. We now know that this phenomenon is not exclusive to Tay–Sachs and related GM2 gangliosidoses, but occurs in many types of lysosomal diseases including MPSs and glycoproteinoses (Walkley 1998). The phenomenon of ectopic dendritogenesis has not, however, been observed in other neurological disorders. One common feature of all neuronal storage diseases exhibiting ectopic dendrite initiation is an abnormal elevation of GM2 ganglioside, with this increase occurring specifically within neurones bearing new dendritic sprouts (Goodman and Walkley 1996; Walkley 1998).

A central question in the apparent association between ectopic dendritogenesis and an abnormal elevation of GM2 ganglioside in mature pyramidal neurones has been whether a similar relationship exists during dendritogenesis of normal development. Examination of normal developing brain for GM2 expression has shown that post-migratory cortical neurones in the cerebral cortex of multiple species (cat, ferret, human, and mouse) express GM2 ganglioside coincident with initiation of dendritogenesis, and after dendritic maturation is complete in the early postnatal period, GM2 drops to negligible levels (Goodman *et al.* 1991; Zervas and Walkley 1999; Walkley *et al.* 2000; Gondré-Lewis *et al.* 2002*a*). Ultrastructural studies showed that GM2 immunoreactivity was localized to vesicles in a manner consistent with Golgi synthesis, exocytic trafficking to the soma-dendritic

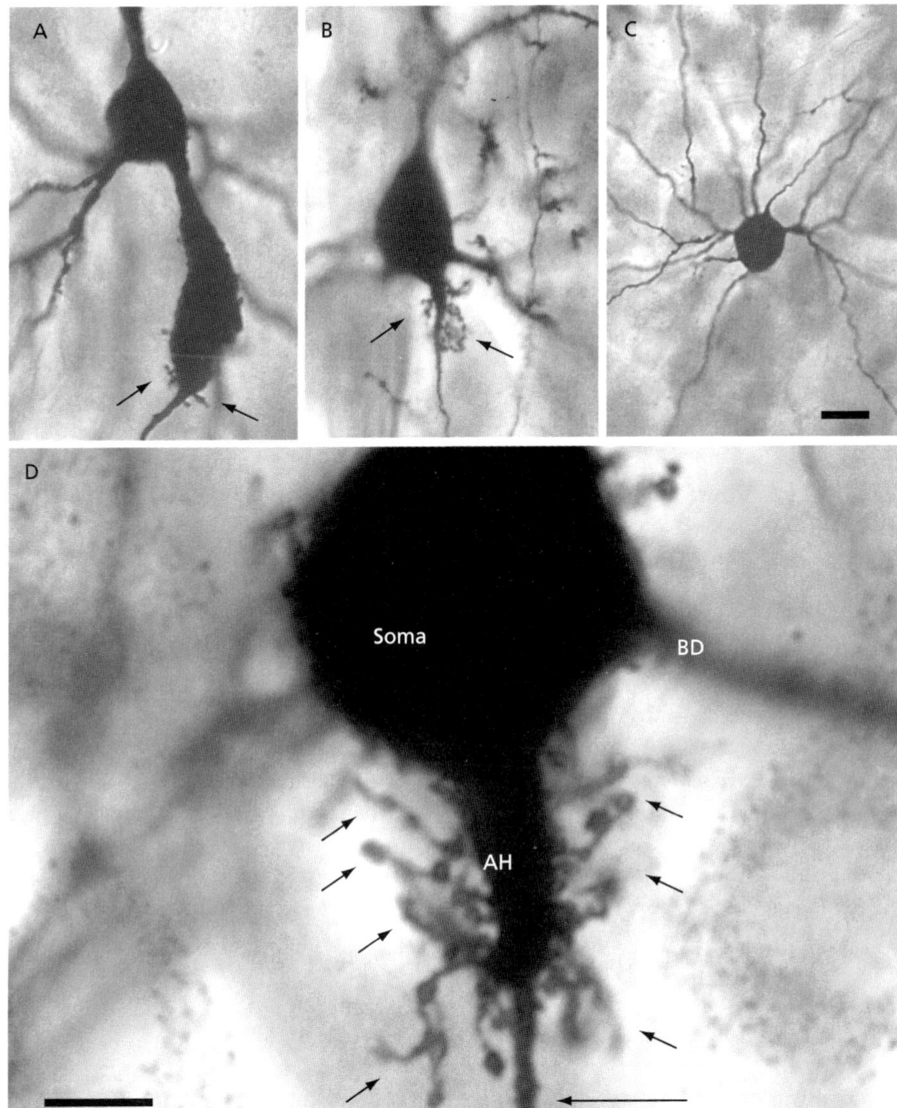

Fig. 12.2 Ectopic dendritogenesis affecting neurones of the cerebral cortex in a feline model of GM2 gangliosidosis. (A) Layer III cortical pyramidal neurone with a large meganeurite and numerous ectopic sprouts at its distal end (arrows). (B) Layer III pyramidal neurone lacking a meganeurite but possessing extensive sprouting of dendritic processes at the axon hillock area (arrows). (C) Non-pyramidal neuron of midlevel cortex which lacks a meganeurite and ectopic dendrites, but whose perikaryon appears rounded and swollen. (D) Higher magnification of the axon hillock of a cortical neurone with ectopic dendritogenesis. Ectopic dendrites (short arrows) sprout prolifically from an enlarged axon hillock (AH) from which also emerges a normal appearing axon (long arrow). Adjacent basilar dendrites (BD) appeared normal. Calibration bar in C equals 15 μm and applies to A-C and in D equals 8 μm.

plasmalemma, endocytic retrieval and lysosomal degradation. No other gangliosides have been found to exhibit a similar correlation with dendritic sprouting, although GD2 ganglioside showed a vesicular staining pattern persisting into adulthood (Zervas and Walkley 1999). As described earlier, the functions of GM2 and other gangliosides remain poorly understood. However, several types of gangliosides have been implicated in modulation of a variety of cell-surface proteins as well as signal-transduction molecules, possibly functioning within specialized membrane microdomains knows as rafts (reviewed in Walkley *et al.* 2000). Candidate proteins linked to mechanisms of dendritogenesis as well as to gangliosides and GSL-containing microdomains include Trk receptors (McAllister *et al.* 1995; Pitto *et al.* 1998; Fukumoto *et al.* 2000), Rho-related GTPases (Threadgill *et al.* 1997; Hakomori 2000; Simons and Toomre 2000), Src-family kinases (Kasahara *et al.* 1997; Prinetti *et al.* 1999) and CaMKII (Zou and Cline 1999; Gondré-Lewis *et al.* 2002*b*). One hypothesis is that the presence of heightened levels of GM2 ganglioside in immature or storage disease-affected cortical pyramidal neurones facilitates the function of dendritogenic agents and/or their second messenger cascades, whereas the replacement of this ganglioside by others which dominate in the normal, mature neurones (e.g. GD2) has neutral or opposite effects on dendritogenesis (Walkley *et al.* 2000).

Ectopic dendrites of storage diseases occur principally at the axon hillock where they emerge either as a prolific tuft of processes or as a component of the larger meganeurite structure. Over time, ectopic dendrites become richly vested with spines and type I synapses and thus resemble normal adjacent basilar dendrites (Walkley *et al.* 1981; Walkley *et al.* 1990*b*; Walkley and Wurzelmann 1995). Studies of elevated GM2 ganglioside expression as a 'stimulus' for ectopic dendritogenesis appears to suggest that GM2 is driving the formation of new dendritic membrane surface area for type 1 (excitatory) synapses rather than for 'neuritogenesis' *per se.* This is based on the observation that meganeurite surfaces lacking ectopic dendrites may nonetheless exhibit ectopic dendritic spines and new synapses. Pyramidal neurones with either axon hillock neurites or spiny meganeurites have been shown to contain abnormal elevations of GM2 ganglioside. In contrast, pyramidal neurones undergoing significant storage that does not include GM2 ganglioside (e.g. the NCL diseases) have meganeurites that are non-spiny, i.e. exhibit smooth surfaces and lack evidence of spines and synapses (Walkley 1998).

Ectopic dendrites and spiny meganeurites have been found in greatest abundance on cortical pyramidal neurones in primary GM2 gangliosidosis (e.g. Sandhoff disease), a disorder in which GM2 elevation is the direct result of a catabolic enzyme defect (Siegel and Walkley 1994). Developmental studies have further shown that intraneuronal elevation of GM2 precedes the outgrowth of ectopic dendrites (Goodman *et al.* 1991). These two findings are consistent with GM2 elevation being the cause, not a consequence, of new dendritogenesis (Walkley 1998). Developmental studies in feline models of ganglioside storage disease have also revealed that ectopic dendrites only begin sprouting after normal dendritogenesis has run its course at 4–6 weeks after birth (Walkley *et al.* 1990a). However, it is also known that ectopic dendrites will sprout from older (as late as one year of age) pyramidal neurones in this species when neuronal storage is induced with the lysosomal enzyme (α-mannosidase) inhibitor, swainsonine (Walkley *et al.* 1988). In spite of their unusual location at the axon hillock of pyramidal neurones, ectopic dendrites appear to become functionally integrated with the overall dendritic arbour. That is, reversal of the storage process, for example by cessation of swainsonine treatment and restoration of normal lysosomal function, does not necessarily lead to their disappearance (Walkley *et al.*

1987; Walkley 1998). Maintenance of ectopic dendrites in normalized neurones may be related to their stabilization by the presence of ample numbers of new synaptic contacts.

Ectopic dendritogenesis exhibits both neurone-type and species-type differences (Walkley 1998, Walkley *et al.* 2000). The neurone type-specificity issue is best illustrated in cerebral cortex where even though all neurones accumulate GM2, it is pyramidal neurones, not GABAergic neurones that sprout ectopic dendrites (Walkley *et al.* 1991). Elsewhere in brain, spiny multipolar cells of the amygdala and claustrum exhibit new dendrites but most other prominent dendritic spine-covered multipolar neurones, like Purkinje cells, do not. Interestingly, the same types of neurones appear susceptible to ectopic dendritogenesis in all storage diseases that exhibit this phenomenon (Walkley 1998). Ectopic dendritogenesis also varies by species, but in this case the difference appears more as a gradient rather than as an absolute difference with human>cat, dog>mouse (Walkley *et al.* 2000). That is, pyramidal neurones in humans with storage diseases often exhibit massive production of new dendritic membrane, whereas the phenomenon is present but less extensive in carnivores, and is only minimally present or absent in mouse models of storage diseases. Why this difference occurs is unknown, but one possible explanation is suggested by the correlation between the capacity for a disease-induced renewal of dendritogenesis and the overall length of time for postnatal maturation prior to adulthood. This period is characterized by critical periods and other types of functional plasticity (Jacobsen 1991), and children with storage diseases are far more likely to experience sustained disease-associated GM2 elevations during this developmental phase than are mice. The suggestion here is that the period between normal pyramidal neurone dendritogenesis and adulthood is characterized by a capacity for dendritic plasticity, including dendritic sprouting, that may disappear or significantly diminish over time. In mice, the brevity of the postnatal developmental period prior to adulthood appears insufficient time in most GM2-accumulating storage diseases to allow GM2 levels to reach threshold and stimulate renewal of dendritogenesis. Determining what factors render neurones in rodents less sensitive to a renewal of dendritic sprouting in storage diseases could provide important insight into postnatal developmental mechanisms controlling dendritic plasticity in higher mammals, including humans.

Axons and myelin

Two prominent abnormalities of axons in neuronal storage diseases are neuroaxonal dystrophy and demyelination. Neuroaxonal dystrophy, also known as axonal spheroid formation, is seen as focal enlargements of various sizes scattered along myelinated and unmyelinated axons in both grey and white matter (Fig. 12.3). Neuroaxonal dystrophy has long been known to be a characteristic feature of storage diseases, although in many early reports spheroids undoubtedly were confused with the more recently defined meganeurites. There are two critically important distinctions between axonal spheroids and meganeurites: Firstly, axonal spheroids occur *distal* to the axonal initial segment and thus are truly axonal in location, whereas meganeurites occur at the axon hillock and may, under appropriate stimulation, be composed of dendritic-like membrane. Secondly, spheroids do *not* contain the characteristic storage bodies observed in neuronal perikarya in a given storage disease, whereas meganeurites do. Spheroids instead contain aggregates of multivesicular and dense bodies, tubulovesicular profiles, mitochondria, and other organelles that would normally be seen scattered singly in axons. Microtubules and neurofilaments generally are not conspicuously increased in number in these enlargements, which distinguishes these granular spheroids

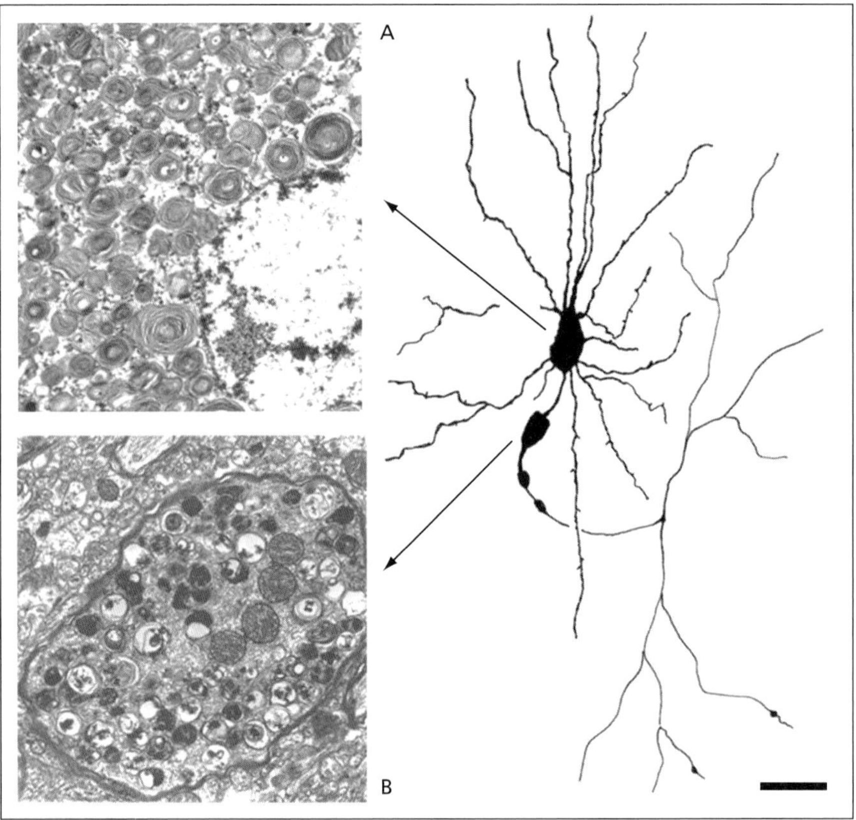

Fig,12.3 Neuroaxonal dystrophy (axonal spheroid formation) affecting a non-pyramidal (GABAergic) neurone of the cerebral cortex in a feline model of GM1 gangliosidosis. As shown in the upper panel (a) the perikaryon of such neurones contains typical storage vacuoles containing swirls of membranous material (membranous cytoplasmic bodies,MCBs), whereas the myelinated axonal spheroid shown in the lower panel (b) contains dense bodies, mitochondria, and tubulovesicular profiles. Calibration bar equals 50 μm for neurone at right and 1 μm for electron micrographs in A and B.

from axonal swellings found in toxic neuropathies and some other diseases, where such filamentous accumulation is characteristic (Schaumburg and Spencer 1984). Interestingly, ultrastructural studies of spheroids from a wide spectrum of storage diseases reveal that they are largely indistinguishable, in contrast to perikaryal storage which does vary by disease type (Walkley 1988). This finding also suggests that a common pathogenic mechanism may underlie spheroid development in all such diseases, as discussed below. Axonal spheroids in storage diseases also are not simple 'retraction bulbs' of dying axons. Rather, they are swellings of significant size that occur along the length of an axon with axonal continuities clearly visible on both the proximal and distal sides of the enlargement (Walkley *et al.* 1991).

Most early studies of axonal spheroid formation in storage diseases considered this phenomenon to be a non-specific degenerative change affecting all types of neurones. Immunocytochemical staining of brain tissue from feline storage disease models using antibodies to neurone type-specific proteins has revealed that spheroids predominate in neurones expressing the inhibitory neurotransmitter, γ-aminobutyric acid (GABA) (Walkley, *et al.*, 1991). Importantly, in terms of understanding the pathogenesis of brain dysfunction in storage diseases, it has been established in these models that the distribution and incidence of axonal spheroids in different CNS populations of GABAergic neurones closely correlates with the type and severity of clinical neurological signs (Walkley 1998). For example, in ganglioside storage diseases, Niemann–Pick diseases and α-mannosidosis spheroids are abundant in basal ganglia, cerebral cortex, and cerebellum and develop coincident with the onset and progression of tremors and ataxia (Walkley *et al.*, 1988, 1991; March *et al.*, 1997). In feline MPS I disease, in contrast, spheroids are not commonly observed in GABAergic or other neurones and these animals lack significant motor system dysfunction (in spite of widespread intraneuronal storage) (Walkley 1998). In murine models, the greatest degree of spheroid development is seen in NPC disease, with changes evident primarily in cerebellar Purkinje cells (Zervas *et al.* 2001*b*). Mice with many storage diseases exhibit striking cerebellar deficits and eventually most Purkinje cells die. Finally, studies of swainsonine-induced (and reversible) α-mannosidosis in cats reveal changes identical to genetic disease and also establish that spheroids persist in brain regions like cerebellum several years after normalization of the perikaryal lysosomal defect (Walkley *et al.* 1987). One interpretation of this finding is that once formed, axonal spheroids are not readily eliminated by parent neurones.

Although no in depth studies on specifically how spheroids affect neurone function have been carried out (but see physiological assessments below), two probable possibilities can be cited. Firstly, spheroids are large enough (at 10–30 micrometre in diameter) to affect action potential propagation down axons. This could occur either as slowing or blocking effects, or possibly by causing retrograde invasion of the action potential into the perikaryon. Given the observation that many spheroids are in GABAergic neurones that supply inhibition to other neurones, including both excitatory and other inhibitory neurones, local increases in both excitation and inhibition (the latter through loss of inhibition to inhibitory neurones) would be anticipated depending on which local circuits are affected. This makes the early functional consequences of such spheroid formation in complex brain regions like cerebral cortex almost impossible to predict. By late disease, however, the loss of inhibition and inhibitory neurones probably would lead to an overall enhancement of excitation and possible seizures. A second consequence of axonal spheroid formation may be a reduction or loss of effective delivery of a retrogradely transported sustaining factor (e.g. a growth factor) from distant synaptic targets to neuronal perikarya. Such loss may cause the affected neurone to be more vulnerable to stress and premature death. One GABAergic cell type with a long projecting axon, the Purkinje cell, may be such an example. Not only do spheroids commonly affect these neurones in many storage diseases, but Purkinje cell loss often dominates brain pathology (and consequently, clinical disease) even when neuronal cell loss elsewhere is minimal.

The ultrastructural appearance of spheroids mentioned above—i.e. as generic accumulations of organelles normally moving along the axon—suggests that a defect in axoplasmic transport may be responsible for their formation. Accumulations of similar heterogeneous organelles have been reported to occur distal to crush or low temperature lesions in axons, indicating that these types of materials are characteristic of a block in retrograde transport (Parton *et al.* 1992; Smith 1980; Tsukita and Ishikawa 1980). On the other hand, there is less evidence to support a defect in anterograde transport in the formation of spheroids. For example, in GABAergic neurones the anterogradely transported enzyme, glutamic acid decarboxylase (GAD), fills the spheroid (hence allowing their identification, see Walkley *et al.* 1991), but GAD immunoreactivity in synaptic terminals of these cells appears to be normal. Exactly why spheroids predominate in GABAergic neurones in storage diseases, as described above, is not clear. It is widely believed that many types of GABAergic neurones have higher firing rates and metabolic activity than other types of neurones (e.g. see Houser *et al.* 1984). This feature may result in a greater turnover in axonal and synaptosomal components, and thus greater reliance on fully intact axoplasmic transport mechanisms.

The presence of lysosomes in axons is controversial (Chapter 1), with numerous studies indicating their apparent exclusion from this neuronal process. Thus, endosomes in axon terminals are generally believed to be retrogradely trafficked and to eventually fuse with lysosomes in neuronal perikarya (Hollenbeck 1993; Nixon and Cataldo 1995). However, some studies do provide support for the presence of at least small numbers of lysosomes (or acidified vacuoles) and lysosomal enzymes in axons (Holtzman and Novikoff 1965; Broadwell *et al.* 1980; Gatzinsky and Berthold 1990; Overly *et al.* 1995). If lysosomes or lysosomal enzymes are transported down axons even in small amounts, they may be combined with retrogradely transported endosomes, with the resulting catabolic processing being initiated well before endosomes reach perikarya. Endosomal–lysosomal engorgement in the perikaryon may thus deprive axons of this input and result in retrograde endosomal organelles that do not undergo acidification/lysosomal fusion. If true, the enlarged tubulo- and multivesicular profiles seen in spheroids may be engorged endosomes. A second possibility is that lysosomal compromise in perikarya may deprive the axon of axon transport-linked molecules like dynein or dynactin, both of which have been shown to be associated with perikaryal endosomes/lysosomes (Lin and Collins 1992; Noda *et al.* 1993). Disruption of the dynein/dynactin complex has been shown to lead to retrograde transport defects, axonal spheroid formation, and axonal degeneration (LaMonte *et al.* 2002). Finally, there may also be retrogradely transported lysosomal hydrolases in axons that have been endocytosed at axon terminals and transported to perikarya in a manner not unlike that shown experimentally for horseradish peroxidase (Broadwell *et al.* 1980), and conceivably this mechanism could also be compromised secondary to a primary lysosomal defect involving these enzymes.

An alternative possibility is that spheroids are due, not to lysosomal-related defects in neuronal perikarya, but to abnormalities in oliogodendroglial–neuronal interactions at specific sites along the axon. This suggestion is based on the discovery that granular axonal spheroids very similar to those seen in storage diseases have been found in mice lacking the myelin membrane proteolipid, PLP (Griffiths *et al.* 1998). Spheroids were not observed in other dysmyelination mutant mice, suggesting a direct connection between oligodendroglial function, PLP, and axonal transport. Axonal spheroids are also known to occur in other types of brain diseases, including Seitelberger, Hallorvoiden–Spatz, and other so-called primary neuroaxonal dystrophies (Seitelberger 1971). The primary metabolic defects in these diseases are unknown, and there is no evidence of direct lysosomal involvement. Interestingly, parallels have been drawn between these disorders and one type of lysosomal disorder known as Schindler disease, a glycoproteinosis secondary to a defect in α-*N*-acetylgalactosaminidase (Desnick and Schindler 2001). This storage disease exhibits little intraneuronal storage but is reported to have large numbers of axonal spheroids.

Another feature of axons often involved in storage diseases is demyelination. Myelin loss is most severe in the leukodystrophies like Krabbe disease and MLD in which disease impact on oligodendroglial cell populations predominates (von Figura *et al.* 2001; Wenger *et al.*

2001). For Krabbe disease, one current hypothesis is that accumulating psychosine, a substrate for the missing galactosylceramidase enzyme, is directly toxic to those cells, the oligodendroglia, that are responsible for myelin production (Miyatake and Suzuki 1972). In addition to the leukodystrophies, mild-to-severe myelin loss is also found in most other types of storage diseases affecting brain. In ganglioside storage diseases, loss of myelin occurs to the greatest extent in cases of infantile onset, whereas later onset types reveal normal myelination (Lake 1997). Whether myelin loss in most storage disease is due to direct effects on oligodendroglia (as appears to be the case in the leukodystophies) or is partly or wholly secondary to loss of axons, has not been thoroughly explored. In most cases, it appears that the myelin abnormalities are caused by a failure to myelinate, rather than by loss of myelin after successful myelination. Some types of storage diseases appear to lack any significant effect on myelination, including many of the MPSs and the glycogen storage disorder, Pompe disease (Lake 1997).

Glia

Lysosomal diseases that cause neuronal storage commonly affect glia as well, either directly because the defective degradative pathway is critical to all cells (leading to storage in its absence), or indirectly in that glia react to disease-induced changes in neurones or other cells, e.g. through phagocytic activity or release of toxic compounds. Glial involvement also occurs in some lysosomal diseases in the absence of widespread or significant neuronal storage. Prominent examples of the latter are the leukodystrophies, Krabbe disease, and MLD, as discussed above in terms of demyelinating events. In these diseases, oligodendroglial involvement occurs as a consequence of the critical importance of the disordered metabolic pathway for handling myelin-related constituents synthesized by these cells. In addition to oligodendroglial involvement, both of these diseases also demonstrate prominent reactions by macrophage-lineage cells in brain and other tissues. The so-called globoid cells of Krabbe disease, for example, are multinucleated cells found along blood vessels of brain apparently in response to massive death of oligodendroglia (Wenger *et al.* 2001). A similar phenomenon occurs during myelin loss in MLD, but in this case the macrophages do not contain multiple nuclei (von Figura *et al.* 2001). Rather, MLD-associated macrophages store large amounts of cerebroside sulfate which appears metachromatic in the analysis of frozen sections, hence the disease name. The role of macrophage infiltration as part of the pathogenic cascade in Krabbe disease was recently emphasized in studies in which oestrogen treatment was administered to female saposin-A-deficient mice (an activator of galactosylceramidase as described in Chapter 8). Treated animals showed dramatic reduction in the neurological phenotype, similar to what had been previously found in pregnant Krabbe disease-affected mice (Matsuda *et al.* 2001). The pathological hallmarks of this disease, demyelination and globoid cell invasion, were dramatically reduced in both circumstances, suggesting a major role of macrophage invasion of the CNS in terms of generating clinical disease. Macrophage infiltration and microglial activation are seen in many other storage diseases as well and may play key roles in pathogenic cascades leading to brain dysfunction (Wada *et al.* 2000; Myerowitz *et al.* 2002; Jeyakumar *et al.* 2003; Ohmi *et al.* 2003).

Astrocytes are intimately involved in maintaining the internal milieu of the brain through structural and metabolic support for neurones, including control of the ionic environment and pH of the extracellular space, neurotransmitter uptake, and metabolism, and so forth. In addition to these functions, recent studies have also suggested that astrocytes directly provide neurones with cholesterol, and that this supply is rate-limiting for the normal development of synapses by neurones (Mauch *et al.* 2001). In disease, astrocytes may respond in a variety of ways, including hypertrophy and proliferation, phagocytosis, and cytokine secretion. Not surprisingly, astrocytes are clearly involved in progressive changes in brain in a variety of storage diseases, either through direct metabolic compromise and storage, or in reaction to neuronal degeneration and death. For example, astrocytic hypertrophy secondary to storage is common in diseases like Fabry and Pompe, with individual astrocytes showing evidence of substantial accumulation of ceramide compounds and glycogen, respectively. In the leukodystrophies, astrocytic hypertrophy secondary to demyelination is commonly described. In diseases like the infantile form of NCL (CLN1) in which there is massive loss of neurones in early life, the cerebral cortex eventually is only composed of large numbers of reactive astrocytes (Santavuori *et al.* 1999). For diseases like NPC, for which some studies have suggested metabolic errors involving cholesterol trafficking, the possible role of astrocytes as a key source of cholesterol for synapse formation have raised new possibilities in terms of pathogenic mechanisms of neurodegeneration.

Cell death

Neurones die in most types of storage disorders affecting brain, but generally speaking cell loss is a conspicuous neuropathological feature in late disease after onset of significant neurological decline. There are some notable exceptions, however, including well-established Purkinje cell death in the cerebellum that affects many storage diseases in which axonal spheroids are found (as discussed above). Neurone loss elsewhere in the CNS may be more scattered in these diseases and typically would not necessarily lead to visible brain atrophy. While in some cases neurone death in the cerebellum and elsewhere in storage diseases has been attributed to apoptosis (Lane *et al.* 1996; Huang *et al.* 1997), the immediate inducers of an apoptotic cascade have yet to be identified. Cell loss in such diseases also is not confined to neurones. One of the clearest examples of cell death in a lysosomal disease in which an inciting agent has been identified is Krabbe disease. Here, there is rapid and widespread death of oligodendroglia, with severe consequences for normal myelination and brain function (Wenger *et al.* 2001). As described above, the abnormal metabolite, psychosine, is believed to accumulate secondary to the galactosylceramidase deficiency. The psychosine hypothesis (Miyatake and Suzuki 1972) posits that large amounts of this compound are generated in oligodendroglia during the early phase of myelination, with the subsequent killing of these cells.

While some degree of cell death may occur in many types of storage diseases, the single most striking example of this phenomenon is in the NCL disease family. Here, death of neurones in select brain regions like cerebral cortex is massive and occurs very early in the disease course. Thus, although manifesting in infants or young children, the degree of cortical atrophy in some NCL disease forms resembles that seen in Alzheimer's dementia (Hofmann and Peltonen 2001). This dramatic death of neurones is most prominent in the infantile form and occurs in graded fashion in the other NCL types according to age of onset (i.e. the later the onset, the slower the neurone loss). Recent studies have indicated that the NCL disorders are appropriately classed as lysosomal proteinoses (based on evidence of lysosomal function for some CLN proteins and on lysosomal storage of the c subunit of mitochondrial ATP synthase and SAPs), the pathogenic cascade affecting neurones nonetheless is clearly unlike that seen in the classic lysosomal hydrolase deficiencies like Tay–Sachs and Hurler diseases (Walkley 1998). For example, as described earlier, the latter disorders often exhibit primary or secondary storage of GSLs within select populations of neurones, and these cells often undergo renewal of dendritogenesis and aberrant synapse formation. GABAergic neuronal populations in the gangliosidoses and other glycosphingolipidoses also exhibit extensive formation of granular spheroidal enlargements along axons. Neither of these features of cellular pathology has been reported to occur to any significant degree in the NCL disorders (March *et al.* 1995; Walkley *et al.* 1995*a*). Even the one key feature of cellular pathology shared by essentially all of these storage diseases, the presence of meganeurites on cortical pyramidal neurones, also appears distinctly different in the NCL disorders. Here, the meganeurites are consistently non-spiny in character, i.e. they lack evidence of ectopic dendrites, spines, and new synapses that characteristically occur on pyramidal neurone meganeurites in the gangliosidoses (Williams *et al.* 1977).

The hallmark of the NCL disorders thus is massive, and selective, neuronal degeneration. Widespread loss of neurones in the cerebral cortex leads to a profound cortical atrophy and dementia/retardation are clinical manifestations. Similarly, in some forms of NCL disease, death of neurones in retina leads to blindness and in cerebellum to ataxia. In trying to explain cell death in the NCL disorders, it is clear that the storage material is itself not universally cytotoxic since many populations of neurones (as well as other cell types) undergo extensive storage but nonetheless survive for many years. While the basis of this selective neuronal vulnerability in NCL diseases remains unknown, recent findings suggest a possible parallel with other human neurodegenerative diseases. Slow or chronic excitotoxicity and accompanying oxidative damage have been hypothesized to contribute to selective neurone death in several of these disorders, including Huntington's, Parkinson's, and Alzheimer's (Novelli *et al.* 1988; Beal 1992; Coyle and Puttfarken 1993; Horowski *et al.* 1994). The so-called 'weakened target cell' or energy-linked excitotoxicity model argues that impaired energy production within neurones possessing abundant NMDA receptors and receiving glutatmatergic input puts them at risk for excitotoxic damage. Since a major storage product in NCL diseases is a component of a key enzyme involved in ATP production (subunit c of mitochondrial ATP synthase), it has been proposed that mitochondrial function in NCL-affected neurones may be suboptimal, with the ensuing mechanism of slow excitotoxicity and resulting oxidative damage leading to selective neurone death (Walkley *et al.* 1996). A variety of studies indicate that mitochondrial function is compromised in NCL neurones (Das *et al.* 1999; Jolly *et al.* 2002). As proposed for other human neurodegenerative diseases, suboptimal mitochondrial function in NCL-affected neurones would be anticipated to lead to chronic membrane depolarization secondary to reduced activity of $Na\text{-}K^{+}$ ATPase, followed by excessive Ca^{++} influx via the NMDA receptor (following a depolarization-induced loss of the Mg^{++} block of these receptors). Further compromise of mitochondrial function would be anticipated, as well as free radical formation and oxidative damage, lipid peroxidation, and cell death, all of which have been implicated in NCL disease (Rider *et al.* 1992; Hofmann and Peltonen 2001).

An excitotoxic process occurring in NCL-affected neurones probably would play out differently in different types of neurones, since mitochondrial characteristics, metabolic requirements for individual types of neurones, and types of synaptic inputs vary widely in the CNS (Wong-Riley 1989). Neurones with high metabolic rates, substantial glutamatergic inputs, and abundant NMDA receptors would be predicted to be the most vulnerable. GABAergic neurones, which have been shown to contain large numbers of mitochondria

(Houser *et al.* 1984), have been directly implicated in NCL disease pathogenesis due in part to the presence of abnormal mitochondria in these cells (Walkley *et al.* 1995*a*, 1996). Recent studies have reported that mice and humans with CLN3 disease exhibit the presence of an autoantibody to the GABA-synthesizing enzyme, GAD65, which may compromise its function and interfere with normal inhibition in brain (Chattopadhyay *et al.* 2002). Regardless of the cause, loss of inhibitory GABAergic inputs to cortical pyramidal neurones would probably increase their base-line activity and enhance their vulnerability to excitotoxic damage if mitochondrial function is suboptimal. If c subunit accumulation in NCL-affected neurones leads to an abnormal distribution of functional 'cationic pores'—as suggested by the work of McGeoch and Palmer (1999)—this event may as a consequence lead to chronic depolarization and exacerbated Ca^{++} entry even if mitochondrial function initially is normal. Thus, there are several plausible scenarios that may underlie a chronic excitotoxic cascade in NCL disease, with each mechanism ultimately targeting neurones with high NMDA receptor expression and providing a final common pathway of selective neuronal destruction.

Functional assessment of brain

A primary tool for evaluating mechanisms of pathogenesis in storage diseases has been the availability of animal models. As described elsewhere (Chapters 10 and 11) numerous model systems ranging from yeast to mammals have been developed. While simple systems (yeast, nematodes, flies) are useful for analysis at the cell biological level, mammalian models allow for direct assessment of CNS function relevant to human neurological disease, and thus will be emphasized here. Genetic, neurophysiological, and functional imaging techniques have been applied to mammalian models of storage diseases with the goal of delineating those specific processes involved in abnormal brain function.

Genomic and proteomic analysis

Evaluation of changes in gene and protein expression in brain cells affected by storage diseases, just as for other brain diseases (Greenberg 2001), offers a tool of enormous potential for understanding the key metabolic pathways incorporated into, and/or deranged by, the initial gene/protein defect. Such analysis also offers a powerful means by which to precisely monitor new treatment strategies for these diseases in experimental animals. While genomic analysis using DNA microarray technology has not yet been extensively applied to the study of storage diseases, it is beginning to reveal novel insights into other brain disorders, including multiple sclerosis (Whitney *et al.* 1999) and Alzheimer's disease (Loring *et al.* 2001). Given the availability of numerous mouse models of storage diseases with neurological involvement, there is every reason to believe that this new technology will eventually provide important insights here as well. The value of this methodology will by no means be limited to brain in terms of its application to storage diseases, since delineation of altered metabolic pathways in other, more homogeneously organized organs, like liver, may readily provide the clearest insights of the disease cascade at the cell biological level. Nonetheless, analysis of brain tissue will be crucial for providing direct insight into those events directly responsible for brain dysfunction. Clearly such analysis is complicated by region to region variations in brain as well by the considerable heterogeneity of neuronal and glial cell types within most individual brain areas. Finally, early-versus late-stage events may also differ widely in brain in a given disease, necessitating analysis over a wide age span.

While proteomic analysis of storage diseases have yet to be described, several recently published reports on the analysis of gene expression changes in Tay–Sachs and Sandhoff diseases provides ample evidence of the importance of this approach (Myerowitz *et al.* 2002; Wada *et al.* 2000). Sandhoff disease mice exhibit GM2 ganglioside storage secondary to a total β-hexosamindase deficiency, with neurological decline beginning at 3 months of age and death by 4–5 months. cDNA microarray analysis of spinal cord tissues of 1–4-month-old mice revealed upregulation of genes related to inflammation and activated microglia, with these changes largely preceding late stage events like cell death. Histological analysis provided parallel evidence of microglial activation in the spinal cord during this time (Wada *et al.* 2000). Studies using serial analysis of gene expression (SAGE) in a children with Tay–Sachs and Sandhoff diseases have similarly revealed elevated gene expression that signify the presence of activated astrocytes, and macrophages/microglia (Myerowitz *et al.* 2002). These two studies provide compelling evidence that glial activation is a significant component of the pathogenic cascade in GM2 gangliosidosis and probably contributes to the neurodegenerative process. This view reinforced by other reports that microglia may act to damage neurones through secretion of inflammatory mediators. Parallel views on the importance of inflammatory processes in neurological progression have emerged for Alzheimer's and other neurodegenerative diseases (Streit *et al.* 2001).

Behavioral and electrophysiological analyses and imaging

A variety of techniques have been applied to animals with storage diseases in order to document behavioural and other phenotype differences. For mice, these include rotarod, balance beam, vertical screen, repeated acquisition and performance chamber (RAPC) analysis, and foot print and open field analysis (e.g. see Brooks *et al.* 2002; Võikar *et al.* 2002), whereas for companion animals more traditional veterinary neurological examinations and routine electrodiagnostic tests have been utilized. Less commonly, modern imaging techniques directed at evaluating specific functional changes, e.g. in cerebral blood flow (Itoh *et al.* 2001) or structural alterations over time, e.g. in brain myelination (Vite *et al.* 2001), have been applied but are not yet routinely used. Generally speaking, the motor, sensory, and overall behavioural changes observed in cats and dogs with storage diseases appear to more closely resemble those in humans than have those in mice, a finding which undoubtedly reflects the greater similarity and complexity of gyrencephalic brains of carnivores and primates versus the considerably simpler lissencephalic brains of rodents. A major component of any behavioural analysis of brain disease in an animal model, whether rodent or carnivore, is clearly the motor system, since dysfunction of movement is a readily detectable behavioural change. Mice with some storage diseases, e.g. NPC, exhibit early-onset enhanced activity featuring tremors and ataxia, whereas others like MPS disease mice typically show a gradual onset of reduced mobility and late-stage gait abnormalities. Storage disease-affected mice exhibiting motor disturbances typically are found to have cerebellar disease consisting of axonal spheroids in cerebellar white matter and loss of Purkinje cells (Suzuki *et al.* 1998). In cats, disordered motor system function is observed as limb and body tremors, titubation, ataxia, and opisthotonus, which may occur singly or in combination. Feline models of GM1 and GM2 gangliosidoses and Niemann–Pick diseases types A and C exhibit these features in striking fashion (Baker *et al.* 1979; March *et al.* 1997). As described earlier, the presence of severe motor system dysfunction along with hyperacusis and seizure tendency is tightly correlated with the incidence and distribution of neuroaxonal dystrophy affecting GABAergic neurones. MPS I disease in cats, in contrast, lacks both the GABAergic neurone defect as well as the motor system signs, consistent with neuroaxonal dystrophy being a major generator of brain dysfunction (Walkley 1998).

While storage diseases in children typically exhibit cognitive deficits and various degrees of mental retardation, studies directed specifically at mechanisms of learning and memory in animal models are uncommon. The application of behavioural paradigms like the Morris water maze for such analysis (e.g. spatial learning) in rodents often is limited by the complicating features of motor system compromise. However, mice with NPC disease have been analysed in this way and are reported to exhibit deficits in learning and memory (Võikar *et al.* 2002). In spite of the relative ease of application to rodents, and their widespread use in normal rats and mice, brain slice and whole-brain electrophysiological studies to analyse long-term potentiation, long-term depression, or other neuronal activity measures believed linked to learning and memory have not been reported in murine models of storage diseases. This is in contrast to other murine models of genetic brain diseases, like Fragile X, which have received significant attention in this way (Godfraind *et al.* 1996; Gu *et al.* 2002). Single-unit electrophysiological studies directed at cortical neurone function have been carried out in cats with ganglioside storage diseases (Purpura *et al.* 1980; Karabelas and Walkley 1985). Results of these studies indicated the presence of abnormalities in integration of excitatory and inhibitory postsynaptic potentials in pyramidal cell somata, although in other respects the neurones appeared much like normal cells.

Multi-unit analysis sampling large ensembles of cortical neurones has also been utilized in feline storage disease models in an attempt to evaluate functional abnormalities within synaptic circuits. Intracortical laminar activity has been evaluated in primary auditory cortex through the use of concomitant field potential, current source density, and multiunit activity profiles sampled from incremental intracortical depths, using linear array multicontact electrodes (March, Walkley, Thrall, and Schroeder, unpublished data). Current source density is an index of local patterns of postsynaptic potentials, while multiunit activity is an index of concomitant action potentials. Cats with different types of storage diseases (GM1 gangliosidosis, NPC disease, and MPS I disease) have been compared to age-similar normal cats (Fig 12.4). Cats with GM1 gangliosidosis and NPC exhibited auditory cortical responses that were atypical in several respects. A GM1 gangliosidosis-affected animal exhibited longer than normal onset latencies and an extended duration of responses, whereas a cat with NPC disease showed more normal response latencies, but had abnormally increased supragranular neuronal activity (Fig. 12.4B). In both of these diseases, the magnitude and extent of cortical activation was abnormal, with initial current sinks being larger and/or longer in duration than their counterparts in normal animals, with this pattern being most exaggerated in superficial cortical laminae. Sink/source pairs were higher in magnitude, more prolonged, and less confined to localized neuronal ensembles than were the corresponding sink/source pairs in normal cats. In contrast to these two diseases, a cat with MPS I disease exhibited overall electrical activity equivalent to that obtained from normal cats. Given that all three of these diseases exhibit some degree of ectopic dendritogenesis and new synapse formation affecting pyramidal neurones (see earlier discussion), but only cats with GM1 gangliosidosis and NPC have neuroaxonal dystrophy affecting GABAergic neurones, the suggestion is that the latter defect in inhibitory circuitry may underlie the observed abnormalities in cortical activity. However, the issue of what the specific contributions of altered excitatory versus inhibitory mechanisms are in overall cortical dysfunction remains unresolved.

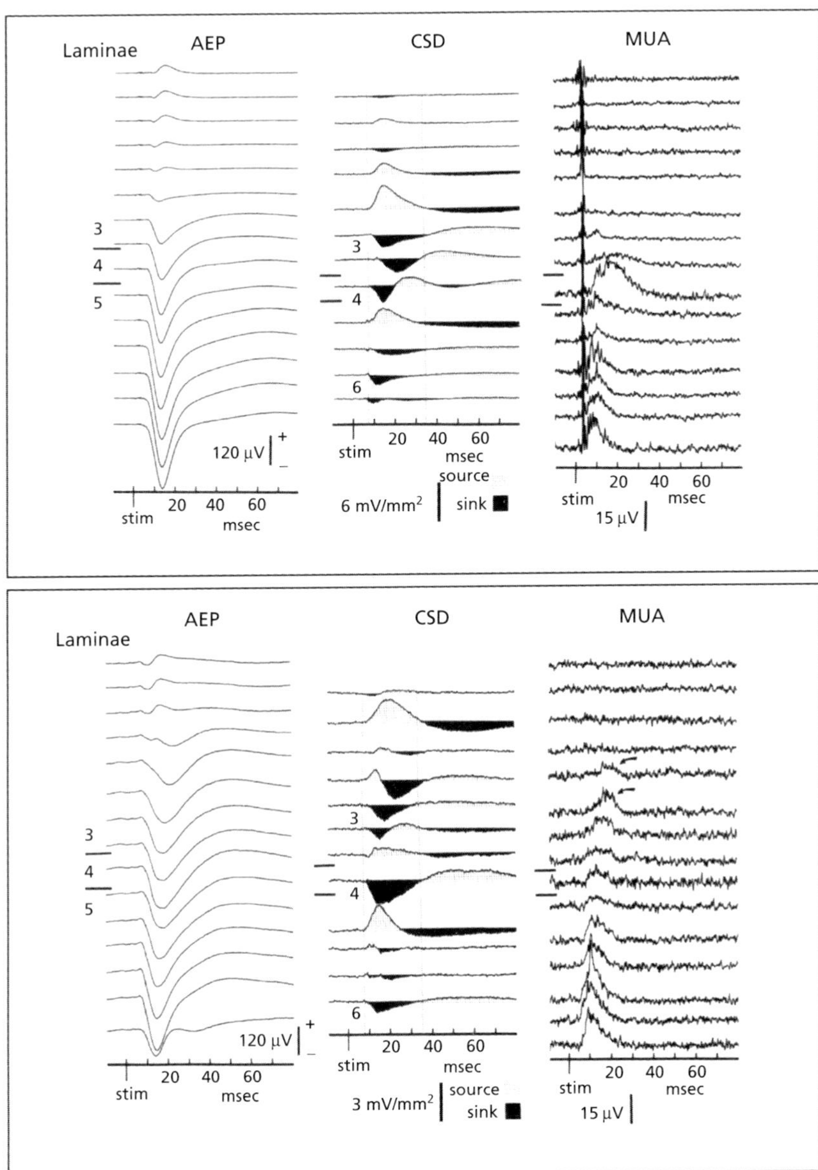

Fig.12.4 Representative laminar activity profiles in cerebral cortex elicited by auditory stimulation in area A1 of a normal cat (upper panel) and a cat with Niemann–Pick disease type C (lower panel). Responses were delayed and prolonged in the cat with NPC disease. Normal onset and termination of lamina 3 current source are denoted by vertical dotted lines in the CSD profiles. Supragranular sources (grey stipple) and sinks (black stipple) were much greater amplitude and duration in the diseased animal when compared to normal. [Note difference in amplitude of CSD setting in the two sets of traces (6mV/mm^2 versus 3mV/mm2)]. For the MUA pattern, curved arrows in NPC disease show areas of increased activity in upper cortical laminae compared to normal cortex. The CSD and MUA patterns in a cat with GM1 gangliosidosis closely resembled those for the cat with NPC disease shown here. AEP, auditory-evoked potential; CSD, current source density; MUA, multi-unit activity.

Summary

Lysosomal diseases begin quite simply as single gene mutations that affect the function of one protein. This protein may be an enzyme critical in the degradative action of the lysosomal system or in the processing and/or trafficking of such enzymes to the lysosome. Alternatively, the defective protein may not be an enzyme but rather a structural or soluble protein critically important for some other event central to the proper functioning of the endosomal–lysosomal system. Regardless, the pathophysiological consequences in brain ultimately play out as an expanding cascade involving multiple substrate accumulation and widespread, but variable, impact on different types of neurones and glia. In some cases these changes may actually *appear* as regenerative, as seen in the new growth of dendrites and formation of synaptic connections in Tay–Sachs disease, but which more likely lead to inappropriate connections and neurone dysfunction. At the other extreme, neurones or glia may die in massive numbers as seen in infantile NCL disease, leading to dramatic loss of grey or white matter and concomitant dysfunction in these brain circuits. While a great deal has been learned about lysosomal storage diseases of brain over the past three decades, in no case is there a complete understanding of the step-by-step demise of individual brain cells and their circuits leading to the array of neurological deficits characterizing these diseases. Such knowledge, when available, will likely provide key insights into new therapeutic interventions and the critical windows when their application would be most beneficial. Current availability of sophisticated techniques for analysis of changes in gene and protein expression and in cellular structure and function, coupled with ideal disease model systems in multiple organisms, bode well for research progress over the next decade. It is likely that what is to be learned will contribute as much or more to our knowledge of the normal cell biology of neurones as to storage diseases *per se*. Finally, that patients with storage diseases typically exhibit a period of normalcy prior to clinical onset of disease provides considerable optimism that if effective therapies could be developed, many of the severest disease-related events in brain could in fact be prevented.

Acknowledgements

This work has been supported by grants from the National Institutes of Health and the Ara Parseghian Medical Research Foundation.

References

Assmann, G. and Seedorf, U. (2001). Acid lipase deficiency: Wolman's disease and cholesterol ester storage disease. In *The metabolic and molecular bases of inherited disease* (Scriver, C. R., Beaudet, A. L., Sly, W. S. and Valle, D., ed.) Vol. 3, 8th edn, pp. 3551–72. New York: McGraw-Hill.

Aula, P., Jalanko, A. and Peltonen, L. (2001). Aspartylglucosaminuria. In *The metabolic and molecular bases of inherited disease* (Scriver, C. R., Beaudet, A. L., Sly, W. S. and Valle, D., ed.) 8th edn, pp. 3535–50. New York: McGraw-Hill.

Avila, J. A. and Convit, J. (1975). Inhibition of leukocyte lysosomal enzymes by glycosaminoglycans *in vitro*. *Biochem J*, **152**, 57–64.

Baker, H. J., Reynolds, G. D., Walkley, S. U., Cox, N. R. and Baker, G. H. (1979). The gangliosidoses: Comparative features and research applications. *Vet Pathol*, **16**, 635–49.

Bandtlow, C. E. and Zimmermann, D. R. (2000). Proteoglycans in the developing brain: New conceptual insights for old proteins. *Physiol Rev*, **80**, 1267–90.

Baumkotter, J. and Cantz, M. (1983). Decreased ganglioside neuraminidase activity in fibroblasts from mucopolysaccharidosis patients. *Biochem Biophys Acta*, **761**, 163–70.

Beal, M. F. (1992). Does impairment of energy metabolism result in excitotoxic neuronal death in neuro-degenerative disease? *Ann Neurol*, **31**, 119–30.

Bevan, A. P., Drake, P. G., Bergeron, J. M. and Posner, B. I. (1996). Intracellular signal transduction: The role of endosomes. *TEM*, **7**, 13–21.

Bielschowsky, M. (1932). Histopathology of nerve cells. In *Cytology and cellular pathology of the nervous system* (Penfield W., ed.), pp. 147–83.

Bovolenta, P. and Fernaud-Espinosa, I. (2000). Nervous system proteoglycans as modulators of neurite outgrowth. *Prog Neurobiol*, **61**, 113–32.

Brdickova, N., Brdicka, T., Anera, L. *et al.* (2001). Interaction between two adaptor proteins, PAG and EBP50: a possible link between membrane rafts and actin cytoskeleton. *FEBS Letters*, **507**, 133–6.

Bremer, E. G. (1994). Glycosphingolipids as effectors of growth and differentiation. *Curr Top Membr*, **40**, 387–411.

Broadwell, R. D., Oliver, C. and Brightman, M. W. (1980). Neuronal transport of acid hydrolases and peroxidase within the lysosomal system of organelles: Involvement of agranular reticulum-like cisterns. *J Comp Neurol*, **190**, 519–32.

Brooks, A. I., Stein, C. S., Hughes, S. M. *et al.* (2002). Functional correction of established CNS deficits in an animal model of lysosomal storage disease using feline immunodeficiency virus-based vectors. *Proc Natl Acad Sci USA*, **99**, 6216–21.

Brown, D. A. and London, E. (1998). Functions of lipid rafts in biological membranes. *Ann Rev Cell Dev Biol*, **14**, 111–36.

Byrd, J. C. and Powers, J. M. (1979). Wolman's disease: Ultrastructural evidence of lipid accumulation in central and peripheral nervous systems. *Pediatrics*, **46**, 431–6.

Cano-Gauci, D. F., Song, H. H., Yang, H. *et al.* (1999). Glypican-3-deficient mice exhibit developmental overgrowth and some of the abnormalities typical of Simpson–Golabi–Behmel syndrome. *J Cell Biol*, **146**, 255–64.

Ceresa, B. P. and Schmid, S. L. (2000). Regulation of signal transduction by endocytosis. *Curr Opin Cell Biol*, **12**, 204–10.

Chattopadhyay, S., Ito, M., Cooper, J. D. *et al.* (2002). An autoantibody inhibitory to glutamic acid decarboxylase in the neurodegenerative disorder Batten disease. *Hum Mol Genet*, **11**, 1421–31.

Chen, Y.-T. (2001). Glycogen storage diseases. In *The metabolic and molecular bases of inherited disease* (Scriver, C. R., Beaudet, A. L., Sly, W. S. and Valle, D., ed.), Vol. 1, 8th edn, pp. 1521–51. New York: McGraw-Hill.

Coyle, J. T. and Puttfarken, P. (1993). Oxidative stress, glutamate, and neurodegenerative disorders. *Science*, **262**, 689–700.

Danon, M. J., Oh, S. J., DiMauro, S. *et al.* (1981). Lysosomal glycogen storage diseases with normal acid maltase. *Neurology*, **31**, 51–7.

Das, A. M., Jolly, R. D. and Kohlschütter, A. (1999). Anomalies of mitochondrial ATP synthase regulation in four different types of neuronal ceroid lipofuscinosis. *Mol Gen Metab*, **66**, 349–55.

Desnick, R. J. and Schindler, D. (2001). α-N-Acetylgalactosaminidase deficiency: Schindler disease. In *The metabolic and molecular bases of inherited disease* (Scriver, C. R., Beaudet, A. L., Sly, W. S. and Valle, D., ed.), Vol. 3, 8th edn, pp. 3483–505. New York: McGraw-Hill.

Desnick, R. J., Thorpe, S. R. and Fiddler, M. (1976). Toward enzyme therapy for lysosomal storage diseases. *Physiol Rev*, **56**, 57–99.

Du, H., Heur, M., Duanmu, M. *et al.* (2001). Lysosomal acid lipase-deficient mice: depletion of white and brown fat, severe hepatosplenomegaly, and shortened life span. *J Lipid Res*, **42**, 489–500.

Dwek, R. A. (1996). Glycobiology: Toward understanding the function of sugars. *Chem Rev*, **96**, 683.

Elleder, M. and Sokolová and Hřebíček, M. (1997). Follow-up study of subunit c of mitochondrial ATP synthase (SCMAS) in Batten disease and in unrelated lysosomal disorders. *Acta Neuropathol*, **93**, 379–90.

Ethell, I. M., Hagihara, K., Miura, Y., Irie, F. and Yamaguchi, Y. (2000). Synbindin, a novel syndecan-2 binding protein in neuronal dendritic spines. *J Cell Biol*, **151**, 53–67.

Ezaki, J., Takeda-Ezaki, M., Kominami, E. *et al.* (2002). Tripeptidyl peptidase I, the late infantile neuronal ceroid lipofuscinosis gene product, initiates the lysosomal degradation of subunit c of ATP synthase. *J Biochem (Tokyo)*, **128**, 509–16.

von Figura, K., Gieselmann, V. and Jaeken, J. (2001). Metachromatic leukodystrophy. In *The metabolic and molecular bases of inherited disease* (Scriver, C. R., Beaudet, A. L., Sly, W. S. and Valle, D., ed.), Vol. 3, 8th edn, pp. 3695–724. New York: McGraw-Hill.

Fukumoto, S., Mutoh, T., Hasegawa, T. *et al.* (2000). *GD3* Synthase gene expression in PPC12 cells results in the continuous activation of TrkA and ERK1/2 and enhanced proliferation. *J Biol Chem*, **275**, 5832–8.

Futerman, A. H. (1995). Inhibition of sphingolipid–GPI-anchored protein microdomains. *Trends Cell Biol*, **5**, 377–80.

Gao, H., Boustany, R. N., Espinola, J. A. *et al.* (2002). Mutations in a novel *CLN6*-encoded transmembrane protein cause variant neuronal ceroid lipofuscinosis in man and mouse. *Am J Hum Gen*, **70**, 324–35.

Garrod, A. (1928). The lessons of rare maladies. *Lancet*, **1**, 1055–9.

Gatzinsky, K. P. and Berthold, C.-H. (1990). Lysosomal activity at nodes of Ranvier during retrograde axonal transport of horseradish peroxidase in alpha-motor neurons of the cat. *J Neurocytol*, **20**, 989–1002.

Godfraind, J. M., Reyniers, E., De Boulle, K. *et al.* (1996). Long-term potentiation in the hippocampus of fragile X knockout mice. *Am J Med Genet*, **64**, 246–51.

Goldman, J. E., Katz, D., Rapin, I., Purpura, D. and Suzuki, K. (1981). Chronic GM1 gangliosidosis presenting as dystonia. I. Clinical and pathological features. *Ann Neurol*, **9**, 465–75.

Gondré-Lewis, M., Dobrenis, K. and Walkley, S. U. (2002*a*). GM2 ganglioside is expressed in murine cortical pyramidal neurons during dendritic differentiation. *Soc Neurosci Abstr.* **27**, Program number 250.6.

Gondré-Lewis, M., Dobrenis, K. and Walkley, S. U. (2002*b*). CaMKII inhibition causes altered GM2 ganglioside expression in cortical neurons. *Soc Neurosci Abstr.* 28, Program number 233.16.

Gondré-Lewis, M., McGlynn, R. and Walkley, S. U. (2003). Cholesterol accumulation in NPC1-deficient neurons is ganglioside dependent. *Current Biology*, **13**, 1324–9.

Goodman, L. A. and Walkley, S. U. (1996). GM2 ganglioside is associated with cortical neurons undergoing active dendritogenesis during normal brain development. *Dev Brain Res*, **93**, 162–71.

Goodman, L. A., Livingston, P. O. and Walkley, S. U. (1991). Ectopic dendrites occur only on cortical pyramidal cells containing elevated GM2 ganglioside in α-mannosidosis. *Proc Natl Acad Sci USA*, **88**, 11330–4.

Greenberg, S. A. (2001). DNA microarray gene expression analysis technology and its application to neurological disorders. *Neurol*, **57**, 755–61.

Griffiths, I., Klugmann, M., Anderson, T. *et al.* (1998). Axonal swellings and degeneration in mice lacking the major proteolipid of myelin. *Science*, **280**, 1610–13.

Gu, Y., McIlwain, K. L., Weeber, E. J. *et al.* (2002). Impaired conditioned fear and enhanced long-term potentiation in Fmr2 knock-out mice. *J Neurosci*, **22**, 2753–63.

Hakomori, S.-I. (2000). Cell adhesion/recognition and signal transduction through glycosphingolipid microdomain. *Glycoconj J*, **17**, 143–51.

Hannun, Y. A. and Luberto, C. (2000). Ceramide in the eukaryotic stress response. *Trends Cell Biol*, **10**, 73–80.

Hers, H. G. (1965). Progress in Gastroenterology: Inborn lysosomal diseases. *Gastroenterology*, **48**, 625–33.

Hers, H. G. and Van Hoof, F. (1973). *Lysosomes and storage diseases.* New York: Academic Press.

Herschkowitz, N. and Schulte, F. J. (1984). The lipidoses: From defect to dysfunction. *Neuropediatrics*, **15**, 110–11.

Hirshhorn and Reuser (2001). Glycogen storage disease type II: Acid glucosidase (acid maltase) deficiency. In *The metabolic and molecular bases of inherited disease* (Scriver, C. R., Beaudet, A. L., Sly, W. S. and Valle, D., ed.), Vol. 3, 8th edn, pp. 3389–420. New York: McGraw-Hill.

Hofmann, S. L. and Peltonen, L. (2001). The neuronal ceroid lipofuscinoses. In *The metabolic and molecular bases of inherited disease* (Scriver, C. R., Beaudet, A. L., Sly, W. S. and Valle, D., ed.), Vol. 3, 8th edn, pp. 3877–94. New York: McGraw-Hill.

Hollenbeck, P. J. (1993). Products of endocytosis and autophagy are retrieved from axons by regulated retrograde organelle transport. *J Cell Biol*, **121**, 305–15.

Holtzman, E. and Novikoff, A. B. (1965). Lysosomes in the rat sciatic nerve following crush. *J Cell Biol*, **27**, 651–68.

Horowski, R., Wachtel, H., Turski, L. and Löschmann, P.-A. (1994). Glutamate excitotoxicity as a possible pathogenetic mechanism in chronic neurodegeneration. In *Neurodegenerative diseases* (Calne, D. B., ed.), pp. 163–75. New York: W.B. Saunders Company.

Houser, C. R., Vaughn, J. E., Hendry, S. H. C., Jones, E. G. and Peters, A. (1984). GABA neurons in the cerebral cortex. In *Cerebral cortex: functional properties of cortical cells* (Jones, E. G. Peter, A., ed.), Vol. 2, pp. 63–89. New York: Plenum.

Huang, J. Q., Trasler, J. M., Igdoura, S., Michaud, J., Hanal, N. and Gravel, R. A. (1997). Apoptotic cell death in mouse models of GM2 gangliosidosis and observations on human Tay–Sachs and Sandhoff diseases. *Hum Mol Genet*, **6**, 1879–85.

Isosomppi, J., Vesa, J., Jalanko, A. and Peltonen, L. (2002). Lysosomal localization of the neuronal ceroid lipofuscinosis CLN5 protein. *Hum Mol Genet*, **11**, 885–91.

Itoh, Y., Takanori, E., Cook, M. *et al.* (2001). Local and global cerebral blood flow and glucose utilization in the α-galactosidase A knockout mouse model of Fabry disease. *J Neurochem*, **79**, 1217–24.

Jacobsen, M. (1991). *Developmental neurobiology*, 3rd edn. NY: Plenum Press.

Jaeken, J. and Matthijs, G. (2001). Congenital disorders of glycosylation. *Ann Rev Genomics Hum Genet*, **2**, 129–51.

Jeyakumar, M., Thomas, R., Elliot-Smith, E. *et al.* (2003). Central nervous system inflammation is a hallmark of pathogenesis in mouse models of GM1 and GM2 gangliosidosis. *Brain*, **126**, 974–87.

Jolly, R. D., Brown, S., Das, A. M. and Walkley, S. U. (2002). Mitochondrial dysfunction in the neuronal ceroid-lipofuscinoses (Batten disease). *Neurochem Internation*, **40**, 565–71.

Kahana, D., Berant, M. and Wolman, M. (1968). Primary familial xanthomatosis with adrenal involvement (Wolman's disease): Report of a further case with nervous system involvement and pathogenetic considerations. *Pediatrics*, **42**, 70.

Kamoshita, S. and Landing, B. H. (1968). Distribution of lesions in myenteric plexus and gastrointestinal mucosa in lipidoses and other neurological disorders of children. *Am J Clin Pathol*, **49**, 312.

Karabelas, A. B. and Walkley, S. U. (1985). Altered patterns of evoked synaptic activity in cortical pyramidal neurons in feline ganglioside storage disease. *Brain Research*, **339**, 329–36.

Kasahara, K. and Sanai, Y. (2000). Functional roles of glycosphingolipids in signal transduction via lipid rafts. *Glycoconj J*, **17**, 153–62.

Kasahara, K., Watanabe, Y., Yamamoto, T. and Sanai, Y. (1997). Association of Src family tyrosine kinase Lyn with ganglioside GD3 in rat brain. Possible regulation of Lyn by glycosphingolipid in caveolae-like domains. *J Biol Chem*, **21**, 29947–53.

Kint, J. A., Dacremont, G., Carton, D., Orye, E. and Hooft, C. (1973). Mucopolysaccharidosis: Secondarily induced abnormal distribution of lysosomal isoenzymes. *Science*, **181**, 352–4.

Kobayashi, T. and Hirabayashi, Y. (2000). Lipid membrane domains in cell surface and vacuolar systems. *Glycoconj J*, **17**, 163–71.

Koike, M., Nakanishi, H., Saftig, P. *et al.* (2000). Cathepsin D deficiency induces lysosomal storage with ceroid lipofuscin in mouse CNS neurons. *J Neurosci*, **20**, 6898–906.

Lake, B. D. (1997). Lysosomal and peroxisomal disorders. *Greenfield's Neuropathol*, **1**, 657–753.

Lake, B. D. and Hall, N. A. (1993). Immunolocalization studies of subunit c in late infantile and juvenile Batten disease. *J Inherit Metab Dis*, **16**, 263–6.

LaMonte, B. H., Wallace, K. E., Holloway, B. A. *et al.* (2002). Disruption of dynein/dynactin inhibits axonal transport in motor neurons causing late-onset progressive degeneration. *Neuron*, **34**, 715–27.

Lane, S., Jolly, R. D., Schmechel, D. E., Alroy, J. and Boustany, R.-M. (1996). Apoptosis as the mechanism of neurodegeneration in Batten's disease. *J Neurochem*, **67**, 677–83.

Ledeen, R. W. (1985). Biology of gangliosides: Neuritogenic and neuronotrophic properties. In *Neurobiology of gangliosides* (Gorio A. and Haber B., ed.), pp. 147–59. New York: Alan R. Liss, Inc. Publisher.

Lehtovirta, M., Kyttala, A., Eskelinen, E. L., Hess, M., Heinonen, O. and Jalanko, A. (2001). Palmitoyl protein thioesterase (PPT) localizes into synaptosomes and synaptic vesicles in neurons: Implications for infantile neuronal ceroid lipofuscinosis (INCL). *Hum Mol Genet*, **10**, 69–75.

Li, C. M., Park, J. H., Simonaro, C. M. *et al.* (2002). Insertional mutagenesis of the mouse acid ceramidase gene leads to early embryonic lethality in homozygotes and progressive lipid storage disease in heterozygotes. *Genomics*, **79**, 218–24.

Lin, S. X. H. and Collins, C. A. (1992). Immunolocalization of cytoplasmic dynein to lysosomes in cultured cells. *J of Cell Sci*, **101**, 125–37.

Loeb, H., Jonnieaxu, G., Resibois, A. *et al.* (1968). Biochemical and ultrastructural studies in Hurler's syndrome. *J Pediatr*, **73**, 860–74.

Loring, J. F., Wen, X., Lee, J. M., Seilhamer, J. and Somogyi, R. (2001). A gene expression profile of Alzheimer's disease. *DNA Cell Biology*, **20**, 683–95.

Lusa, S., Blom, T., Eskelinen, E.-L. *et al.* (2001). Depletion of rafts in late endocytic membranes is controlled by NPC1-dependent recycling of cholesterol to the plasma membrane. *J Cell Sci*, **114**, 1893–900.

McAllister, A. K., Lo, D. C. and Katz, L. C. (1995). Neurotrophins regulate dendritic growth in developing visual cortex. *Neuron*, **15**, 791–803.

McGeoch, J. E. and Palmer, D. N. (1999). Ion pores made of mitochondrial ATP synthase c in the neuronal plasma membrane and Batten disease. *Mol Gen Metabol*, **66**, 387–92.

McGlynn, R., Dobrenis, K. and Walkley, S. U. (2003). Differential accumulation of cholesterol and gangliosides accompanies glycosaminoglycan storage in mucopolysaccharide storage disorders (submitted).

March, P. A., Walkley, S. U. and Wurzelmann, S. (1995). Morphological alterations in neocortical and cerebellar GABAergic neurons in canine Batten's disease. *Am J Med Genet*, **57**, 204–12.

March, P. A., Thrall, M. A., Wurzelmann, S., Brown, D. and Walkley, S. U. (1997). Dendritic and axonal abnormalities in feline Niemann–Pick disease type C. *Acta Neuropathol*, **94**, 164–72.

Marks, D. L. and Pagano, R. E. (2002). Endocytosis and sorting of glycosphingolipids in sphingolipid storage disease. *Trends in Cell Biology*, **12**, 605–13.

Martin, J. J., De Barsy, T., Van Hoof, F. and Palladini, G. (1973). Pompe's disease: An inborn lysosomal disorder with storage of glycogen. A study of brain and striated muscle. *Acta Neuropathol (Berl)*, **23**, 229.

Matsuda, J., Vanier, M. T., Saito, Y., Suzuki, K. and Suzuki, K. (2001). Dramatic phenotypic improvement during pregnancy in a genetic leukodystrophy: estrogen appears to be a critical factor. *Hum Mol Genet*, **10**, 2709–15.

Mauch, D. H., Nägler, K., Schumacher, S. *et al.* (2001). CNS synaptogenesis promoted by glia-derived cholesterol. *Science*, **294**, 1354–57.

Miyatake, T. and Suzuki, K. (1972). Globoid cell leukodystrophy: Additional deficiency of psychosine galactosidase. *Biochem Biophys Res Commun*, **45**, 1363.

Mutoh, T., Tokuda, A., Miyadai, T., Hamaguchi, M. and Fujiki, N. (1995). Ganglioside GM1 binds to the TRK protein and regulates receptor function. *Proc Natl Acad Sci USA*, **92**, 5087–91.

Myerowitz, R., Lawson, D., Mizukami, H., Mi, Y., Tifft, C. J. and Proia, R. L. (2002). Molecular pathophysiology in Tay-Sachs and Sandhoff diseases as revealed by gene expression profiling. *Hum Mol Genet*, **11**, 1343–50.

Neufeld, E. and Muenzer, J. (2001). The metabolic and molecular bases of inherited disease. In *The mucopolysaccharidoses* (Scriver *et al.*, ed.), Chapter 136, 8th edn. NewYork: McGraw-Hill.

Nishino, I., Fu, J., Tanji, K. *et al.* (2000). Primary LAMP-2 deficiency causes X-linked vacuolar cardiomyopathy and myopathy (Danon disease). *Nature*, **406**, 906–10.

Nixon, R. A. and Cataldo, A. M. (1995). The endosomal-lysosomal system of neurons: new roles. *Trends Neurosci*, **18**, 489–96.

Noda, Y., Nakata, T. and Hirokawa, N. (1993). Localization of dynamin: Widespread distribution in mature neurons and association with membranous organelles. *Neuroscience*, **55**, 113–27.

Novelli, A., Reilly, J. A., Lysko, P. G. and Henneberry, R. C. (1988). Glutamate becomes neurotoxic via the *N*-methyl-D-aspartate receptor when intracellular energy levels are reduced. *Brain Res*, **451**, 205–12.

Ohmi K., Greenberg D. S., Rajavel K. S., Ryazantsev S., Li H. H., Neufeld E. F. (2003). Activated microglia in cortex of mouse models of mucopolysaccharidoses I and IIIB. *Proc Natl Acad Sci USA*, **100**, 1902–7.

Overly, C. C., Lee, K., Berthiaume, E. and Hollenbeck, P. J. (1995). Quantitative measurement of intra-organelle pH in the endosomal-lysosomal pathway in neurons by using ratiometric imaging with pyranine. *Proc Natl Acad Sci USA*, **92**, 3156–60.

Pagano, R. E., Puri, V., Dominguez, M. and Marks, D. L. (2000). Membrane traffic in sphingolipid storage diseases. *Traffic*, **1**, 807–15.

Palmer, D. N., Fearnley, I. M., Walker, J. E. *et al.* (1992). Mitochondrial ATP synthase subunit *c* storage in the ceroid lipofuscinoses (Batten disease). *Am J Med Gen*, **42**, 561–7.

Parton, R. G. and Dotti, C. G. (1993). Cell biology of neuronal endocytosis. *J Neurosci Res*, **36**, 1–9.

Parton, R. G., Simons, K. and Dotti, C. G. (1992). Axonal and dendritic endocytic pathways in cultured neurons. *J Cell Biol*, **119**, 123–37.

Patterson, M. C., Vanier, M. T., Suzuki, K. *et al.* (2001). Niemann-Pick disease Type C: A lipid trafficking disorder. In *The metabolic and molecular bases of inherited disease* (Scriver, C. R., Beaudet, A. L., Sly, W. S. and Valle, D., ed.), Vol. 3, 8th edn, pp. 3611–33. New York: McGraw-Hill.

Peltonen, L., Savukoski, M. and Vesa, J. (2000). Genetics of the neuronal ceroid lipofuscinoses. *Curr Opin Genet Dev*, **10**, 299–305.

Pentchev, P. G., Comly, M. E., Kruth, H. S. *et al.* (1985). A defect in cholesterol esterification in Niemann–Pick disease (type C) patients. *Proc Natl Acad Sci USA*, **82**, 8247–51.

Pitto, M., Mutoh, T., Kuriyama, M., Ferraretto, A., Palestini, P. and Masserini, M. (1998). Influence of endogenous GM1 ganglioside on TrkB activity, in cultured neurons. *FEBS Letters*, **439**, 93–6.

Prinetti, A., Kazuhisa, I. and Hakomori, S. (1999). Glycosphingolipid-enriched signaling domain in mouse neuroblastoma Neuro2a cells. *J Biol Chem*, **274**, 20916–24.

Puri, V., Watanabe, R., Dominguez, M. *et al.* (1999). Cholesterol modulates membrane traffic along the endocytic pathway in sphingolipid-storage diseases. *Nat Cell Biol*, **1**, 386–8.

Purpura, D. P. (1978). Ectopic dendritic growth in mature pyramidal neurons in human ganglioside storage disease. *Nature*, **276**, 520–1.

Purpura, D. P. and Suzuki, K. (1976). Distortion of neuronal geometry and formation of aberrant synapses in neuronal storage disease. *Brain Res*, **116**, 1–21.

Purpura, D. P., Highstein, S. M. and Karabelas, and Walkley, S. U. (1980). Intracellular recording and HRP-staining of cortical neurons in feline ganglioside storage disease. *Brain Res*, **181**, 446–9.

Rabin, S. J. and Mocchetti, I. (1995). GM1 ganglioside activates the high-affinity nerve growth factor receptor TRKA. *J Neurochem*, **65**, 347–54.

Rapraeger, A. C. (2001). Molecular interaction of syndecans during development. *Cell Dev Biol*, **12**, 107–16.

Rider, J. A., Dawson, G. and Siakotos, A. N. (1992). Perspective of biochemical research in the neuronal ceroid-lipofuscinosis. *Am J Med Gen*, **42**, 519–24.

Sachs, B. (1887). On arrested cerebral development, with special reference to its cortical pathology. *J Nerv Ment Dis*, **14**, 541–53.

Sachs, B. (1903). On amaurotic family idiocy. A disease chiefly of the gray matter of the central nervous system. *J Nerv Ment Dis*, **30**, 1–13.

Sachs, B. and Strauss, I. (1910). The cell changes in amaurotic family idiocy. *J Exp Med*, **12**, 685–95.

Samuels, S., Korey, S. R., Gonatas, J., Terry, R. D. and Weiss, D. (1963). Studies on Tay–Sachs disease. IV. Membranous cytoplasmic bodies. *Biochem J Neuropathol Exp Neurol*, **22**, 81–91.

Sandhoff, K. and Echten, G. (1994). Ganglioside metabolism: Enzymology, topology, and regulation. *Prog Brain Res*, **101**, 17–30.

Sandhoff, K. and Kolter, T. (1996). Topology of glycosphingolipid degradation. *Trends Cell Biol*, **6**, 98–103.

Sandhoff, K. and Schwarzmann, G. (1989). Dynamics of gangliosides in neuronal membranes. In Prog. In *Fundamentals of memory formation; neuronal plasticity and brain function* (Zoology, Rahmann, H., ed.), Vol. 37, pp. 229–39. New York: VCH Publishers.

Santavuori, P., Gottlob, I., Haltia, M. *et al.* (1999). CLN1: Infantile and other types of NCL with GROD. In *The neuronal ceroid lipofuscinoses (Batten disease)* (Goebel, H. H., Mole, S. E. and Lake, B. D., ed.), pp. 16–36. Amsterdam: IOS Press.

Schachter, H. (2001). The clinical relevance of glycobiology. *J Clin Invest*, **108**, 1579–82.

Schaumburg, H. H. and Spencer, P. S. (1984). Human toxic neuropathy due to industrial agents. In *Peripheral Neuropathy* (Dyck, P. J., Thomas, P. K., Lambert, E. H. and Bunge, R., ed.), 2nd edn, pp. 2124. Philadelphia: W.B. Saunders.

Schwarzmann, G. and Sandhoff, K. (1990). Metabolism and intracellular transport of glycosphingolipids. *Biochemistry*, **29**, 10865–70.

Seitelberger, F. (1971). Neuropathology conditions related to neuroaxonal dystrophy. *Acta Neuropathol*, Suppl. V, 17–29.

Siegel, D. A. and Walkley, S. U. (1994). Growth of ectopic dendrites on cortical pyramidal neurons in neuronal storage diseases correlates with abnormal accumulation of GM2 ganglioside. *J Neurochem*, **62**, 1852–62.

Simons, K. and Gruenberg, J. (2000). Jamming the endosomal system: lipid rafts and lysosomal storage diseases. *Trends Cell Biol*, **10**, 459–62.

Simons, K. and Toomre, D. (2000). Lipid rafts and signal transduction. *Nat Rev*, **1**, 31–41.

Smith, R. S. (1980). The short term accumulation of axonally transported organelles in the region of localized lesions of single myelinated axons. *J Neurocytol*, **9**, 39–65.

Sonderfeld, S., Conzelmann, E., Schwarzmann, G., Burg, J., Hinrichs, U. and Sandhoff, K. (1985). Incorporation and metabolism of ganglioside GM1 in skin fibroblasts from normal and GM2 gangliosidosis subjects. *Eur J Biochem*, **149**, 247–55.

Stern, C. A. and Tiemeyer, M. (2001). A ganglioslide-specific sialyltransferase localizes to axons and non-Golgi structures in neurons. *J Neurosci*, **21**, 1434–43.

Streit, W. J., Conde, J. R. and Harrison, J. K. (2001). Chemokines and Alzheimer's disease. *Neurobiol Aging*, **22**, 909–13.

Suzuki, K. (1976). Neuronal storage diseases. In *Progress in neuropathology. A Review* (Zimmerman, H. M., ed.), Vol. 3, pp. 173–202. New York: Grune & Straton.

Suzuki, K., Proia, R. L. and Suzuki, K. (1998). Mouse models of human lysosomal diseases. *Brain Pathol*, **8**, 195–215.

Tai, T., Paulson, J. C., Cahan, L. D. and Irie, R. F. (1983). Ganglioside GM2 as a human tumor antigen (OF A-I-1). *Proc Natl Acad Sci USA*, **80**, 5392–6.

Tanaka, Y., Guhde, G., Suter, A. *et al.* (2000). Accumulation of autophagic vacuoles and cardiomyopathy in LAMO-2-deficient mice. *Nature*, **406**, 902–6.

Terry, R. and Weiss, M. (1963). Studies in Tay–Sachs disease II. Ultrastructure of the cerebrum. *J Neuropathol Exp Neurol*, **22**, 18–55.

Thomas, G. H. (2001). Disorders of glycoprotein degradation: α-mannosidosis, α-mannosidosis, fucosidosis, and sialidosis. In *The metabolic and molecular bases of inherited disease* (Scriver, C. R., Beaudet, A. L., Sly, W. S. and Valle, D., ed.), Vol, 3, pp. 3507–33, 8th edn. New York: McGraw-Hill.

Threadgill, R., Bobb, K. and Ghosh, A. (1997). Regulation of dendritic growth and remodeling by Rho, Rac, and Cdc42. *Neuron*, **19**, 625–34.

Trinchera, M. and Ghidoni, R. (1990). Precursor-product relationship between GM1 and GD1a biosynthesized from exogenous GM2 ganglioside in rat liver. *J Biochem*, **107**, 619–23.

Trinchera, M., Ghidoni, R., Greggia, L. and Tettamanti, G. (1990). The N-acetylgalactosamine residue of GM2 ganglioside is recycled for glycoconjugate biosynthesis in rat liver. *Biochem J*, **266**, 103–6.

Tsukita, S. and Ishikawa, H. (1980). The movement of membranous organelles in axons: Electron microscopic identification of anterogradely and retrogradely transported organelles. *J Cell Biol*, **84**, 513–30.

Vesa, J., Chin, M. H., Oelgeschläger, K. *et al.* (2002). Neuronal ceriod lipofuscinoses are connected at molecular level: Interaction of CLN5 protein with CLN2 and CLN3. *Mol Biol Cell*, **13**, 2410–20.

Vite, C. H., McGowen, J. C., Braund, K. G. *et al.* (2001). Histopathology, electrodiagnostic testing, and magnetic resonance imaging show significant peripheral and central nervouse system myelin abnormalities in the cat model of alpha-mannosidosis. *J Neuropathol Exp*, **60**, 817–28.

Võikar, V., Rauvala, H. and Ikonon, E. (2002). Cognitive deficit and development of motor impairment in a mouse model of Niemann-Pick type C disease. *Behav Brain Res*, **132**, 1–10.

Wada, R., Tifft, C. J. and Proia, R. L. (2000). Microglial activation precedes acute neurodegeneration in Sandhoff disease and is suppressed by bone marrow transplantation. *Proc Natl Acad Sci USA*, **97**, 10954–9.

Walkley, S. U. (1988). Pathobiology of neuronal storage disease. *Int Rev Neurobiol*, **29**, 191–244.

Walkley, S. U. (1995). Pyramidal neurons with ectopic dendrites in storage diseases contain elevated levels of GM2 ganglioside. *Neuroscience*, **68**, 1027–35.

Walkley, S. U. (1998). Cellular pathology of lysosomal storage diseases. *Brain Pathol*, **8**, 175–93.

Walkley, S. U. and Pierok, A. L. (1986). Ferric ion-ferrocyanide staining in ganglioside storage disease establishes that meganeurites are of axon hillock origin and distinct from axonal spheroids. *Brain Res*, **382**, 379–86.

Walkley, S. U. and Wurzelmann, S. (1995). Alterations in synaptic connectivity in cerebral cortex in neuronal storage diseases. *Ment Retard Dev Disabil Res Rev*, **1**, 183–92.

Walkley, S. U., Wurzelmann, S. and Purpura, D. P. (1981). Ultrastructure of neurites and meganeurites of cortical pyramidal neurons in feline gangliosidosis as revealed by the combined Golgi-EM technique. *Brain Res*, **211**, 393–98.

Walkley, S. U., Wurzelmann, S. and Siegel, D. A. (1987). Ectopic axon hillock-associated neurite growth is maintained in metabolically reversed swainsonine-induced neuronal storage disease. *Brain Res*, **410**, 89–96.

Walkley, S. U., Siegel, D. A. and Wurzelmann, S. (1988). Ectopic dendritogenesis and associated synapse formation in swainsonine-induced neuronal storage disease. *J Neurosci*, **8**, 445–57.

Walkley, S. U., Baker, H. J. and Rattazzi, M. C. (1990*a*). Initiation and growth of ectopic neurites and meganeurites during postnatal brain development in ganglioside storage disease. *Dev Brain Res*, **51**, 167–78.

Walkley, S. U., Wurzelmann, S., Rattazzi, M. C. and Baker, H. J. (1990*b*). Distribution of ectopic neurite growth and other geometrical distortions of neurons in feline GM2 gangliosidosis. *Brain Research*, **510**, 63–73.

Walkley, S. U., Baker, H. J., Rattazzi, M. C., Haskins, M. and Wu, J.-Y. (1991). Neuroaxonal dystrophy in neuronal storage disorders: Evidence for major GABAergic neuron involvement. *J Neurol Sci*, **104**, 1–8.

Walkley, S. U., March, P. A., Schroeder, C. E., Wurzelmann, S. and Jolly, R. D. (1995*a*). Pathogenesis of brain dysfunction in Batten's disease. *Am J Med Genet*, **57**, 196–203.

Walkley, S. U., Siegel, D. A. and Dobrenis, K. (1995*b*). GM2 ganglioside and pyramidal neuron dendritogenesis. *Neurochem Res*, **20**, 1287–99.

Walkley, S. U., Siegel, D. A. and Dobrenis, K. (1996). Batten disease: A typical neuronal storage disease or a genetic neurodegenerative disorder characterized by excitotoxicity?. In *Neurodegenerative diseases* (Fiskum G., ed.), pp. 217–24. New York: Plenum.

Walkley, S. U., Zervas, M. and Wiseman, S. (2000). Gangliosides as modulators of dendritogenesis in storage disease-affected and normal pyramidal neurons. *Cerebral Cortex*, **10**, 1028–37.

Weis, F. M. B. and Davis, R. J. (1990). Regulation of epidermal growth factor receptor signal transduction: role of gangliosides. *J Biol Chem*, **265**, 12059–66.

Wenger, D. A., Suzuki, K., Suzuki, Y. and Suzuki, K. (2001). Galactosylceramide lipidosis: Globoid cell leukodystrophy (Krabbe disease). In *The metabolic and molecular bases of inherited disease* (Scriver, C. R., Beaudet, A. L., Sly, W. S. and Valle, D., ed.), Vol. 3, 8th edn, pp. 3669–94. New York: McGraw-Hill.

Whitney, L. W., Becker, K. G., Tresser, N. J. *et al.* (1999). Analysis of gene expression in multiple sclerosis lesions using cDNA microarrays. *Ann Neurol*, **46**, 425–8.

Williams, R. S., Lott, I. T., Ferrante, R. J. and Caviness, V. S. (1977). The cellular pathology of neuronal ceroid-lipofuscinosis. *Arch Neurol*, **34**, 298–305.

Winchester, B. G. (1996). Lysosomal Metabolism of glycoconjugates. In *Subcellular biochemistry biology of the lysosome*, Vol. 27, pp. 191–238. New York: Plenum Press.

Wong-Riley, M. T. T. (1989). Cytochrome oxidase: an endogenous metabolic marker for neuronal activity. *Trends Neurosci*, **12**, 94–101.

Yamaguchi, Y. (2001). Heparan sulfate proteoglycans in the nervous system: their diverse roles in neurogenesis, axon guidance, and synaptogenesis. *Cell Dev Biol*, **12**, 99–106.

Yates, A. J. (1986). Gangliosides in the nervous system during development and regeneration. *Neurochem Pathol*, **5**, 309–29.

Yates, A. J., Saqr, H. E. and Van Brocklyn, J. (1995). Ganglioside modulation of the PDGF receptor: a model for ganglioside functions. *J Neurooncol*, **24**, 65–73.

Yu R. K., Macala, L. J., Taki, T., Winfield, H. M. and YuF. S. (1988). Developmental changes in ganglioside composition and synthesis in embryonic rat brain. *J Neurochem*, **50**, 1825–9.

Yu R. K. (1994). Developmental regulation of ganglioside metabolism. *Prog Brain Res*, **101**, 31–44.

Yusuf, H. K. M., Pohlentz, G. and Sandhoff, K. (1984). Ganglioside biosynthesis in Golgi apparatus: New perspectives on its mechanism. *J Neurosci Res*, **12**, 161–78.

Zeman, W. and Donahue, S. (1963). Fine structure of the lipid bodies in juvenile amaurotic idiocy. *Acta Neuropathol (Berl)*, **3**, 144–9.

Zemen, W. (1976). The neuronal ceroid-lipofuscinoses. *Prog Neuropathol*, **3**, 203–23.

Zemen, W. and Dyken, P. (1969). Neuronal ceroid-lipofuscinoses (Batten's disease). Relationship to amaurotic familial idiocy? *Pediatrics*, **44**, 570–83.

Zervas, M., Somers, K., Thrall, M. A. and Walkley, S. U. (2001*a*). Critical role for glycosphingolipids in Niemann–Pick disease type C. *Current Biol*, **11**, 1283–7.

Zervas, M., Dobrenis, K. and Walkley, S. U. (2001*b*). Neurons in Niemann–Pick disease type C accumulate gangliosides and cholesterol and undergo dendritic and axonal alterations. *J Neuropathol Exp Neurol*, **60**, 49–64.

Zervas, M. and Walkley, S. U. (1999). Ferret pyramidal cell dendritogenesis: Changes in morphology and ganglioside expression during cortical development. *J Comp Neurol*, **413**, 429–48.

Zou, D. J. and Cline, H. T. (1999). Postsynaptic calcium/calmodulin-dependent protein kinase II is required to limit elaboration of presynaptic and postsynaptic neuronal arbors. *J Neurosci*, **19**, 8909–18.

Section IV

Treatment of storage diseases

Chapter 13

Enzyme replacement therapy

Elizabeth F. Neufeld

Introduction

The discoverer of lysosomes, Christian de Duve, provided the conceptual basis of enzyme replacement for lysosomal storage diseases in this short statement:

> 'In our pathogenic speculations and in our therapeutic attempts, it may be well to keep in mind that any substance which is taken up intracellularly in an endocytic process is likely to end up within lysosomes. This obviously opens up many possibilities for interaction, including replacement therapy' (de Duve 1964).

Bringing this simple concept to effective therapy for patients with lysosomal storage diseases has taken over three decades. First, the cell biology of endocytosis of lysosomal enzymes had to be elucidated. Then, tools had to be developed and reagents acquired—cloned genes, recombinant enzymes, and animal models. Biotechnology companies had to become interested in the treatment of lysosomal storage diseases, most of which are individually rare, though together they constitute a significant burden of illness. Lysosomal enzymes made their appearance as pharmaceuticals only in the last decade but are in the process of development and testing for an increasing number of lysosomal storage diseases.

This chapter will trace the development of the field of enzyme replacement and explore the major remaining problem—i.e. treatment of lysosomal storage diseases with a major neurologic component, because of insulation of the brain from the therapeutic enzyme by the blood–brain barrier.

Enzyme replacement therapy is based on the process of endocytosis

Working together at the University of Louvain, Christian de Duve and Henry-Gery Hers (the discoverer of lysosomal storage disease) (see Foreword) noted that molecules taken up by cells from the extracellular milieu would appear in lysosomes. They predicted, rather optimistically, that it should be possible to take advantage of this biological system for therapeutic purposes and to treat lysosomal storage disease by administration of exogenous enzyme (Baudhuin *et al.* 1964; de Duve 1964). This concept was soon supported by experimental systems, such as loading macrophages with sucrose and then rapidly clearing the distended lysosomes by the incubation of the cells with invertase (Cohn and Ehrenreich 1969).

Further support for a therapeutic potential came from the finding that the abnormal glycosaminoglycan catabolism of fibroblasts cultured from patients with the Hurler or Hunter syndrome could be normalized by the addition of 'corrective factors' to the medium (Fratantoni *et al.* 1968; Fratantoni *et al.* 1969; Neufeld and Fratantoni 1970). From the start, the corrective factors were presumed to be the missing enzymes for the respective diseases, and correction was viewed as enzyme replacement, although proof came only a few years later. In the meantime, a known lysosomal enzyme, arylsulfatase A, was shown capable of degrading stored cerebroside sulfate in fibroblasts cultured from a patient with metachromatic leukodystrophy, in which arylsulfatase A is deficient (Porter *et al.* 1971).

The corrective factors for Hurler and Hunter syndrome were subjected to purification as though they were enzymes, although the assay was based on reducing the accumulation of [^{35}S]-labelled glycosaminoglycans in intact cells (Barton and Neufeld 1971). Eventually, the 'Hurler corrective factor' was identified as the enzyme α-L-iduronidase, and the 'Hunter corrective factor' was identified as the enzyme iduronate sulfatase—both required for the degradation of dermatan sulfate and heparan sulfate and missing in the respective disorders (Bach *et al.* 1972; Bach *et al.* 1973). Correction of fibroblasts from Hurler patients was accompanied by the uptake of the corrective factor/α-L-iduronidase, as predicted by the hypothesis that correction was a form of enzyme replacement (Bach *et al.* 1972).

Endocytosis of lysosomal enzymes is receptor-mediated

But there was a complication: the α-L-iduronidase enzymatic activity and the Hurler-corrective activity were not precisely co-eluted from a chromatography column (Bach *et al.* 1972). Two forms of α-L-iduronidase could be separated from each other, one corrective and the other not; moreover, these two forms differed by their ability to be taken up by endocytosis (Shapiro *et al.* 1976). Similar studies of β-glucuronidase also showed the existence of 'high uptake' and 'low uptake' forms of that enzyme (Brot *et al.* 1974; Glaser *et al.* 1975). It seemed that uptake required some feature on a lysosomal enzyme, other than its catalytic activity, that could function as a signal for endocytosis.

The requirement for such a signal was confirmed by the discovery that fibroblasts from a patient with I-cell disease secreted enzymatically active α-L-iduronidase with little corrective activity as well as other lysosomal enzymes that were poorly endocytosed (Hickman and Neufeld 1972). The sensitivity of the signal to periodate oxidation suggested that it was a carbohydrate (Hickman *et al.* 1974). The eventual characterization of this signal showed it to be something never previously seen in mammalian cells—namely, mannose-6-phosphate on the carbohydrate chains of lysosomal enzymes (Kaplan *et al.* 1977) (Chapter 6). Subsequently, mannose-6-phosphate was shown also to be the signal for intracellular targeting of newly made soluble hydrolases to lysosomes (Fischer *et al.* 1980*a*).

The synthesis of the signal was found to occur in two steps (transfer of phospho-*N*-acetylglucosamine to mannose residues on the nascent lysosomal enzyme, followed by cleavage of the phosphodiester bond to uncover the mannose-6-phosphate). Patients with I-cell disease were found deficient in the enzyme catalyzing the first reaction (reviewed by von Figura and Hasilik 1986; Kornfeld 1987; Kornfeld and Sly 2000). Therefore, their soluble lysosomal enzymes, lacking the mannose-6-phosphate signal, do not reach lysosomes either intracellularly or by endocytosis (Chapter 6).

The presence of a signal implied the existence of a specific and saturable receptor, which was first demonstrated in cultured fibroblasts (Sando and Neufeld 1977; Rome *et al.* 1979;

Fischer *et al.* 1980*b*). The biology of the mannose-6-phosphate receptor has proved to be a large and fascinating field in itself (for reviews, see von Figura and Hasilik 1986; Kornfeld 1987; Hille-Rehfeld 1995) (Chapter 6). There are two receptors with very different properties. The larger one of the two and the first to be discovered (approximately 300 kDa), not only participates in the targeting of endogenous and extracellular lysosomal enzymes by binding to mannose-6-phosphate residues, but has the additional and unrelated property of binding insulin growth factor II for endocytosis and clearance from the cell surface. The smaller of the two mannose-6-phosphate receptors (46 kDa) participates in the endogenous sorting and targeting of enzymes to lysosomes, but does not appear to participate in endocytosis unless overexpressed (Watanabe *et al.* 1990). Therefore, proteins containing mannose-6-phosphate are most likely to be endocytosed by the 300 kDa mannose-6-phosphate/insulin-like growth factor (IGF) II receptor, which is nearly ubiquitous on the surface of cells.

The discovery of the mannose-6-phosphate system for receptor-mediated uptake of lysosomal enzymes was preceded (and strongly influenced) by the work of Ashwell and colleagues on the uptake of glycoproteins by terminal galactose or *N*-acetylgalactosamine residues (Ashwell and Morell 1974; Ashwell and Harford 1982). This receptor (known as the asialoglycoprotein receptor because galactose residues of glycoproteins are generally covered by sialic acid and must be uncovered for receptor binding) is found on the surface of hepatocytes. Another important carbohydrate receptor system for endocytosis is the one recognizing terminal mannose residues (reviewed in Pontow *et al.* 1992). This receptor appears specific to cells of the monocyte/macrophage lineage; it was probably involved in the uptake of yeast invertase (a glycoprotein with mannan chains) by the macrophages mentioned above (Cohn and Ehrenreich 1969). The mannose receptor has been the receptor of choice for targeting enzyme in Gaucher type I disease, in which the storage cells are of the macrophage lineage (see below). A comparison of β-glucuronidase targeted to the mannose and the mannose-6-phosphate receptors in the mucopolysaccharidosis (MPS) VII mouse showed that both forms of the enzyme were taken up avidly, the former by cells of the macrophage lineage and the latter by a wide assortment of cells (Sands *et al.* 2001). The cells to be targeted and the signal to be used are therefore important considerations in the development of therapeutic enzyme.

Early attempts at enzyme replacement were unsuccessful

Enzyme replacement for lysosomal storage disease was tried immediately after the suggestion of de Duve and Hers (see above). Administration of an α-glucosidase of fungal origin to a patient with Pompe disease (Lauer *et al.* 1968), though quite unsuccessful for the desired goal, at least led to the realization that therapeutic enzyme would have to be of human origin in order to avoid major immune complications. But subsequent administration of α-glucosidase purified from placenta did not lead to morphologic or clinical improvement either (De Barsy *et al.* 1973). Other investigators used preparations of leucocytes or plasma for enzyme replacement in Hurler and Hunter syndromes in the hope that these biological materials would contain the required though as yet unidentified enzymes (e.g. Di Ferrante *et al.* 1971; Knudson *et al.* 1971). β-Hexosaminidase A was administered directly into the ventricles of a child with Tay–Sachs disease, with no discernible effect on storage or clinical progression of the disease (Von Specht *et al.* 1979). These experiments were performed before the need for signals for receptor-mediated endocytosis of lysosomal enzymes was understood. Subsequently, when plasma (a source of iduronate sulfatase) was again used in a well-controlled, but unsuccessful, attempt at therapy for Hunter syndrome (Brown *et al.* 1982), the importance of carbohydrate signals for clearance from plasma was already well known. However, it was not appreciated that lysosomal enzymes present in plasma would probably be devoid of a signal for endocytosis, the ones with a signal having already been cleared by one of the receptor systems.

The first successful enzyme replacement therapy was treatment of type I Gaucher disease with macrophage-targeted glucocerebrosidase

The most prevalent form of Gaucher disease, type I, is a deficiency of the enzyme glucocerebrosidase that affects cells of the monocyte/macrophage lineage, with no involvement of the central nervous system. Undegraded glucocerebroside is stored in the macrophage system of numerous organs, most prominently in the spleen, liver, and bone marrow; enlargement of liver and spleen, haematological abnormalities, and debilitating bone disease are major clinical manifestations (reviewed by Beutler and Grabowski 2000) (Chapter 3). Early attempts at enzyme replacement were disappointing, since the need for targeting the enzyme to macrophages via the mannose receptor was not yet understood. It was only after glucocerebrosidase was modified to uncover the signalling mannose residues that efficient endocytosis was observed, first in cultured cells (Furbish *et al.* 1978) and soon thereafter, in human patients (Barton *et al.* 1990; Barton *et al.* 1991). The targeted enzyme produced objective clinical improvement and improved the quality of life. Commercial production of human glucocerebrosidase purified from placenta (Ceredase®) was followed by the production of recombinant human glucocerebrosidase made by Chinese hamster ovary (CHO) cells (Cerezyme®). Native and recombinant forms of the enzyme have been found to be equally effective (Grabowski *et al.* 1995; Grabowski *et al.* 1998). The enzyme can be used to reverse the clinical manifestations after these develop or, preferably, to prevent their occurrence. Enzyme replacement therapy for type I Gaucher disease serves as a model for other diseases.

Enzyme replacement therapy is at various stages of development for several other lysosomal storage diseases

Fabry disease and α-galactosidase

α-Galactosidase was the next enzyme to be produced commercially for therapy of a lysosomal storage disease. Deficiency of α-galactosidase and the resulting accumulation of glycolipids with terminal α-galactosyl group are the cause of Fabry disease. Excruciating pain in the extremities, cardiovascular disease, and renal impairment are the most prominent clinical manifestations (Chapter 3). Pre-clinical experiments in α-galactosidase-deficient mice showed uptake of the recombinant enzyme and reduction of the accumulated substrate in a dose-dependent manner (Ioannou *et al.* 2001). Recombinant α-galactosidase made by CHO cells is modified by a heterogeneous mixture of carbohydrate chains including some with mannose-6-phosphate (Matsuura *et al.* 1998), and the enzyme administered to patients is thought to be endocytosed by the mannose-6-phosphate receptor, although the mannose receptor may also be involved (Schiffmann *et al.* 2000). Clinical trials have shown objective clinical improvement as well as safety (Schiffmann *et al.* 2000; Eng *et al.* 2001; Ioannou *et al.*

2001; Schiffmann *et al.* 2001). There are currently two pharmaceutical preparations of recombinant α-galactosidase, produced in different cells by two competing biotechnology companies. Both Replagal® and Fabrazyme® have been approved in a number of countries and Fabrazyme® has also been approved in the United States.

Mucopolysaccharidosis and α-L-iduronidase

As described above, the early work on α-L-iduronidase, initially discovered as 'Hurler factor' for its ability to correct defective glycosaminoglycan catabolism in cells from patients with Hurler syndrome, gave impetus to the development of enzyme replacement therapy. The Hurler syndrome is the most severe of the α-L-iduronidase deficiency diseases, which are collectively known as MPS I, with the milder end of the clinical spectrum known as Scheie syndrome and the intermediate forms as Hurler/Scheie (reviewed by Neufeld and Muenzer 2001) (Chapter 3). Deficiency of α-L-iduronidase causes lysosomal accumulation of dermatan sulfate and heparan sulfate in numerous organs, including liver, spleen, heart, skeleton, and brain. All forms of MPS I show cloudy corneas, organomegaly, skeletal deformities, limitation of joint motion, and heart and respiratory difficulties, but only the Hurler syndrome manifests severe mental retardation. Pre-clinical tests of recombinant α-L-iduronidase in a canine model of MPS I gave promising results with respect to uptake of enzyme, reduction of storage, and general well being of the animal (Shull *et al.* 1994; Kakkis *et al.* 1996). Similar, though somewhat less impressive, results were obtained with a feline model of MPS I (Kakkis *et al.* 2001*a*). The recombinant enzyme made in CHO cells has mannose-6-phosphate residues (Zhao *et al.* 1997), and its uptake is presumed to occur *in vivo* through the mannose-6-phosphate receptor system. The first clinical trial showed that the treatment of 10 MPS I patients (mostly with the intermediate form) with recombinant α-L-iduronidase produced biochemical and clinical improvement, as well as improvement in the quality of life (Kakkis *et al.* 2001*b*). A larger, multicentre clinical trial was subsequently conducted and a recombinant α-L-iduronidase (Aldurazyme®) has been approved for use in the United States and Europe.

Pompe disease and α-glucosidase

While α-glucosidase deficiency (Pompe disease) is characterized by lysosomal deposits of glycogen in most organs, muscle is especially affected. In the severe form of the disease, infants usually die of cardiac failure before 1 year of age. It is only fitting that Pompe disease, from which the concept of lysosomal storage disease had emerged (Foreword) (Baudhuin *et al.* 1964), should be a serious candidate for enzyme replacement. In pre-clinical experiments, recombinant α-glucosidase was shown to deplete lysosomal glycogen stores in mouse and quail models of Pompe disease (Kikuchi *et al.* 1998; Bijvoet *et al.* 1999). Two small clinical trials in human patients have provided encouraging results (Van den Hout *et al.* 2000; Amalfitano *et al.* 2001), as determined by cardiac function and survival. The development of α-glucosidase as a pharmaceutical product for the treatment of Pompe disease is in progress.

Other lysosomal enzyme deficiency diseases

The first mouse model of a lysosomal storage disease to be publicly available, the β-glucuronidase-deficient mouse (MPS VII, Sly syndrome), has been the subject of numerous enzyme replacement studies (Vogler *et al.* 1993; Sands *et al.* 1994; Vogler *et al.* 1996; Vogler *et al.*

1999; O'Connor *et al.* 1998; Sands *et al.* 2001) (Chapter 11). Additional mouse models used for testing enzyme replacement include knock-out mice for α-*N*-acetylglucosaminidase deficiency (MPS IIIB, Sanfilippo syndrome type B) (Yu *et al.* 2000), sphingomyelinase deficiency (Niemann–Pick disease) (Miranda *et al.* 2000), and acid lipase deficiency (Wolman disease) (Du *et al.* 2001) (Chapter 11). Pre-clinical trials of enzyme replacement have been reported for arylsulfatase B deficiency (MPS VI, Maroteaux–Lamy syndrome) in cats (Crawley *et al.* 1996; Byers *et al.* 2000). On the basis of promising experiments in animals, clinical trials are planned or are ongoing for the administration of sphingomyelinase to patients with Niemann–Pick disease type B, arylsulfatase B to patients with MPS VI, and iduronate sulfatase to patients with MPS II (Hunter syndrome), but results are not yet available.

General considerations for enzyme replacement in lysosomal storage disorders

In addition to efficient uptake by receptor-mediated endocytosis, lysosomal enzymes have properties that bode well for therapeutic usage. There is no need for the administered enzyme to reach a normal level of activity, as even a very low level can be beneficial to organs. Nor is a very high level of activity likely to be harmful. As lysosomal enzymes generally have long intracellular half-lives, they can be administered on schedules that are reasonably convenient for patients; depending on the enzyme, the schedules range from twice a week to once every other week.

On the other hand, there are some general concerns related to efficacy and safety of enzyme replacement. While some tissues and organs (e.g. liver, spleen, and kidney) are readily helped by intravenous administration of lysosomal enzymes, others are essentially avascular (e.g. cornea and cartilage) and therefore are unlikely to benefit from circulating enzyme. And in spite of its large bed of capillaries, the brain presents a particular problem because the blood–brain barrier does not permit the therapeutic enzyme to enter the brain parenchyma (see below).

Antigenicity of the therapeutic enzymes is another major concern. Predictably, antibodies will develop when the recipient makes no protein whatsoever due to deletion, frameshift, or nonsense mutations on both alleles. Such mutations are most likely to be found in patients at the more severe end of the clinical spectrum for a given disease. But antibodies may be formed even when the recipient makes an altered protein because of missense mutation. Potential antigenic reactions range from very severe (e.g. anaphylaxis) to benign (e.g. hives). To date, the problem of antigenicity has been successfully managed by cautious administration of enzyme and pre-medication; fortunately, enzyme infusion can be stopped if an adverse immune reaction occurs.

Antigenicity of the therapeutic enzyme has also been observed in animal experiments. Complement-activating antibodies were formed in dogs receiving either human or canine α-L-iduronidase (Shull *et al.* 1994; Kakkis *et al.* 1996). In order to remove possibly confounding effects of antibodies on the interpretation of therapeutic experiments, Sly *et al.* (2001) made an MPS VII mouse tolerant of β-glucuronidase by introducing an active-site mutant transgene.

Antibodies to lysosomal enzymes generally do not inactivate catalytic activity, probably because the enzyme–antibody complex dissociates at the acidic pH of lysosomes; in rare cases, neutralizing antibodies against glucocerebrosidase were observed in Gaucher patients

(Ponce *et al.* 1997; Germain *et al.* 2001). On the other hand, antibodies may alter the targeting of the therapeutic enzyme, since the enzyme–antibody complex may be taken up by the Fc receptor on cells of the reticuloendothelial system. The extent of altered targeting differs between enzymes, since it was prominent for *N*-acetylgalactosamine-6-sulfatase (Brooks *et al.* 1997) but not for α-L-iduronidase (Turner *et al.* 2000). It is clear that the field of enzyme replacement would benefit from better understanding of the immune response as well as of technology to induce tolerance to the therapeutic enzyme.

Another concern about enzyme replacement is an economic one: this therapy is expensive. Because each lysosomal storage disease is rare, each recombinant enzyme must be developed for eventual use by relatively few people. Families with affected members clearly cannot bear the cost of enzyme replacement, and the extent to which insurance companies or governments might be willing to do so is unpredictable in a climate of cost containment. But another potential problem fortunately has not materialized. Though it was feared that the private sector would not want to invest the resources necessary to produce lysosomal enzymes as pharmaceuticals, biotechnology companies are actually competing with each other for the niche markets.

Can the blood–brain barrier be circumvented?

Of the approximately 50 known lysosomal storage disorders (Wraith 2002), most have marked involvement of the central nervous system. The few that do not are the exception, which include Gaucher disease type I, Fabry disease, Niemann–Pick disease type B (the milder form of sphingomyelinase deficiency), Wolman disease, Pompe disease, MPS IV (Morquio syndrome), MPS VI (Maroteaux–Lamy syndrome), as well as the milder forms of MPS I (Hurler/Scheie and Scheie syndromes), MPS II (Hunter syndrome), and MPS VII (Sly syndrome). Not surprisingly, these are the disorders for which enzyme replacement is available, under development, or at least being considered.

It is generally accepted that because of the blood–brain barrier, enzyme administered intravenously will be therapeutic for somatic organs but not for the brain. The blood–brain barrier is a system of very tight junctions between vascular endothelial cells in brain capillaries, which protects the brain by keeping out potentially toxic substances (Drewes 1999; Drewes 2001). In mice, the blood–brain barrier is not fully formed at birth, and it is possible to introduce enzyme into the brain of newborn or very young pups by intravenous injection. This has been demonstrated by administration of β-glucuronidase to MPS VII mice between birth and 5 days after birth (Vogler *et al.* 1993; O'Connor *et al.* 1998; Vogler *et al.* 1999; Vogler *et al.* 2001). Not only was the morphology of neurones and other neural cells improved by such early administration, but so was learning in the Morris water maze. But by 2 weeks of age, intravenous administration of β-glucuronidase was no longer effective, indicating that the blood–brain barrier had closed (Vogler *et al.* 1999). In other studies involving adult dogs with MPS I, administration of α-L-iduronidase resulted in only minuscule enzyme activity in the brain (Shull *et al.* 1994; Kakkis *et al.* 1996).

A number of ways have been tried in experimental animals to circumvent the blood–brain barrier (Miller 2002). The blood–brain barrier can be disrupted by hyperosmolar mannitol, allowing the entry of drugs and even lysosomal enzymes (Neuwelt *et al.* 1984; Kroll and Neuwelt 1998; Neuwelt *et al.* 1999). But this invasive procedure is not suited for repeated use, such as would be required for enzyme replacement therapy. Stereotactic injection is often used to introduce therapeutic genes into the brain of animal models, including genes encoding lysosomal enzymes (see Chapter 16), but this method is also inappropriate for repeated administration.

Since many molecules gain access to the brain through receptor-mediated endocytosis or transcytosis, therapeutic agents can potentially be targeted to the brain by way of such receptors. The earliest use of this concept was the attachment of a lysosomal enzyme (β-hexosaminidase A) to fragment C of tetanus toxin (Dobrenis *et al.* 1992), but this system was tested in cell culture only. A related approach is to fuse a protein of interest to melanotransferrin, a protein that undergoes transcytosis through an as yet unknown receptor, possibly of the lipoprotein receptor-related (LRP) family (Demeule *et al.* 2002) (T. Zankel, personal communication). A different delivery system suitable for application in mice or rats uses transferrin or insulin receptors as transcytosis carriers (Pardridge 2002). Monoclonal antibodies to the transferrin or insulin receptor are selected for undergoing transcytosis with the receptor. Such antibodies have been linked to peptides of interest by avidin/biotin (Song *et al.* 2002). Alternatively, the monoclonal antibodies can be attached to liposomes containing molecules to be carried to the brain, with polyethylene glycol as linker of antibody to liposome as well as stabilizer of the structure (Shi and Pardridge 2000; Shi *et al.* 2001). Because the harsh conditions used in making the liposomes may denature proteins, the cargo is more likely to be a gene than an enzyme. The monoclonal antibody allows transport across the blood–brain barrier by transcytosis and also permits uptake by neurons, which carry both transferrin and insulin receptors. A chimeric antibody has been produced that reacts with the human insulin receptor and could in principle be used to target macromolecules to the human brain (Coloma *et al.* 2000). All of these approaches need to be developed specifically for lysosomal storage diseases.

Is there currently any role for enzyme replacement for lysosomal disorders with a neurologic component?

Even though intravenously administered enzyme may not pass through the blood–brain barrier, it may improve CNS function indirectly in some instances. For example, the clinical trial of α-L-iduronidase in MPS I indicated that reduced storage in liver and airways resulted in improved breathing and decreased sleep apnea, both of which are expected to have positive effects on cognitive function (Kakkis *et al.* 2001*b*). Likewise, the reduction of storage in the meninges should result in improved flow of cerebrospinal fluid, reduced pressure, and decreased risk of hydrocephalus. In some cases, reduction of the body burden of undegraded substrate may reduce the amount that is carried to the brain. But these considerations are not likely to apply to the many lysosomal disorders in which the neurological damage is primary and severe.

Summary

Three decades of basic science exploration have shown that many lysosomal storage diseases can be treated in cell culture and in animal models by receptor-mediated endocytosis of exogenous lysosomal enzymes. The enzymes are generally targeted for uptake by the mannose-6-phosphate receptor system present on the surface of nearly all cells. They may also be targeted to the mannose receptor of cells of the macrophage lineage. The research moved to the clinic a decade ago, with the successful use of glucocerebrosidase for enzyme replacement therapy of Gaucher disease. Several other recombinant lysosomal enzymes (α-galactosidase, α-L-iduronidase, α-glucosidase, iduronate sulfatase and arylsulfatase B) are in various stages of development as pharmaceuticals for the respective deficiency diseases. A limitation of enzyme replacement is the blood–brain barrier, which prevents therapeutic enzymes from reaching neural cells. Development of methods to bypass this barrier constitutes the major challenge for the treatment of lysosomal storage diseases, most of which affect the central nervous system.

Acknowledgements

Work from the author's laboratory at UCLA was supported in part by grants from the National Institutes of Health, DK 38857 and NS 22376, as well as from the Children's Medical Research Foundation. I thank members of my laboratory, especially Dr. K.W. Zhao, for their helpful review of the manuscript.

References

Amalfitano, A., Bengur, A. R., Morse, R. P. *et al.* (2001). Recombinant human acid alpha-glucosidase enzyme therapy for infantile glycogen storage disease type II: results of a phase I/II clinical trial. *Gen Med*, **3**, 132–8.

Ashwell, G. and Harford, J. (1982). Carbohydrate-specific receptors of the liver. *Ann Rev Biochem*, **51**, 531–4.

Ashwell, G. and Morell, A. G. (1974). The role of surface carbohydrates in the hepatic recognition and transport of circulating glycoproteins. *Adv EnzyMol Relat Areas Mol Biol*, **41**, 99–128.

Bach, G., Friedman, R., Weissmann, B. and Neufeld, E. F. (1972). The defect in the Hurler and Scheie syndromes: deficiency of α-L-iduronidase. *Proc Natl Acad Sci USA*, **69**, 2048–51.

Bach, G., Eisenberg, F. Jr, Cantz, M. and Neufeld, E. F. (1973). The defect in the Hunter syndrome: deficiency of sulfoiduronate sulfatase. *Proc Natl Acad Sci USA*, **70**, 2134–8.

Barton, R. W. and Neufeld, E. F. (1971). The Hurler corrective factor. Purification and some properties. *J Biol Chem*, **246**, 7773–9.

Barton, N. W., Furbish, F. S., Murray, G. J., Garfield, M. and Brady, R. O. (1990). Therapeutic response to intravenous infusions of glucocerebrosidase in a patient with Gaucher disease. *Proc Natl Acad Sci USA*, **87**, 1913–16.

Barton, N. W., Brady, R. O., Dambrosia, J. M. *et al.* (1991). Replacement therapy for inherited enzyme deficiency—macrophage-targeted glucocerebrosidase for Gaucher's disease. *N Engl J Med*, **324**, 1464–70.

Baudhuin, P., Hers, H. G. and Loeb, H. (1964). An electron microscopic and biochemical study of Type II glycogen. *Lab Invest*, **13**, 1139–52.

Beutler, E. and Grabowski, G. A. (2000). Gaucher disease. In *The metabolic and molecular bases of inherited disease* (Scriver, C. R., Beaudet, A. L., Sly, W. S. and Valle, D., ed.), pp. 3635–68. New York: McGraw-Hill.

Bijvoet, A. G., Van Hirtum, H., Kroos, M. A. *et al.* (1999). Human acid alpha-glucosidase from rabbit milk has therapeutic effect in mice with glycogen storage disease type II. *Hum Mol Genet*, **8**, 2145–53.

Brooks, D. A., King, B. M., Crawley, A. C., Byers, S. and Hopwood, J. J. (1997). Enzyme replacement therapy in mucopolysaccharidosis VI: evidence for immune responses and altered efficacy of treatment in animal models. *Biochem Biophys Acta*, **1361**, 203–16.

Brot, F. E., Glaser, J. H., Roozen, K. J., Sly, W. S. and Stahl, P. D. (1974). In vitro correction of deficient human fibroblasts by beta-glucuronidase from different human sources. *Biochem Biophys Res Commun*, **57**, 1–8.

Brown, F., Rd, Hall, C. W., Neufeld, E. F. *et al.* (1982). Administration of iduronate sulfatase by plasma exchange to patients with the Hunter syndrome: a clinical study. *Am J Med Genet*, **13**, 309–18.

Byers, S., Crawley, A. C., Brumfield, L. K., Nuttall, J. D. and Hopwood, J. J. (2000). Enzyme replacement therapy in a feline model of MPS VI: modification of enzyme structure and dose frequency. *Pediatr Res*, **47**, 743–9.

Cohn, Z. A. and Ehrenreich, B. A. (1969). The uptake, storage, and intracellular hydrolysis of carbohydrates by macrophages. *J Exp Med*, **129**, 201–25.

Coloma, M. J., Lee, H. J., Kurihara, A. *et al.* (2000). Transport across the primate blood–brain barrier of a genetically engineered chimeric monoclonal antibody to the human insulin receptor. *Pharm Res*, **17**, 266–74.

Crawley, A. C., Brooks, D. A., Muller, V. J. *et al.* (1996). Enzyme replacement therapy in a feline model of Maroteaux–Lamy syndrome. *J Clin Invest*, **97**, 1864–73.

De Barsy, T., Jacquemin, P., Van Hoof, F. and Hers, H. G. (1973). Enzyme replacement in Pompe disease: an attempt with purified human acid alpha-glucosidase. *Birth Defect Original Article Series*, **9**, 184–90.

Demeule, M., Poirier, J., Jodoin, J. *et al.* (2002). High transcytosis of melanotransferrin across the blood–brain barrier: a possible new drug carrier to the brain. *J Neurochem* (in press).

Di Ferrante, N., Nichols, B. L., Donnelly, P. V., Neri, G., Hrgovcic, R. and Berglund, R. K. (1971). Induced degradation of glycosaminoglycans in Hurler's and Hunter's syndromes by plasma infusion. *Proc Natl Acad Sci USA*, **68**, 303–7.

Dobrenis, K., Joseph, A. and Rattazzi, M. C. (1992). Neuronal lysosomal enzyme replacement using fragment C of tetanus toxin. *Proc Natl Acad Sci USA*, **89**, 2297–301.

Drewes, L. R. (1999). What is the blood–brain barrier? A molecular perspective. Cerebral vascular biology. *Adv Exp Med Biol*, **474**, 111–22.

Drewes, L. R. (2001). Molecular architecture of the brain microvasculature: perspective on blood–brain transport. *J Mol Neurosci*, **16**, 93–8 [Discussion 151–7].

Du, H., Schiavi, S., Levine, M., Mishra, J., Heur, M. and Grabowski, G. A. (2001). Enzyme therapy for lysosomal acid lipase deficiency in the mouse. *Hum Mol Genet*, **10**, 1639–48.

de Duve, C. (1964). From cytases to lysosomes. *Fed Proc*, **23**, 1045–9.

Eng, C. M., Banikazemi, M., Gordon, R. E. *et al.* (2001). A phase 1/2 clinical trial of enzyme replacement in Fabry disease: pharmacokinetic, substrate clearance, and safety studies. *Am J Hum Genet*, **68**, 711–22.

von Figura, K. and Hasilik, A. (1986). Lysosomal enzymes and their receptors. *Ann Rev Biochem*, **55**, 167–93.

Fischer, H. D., Gonzalez-Noriega, A., Sly, W. S. and Morre, D. J. (1980*a*). Phosphomannosyl-enzyme receptors in rat liver. Subcellular distribution and role in intracellular transport of lysosomal enzymes. *J Biol Chem*, **255**, 9608–15.

Fischer, H. D., Gonzalez-Noriega, A. and Sly, W. S. (1980*b*). Beta-glucuronidase binding to human fibroblast membrane receptors. *J Biol Chem*, **255**, 5069–74.

Fratantoni, J. C., Hall, C. W. and Neufeld, E. F. (1968). Hurler and Hunter syndromes: mutual correction of the defect in cultured fibroblasts. *Science*, **162**, 570–2.

Fratantoni, J. C., Hall, C. W. and Neufeld, E. F. (1969). The defect in Hurler and Hunter syndromes. II. Deficiency of specific factors involved in mucopolysaccharide degradation. *Proc Natl Acad Sci USA*, **64**, 360–6.

Furbish, F. S., Steer, C. J., Barranger, J. A., Jones, E. A. and Brady, R. O. (1978). The uptake of native and desialylated glucocerebrosidase by rat hepatocytes and Kupffer cells. *Biochem Biophys Res Commun*, **81**, 1047–53.

Germain, D. P., Kaneski, C. R. and Brady, R. O. (2001). Mutation analysis of the acid beta-glucosidase gene in a patient with type 3 Gaucher disease and neutralizing antibody to alglucerase. *Mutat Res*, **483**, 89–94.

Glaser, J. H., Roozen, K. J., Brot, F. E. and Sly, W. S. (1975). Multiple isoelectric and recognition forms of human beta-glucuronidase activity. *Arch of Biochem Biophys*, **166**, 536–42.

Grabowski, G. A., Barton, N. W., Pastores, G. *et al.* (1995). Enzyme therapy in type 1 Gaucher disease: comparative efficacy of mannose-terminated glucocerebrosidase from natural and recombinant sources. *Ann Intern Med*, **122**, 33–9.

Grabowski, G. A., Leslie, N. and Wenstrup, R. (1998). Enzyme therapy for Gaucher disease: the first 5 years. *Blood Review*, **12**, 115–33.

Hickman, S. and Neufeld, E. F. (1972). A hypothesis for I-cell disease: defective hydrolases that do not enter lysosomes. *Biochem Biophys Res Commun*, **49**, 992–9.

Hickman, S., Shapiro, L. J. and Neufeld, E. F. (1974). A recognition marker required for uptake of a lysosomal enzyme by cultured fibroblasts. *Biochem and Biophys Res Commun*, **57**, 55–61.

Hille-Rehfeld, A. (1995). Mannose 6-phosphate receptors in sorting and transport of lysosomal enzymes. *Biochem Biophys Acta*, **1241**, 177–94.

Ioannou, Y. A., Zeidner, K. M., Gordon, R. E. and Desnick, R. J. (2001). Fabry disease: preclinical studies demonstrate the effectiveness of alpha-galactosidase A replacement in enzyme-deficient mice. *Am J Hum Gen*, **68**, 14–25.

Kakkis, E. D., McEntee, M. F., Schmidtchen, A. *et al.* (1996). Long-term and high-dose trials of enzyme replacement therapy in the canine model of mucopolysaccharidosis I. *Biochem Mol Med*, **58**, 156–67.

Kakkis, E. D., Schuchman, E., He, X. *et al.* (2001*a*). Enzyme replacement therapy in feline mucopolysaccharidosis I. *Mol Genet Metab*, **72**, 199–208.

Kakkis, E. D., Muenzer, J., Tiller, G. E. *et al.* (2001*b*). Enzyme-replacement therapy in mucopolysaccharidosis I. *N Engl J Med*, **344**, 182–8.

Kaplan, A., Achord, D. T. and Sly, W. S. (1977). Phosphohexosyl components of a lysosomal enzyme are recognized by pinocytosis receptors on human fibroblasts. *Proc Natl Acad Sci USA*, **74**, 2026–30.

Kikuchi, T., Yang, H. W., Pennybacker, M. *et al.* (1998). Clinical and metabolic correction of Pompe disease by enzyme therapy in acid maltase-deficient quail. *J Clin Invest*, **101**, 827–33.

Knudson, A. G. Jr., Di Ferrante, N. and Curtis, J. E. (1971). Effect of leukocyte transfusion in a child with type II mucopolysaccharidosis. *Proc Natl Acad Sci USA*, **68**, 1738–41.

Kornfeld, S. (1987). Trafficking of lysosomal enzymes. *FASEB J*, **1**, 462–68.

Kornfeld, S. and Sly, W. S. (2000). I-Cell disease and pseudo-Hurler polydystrophy: disorders of lysosomal enzyme phosphorylation and localization. In *The metabolic and molecular bases of inherited disease* (Scriver, C. R., Beaudet, A. L., Sly, W. S. and Valle, D., ed.). pp. 3469–82. New York: McGraw-Hill.

Kroll, R. A. and Neuwelt, E. A. (1998). Outwitting the blood–brain barrier for therapeutic purposes: osmotic opening and other means. *Neurosurgery*, **42**, 1083–99 [Discussion 1099–100].

Lauer, R. M., Mascarinas, T., Racela, A. S., Diehl, A. M. and Brown, B. I. (1968). Administration of a mixture of fungal glucosidases to a patient with type II glycogenosis (Pompe's disease). *Pediatrics*, **42**, 672–6.

Matsuura, F., Ohta, M., Ioannou, Y. A. and Desnick, R. J. (1998). Human alpha-galactosidase A: characterization of the *N*-linked oligosaccharides on the intracellular and secreted glycoforms overexpressed by Chinese hamster ovary cells. *Glycobiology*, **8**, 329–39.

Miller, G. (2002). Breaking down barriers. *Science*, **297**, 1116–18.

Miranda, S. R., He, X., Simonaro, C. M. *et al.* (2000). Infusion of recombinant human acid sphingomyelinase into Niemann–Pick disease mice leads to visceral, but not neurological, correction of the pathophysiology. *FASEB J*, **14**, 1988–95.

Neufeld, E. F. and Fratantoni, J. C. (1970). Inborn errors of mucopolysaccharide metabolism. *Science*, **169**, 141–46.

Neufeld, E. F. and Muenzer, J. (2001). The mucopolysaccharidoses. In *The metabolic and molecular bases of inherited disease* (Scriver, C. R., Beaudet, A. L., Sly, W. S. and Valle, D., ed.), pp. 3421–52. New York: McGraw-Hill.

Neuwelt, E. A., Barranger, J. A., Pagel, M. A., Quirk, J. M., Brady, R. O. and Frenkel, E. P. (1984). Delivery of active hexosaminidase across the blood–brain barrier in rats. *Neurology*, **34**, 1012–19.

Neuwelt, E. A., Abbott, N. J., Drewes, L. *et al.* (1999). Cerebrovascular Biology and the various neural barriers: challenges and future directions. *Neurosurgery*, **44**, 604–8 [Discussion 608–9].

O'Connor, L. H., Erway, L. C., Vogler, C. A. *et al.* (1998). Enzyme replacement therapy for murine mucopolysaccharidosis type VII leads to improvements in behavior and auditory function. *J Clin Invest*, **101**, 1394–400.

Pardridge, W. M. (2002). Drug and gene targeting to the brain with molecular Trojan horses. *Nat Rev Drug Discov*, **1**, 131–9.

Ponce, E., Moskovitz, J. and Grabowski, G. (1997). Enzyme therapy in Gaucher disease type 1: effect of neutralizing antibodies to acid beta-glucosidase. *Blood*, **90**, 43–8.

Pontow, S. E., Kery, V. and Stahl, P. D. (1992). Mannose receptor. *Int Rev Cytol*, **137B**, 221–4.

Porter, M. T., Fluharty, A. L. and Kihara, H. (1971). Correction of abnormal cerebroside sulfate metabolism in cultured metachromatic leukodystrophy fibroblasts. *Science*, **172**, 1263–5.

Rome, L. H., Weissmann, B. and Neufeld, E. F. (1979). Direct demonstration of binding of a lysosomal enzyme, alpha-L-iduronidase, to receptors on cultured fibroblasts. *Proc Natl Acad Sci USA*, **76**, 2331–4.

Sando, G. N. and Neufeld, E. F. (1977). Recognition and receptor-mediated uptake of a lysosomal enzyme, alpha-L-iduronidase, by cultured human fibroblasts. *Cell*, **12**, 619–27.

Sands, M. S., Vogler, C., Kyle, J. W. *et al.* (1994). Enzyme replacement therapy for murine mucopolysaccharidosis type VII. *J Clin Invest*, **93**, 2324–31.

Sands, M. S., Vogler, C. A., Ohlemiller, K. K. *et al.* (2001). Biodistribution, kinetics, and efficacy of highly phosphorylated and non-phosphorylated beta-glucuronidase in the murine model of mucopolysaccharidosis VII. *J Biol Chem*, **276**, 43160–5.

Schiffmann, R., Kopp, J. B., Austin, H. A. 3rd *et al.* (2001). Enzyme replacement therapy in Fabry disease: a randomized controlled trial. *JAMA*, **285**, 2743–9.

Schiffmann, R., Murray, G. J., Treco, D. *et al.* (2000). Infusion of alpha-galactosidase A reduces tissue globotriaosylceramide storage in patients with Fabry disease. *Proc Natl Acad Sci USA*, **97**, 365–70.

Shapiro, L. J., Hall, C. W., Leder, I. G. and Neufeld, E. F. (1976). The relationship of alpha-L-iduronidase and Hurler corrective factor. *Arch Biochem Biophys*, **172**, 156–61.

Shi, N. and Pardridge, W. M. (2000). Noninvasive gene targeting to the brain. *Proc Natl Acad of Sci USA*, **97**, 7567–72.

Shi, N., Boado, R. J. and Pardridge, W. M. (2001). Receptor-mediated gene targeting to tissues in vivo following intravenous administration of pegylated immunoliposomes. *Pharm Res*, **18**, 1091–5.

Shull, R. M., Kakkis, E. D., McEntee, M. F., Kania, S. A., Jonas, A. J. and Neufeld, E. F. (1994). Enzyme replacement in a canine model of Hurler syndrome. *Proc Natl Acad Sci USA*, **91**, 12937–41.

Sly, W. S., Vogler, C., Grubb, J. H. *et al.* (2001). Active site mutant transgene confers tolerance to human beta-glucuronidase without affecting the phenotype of MPS VII mice. *Proc Natl Acad Sci USA*, **98**, 2205–10.

Song, B. W., Vinters, H. V., Wu, D. and Pardridge, W. M. (2002). Enhanced neuroprotective effects of basic fibroblast growth factor in regional brain ischemia after conjugation to a blood–brain barrier delivery vector. *J Pharm Exp Ther*, **301**, 605–10.

Turner, C. T., Hopwood, J. J. and Brooks, D. A. (2000). Enzyme replacement therapy in mucopolysaccharidosis I: altered distribution and targeting of α-L-iduronidase is immunized rats. *Mol Genet Metab*, **69**, 277–85.

Van den Hout, H., Reuser, A. J., Vulto, A. G., Loonen, M. C., Cromme-Dijkhuis, A. and Van der Ploeg, A. T. (2000). Recombinant human alpha-glucosidase from rabbit milk in Pompe patients [Letter]. *Lancet*, **356**, 397–8.

Vogler, C., Sands, M., Higgins, A. *et al.* (1993). Enzyme replacement with recombinant beta-glucuronidase in the newborn mucopolysaccharidosis type VII mouse. *Pediatr Res*, **34**, 837–40.

Vogler, C., Sands, M. S., Levy, B., Galvin, N., Birkenmeier, E. H. and Sly, W. S. (1996). Enzyme replacement with recombinant beta-glucuronidase in murine mucopolysaccharidosis type VII: impact of therapy during the first six weeks of life on subsequent lysosomal storage, growth, and survival. *Pediatr Res*, **39**, 1050–54.

Vogler, C., Levy, B., Galvin, N. J. *et al.* (1999). Enzyme replacement in murine mucopolysaccharidosis type VII: neuronal and glial response to beta-glucuronidase requires early initiation of enzyme replacement therapy. *Pediatr Res*, **45**, 838–44.

Vogler, C., Barker, J., Sands, M. S., Levy, B., Galvin, N. and Sly, W. S. (2001). Murine mucopolysaccharidosis VIL: impact of therapies on the phenotype, clinical course, and pathology in a model of a lysosomal storage disease. *Pediatr Dev Pathol*, **4**, 421–33.

Von Specht, B. U., Geiger, B., Arnon, R. *et al.* (1979). Enzyme replacement in Tay–Sachs disease. *Neurology*, **29**, 848–54.

Watanabe, H., Grubb, J. H. and Sly, W. S. (1990). The overexpressed human 46-kDa mannose 6-phosphate receptor mediates endocytosis and sorting of beta-glucuronidase. *Proc Natl Acad of Sci USA*, **87**, 8036–40.

Wraith, J. E. (2002). Lysosomal disorders. *Semin Neonatol*, **7**, 75–83.

Yu W. H., Zhao, K. W., Ryazantsev, S., Rozengurt, N. and Neufeld, E. F. (2000). Short-term enzyme replacement in the murine model of Sanfilippo syndrome type B. *Mol Genet Metab*, **71**, 573–80.

Zhao, K. W., Faull, K. F., Kakkis, E. D. and Neufeld, E. F. (1997). Carbohydrate structures of recombinant human α-L-iduronidase secreted by Chinese hamster ovary cells. *J Biol Chem*, **272**, 22758–65.

Chapter 14

Cell-mediated delivery systems

Kostantin Dobrenis

Introduction

Diseases that involve the central nervous system (CNS) pose one of the most difficult challenges in human therapy. Cell-mediated therapy (CMT) is a uniquely complex and powerful approach that offers an unparalleled advantage. The use of a cell as the therapeutic agent provides a multifaceted tool that can be utilized to deal with the multiple hurdles of CNS treatment and to achieve efficacious treatment by incorporating several complementary mechanisms. While the promise of 'stem cells' for therapy has drawn much attention in recent years, there is already an extensive record of varied cell-mediated approaches tested in the context of CNS storage diseases. *In vitro* studies have helped us recognize the ability to obtain 'cross-correction' through secretion and uptake from cells expressing lysosomal enzyme to enzyme-deficient cells, and pointed to other potentially valuable mechanisms (Chapter 13). Many *in vivo* studies on animal models (Chapter 11) have been performed utilizing approaches that include the use of haematopoietic cells that can migrate into the CNS or the introduction of other cell types directly into the CNS. Genetic manipulation has been used to improve the corrective power of cells to be delivered (Chapter 16), and *in vivo* gene replacement has revealed the importance of transduced resident cells cross-correcting their neighbours. Finally, the outcome of therapeutic studies has also contributed to our understanding of pathogenetic mechanisms, and hence provided additional ideas on how to use CMT effectively. Below, the work in this area is reviewed with a bias towards understanding the critical mechanisms that underlie successful CMT for CNS storage disease and highlights the advantages offered by employing cells as the therapeutic agent.

Basic principles of cell-mediated therapy

A cell-mediated approach to therapy may address storage disorders in more than one fundamental way. The first is to replace or compensate for defective cell populations with normal equivalents. If this is done early enough, or if there is sufficient delivery of healthy populations, normal tissue or organ function might be recovered. Examples of this approach include bone marrow transplantation (BMT) and the use of neural progenitor cells.

A second way to obtain therapeutic benefit can be through 'cross-correction'. The nature of storage diseases makes them particularly amenable to this. In this scenario, deficient cells acquire lysosomal enzyme from cells that produce active enzyme (Chapter 13). This primarily relies on two cellular mechanisms: the ability of cells to secrete functional soluble lysosomal enzymes and the existence of natural vesicular endocytic pathways that can deliver extracellular constituents to lysosomal compartments. In this way, 'donor' or 'supply' cells releasing enzyme can be utilized *in situ* as a chronic provider of extracellular enzyme for subsequent capture. Greater levels of secretion, which can be genetically engineered, will produce a higher extracellular concentration and result in proportionately greater enzyme uptake by neighbouring deficient cells through constitutive fluid-phase endocytosis. In addition, through diffusion, greater local secretion may provide effective concentrations of extracellular enzyme to more distal, deficient cells.

The type of endocytic mechanism involved will also play a significant role, essentially as discussed in the context of enzyme replacement therapy (ERT) (see Chapter 13). While enzymes will be taken up by fluid-phase endocytosis and in part delivered to lysosomes, far superior results are obtained if the target cells express surface receptors, or acceptors, able to recognize the secreted enzyme. Through capture by high-affinity binding sites on the plasma membrane, the efficiency of enzyme uptake is enhanced, and therapeutic efficacy may be achieved with extracellular concentrations that are insufficient to be effective using fluid-phase endocytosis. Cell-mediated therapy is unlikely to produce the high extracellular enzyme concentrations obtained, at least initially, after enzyme infusion in ERT. Thus, the extent of enzyme replacement achieved through fluid-phase endocytosis may be quite limited for CMT. Conversely, lower extracellular concentrations would not probably saturate receptor-mediated pathways and hence be fully subject to improved uptake by this mechanism, arguing that this may be a critical component of successful CMT.

Thirdly, CMT may produce improvement through indirect depletion of storage substrate, a mechanism that has not been adequately studied. Cells expressing lysosomal enzymes could take up and catabolize circulating *extracellular* substrate. This would then reduce the burden on those enzyme-deficient cells that are accumulating substrate, at least in part, through endocytosis. The potential impact of this mechanism would depend on the specific disease, as significant levels of extracellular substrate are not always present.

Finally, the mechanisms employed in CMT must be considered with respect to anatomic variables. For example, if cross-correction is pursued, deficient cells must have reasonable access to the enzyme. The extent of cellular involvement, organ cytoarchitecture, and fluid dynamics can all influence this need. Thus, appropriate placement and distribution of supply cells can become a critical factor. This is especially the case for treating the CNS which also imposes a barrier to circulating enzyme, as discussed below.

The challenges of the CNS and how CMT can address them

Successful therapy must effectively address a number of challenges posed by the CNS. Introduction of the therapeutic tool must deal with the blood–brain barrier (BBB) which prevents the entry of lysosomal enzymes and DNA. The BBB is created by formation of tight junctions between and low rates of transcytosis in the specialized endothelial cells of the CNS (Bradbury 1993; Janzer 1993; Staddon and Rubin 1996). Beyond this, additional barriers are present. Perivascular spaces are patrolled by phagocytes that can sequester foreign compounds (Kida *et al.* 1993) and by cells that can activate an immune response (reviewed in Dobrenis 1998). Furthermore, layers of basal laminae, macromolecular meshes of protein, lie between the vasculature and CNS parenchyma (Wolburg and Risau 1995). After this, the *glia limitan*, a sheath made up of the end feet of astroglia and microglia, forms another physical barrier (Lassmann *et al.* 1991). Finally, solutes beyond the endothelial barrier are also subject to an outward bulk fluid flow through contiguous spaces. Interstitial fluid from the

CNS parenchyma moves partly into the ventricular system and perivascular spaces, and subsequently solutes are carried to the subarachnoid spaces from which soluble constituents return to the bloodstream (Brightman 1965; Wood 1980; Rennels *et al.* 1985; Cserr 1988; Rattazzi and Dobrenis 1991*a*). Thus, multiple barriers exist that limit and regulate the entry of elements from the blood circulation. While methods to temporarily open the BBB have been used to introduce enzymes or gene constructs (see Chapters 13 and 16), they do not sufficiently address the other barriers. On the other hand, appropriate cell types offer the ability to not only cross the endothelial barrier from the blood, but to actively migrate into the parenchyma and take up residence within the milieu of target diseased cells. As the CNS is extensively invested in vasculature, this route is actually attractive as it can facilitate widespread delivery of cells to address the global involvement present in CNS storage disease. As will be detailed later, cells of haematopoietic origin provide these capabilities. Some of the same hurdles are faced with intraventricular or intra-subarachnoid injections, which result in limited parenchymal entry of macromolecules unless attempts to alter fluid flow are made (Rattazzi and Dobrenis 1991*a*, 1991*b*; Ghodsi *et al.* 1999). Once again, successful results with cells introduced into the ventricular system (e.g. Snyder *et al.* 1995) suggest migratory capability, and appropriate extrinsic cues allow a cell-mediated approach to be a more effective delivery mechanism also through this route.

The compendium of barriers could be largely circumvented by directly injecting therapeutic agents into the CNS parenchyma. It is also fortuitous that foreign agents are better tolerated immunologically within the CNS relative to most other tissues and organs. Nevertheless, this invasive approach must contend with cellular destruction and BBB compromise, and subsequent deleterious cellular responses that can include inciting a greater immune response. These consequences might be argued acceptable and manageable if the therapeutic strategy is worthy. Focal introduction is a reasonable approach in diseases such as Parkinson's where sites of pathology are relatively contained, but appears inadequate in the face of global CNS involvement seen in storage diseases. However, even with this method of introduction, the active migration of injected cellular agents compared to macromolecular agents can offer an improved penumbra of therapeutic targeting.

Once extracellular enzyme is made available, one is faced with issues regarding the endocytic behaviour of neural cells. For neurones, a key target for therapy, endocytic pathways leading to the lysosomal compartment are poorly defined but likely to be complex and to arise only from specific membrane regions, given the polarized nature and functions of neurones (Broadwell *et al.* 1980; Sudhof and Jahn 1991; Parton *et al.* 1992; Yin and Yang 1992; Kelly 1993; Nixon and Cataldo 1995; Overly and Hollenbeck 1996; Buckley *et al.* 2000). It is also evident that constitutive fluid-phase endocytosis leading to accumulation of extracellular compounds in neurones is very low as compared to other cell types (Klatzo and Miquel 1960; Rattazzi *et al.* 1987; Ohata *et al.* 1990; Dobrenis *et al.* 1992; Matteoli *et al.* 1996; Kyttala *et al.* 1998; Rattazzi and Dobrenis 2001). The potential for appropriately localized and chronic supply offered by CMT may help in dealing with these problems. However, CMT, like ERT, will be most effective if suitable acceptors/receptor systems for neural uptake are better defined and appropriately utilized.

The additional potential of CMT to substitute normal cells for affected cell populations may be particularly useful in diseases involving severe compromise of cells, such as oligodendrocytes in Krabbe disease or where neuronal death is rampant as in the neuronal ceroid lipofuscinoses. Early intervention can permit normal neural progenitors to partake in ongoing developmental pathways fostering delivery to appropriate anatomic locations and to compete with endogenous equivalents for survival during normal programmed cell death. Growing recognition that the adult mammalian CNS harbours considerable turnover of neural populations, including some neuronal types, from intrinsic stem or progenitor cells indicates that permissive conditions also exist post development for neural replacement. The challenge that the CNS presents for this approach lies in the extreme complexity of cellular specialization and interactions found in the nervous system, and the difficulty in substantiating that genuine integration of exogenous populations has been obtained.

Cross-correction in a dish

Early seminal and follow-up studies laid what we can now view as a cornerstone in CMT for storage diseases: the concept of cellular metabolic cross-correction (Fratantoni *et al.* 1968; Neufeld and Fratantoni 1970; Bach *et al.* 1972; Hickman and Neufeld 1972; Kresse and Neufeld 1972; von Figura and Kress 1972, 1974; Kaplan *et al.* 1977; Neufeld *et al.* 1977; Rome *et al.* 1979; Vladutiu and Rattazzi 1979; Neufeld 1991) (Chapter 13). Studies primarily using fibroblasts demonstrated that upon co-culturing with enzyme-expressing cells, activity became detectable within enzyme-deficient cells and could lead to catabolism of storage substrates, provided that the protein was not an integral or tightly bound membrane component. That secretion and subsequent endocytosis was involved was supported further by the observation that incubation with conditioned medium from donor cell cultures could also correct enzyme-deficient cells. Uptake of several enzymes was found to depend heavily on receptor-mediated endocytosis obtained through recognition of secreted enzyme-bearing phosphohexosyl moieties by plasma membrane mannose-6-phosphate (M6P) receptor. The critical importance of this receptor to realizing effective enzyme delivery for numerous cell types is now widely accepted (Chapter 6). Subsequent studies demonstrated that similar enzyme transfer phenomena could occur with other cell types as donors, such as peripheral macrophages or lymphocytes (Jessup and Dean 1982; McNamara *et al.* 1985; Olsen *et al.* 1993), pertinent to BMT as a therapeutic approach. More recent research has confirmed that transfer of enzymes is possible also between initially deficient fibroblasts when transgenes are inserted to convert deficient cells into supply cells (Taylor and Wolfe 1994; Francesco *et al.* 1997; Sangalli *et al.* 1998; Sun *et al.* 1999; Sena-Esteves *et al.* 2000; Teixeira *et al.* 2001).

A series of early studies revealed that efficient transfer of lysosomal enzymes to fibroblasts could be obtained by another mechanism referred to as 'contact-dependent' or 'direct' enzyme transfer. This transfer, largely explored using lymphocytes as donors and fibroblasts as recipients, was not inhibited by the addition of exogenous competing M6P to block receptor-mediated uptake, and the magnitude of transfer could not be replicated by using only conditioned medium from donor cells or when donor and recipient cells were physically separated by a membrane permeable to soluble enzyme (Olsen *et al.* 1981, 1982, 1983, 1986; Abraham *et al.* 1985). The full details of this mechanism are lacking, but secretion and endocytosis, possibly fluid-phase, are probably still responsible, as membrane-bound lysosomal enzymes and cytosolic enzymes were not found to be transferred in these studies (Olsen *et al.* 1983). The apparently high transfer efficiency may have been achieved through the benefit of close proximity (Olsen *et al.* 1986; Abraham *et al.* 1988), yielding enhanced extracellular enzyme concentrations within the micro-environment between cells. Indeed, the *total* amount of secreted enzyme that can be measured in recovered culture medium from the type of lymphocytes used is very low-to-undetectable yet 'direct' transfer substantial (Olsen *et al.* 1982, 1983, 1993; Sangalli *et al.* 1998). In a case where secreted enzyme was measurable in 2-day direct co-cultures, the total amount of aspartylglucosaminidase transferred to deficient fibroblasts was three times that found in the extracellular fluid (Enomaa *et al.* 1995). Two additional observations provide further insight. Studies on direct transfer of acid α-D-mannosidase, which produced significant reduction of mannose-terminal oligosaccharides in deficient fibroblasts (Abraham *et al.* 1985), revealed that cell contact heightened the synthesis of enzyme by donor cells (Olsen *et al.* 1988). Second, microscopy analyses on β-glucuronidase transfer suggested that cell contact may have enhanced the rate of pinocytosis in recipient fibroblasts (Olsen *et al.* 1986). Collectively, the studies on direct transfer suggest added merit to employing cells to deliver enzyme within a target organ and argue that the specific cellular distribution and localization in the target tissue might play a significant role in the efficacy of CMT. This is not to say that diffusion of secreted enzyme followed by M6P receptor-mediated uptake is unimportant, nor that this and direct transfer are self-exclusive, as plasma cells (Olsen *et al.* 1993) and macrophages (McNamara *et al.* 1985) have been shown to correct fibroblasts through both mechanisms.

In comparison to fibroblasts, cross-correction studies on neural cells have been limited, given the greater difficulty of culturing them and the relative scarcity of suitable neural cell lines. Nevertheless, experiments suggest that the three major CNS lineages, neurones, astrocytes, and oligodendrocytes, are not so fundamentally different and are amenable to uptake of cell-secreted enzyme and able to serve as supply cells. For example, primary neuronal cell cultures have been shown to internalize β-hexosaminidase A (Flax *et al.* 1998), α-L-iduronidase (Stewart *et al.* 1997), aspartylglucosaminidase (Kyttala *et al.* 1998), and β-glucuronidase (Kosuga *et al.* 2001) either following co-culture with or exposure to conditioned medium from enzyme-secreting cells. The majority of uptake was compatible with M6P receptor-mediated endocytosis assessed in the latter two studies. Using neural cells from a Tay–Sachs mouse model, evidence for reduction of ganglioside storage was also provided (Flax *et al.* 1998). Transfer of human enzyme to rodent neurone-like cell lines has also been demonstrated (Enomaa *et al.* 1995; Stewart *et al.* 1997; Kyttala *et al.* 1998). The use of neuronal cell lines facilitates *in vitro* testing, but results must be interpreted cautiously, given most lines generate poorly differentiated neurons. Dramatic differences in the extent of enzyme uptake have been found, at least for α-L-iduronidase and aspartylglucosaminidase, between primary neurons and Neuro2a (Stewart *et al.* 1997) or PC12 and N18 (Kyttala *et al.* 1998) cell lines. Examples of enzyme transfer to astroglial and oligodendroglial lineage cells have been reported for arylsulfatase A (Sangalli *et al.* 1998; Matzner *et al.* 2000*a*, 2001; Muschol *et al.* 2002), aspartylglucosaminidase (Enomaa *et al.* 1995), α-L-iduronidase (Stewart *et al.* 1997), galactocerebrosidase (Luddi *et al.* 2001), and β-hexosaminidase A (Flax *et al.* 1998) and included evidence supporting lysosomal substrate catabolism (Flax *et al.* 1998; Matzner *et al.* 2000*a*, 2001). In addition, co-culture with secreting fibroblasts was found to correct an abnormal morphologic phenotype displayed by oligodendrocytes cultured from a mouse model of Krabbe disease (Luddi *et al.* 2001). Uptake of secreted arylsulfatase A and α-L-iduronidase by astrocyte-like cell lines 17−/− A1 (Matzner *et al.* 2001) and C6 (Stewart *et al.* 1997), respectively, was largely inhibited by excess free M6P, suggesting receptor-mediated endocytosis.

Relevant to strategies involving replacement of diseased neural cells with enzyme-expressing equivalents, co-culture studies have tested the capacity of multipotent neural progenitor, astroglial lineage, and oligodendroglial lineage cells to transfer enzyme. Neural stem cells, including ones from human telencephalon, produced measurable reduction of ganglioside storage in Tay–Sachs disease brain cells after 10 days of co-culture without direct contact

(Flax *et al.* 1998). Neural progenitors overexpressing galactocerebosidase led to almost complete cross-correction of substrate-loaded fibroblasts from twitcher mice after 3 days in co-culture (Torchiana *et al.* 1998). Galactocerebosidase transfer has also been demonstrated from astroglia and oligodendroglial progenitors to their respective counterparts, obtained from twitcher mice, in 4-day co-culture studies (Luddi *et al.* 2001).

In summary, the cell-culture studies demonstrate the principle of cross-correction, yielding evidence of both enzyme transfer to and depletion of storage in diseased cells. In the absence of the many uncontrolled variables faced *in vivo*, they are able to reveal and quantify specific mechanisms that support the potential of the CMT approach. However, it is difficult to accurately extrapolate these findings to outcome *in vivo*, given inevitable extrinsic differences. Biologically active factors absent from the culture system may well modulate phenomena underlying enzyme transfer. In addition, cell-culture studies do not take into account fluid volume and flow dynamics of intact tissue. The typically large extracellular volume to cell ratio in culture may lead to some underestimation of potential long-distance enzyme transfer by diffusion, while the relatively stagnant fluid flow *in vitro* may favour overestimation of transfer between cells in closer proximity than possible *in vivo*. It should also be noted that co-culture studies have rarely used less than a 1 : 1 ratio of supply-to-demand cells and typically required arguably unrealistic ratios to obtain meaningful cross-correction. Only in rare cases, lower ratios did result in substantial impact by using transgenic 'hyper-secreting' cell lines as donors for neural cells (e.g. Luddi *et al.* 2001). Thus in addition to establishing principle, culture studies argue the importance of maximizing supply-cell number, enzyme release, and efficiency of uptake.

Secretion studies *in vitro*

Variables of secretion

While few examples of mammalian cells specialized to actively release lysosomal enzymes exist (Holtzman 1989), numerous cell types examined in culture studies appear to release or leak at least modest amounts. Studies with skin fibroblasts have led to a view that this release is the consequence of a default exocytic pathway. Partially processed yet active enzymes from Golgi and subsequent endosomal compartments diverge from their lysosomal destination and are released to the extracellular fluid. This is supported by the common finding of intermediate rather than lysosomally mature forms in extracellular fluids and fortunately for cross-correction, this can include enzyme bearing M6P moieties. However, release of enzymes from the lysosome proper can also occur even from fibroblastic and other cells not commonly viewed as secretory, following stimuli eliciting increases in intracellular Ca^{++} (Koenig *et al.* 1978; Rodriguez *et al.* 1997). Several cell types derived from the haematopoeitic system, and so relevant to BMT-mediated therapy, may possess specialized 'secretory' lysosomal compartments also subject to regulated exocytosis (Griffiths 1996; Claus *et al.* 1998). The relatively high release of enzyme that can be obtained from macrophages (Schnyder and Bagglioni 1978) is subject to Ca^{++} levels (Schneider *et al.* 1978; Ho and Klempner 1985; Griffiths 1996; Rodriguez *et al.* 1997) and may involve direct lysosome extrusion or premature phagosome–lysosome fusion (Schnyder and Bagglioni 1978; Griffiths 1996; Holtzman 1989).

Reported values for secretion of different enzymes or by different cell types widely vary. (In very general terms, the amount released in a period of 24 hr often corresponds to 10%

or less of that found within the cells.) It can be argued that experimental diversity, varying cell lysis, dissimilar reuptake, and varied instability of extracellular enzymes all contribute to exaggeration of actual secretion differences. Nonetheless, sufficiently controlled studies indicate that genuine heterogeneity in this regard does exist between cell types. Differing rates of enzyme production affecting levels released and alternative compartmental modes of release, as discussed above, no doubt contribute to this. The details of intracellular trafficking pathways may also play a role. For example, lymphocytes which release lower amounts of several lysosomal enzymes than fibroblasts (Olsen *et al.* 1982, 1983, 1993; Sangalli *et al.* 1998) also appear to rely to a greater extent on M6P-independent pathways for lysosomal delivery (DiCioccio and Miller 1991; Glickman and Kornfeld 1993) than fibroblasts (Ludwig *et al.* 1994; Dittmer *et al.* 1999). In the genetic absence of M6P-mediated trafficking, additional differences become apparent in the use of alternate pathways and release of cathepsin D between thymocytes, hepatocytes, and fibroblasts (Dittmer *et al.* 1999). Differences in trafficking also exist between varied lysosomal enzymes (see Chapter 6) and this could contribute to a ranging enzyme secretion profile for an individual cell type. Furthermore, studies with a macrophage cell line suggest that differential release may relate to the differential distribution of lysosomal enzymes in endosomal–lysosomal compartments (Claus *et al.* 1998). Finally, despite the 'housekeeping' view of lysosomal enzymes, studies show that extrinsic conditions can substantially affect secretion. For example, B-cell maturation (Olsen *et al.* 1993) or macrophage activation can lead to enhanced release of lysosomal enzymes (e.g. Davies *et al.* 1974; Schnyder and Bagglioni 1978; Dean *et al.* 1979; Jessup and Dean 1980; Petanceska *et al.* 1996; Liuzzo *et al.* 1999*b*). In summary, these observations indicate that the potential of CMT for storage disorders cannot be generalized in that the choice of supply cell type, the particular enzyme involved, and the ambient disease-induced conditions can all have deterministic influence on the level of secretion, and thus each disease may demand appropriate modification of strategic elements. Studies with cells particularly relevant to the CNS further support this, as described next.

Secretion by microglial and neural cells

Microglia, the parenchymal macrophages of the CNS, and several related brain macrophages found in perivascular, meningeal, and ventricular regions, have been shown to arise from donor cells in BMT studies. As potential enzyme donors, these cells are promising since they are relatively rich in lysosomes and lysosomal enzymes (e.g. Rio-Hortega 1932; Davidoff and Galabov 1976; Ling 1976, 1977; Peters *et al.* 1991; Banati *et al.* 1993; Nakajima and Kohsaka 1993; Petanceska *et al.* 1996) and are commonly viewed as highly secretory, releasing a wide variety of compounds (Dobrenis 1998). Most importantly, reported studies have verified that microglia have the capacity to release a number of acid glycosidases (Dobrenis *et al.* 1994, 1996) and cathepsins (Petanceska *et al.* 1996; Liuzzo *et al.* 1999*a,b*; Muschol *et al.* 2002). Little is known about the oligosaccharide structure of microglial secreted enzymes, but cathepsin D released by a murine microglial line was phosphate poor (Muschol *et al.* 2002).

As discussed for other cells, the amount of activity accumulating in culture medium of microglia/brain macrophages can widely differ between enzymes. For example, in cultures of purified cat microglia (Dobrenis 1998), enzyme activity accumulating in the extracellular fluid was found to be strikingly substantial for α-mannosidase and minimal for β-hexosaminidase and β-galactosidase (Dobrenis *et al.* 1994). In 24 h incubations, these amounted to 300, 40, and 4 nmol substrate cleaved/h/1 $\times$ 10^6 cells. This difference was not simply due to differences in substrate-specific kinetics. Taken as a percentage of intracellular activity of the respective enzymes, values corresponded to 30% for α-mannosidase and < 1% for β-hexosaminidase and β-galactosidase, implying differences in relative secretion (Dobrenis *et al.* 1996). Beyond providing another example of enzyme-specific variance, the significance of these differences is made clearer when the potential demand of target cells is considered. The β-hexosaminidase activity measured by standard assay methods is prominently higher in many cells and tissues, compared to α-mannosidase, β-galactosidase, and others, and this appears to be true also for neurones and macroglia (Raghavan *et al.* 1972; Bradel and Sloan 1988; Hirayama *et al.* 2001). Thus, with supply and demand considered together, the findings argue that there would be far greater potential for effective cross-correction in α-mannosidosis than for GM2 gangliosidosis in particular. Indeed, *in vivo* findings support this as will be discussed later. There is also evidence for relevant differences between microglia from different animal species. For example, comparison of mouse and cat microglia showed that for β-hexosaminidase, the ratio of extracellular to intracellular activity after 24 h was dramatically different. In contrast to near zero for the cat, it was over 10% for mouse microglia, and the absolute extracellular activity measured was almost two orders of magnitude higher in mouse cultures (Dobrenis *et al.* 1996). Further studies revealed that the apparent differences in release between cat α-mannosidase, β-galactosidase, and β-hexosaminidase, and between mouse and cat β-hexosaminidase may not simply be due to rates of secretion. Instead, assessments on enzyme in the culture medium suggest that the differences can at least in part be explained by differences in stability of the lysosomal enzymes at 37 °C in the physiological neutral pH of extracellular fluid (Dobrenis *et al.* 1996). This raises the point that xenogeneic selection of lysosomal enzymes may offer advantages to transgenic CMT strategies. The apparent release of murine compared to human β-galactosidase was also strikingly higher when the two were transgenically expressed in fibroblasts. The reason for this remained unclear and did not appear related to mRNA levels, but stability in the medium was not investigated (Sena-Esteves *et al.* 2000). Stability can also prove to be the same as demonstrated for rat versus human glucuronidase secreted by fibroblasts (Taylor and Wolfe 1994), again underscoring that enzymes must be weighed on an individual basis.

Considering the fact that microglia are highly responsive to pathologic conditions, transforming into activated macrophages (reviews, Moore and Thanos 1996; Streit *et al.* 1999), the possibility that enzyme release may be both significantly and differentially affected by ambient disease conditions should not be ignored. Upregulation of some agents active on microglia were noted in the CNS of a Sandhoff mouse model (Wada *et al.* 2000). Initial culture studies with physiological factors that may be elevated under disease conditions, granulocyte–macrophage colony stimulating factor and macrophage colony stimulating factor (M-CSF), have shown significant effects can transpire. Selective alterations in intracellular and extracellular levels of α-mannosidase, β-glucuronidase, and β-hexosaminidase were found in cultures of murine primary microglia and immortalized microglia. The most striking was a 100-fold increase in secreted α-D-mannosidase activity following M-CSF treatment (Earley *et al.* 1999). Other studies also show modulation by relevant factors. Intracellular increases in acid phosphatase levels in primary rodent microglia were found following M-CSF-mediated activation (Sawada *et al.* 1990) and neurotrophin stimulation (Nakajima *et al.* 1998). Similarly, intracellular and secreted levels of cathepsin S increased with basic fibroblast growth factor treatment of a murine microglial line (Liuzzo *et al.* 1999*a*). Microglial activation can also lead to *reduction* of intracellular levels, as demonstrated for β-hexosaminidase (Beccari *et al.* 1997) and for cathepsins S, B, and L (Liuzzo *et al.* 1999*b*) in microglial cell lines exposed to lipopolysaccharide (LPS) and to LPS or selected cytokines, respectively. This does not necessarily mean that secretion is reduced, as in the latter case, the same cytokines enhanced cathepsin S secreted levels (Liuzzo *et al.* 1999*b*). We are far from fully understanding the concert of cellular mechanisms that underlie such differential changes in microglia, but they probably operate on more than just the transcriptional level (Liuzzo *et al.* 1999*b*) and hence will also be relevant to enzymes expressed by inserted transgenes with foreign promoters.

Culture studies have shown that secretion of acid hydrolases is detectable from normal neuroectodermal lineage cells (Lacorraza *et al.* 1996; Taylor and Wolfe 1997*a*; Flax *et al.* 1998; Heuer *et al.* 2001; Luddi *et al.* 2001; Buchet *et al.* 2002; Fu *et al.* 2002). The data are too limited to comment reliably on how neural cells compare to non-neural cells in this capacity. Nevertheless, the evidence supports the idea that *cross-correction* can also add to the benefits obtained through transplantation of neural cells or *in vivo* gene replacement targeted at neural cells.

Enhancement of secretion

Secretion of lysosomal enzymes has been enhanced through genetic manipulation, commonly by 'overexpression'. Increased intracellular levels in a given cell type attained through extranumerary genes in normal and/or strong promotor-driven genes in mutant cells produce greater extracellular accumulation and often do so in a roughly proportional manner—more expression yields more secretion. Overexpression of enzymes normally bearing M6P do not appear to overwhelm the receptor, and other lysosomal enzymes are not by default also secreted at higher levels. While overexpression may result in some alterations in post-translational modifications, a significant portion of secreted enzyme retains M6P moieties (Ioannou *et al.* 1992; Francesco *et al.* 1997; Huang *et al.* 1997; Stewart *et al.* 1997; Matsuura *et al.* 1998; Sun *et al.* 1999; Sena-Esteves *et al.* 2000; Muschol *et al.* 2002). Transgenic expression has resulted in a wide range of enhanced intracellular enzyme values, from matching equivalent normal values to even 100-fold enhancements, and similarly varied improvements in secretion have been reported. For example, in studies relevant to CNS therapy, deficient bone marrow cells transduced *in vitro* produced extracellular α-L-iduronidase activity 10-fold greater than normal cells (Fairbairn *et al.* 1996), while ones transduced with a α-galactosidase A gene at best matched that secreted by normal cells (Takenaka *et al.* 2000). MPS VII fibroblasts transduced with a double-copy vector secreted up to 10 times the normal amount of glucuronidase (Wolfe *et al.* 1995), and 30-fold more acid sphingomyelinase secretion was obtained when mouse bone-derived mesenchymal stem cells expressing normal murine enzyme were transduced with DNA encoding the human enzyme (Jin *et al.* 2002). A striking elevation of secreted activity, approximately 100-fold greater than normal, was obtained with human β-glucuronidase expression in amniotic epithelial cells (AECs) derived from normal rats (Kosuga *et al.* 2001). Neural cells have also been transduced with appropriate constructs, yielding replacement or enhancement of enzyme expression (Torchiana *et al.* 1998; Enomaa *et al.* 1995; Luddi *et al.* 2001). When secretion was analysed in transduced neural progenitor cells from MPS VII mice, it was found to be double that of normal cells, and secretion continued following differentiation into progeny that included neurones (Heuer *et al.* 2001). Expression of human β-hexosaminidase α-subunit in murine progenitor cells yielded similar or better results in one subclone (Lacorazza *et al.* 1996). Transduction of primary brain cell cultures from MPS VII (Taylor and Wolfe 1997*a*) or from MPS IIIB (Fu *et al.* 2002) mice yielded secretion similar to analogous cultures from normal mice. Secretion by neurones of overexpressed palmitoyl protein thioesterase, deficient in infantile neuronal ceroid lipofuscinosis, has also been reported (Heinonen *et al.* 2000). Notably, transduction of normal human neural progenitor cells with an additional human glucuronidase copy resulted in almost 100-fold increase in secretion, if cells were switched to media promoting differentiation of the cells (Buchet *et al.* 2002). Thus, significant elevation of secreted enzyme by these methods bring us closer to achieving enzyme replacement with realistic numbers of donor cells in CMT. Based on results of secretion of transgenic overexpressed glucuronidase, it was speculated that 2×10^9 cells would be sufficient to attain corrective enzyme levels in a young child (Taylor and Wolfe 1994). It is also important to point out that it is possible to obtain normal or enhanced levels of secretion with transgene expression even when corresponding mutant protein subunits are present (e.g. Taylor and Wolfe 1994; Teixera *et al.* 2001), further qualifying the utility of the technique as an *in vivo* and *ex vivo* CMT strategy. In addition, in the case of an enzyme produced by two subunits coded by different genes, such as β-hexosaminidase A, overexpression of one gene can fortuitously be accompanied by upregulation of the second (Lacorazza *et al.* 1996; Martino *et al.* 2002), although the ability to cross-correct is greatly heightened by concomitant overexpression of the second gene (Guidotti *et al* 1999).

Given that many enzymes are shuttled to lysosomes *via* M6P receptors, another approach to enhance secretion is through engineering reduction in phosphate-bearing residues, simulating the condition found in I-cell disease where many enzymes are uncontrollably released. This was done by transgenic expression of a mutant form of arylsulfatase A lacking M6P residues and produced approximately twice as much secretion as that obtained with the normal enzyme when expressed in an otherwise enzyme-deficient astrocytoma cell line. However, this sacrifices the benefit provided by M6P receptor-mediated endocytosis. Indeed, the secreted mutant enzyme was four-fold less effective than wild type in cross-correcting deficient astrocytoma cells (Matzner *et al.* 2001). Finally, CMT strategies employing *in vitro* or *ex vivo* gene insertion can benefit from selection techniques geared to isolate favourable stable subpopulations. For example, fluorescent substrate-based vital cell sorting *in vitro*, or following a period of *in vivo* graft survival, has been used to select optimal transduced subpopulations for subsequent transplantation (Lorinez *et al.* 1999).

Uptake and storage depletion

Our understanding of available receptor pathways in neural cells for effective uptake is relatively limited yet critically important to pursue, particularly for neurones which have relatively low rates of fluid-phase endocytosis leading to lysosomes. Several studies do indicate that neurones can express M6P receptor (Lesniak *et al.* 1988; Nielsen and Gammeltoft 1990; Nielsen *et al.* 1991; Couce *et al.* 1992; Dore *et al.* 1997; Stewart *et al.* 1997; Kyttala *et al.* 1998), and cell-culture studies have reported evidence of M6P-mediated uptake in primary neuronal cultures of β-glucuronidase (Kosuga *et al.* 2001) and aspartylglucosaminidase (Kyttala *et al.* 1998). Little-to-no enzyme uptake was observed when competed with free M6P sugar. However, these and other studies (Nielsen and Gammeltoft 1990; Nielsen *et al.* 1991; Dore *et al.* 1997) reporting binding to and endocytosis of ligands by the M6P/IGFII receptor have used cultures of relatively immature neurones. It remains unclear the extent to which mature neurones express the receptor on the surface. Studies have indicated that levels decline with development and may be highly downregulated in the adult (Ocrant *et al.* 1988; Stewart *et al.* 1997; Walter *et al.* 1999), though contrasting evidence has also been reported for some neuronal populations (Couce *et al.* 1992; Kyttala *et al.* 1998).

Astrocytes also can express M6P receptor (Ocrant *et al.* 1988; Stewart *et al.* 1997) and this may be low or restricted to specific subpopulations in the adult brain (Ocrant *et al.* 1988; Couce *et al.* 1992; Walter *et al.* 1999). Upregulation of the receptor in astrocytes has been found in lesioned brain and whether similar events may occur in storage disease may be worth investigating (Walter *et al.* 1999). Culture studies show that substantial uptake of lysosomal enzymes *via* M6P moieties can be obtained in astrocytes or in astroglial-like cell lines (Kiess *et al.* 1989; Kessler *et al.* 1992; Stewart *et al.* 1997; Muschol *et al.* 2002), and provide evidence for subsequent lysosomal localization (Hill *et al.* 1985; Matzner *et al.* 2001). Available receptor for enzyme uptake in oligodendrocytes is probably low at best (Luddi *et al.* 2001).

The mannose receptor is expressed by astrocytes as well as by microglia and can mediate efficient internalization of mannosylated ligands in these cells (Burudi *et al.* 1999; Linehan *et al.* 1999; Marzolo *et al.* 1999). Expression of the receptor is subject to modulation by numerous agents such as cytokines that may be elevated under pathologic conditions and hence may prove to contribute differentially in varied storage diseases. If enzyme-donor cells like microglia secrete phosphate-poor enzyme as shown in some cases, it is conceivable that deficient microglia and astrocytes will still effectively capture it (Matzner *et al.* 2001; Muschol *et al.* 2002).

A greater understanding of the availability of these receptors and other possible glycosyl receptors (Naoi *et al.* 1987; Jenkins *et al.* 1988) that are available in CNS cells for enzyme uptake will be valuable, as will further exploration of novel approaches to enhance uptake as shown with incorporation of tetanus toxin C fragment or TAT peptides (Dobrenis *et al.* 1992; Xia *et al.* 2001). In doing so, the actual extent of lysosomal delivery should not be ignored. While there is considerable evidence that M6P receptors will send extracellular enzyme to storage-laden lysosomes, quantitative assessments of enzyme replacement typically measure total cellular activity and do not provide a direct evaluation of activity localized to lysosomes. Given the relative unfamiliarity with such pathways in neurones and the complexity of neuronal vesicular trafficking (Sudhof and Jahn 1991; Parton *et al.* 1992; Kelly 1993; Nixon and Cataldo 1995; Overly and Hollenbeck 1996; Nakata *et al.* 1998; Buckley *et al.* 2000), it remains important to verify the degree to which internalized enzymes accumulate in the lysosomal compartment. A sobering and surprising example comes from recent cross-correction studies with Tay–Sachs *fibroblasts.* Despite the majority of uptake accounted for by M6P receptor mediation, only a small proportion of internalized enzyme was localized to lysosomal fractions, and degradation of exogenously loaded radioactive ganglioside was undetectable (Martino *et al.* 2002). This raises another point. Cell-culture studies have often employed normal cells and/or cells exogenously loaded with 'storage' substrate as test subjects. We cannot reliably conclude that uptake and storage depletion will be similarly achieved in diseased neural cells. Alteration in endocytic membrane traffic using lipid probes has been reported for a number of sphingolipid storage disorders (Pagano *et al.* 2000; Marks and Pagano 2002), and the presence of some substrates may affect the formation of lysosomes and their intravesicular environment (Schmid *et al.* 1999). Therefore, *in vitro* studies using appropriate target cells with intrinsic storage may be imperative, as enzyme internalization and fate of exogenously loaded substrates may be altered.

Delivery of cells to the CNS

A significant challenge for CMT is adequate delivery of cells to the CNS. For storage diseases, BMT has been employed extensively and its relevance to the CNS stems from the realization that haematopoietic cells contribute to the macrophage population of the CNS. Intraparenchymal and intraventricular injections have also been used to directly deliver cell suspensions into the CNS, and a major issue here is achieving adequately widespread dispersion of cells. (See Table 14.1 for summary of approaches and cells used in disease models.) In comparison to BMT, these latter approaches are still in their infancy for storage diseases despite the common use of grafting as an experimental tool in basic neuroscience studies and its application in other selected human pathologies such as Parkinson's disease. In particular, the wealth of information on oligodendroglial developmental biology, the array of well-characterized heritable disorders of and traumatic insults to myelin, and well-defined criteria of evaluation have led to considerable CMT research on myelin pathology (Franklin and Blakemore 1998; Billinghurst *et al.* 1998; Brustle *et al.* 1999). Relevant to storage disease, the twitcher mouse, a model of Krabbe disease that primarily affects white matter, received intraparenchymal injections of fetal brain cells at 7 days of age into forebrain or cerebellum. Donor-derived allogeneic oligodendrocytes were later identified by *in situ* hybridization and said to be considerably widespread with enrichment in white matter. Of tissue sections analysed, 6% of oligodendrocytes were found to originate from injected cells while no such glia were detected in transplanted normal littermates, suggesting potential disease-dependent determination of cell fate (Huppes *et al.* 1992). Availability of neural stem cell lines and experience with other myelin pathologies will probably yield significant advances in treating this disease (Billinghurst *et al.* 1998). Intra-neocortical injections of glucuronidase-expressing fibroblasts into adult MPS VII mice in contrast produced minimal migration. While cell survival was evident even at 5 months post-transplant, the fibroblasts persisted as focal grafts which became consolidated over time and surrounded by astrocytes (Taylor and Wolfe 1997*b*). Given experience with adult astroglial responses in other grafting scenarios, it is possible that these glia impeded migration. Transplantation of rat AECs over-expressing human β-glucuronidase was tested in young adult normal and MPS VII mice (Kosuga *et al.* 2001). Amniotic epithelial cells, a relatively accessible human resource, are attractive due to reduced expression of histocompatibility markers and evidence of neural cell potentiality. Following injection into the striatum, cells survived for at least 30 weeks. Some migrant cells identified based on a vital fluorescent tag, were evident in neighbouring regions by 9 weeks but not in contralateral cortex. The most remarkable dispersion of cells injected into CNS was obtained with murine neural progenitor cell lines introduced into the lateral ventricles of fetal or newborn mice (Snyder *et al.* 1995; Lacorazza *et al.* 1996). In MPS VII recipients, cells identified by transgenic lacZ expression were widely evident including within the olfactory bulb, cerebral cortex, sub-cortical regions, and midbrain, and persisted at least 8 months, suggesting permanent integration (Snyder *et al.* 1995). While studies in models of storage disease are few, they at least verify that survival and migration of foreign cells can be attained in relevant pathologies. Taken together with studies on normal recipients and unrelated disorders, it is evident that age, site of introduction, and donor cell type are important determinants of cell dispersion, a critical factor for addressing the global involvement of CNS in storage disease. Future research will have to further explore these variables and how extrinsic conditions instigated by individual storage disorders may affect migration, survival, and differentiation.

Table 14.1 Examples of cell types tested for central nervous system (CNS) correction in animal models of storage disease*

Cell type	Delivery to CNS	Key findings	Model and reference
Haematopoietic lineage bone marrow cells	From periphery following irradiation and BMT	Widespread CNS delivery of microglia/macrophages Long-lived within CNS	
		Significant reduction of neural storage Significant neurologic improvement Direct evidence of active enzyme in neurones (Walkley)	MPS I dog (Shull *et al*. 1988) α-Fucosidosis dog (Taylor *et al*. 1992) α-Mannosidosis cat (Walkley *et al*. 1994*a*)
		Definitive evidence of donor-derived brain macrophages Improved myelination and lifespan Some locomotor improvement Oligodendroglial storage persists	Twitcher mouse (globoid cell leukodystropy) (Hoogerbrugge *et al*. 1988; Suzuki *et al*. 1988; Wu *et al*. 2000)
		No (BMT on adult) or limited reduction of neuronal storage (BMT on neonate) Perivascular and meningeal storage reduction, some with detectable enzyme activity Extended lifespan and better mobility	MPS VII mouse (Birkenmeier *et al*. 1991; Sands *et al*. 1993)
		No neuronal enzyme activity or storage reduction Many putative donor-derived macrophages/microglia No neurologic improvement	Sandhoff GM2 gangliosidosis cat (Walkley *et al*. 1994*b*, 1996)

Table 14.1 *(continued)*

Cell type	Delivery to CNS	Key findings	Model and reference
		No neuronal enzyme activity or storage reduction Putative donor-derived macrophages/microglia present Delayed neurologic symptoms (attributed to microglial turnover) and increased lifespan	Sandhoff GM2 gangliosidosis mouse (Norflus *et al*. 1998; Oya *et al*. 2000; Wada *et al*. 2000)
		No CNS neuronal improvement Some motor and behavioural improvement	GM1 gangliosidosis dog (O'Brien *et al*. 1990; Haskins *et al*. 1991; Walkley *et al*. 1996)
Haematopoietic lineage bone marrow cells (overexpressing)	From periphery following irradiation and BMT	Some immunodetectable enzyme in neurones Delayed Purkinje cell degeneration Disappearance of tremor and ataxia up to 10 months after BMT	Galactosialidosis mouse (Leimig *et al*. 2002)
		Definitive evidence of donor-derived cells in CNS Minimal improvement in CNS storage Modest improvement in neuromotor behaviour	Metachromatic leukodystrophy mouse (Matzner *et al*. 2000*b*, 2002)
Fetal liver cells	*In utero* injection into fetal liver	Donor-derived perivascular cells detected but only in older animals Slight reduction in neuronal and glial storage	MPS VII ('kit'-genetically myeloablated) mouse (Barker *et al*. 2001)

Peripheral macrophages	Intravenous injection	Some perivascular and parenchymal localization by 24 h Enzyme activity still present after 3 weeks No cross-correction	Newborn MPS VII mouse (Freeman *et al.* 1999)
Bone marrow mesenchymal stem cells (overexpressing)	Intraparenchymal injection	Distance-dependent Purkinje cell rescue after cerebellar injection Improved motor behaviour	3-week-old Niemann–Pick A/B (Jin *et al.* 2002)
Amniotic epithelial cells	Intraparenchymal injection	Cells survive $\geq$ 30 weeks Migration into neighbouring regions Ipsilateral storage clearance	Adult MPS VII mouse (Kosuga *et al.* 2001)
Fibroblasts (overexpressing)	Intraparenchymal injection	5-month survival Mostly proximal cross-correction	Adult MPS VII mouse (Taylor and Wolfe 1997*b*)
Fetal brain cells	Intraparenchymal injection	Migration into white matter Oligodendroglial replacement Extended lifespan combined with haematopoeitic transplant; motor deficit persisted	1-week-old Twitcher (Krabbe disease) mouse (Huppes *et al.* 1992)
Neural progenitor cell lines	Intraventricular injection	Long-term cell survival Reach multiple CNS regions Evidence for cross-correction of neurones	Newborn MPS VII mouse (Snyder *et al.* 1995)

Table 14.1 *(continued)*

Cell type	Delivery to CNS	Key findings	Model and reference
Resident neural cells	Transduced *in situ* by focal gene delivery	Enzyme replacement and storage depletion of non-transduced cells	Adult MPS VII mouse (Ghodsi *et al.* 1998; Brooks *et al.* 2002; Sferra *et al.* 2000)
		Cross-correction highly distance (100s μm to > 1 mm) and time dependent (weeks to months)	Adult metachromatic leukodystrophy mouse (Consiglio *et al.* 2001)
		Improved learning/memory behaviour (Brooks; Consiglio)	4-week-old MPS IIIB mouse (Fu *et al.* 2002)
		Distal cross-correction through axonal retrograde transport of secreted enzyme	Adult MPS VII mouse (Passini *et al.* 2002)
		Multifocal injection-enhanced multi-region cross-correction Improved spatial learning behaviour (Frisella)	Newborn (Frisella *et al.* 2001) or adult (Skorupa *et al.* 1999; Bosch *et al.* 2000) MPS VII mouse

*Other cell types being developed for use include oligodendroglia, astroglia, and human neural progenitor cells. See text for details.

Studies employing BMT have demonstrated that unparalleled widespread delivery of donor cells to the CNS can be obtained by this approach (Walkley *et al.* 1996; Dobrenis 1998). Combined with autologous transplantation and appropriate *ex vivo* genetic manipulation, this has the potential to address the CNS in a relatively safe manner while also treating peripheral organs. The principle limitation and considerable variable is the total number of donor-derived cells that circumvent the endothelial barrier and the extent to which they enter the parenchyma. The cell types in question are primarily microglia, a term often restricted to those cells that under normal conditions reside within the parenchyma-proper, and their cousins, 'brain macrophages' which are normally found in perivascular, meningeal, subarachnoid, and intraventricular sites.

Microglia constitute a significant proportion of cells in the adult mammalian CNS, in the range of 5–20% (Lawson *et al.* 1990; Peters *et al.* 1991; McKanna 1993). Basic studies on the origin of microglia and brain macrophages indicate that these cells are of haematopoietic lineage, probably related to the myelomonocytic lineage as are many other tissue macrophages (Kennedy and Abkowitz 1998; also see reviews Dobrenis 1998; Cuadros and Navascues 1998). Use of embryonic animal chimeras argue that microglial progenitors enter the rudimentary CNS during fetal development (Cuadros *et al.* 1992, 1993; Kurz and Christ 1998; Alliot *et al.* 1999). Immunohistochemical studies with human fetuses also point to early invasion (Andjelkovic *et al.* 1998; Rezaie *et al.* 1999). While this fetal population, through subsequent proliferation and differentiation, may account for the bulk of microglial cells in the postnatal animal (DeGroot *et al.* 1992; Alliot *et al.* 1999), the resident population in the adult is sustained in part through turnover by newly invading haematopoietic cells (Lawson *et al.* 1992). Existence of turnover in the human brain is supported by post-mortem studies on individuals that had received sex-mismatched bone marrow transplants (Unger *et al.* 1993; Krivit *et al.* 1995*b*). BMT studies carried out in rodents and employing identifiable allogenetic markers consistently show significant replacement of meningeal and non-parenchymal, perivascular macrophage populations in postnatal or adult animals, in the vicinity of 30% or more in 3 months (e.g. Lassmann *et al.* 1991; DeGroot *et al.* 1992; Hickey *et al.* 1992; Kennedy and Abkowitz 1997; Hickey and Kimura 1988). In contrast, the same and other studies show the rate of turnover of (parenchymal) microglia to be very slow and perhaps only involve subpopulations (DeGroot *et al.* 1992; Kennedy and Abkowitz 1998; Ono *et al.* 1999; review Dobrenis 1998). Even after extended periods of time such as 1 year, detectable donor-derived microglia are relatively rare, often representing 1–10% of the estimated population, with variations partly attributed to use of different detection methods (Priller *et al.* 2001). As these studies typically involve irradiation of recipients, it has been argued that even low estimates may over-represent what actually occurs naturally, an issue difficult to resolve. Nevertheless, as conducted, BMT can lead to delivery of cells to the CNS from the periphery. Fortuitously, it also appears that depending on the particulars of pathologic conditions at hand, invasion can become heightened (review Walkley *et al.* 1996). For example, recent comparative BMT studies have clearly demonstrated that greater numbers of donor-derived parenchymal ramified microglia arise after ischemia, axotomy, or autoimmune disease than in healthy animals (Flugel *et al.* 2001; Priller *et al.* 2001). Similarly, significantly higher numbers were found for animal models of Krabbe disease (Wu *et al.* 2000) and for Niemann–Pick types A and B (Miranda *et al.* 1997) when compared to transplanted normal mice. Thus pathology, including that arising in storage diseases, can enhance the extent of microglial/macrophage invasion.

Experiments on the twitcher mouse provided some of the earliest compelling evidence that macrophages in the CNS were haematopoietically derived and that BMT could be used to obtain CNS improvements in a storage disease (Hoogerbrugge *et al.* 1988; Suzuki *et al.* 1988). The origin of invading macrophage populations was confirmed using histocompatibility markers (Hoogerbrugge *et al.* 1988) and again more recently with GFP-expressing cells (Wu *et al.* 2000). Virtually all BMT studies on storage disease have, when examined, found evidence consistent with cellular invasion of CNS. In most cases, assessments of invasion have been indirectly estimated on the basis of enzyme assays on brain homogenates or relied on semi-quantitative histochemical techniques providing approximate measures. However, a few have employed polymerase chain reaction-based analyses to detect donor-specific DNA in extracts of CNS tissue and yielded positive evidence (Krall *et al.* 1994; Learish *et al.* 1996; Matzner *et al.* 2000*b*). When quantified, donor cell numbers were estimated to represent 0.1–0.3% of brain cells 7–12 months after BMT of arylsulfatase A-deficient mice (Matzner *et al.* 2000*b*), and 0.02 and 0.04% in brain and spinal cord, respectively, of normal mice 6–8 months after receiving bone marrow cells carrying a human glucocerebrosidase gene (Krall *et al.* 1994). A time course study in the latter verified previous views that CNS infiltration is a slow process.

In as much as separate studies, often with different techniques, can be compared, it does appear that storage diseases differ in permitting invasion and persistence of donor cells in the CNS (reviews Walkley *et al.* 1996; Dobrenis 1998). BMT studies on the fucosidosis dog model (Taylor *et al.* 1986, 1992) and GM2 gangliosidosis cat model (Walkley *et al.* 1994*b*, 1995, 1996) reported particularly high parenchymal invasion of putative haematopoietic-derived cells. Most studies with storage diseases, similar to BMT studies with normal recipients, detect relatively few donor cells in CNS, and the majority are found to be perivascular or meningeal macrophages (e.g., Birkenmeier *et al.* 1991; Sands *et al.* 1993; Krall *et al.* 1994; Hahn *et al.* 1998). Thus, pathologic conditions produced by different storage diseases may dictate both the quantity of cell delivery and the extent of migration into CNS parenchyma. One cannot exclude the possibility that differences also lie between species, as invasion did appear greater in the cat (Walkley *et al.* 1994*b*, 1995, 1996) than in the mouse model of Sandhoff disease (Oya *et al.* 2000). This again may relate to disease severity, as the same defect in different species can produce distinct phenotypes owing to other species-specific metabolic differences (Sango *et al.* 1995; Phaneuf *et al.* 1996) or may indicate fundamental distinctness in microglial/macrophage trafficking. Another point is that though widespread seeding is typically seen, different CNS regions can vary in the concentration of donor cell numbers, as demonstrated in BMT studies on murine GM2 gangliosidosis (Oya *et al.* 2000). Further insights into how regional differences in pathology or into the underlying turnover demands of the resident microglia (Lawson *et al.* 1990; Oya *et al.* 2000; Priller *et al.* 2001) may conspire to affect these numbers could help better address the specific limitations of individual storage diseases.

Finally, do variables in the BMT protocol itself substantially affect the delivery of cells to the CNS in storage diseases? These variables include irradiative conditioning, immunologic aspects, and recipient age, but the data in the context of storage diseases are minimal. In most cases, to deplete the original haematopoietic system, experimental animals have received total body irradiation, unlike most human patients undergoing BMT, but total lymphoid irradiation has also led to successful engraftment and evidence supporting substantial brain infiltration (Taylor *et al.* 1986, 1988, 1992). With total body irradiation, increasing dosage levels seem to increase brain delivery, but this may simply parallel the extent of blood cell engraftment that is obtained (Birkenmeier *et al.* 1991; Sands *et al.* 1993; Miranda *et al.* 1997). Doses *above* that necessary to achieve maximal blood engraftment did not appear to further increase numbers of cells found in brain, at least when early transplants were performed (Miranda *et al.* 1997). It is worth noting that experiments with MPS VII mice did reveal cells in the brain, primarily meningeal or perivascular and some parenchymal, even in the absence of preparative radiation (Soper *et al.* 1999, 2001) and despite low-level chimerism in bone marrow and peripheral blood cells (Soper *et al.* 2001). How immunologic conditions in recipients may play a role deserves more attention, as one may well expect that histocompatibility differences together with disease state could modulate the extent of CNS invasion (Matsushima *et al.* 1994) since microglia are both strongly subject to and effectors of the immune system (Gehrmann *et al.* 1995). With regard to age, there is general acceptance that given the often infantile or juvenile clinical onset and progressive nature of these diseases, the earlier the intervention the better, as invasion of brain is also protracted relative to other organs. However, the growing view that the majority of microglial progenitors have entered the mammalian brain prenatally suggests that neonatal, juvenile, and young adult transplants may not produce very dramatic differences in ultimate numbers of donor-derived microglia. Indeed, using detection by *in situ* hybridization, a study with normal mice transplanted at various postnatal ages and analysed at several post-transplant periods, suggested only a limited fraction of microglia could ever be replaced, and this was not different when BMT was carried out in neonates versus young adults (DeGroot *et al.* 1992). On the other hand, experiments with MPS VII mice revealed histochemical evidence of some donor-derived cells in the CNS following neonatal transplant (Sands *et al.* 1993) but none with adult recipients (Birkenmeier *et al.* 1991). Similar results were obtained with *in situ* hybridization techniques applied to newborn versus adult sex-mismatched transplants of sphingomyelinase-deficient mice (Miranda *et al.* 1997). As radiation and other conditioning regimens may affect the newborn more than the adult (Sands *et al.*, 1993; Miranda *et al.* 1997), different results with normal and disease animals may in part relate to how the diseased versus normal newborn animal responds to such treatments. More studies with sensitive, quantitative, and consistent methods are needed to achieve a reliable perspective on the variable of postnatal age of transplant. Nevertheless, the speculation remains that *in utero* transplants should ultimately provide a far greater boost to seeding the CNS with donor-derived cells. Although initial studies with MPS VII mice have been somewhat disappointing (Barker *et al.* 2001; Casal and Wolfe 2001), further refinement of methodologies to improve competitive cell engraftment and clarification of fetal origin of microglial progenitors is still pending.

Results of BMT experiments have spurred interest in understanding and exploring further the potential of macrophage populations. A question that arises is whether instead of BMT one could employ selected cells of this microglial/macrophage lineage(s) as vehicles to treat the CNS. Classic studies have shown that tagged monocytes introduced into the blood will enter the CNS taking on microglial characteristics (Ling *et al.* 1980), and more recent studies suggest that it is a mature subpopulation of monocytes that enter the CNS (Kennedy and Abkowitz 1998), although the number of cells found in both cases was very low. To explore the potential of peripherally injected cells in a therapeutic setting, stimulated peritoneal or bone marrow macrophages were intravenously injected into MPS VII mice. Following neonatal injections, numerous cells as identified by a histochemical stain for β-glucuronidase, were found in the brain, but were relatively rare in adult recipients (Freeman *et al.* 1999). Microglial populations introduced into the circulation can also enter the CNS

(Dobrenis *et al.* 1998, 2000; Suzuki *et al.* 2001) and may ultimately prove more advantageous than peripheral macrophages (Imai *et al.* 1997).

While microglia and macrophages have received much attention, lymphocytes also traverse the brain even under normal circumstances (Hickey *et al.* 1991) but have been largely ignored as potential CMT mediators in the CNS. The number of lymphocytes in the CNS is normally low and yet following BMT in normal animals donor-derived lymphocytes may outnumber donor-derived microglia in the parenchyma, at least in the short term (Hickey *et al.* 1992). This number can become significant under the right pathologic condition as shown under autoimmune conditions (Lassmann *et al.* 1993). Given studies of direct enzyme transfer involving lymphocytes, further evaluation of their presence in storage disease CNS may be worthwhile in understanding whether they may contribute to cross-correction (Bou-Gharios *et al.* 1993*a*, 1993*b*). Furthermore, like monocytes and macrophages, when T cells are intravenously injected they can subsequently be found in CNS. This occurs rapidly, by 3 h, but the number is low. One per 2 mm^2 area in cryostat sections of spinal cord was found following intravenous injection of 5×10^5 cells in rats (Hickey *et al.* 1991). If the cells recognize local antigen they appear to persist (or continue to return). A clever therapeutic use was demonstrated with peripheral myelin-specific T cells that were engineered to over-secrete NGF and shown to target to sciatic nerve and locally release the NGF, a potential tool for treatment of peripheral neurodegenerative disease (Kramer *et al.* 1995).

Evidence of cross-correction within the CNS

As predicted by principle and by demonstration in cell culture, it is now clear that cross-correction can also take place within the CNS. Results of directly injected supply cell populations, of resident cells transduced *in vivo* and of BMT-derived invading cells all confirm that enzyme transfer to deficient cells *in situ* is possible and can yield a therapeutic outcome (see also Table 14.1).

Results from cells injected into the central nervous system

Direct parenchymal introduction of supply cells was applied in the neocortex of adult MPS VII mice by injection of 2–3 × 10^5 over-secreting fibroblasts (Taylor and Wolfe 1997*b*). Otherwise absent β-glucuronidase activity was detectable in the thalamus at levels of 1–4% of normal, despite the fact that the fibroblasts formed largely consolidated grafts and showed little cellular migration. Some distal cells were noted, including a substantial number associated with the ventricles, but most of these probably arose by dispersion during injection, as they were detectable by 24 h. Thus, it is possible that some thalamic enzyme activity arose from relatively nearby cells, particularly as it was highest in the first few days following injection. Importantly, by histologic examination 1 month after implant, most neurones and glia appeared to be free of storage within a 2 mm distance from the grafts, providing strong evidence of cross-correction mediated presumably by enzyme release and subsequent uptake beyond the immediate vicinity of donor cells.

Injection of one million over-secreting AECs into MPS VII adult mouse striatum resulted in findings similar in concept but with apparently greater impact (Kosuga *et al.* 2001). Evidence suggested migration of cells, tagged with a fluorescent marker, into overlying cortex by 9 weeks but not into contralateral cortex. Brain tissue was divided into quandrants, and homogenates were quantitatively assayed for β-glucuronidase activity. The quarter containing the injection site had enzyme activity corresponding to 100% that of normal levels, the ipsilateral non-injected quarter had 50% of normal, the proximal contralateral had 20%, and the distal contralateral had 10%. The remarkably high values in all cases probably relate to the fact that very high levels of overexpression (up to 900-fold above normal) were achieved in the AECs by transduction with human β-glucuronidase gene, as evaluated in initial cell-culture studies. The substantial activity in the contralateral brain was probably the product of cumulative distribution of high levels of secretion, which had also been demonstrated *in vitro*. These results appropriately contrasted with those obtained using non-transduced AEC which produced much lower values in all quandrants. Histologic examination showed clearance of storage vacuoles in ipsilateral cortex and some reduction in contralateral cortex, even though histochemical staining for β-glucuronidase did not reveal positive neural cells in the latter. Presumably, sufficient enzyme was taken up to have an impact on storage but was below the level of histochemical detection. This study suggests that remarkable correction can occur with modestly disseminated over-secreting cells and that with very high levels of secretion a penumbra of correction can be obtained well beyond the vicinity of donor cells. Conversely, extensive migration of cells obtained by intraventricular injection of neural progenitor cells into the newborn may afford widespread cross-correction even in the absence of overexpression, as suggested by experiments on MPS VII mice (Snyder *et al.* 1995).

Injection of 50,000 mesenchymal stem cells overexpressing acid sphingomyelinase into the cerebellum of 3-week old deficient mice produced more localized but nonetheless important results (Jin *et al.* 2002). Purkinje neurones are prominently affected and lost in several storage disorders and have previously proven difficult to rescue. However, in this study, Purkinje cell survival was significantly above that of untreated animals up to the 24 weeks examined, and the neurones that persisted demonstrated reduced storage and histochemical evidence of enzyme activity. Furthermore, a decreasing gradient of survival with distance from the site of injection was revealed in sagittal sections taken up to 300 microns away. As mesenchymal cells obtained from bone marrrow have been shown to have multipotent differentiative capacity including generation of neuronal phenotypes, the possibility that the transplanted cells gave rise to new Purkinje cells could not be fully dismissed, although collectively the results were more compatible with cross-correction.

Results from resident cells transduced *in situ*

Studies on gene replacement directed at the CNS have been reviewed elsewhere (Chapter 16), but several points are relevant in the present context. First, transduction of resident neural cells can also lead to cross-correction of deficient cells. Significant enzyme uptake and/or depletion of storage vacuoles can be detected where transduced cells are rare or absent. Second and related, a single site of transduction does not produce global improvement, but clearance of storage vacuoles is observed at considerable distance, often 1–2 mm away or sometimes more (Ghodsi *et al.* 1998; Bosch *et al.* 2000; Sferra *et al.* 2000; Fu *et al.* 2002). Third, when assessed over time (and provided gene expression is sustained), distal cross-correction is found to be a slow process, with improvements in some sites only evident weeks to months after initial transduction (Consiglio *et al.* 2001; Brooks *et al.* 2002). This delay may arise from temporally dependent migration of transduced donor cells or indicate that equilibration of interstitial fluid concentration of enzyme (Bosch *et al.* 2000) in this setting takes longer than predicted by CSF turnover rates. Perhaps the simplest explanation, supported by findings in MPS VII mice where disappearance of storage vacuoles is evident distal to *detectable* enzyme (Bosch *et al.* 2000; Frisella *et al.* 2001), is that there is a spatial margin in which a low level of enzyme replacement is achieved that minimally overcomes the rate of storage such that overt clearance of vacuoles becomes evident only after extended periods of time. Both the temporal and spatial limitations argue the fourth point, the predicted importance of providing widespread *sources* of enzyme to treat these global diseases. It is not surprising that far broader correction has been obtained with multi-focal than with single-site injections of gene constructs. However, these studies also suggest that enzyme contributed from multiple sites of origin may overlap to achieve effective cross-correction at distances not otherwise possible (Skorupa *et al.* 1999; Bosch *et al.* 2000). Fifth, recent work more carefully examining the anatomic patterns of enzyme distribution relative to transduced cells intimates that retrograde axonal transport may underlie much of the cross-correction of distal neuronal cell bodies (Passini *et al.* 2002). This serves to remind us that a diffusion gradient of enzyme through a complex structure will not be a simple function of radial distance. Therefore, educated selection of injection sites may yield significantly more effective results. Finally, the collective observations from gene replacement studies make it clear that cell-mediated cross-correction is an integral part of gene therapy today.

Results from bone marrow transplantation

BMT as a therapy for storage disorders provides a large body of work from which to evaluate approaches involving cell-mediated correction. Indeed, BMT studies on different animal models can offer insight into critical mechanisms that underlie success through analysis of the wide spectrum of results that have been obtained. For example, highly successful reduction of neuronal and macroglial storage has been reported for feline α-mannosidosis (Walkley *et al.* 1994*a*), canine fucosidosis (Taylor *et al.* 1992), and canine MPS type I (Shull *et al.* 1988), which without treatment display high degree of substrate accumulation. The twitcher mouse (globoid cell leukodystrophy) was intermediate, with elimination of globoid macrophages and evidence of some remyelination, but oligodendrocytes still continued to display considerable storage (Hoogerbrugge *et al.* 1988; Suzuki *et al.* 1988). MPS VII mouse showed no neuronal improvement (Birkenmeier *et al.* 1991), unless BMT was performed neonatally which resulted in some modest storage reduction (Sands *et al.* 1993). Some decrease in glial and neuronal storage was detected after *in utero* haematopoietic transplants using fetal liver cells (Barker *et al.* 2001). Canine and feline GM1 gangliosidosis, as well as feline and murine (Sandhoff variant) GM2 gangliosidosis (Haskins *et al.* 1991; Walkley *et al.* 1994*b*, 1996; Norflus *et al.* 1998), all marked by severe neuronal storage showed no detectable improvement in CNS neurones. Syngeneic transplants with bone marrow cells transduced to overexpress arylsulfatase A produced little-to-no impact on CNS storage in metachromatic leukodystrophy model mice (Matzner *et al.* 2002).

Interpretation of BMT findings in the CNS is confounded more than for other CMT approaches, as BMT simultaneously effects variable impact on numerous non-CNS tissues and organs. In as much as the peripheral changes can influence neuropathology and its clinical assessment, distinguishing between mechanistic contributions dependent on donor-derived microglia or macrophages and those from outside the CNS is problematic. Nevertheless, findings to date have not made a case for correlation between peripheral improvements and correction of CNS in terms of neural enzyme replacement or histopathology. There are ample examples of significant therapy of visceral organs with little-to-no CNS improvement (Birkenmeier *et al.* 1991; Walkley *et al.*, 1994*b*; Takenaka *et al.* 2000; Matzner *et al.* 2002), and those with marked CNS changes are not necessarily exceptional in their non-CNS findings (reviews Haskins *et al.* 1991; Walkley *et al.* 1996). As discussed earlier, the blood-brain barrier prevents entry of lysosomal enzymes from the circulation. Despite debate on radiative damage to the barrier and its possible disease-related leakiness (Biswas *et al.* 2001), CNS improvement seems unrelated to enzyme serum levels following BMT (Matzner *et al.* 2000*b*) and can also be obtained following *in utero* haematopoietic cell transplants in the absence of irradiation (Barker *et al.* 2001). In the face of many concomitant and uncertain variables presented by BMT and disease, it is appropriate to still keep an open mind to extravasated enzyme making some contribution, but the consensus is that CNS improvement is predominantly dependent on immigration of donor-derived cell populations. Studies that have shown reduction in storage of resident neural cells also consistently find evidence supporting the infiltration of bone marrow-derived microglial/macrophage cells in the CNS (Taylor *et al.* 1986, 1992; Shull *et al.* 1987, 1988; Breider *et al.* 1989; Walkley *et al.* 1994*a*; Leimig *et al.* 2002). Furthermore, a distinctive result of BMT is that when many CNS regions are examined, storage depletion is found throughout along with widespread seeding of putative or confirmed donor microglia (Shull *et al.* 1988; Taylor *et al.* 1992; Walkley *et al.* 1994*a*; Leimig *et al.* 2002). Strong support of the idea that macrophage lineage cells play a key role comes from comparison of BMT results on galactosialidosis mice to results obtained when the disease mice were cross-bred with transgenic mice that carried a gene for the missing enzyme under the control of the CSF-1 receptor promoter. The resulting hybrid mouse, which expressed enzyme only in macrophage populations and did not undergo preparative irradiation and BMT, was similar to and in some ways more "corrected" than the transplanted disease mouse. Purkinje cells which die in the disease and are not rescued by postnatal BMT were partially rescued possibly due to early enzyme delivery from expressing microglia and perivascular macrophages present (Hahn *et al.* 1998).

Bone marrow transplantation typically leads to the appearance of enzyme activity in the CNS, and the levels determined biochemically in homogenates of recipient CNS can be quite significant. While this is often used as a measure of 'enzyme replacement', clearly a portion of this represents activity within immigrated donor cells. In BMT experiments on galactosialidosis that showed some CNS improvement, immunocytochemistry revealed enzyme-positive cells that indeed included macrophages but also some that were neurones, supporting the idea that enzyme transfer had occurred (Leimig *et al.* 2002). In some instances, suitable histochemical substrates have been available allowing *in situ* testing for neural localization of *active* enzyme, and these provide further instructive results. In MPS VII experiments where reduction in neuronal storage was minimal at best, β-glucuronidase activity in neurones was essentially absent (Sands *et al.* 1993). On the other hand, striking positive neurones were demonstrated in BMT studies on feline α-mannosidosis where CNS neuronal correction of storage was exceptionally effective. The study confirmed the presence of enzyme activity in neurones throughout regions examined and again provided evidence suggesting the presence of donor cells, largely perivascular but also in parenchymal locations (Walkley *et al.* 1994*a*). This finding spurred studies on microglial secretion, as discussed earlier, that support a link between local donor-derived cells and correction of CNS cells. In purified cultures of primary feline microglia, exceptional amounts of α-mannosidase with retention of activity were found to be released, more than any other acid glycosidase evaluated (Dobrenis *et al.* 1994, 1996). Relatively minor amounts of extracellular β-hexosaminidase and β-galactosidase accumulated in the same cultures (Dobrenis *et al.* 1994, 1996). These results correlated with the success of

BMT on feline α-mannosidosis (Walkley *et al.* 1994*a*) and the fact that BMT on the feline disease models deficient in the latter two enzymes failed to show histopathologic improvement in CNS neurones (Haskins *et al.* 1991; Walkley *et al.* 1994*b*, 1996; Walkley and Dobrenis 1995). Indeed, this may resolve what were initially surprising findings in the feline GM2 gangliosidosis BMT studies, where using a histochemical substrate for β-hexosaminidase an enormous number of positive putative donor-derived perivascular macrophages and parenchymal microglia were present and yet no activity could be detected in neurones (Walkley *et al.* 1994*b*, 1996; Walkley and Dobrenis 1995). Although secretion studies extended to murine microglia showed more extracellular β-hexosaminidase activity than for feline cells (Dobrenis *et al.* 1996), enzyme activity by histochemistry was not detected in neurones following BMT in a mouse model of GM2 gangliosidosis (Norflus *et al.* 1998). One might speculate this is due to a combination of insufficient numbers of donor-derived cells and still not enough secretion to attain adequate extracellular enzyme. The possibility cannot be dismissed that GM2 gangliosidosis neurones are simply more refractory to uptake, but this was not evident in enzyme replacement studies with the analogous feline disease neurones in culture (Dobrenis *et al.* 1992).

The impact of enhancing secretion was tested in arylsulfatase A-deficient mice by transducing donor bone marrow cells with a mutant gene that produced active enzyme in a form that was poorly retained by cells, resulting in the doubling of secretion levels assessed *in vitro* (Matzner *et al.* 2001). This was not more effective in reducing CNS storage or in improving on neurologic behavioural tests than BMT using the native form of the enzyme (Matzner *et al.* 2000*b*, 2002). Indeed, although enhanced serum levels were compatible with enhanced secretion, enzyme activity in CNS and other tissues was considerably reduced. Interpretation is confounded by the fact that the mutant enzyme was secreted more due to lack of two of three glycosylation sites, resulting in the abrogation of binding to M6P receptors. At least, this argued that doubling secretion did not outweigh the advantage of M6P receptor endocytosis. Interestingly, when using the mutant versus normal gene construct, enzyme levels in CNS were proportionally less reduced than in liver or spleen. This could relate to the finding that in contrast to other cell types, *normal* macrophages and possibly microglia release arylsulfatase A in a form that is *already* poor in M6P moieties (Muschol *et al.* 2002). Therefore, if enzyme delivery to CNS is more dependent on colonizing macrophages/microglia compared to other tissues which can acquire enzyme from the circulation (which could also arise from non-macrophage cells and normally bear M6P residues), it makes sense that the CNS values were reduced less than those of other organs when using the mutant enzyme. Furthermore, limited uptake by CNS target cells may help explain the finding that BMT studies with normal arylsulfatase A did result in substantial *total* enzyme activity in the CNS, up to 33% of normal because of immigrated cells, yet had minor impact on neuropathology (Matzner *et al.* 2000*b*, 2002). Collectively, BMT studies examining enzyme activity and its distribution in the CNS argue the quantity of locally provided enzyme is important. However, there is a clear need to better understand what uptake mechanisms are available in each case as well as determining the enzyme activity needs of the target cells involved.

A wholly unanswered question in BMT studies is the relevance of location of immigrated cells relative to the parenchyma. As discussed earlier, beyond the endothelial barrier, there are additional potential impediments for enzyme delivery to parenchymal cells, and yet the bone marrow-derived cells are primarily found in perivascular spaces. From this location, secreted enzyme must still get past basal laminae and might be directed outward to the subarachnoid by bulk fluid flow. The perivascular cell population itself would have ample opportunity to sequester much of the released enzyme. So, how much enzyme reaches neurones from this location and are they in fact critically dependent on intraparenchymal donor cells? Does the *glia limitan* formed by glial end-feet also block entry from perivascular sites or provide an opportunity for selected glia to endocytose extracellular enzyme from perivascular spaces? Resolving these questions and modifying strategies accordingly is a significant challenge, but it may allow substantial improvements in therapy even in the absence of enhancing donor cell number.

In addition to providing a source of enzyme, the BMT approach is after all a cell replacement strategy. The direct substitution of members of the microglial/brain macrophage population with 'normal' cells may thus contribute to CNS improvement independent of enzyme transfer. Neurologic improvements seen in α-fucosidosis dog (Taylor *et al.* 1992) and the twitcher mouse (Hoogerbrugge *et al.* 1988; Suzuki *et al.* 1988), disease models that both demonstrate large numbers of storage laden macrophages, may well derive from replacement of these undesirable populations with new bone marrow-derived cells. Furthermore, neuronal viability and function may be influenced by the 'activation' state of microglia, the importance of which has been recognized in numerous other CNS pathologies. For storage diseases, a strong case was made in explaining BMT results on a Sandhoff mouse model that demonstrated significant behavioural improvements but neither enzyme transfer to neurons or improvement of CNS storage (Norflus *et al.* 1998). Studies suggested that neuronal compromise and death was in large part instigated by neurotoxic compounds arising from microglia which were activated in part due to their own enzyme deficiency. Partial replacement of this activated population by normal bone marrow-derived cells helped alleviate this element and slow neurologic deterioration (Wada *et al.* 2000).

In summary, the complexity of BMT involving multiple organ effects, replacement of numerous cell types, and radiative and immunologic variables provide a puzzling array of potential mechanisms that may impact on CNS therapy. Nevertheless, most data indicate that donor-derived brain macrophages and microglia play a key role, both as local enzyme providers and possibly through their substitution of deleterious counterparts. This lineage of cells represents a powerful tool for CMT by providing a convenient route to the CNS that can result in widespread seeding and therapy, if appropriately maximized. The profound success of BMT in some animal models, where it also provides multi-region correction in the CNS, supports this idea.

Neurologic outcome and human therapy

The field of cellular implantation in CNS for storage diseases is still young and behavioural studies limited, hence a picture on neuroclinical improvements has not emerged. However, there is some evidence of impact even with relatively small cell numbers. Injection of 50,000 overexpressing mesenchymal stem cells into hippocampus and cerebellum of a mouse model for Niemann–Pick type A and B did result in improved motor behaviour (Jin *et al.* 2002). Partial oligodendroglial cell replacement in twitcher mice was said not to result in gross improvement of motor behaviour but did significantly enhance survival time when coupled with BMT (Huppes *et al.* 1992). Intraparenchymal gene therapy in MPS VII (Frisella *et al.* 2001; Brooks *et al.* 2002) and metachromatic leukodystrophy (Consiglio *et al.* 2001) mice yielded significant cross-correction *via* transduced cells and treated mice showed reduction of learning deficits. BMT studies have been quite extensive and like the histopathologic findings also variable in neurologic outcome (Haskins *et al.* 1991; Walkley *et al.* 1996). For example, treated α-fucosidosis dogs (Taylor *et al.* 1992) and α-mannosidosis cats (Walkley *et al.* 1994*a*) developed almost no behavioural or motor signs. On the other hand, GM2 gangliosidosis and GM1 gangliosidosis in domestic animals showed no neurologic benefit (O'Brien *et al.* 1990; Haskins *et al.* 1991; Walkley *et al.* 1994*b*, 1996), while a GM2 gangliosidosis mouse did show significant improvements in behavioural motor tests (Norflus *et al.* 1998). BMT with *ex vivo* transduced stem cells for overexpression resulted in only modest improvement in neuromotor behaviour of metachromatic leukodystrophy mice (Matzner *et al.* 2002), but in significant delay of onset of tremor and cerebellar ataxia in galactosialidosis mice (Leimig *et al.* 2002). Underlying reasons for the different outcomes based on detailed analyses have been discussed earlier. BMT in humans has also resulted in highly variable outcomes, but they are more difficult to interpret reliably.

Several hundred patients with storage diseases have undergone haematopoietic stem cell transplants, largely by heterologous BMT, but also utilizing cord blood, mobilized stem cells, and fetal liver cells. As early intervention is viewed as particularly critical, some attempts at *in utero* transplants have been made but have been disappointing. Heterologous BMT continues to be a high-risk procedure despite technical improvements in preparative regimens and post-transplant management, and autologous approaches and strategies for immune tolerance are being pursued. Nonetheless, BMT has been able to improve the course of neuropathology in several forms of storage disease with mental retardation (Walkley *et al.* 1996; Krivit *et al.* 1999; Krivit 2002). Many Hurler patients (MPS IH) have undergone BMT. Patients often show stabilization of IQ and neuropsychologic profile, or increases if transplanted before 2 years, and significant improvement in storage-induced anatomic changes in CNS assessed by magnetic resonance imaging (MRI) (Whitley *et al.* 1993; Hoogerbrugge *et al.* 1995; Krivit *et al.* 1995*a*; Shapiro *et al.* 1995; Vellodi *et al.* 1997; Krivit *et al.* 1999; Neufeld and Muenzer 2001; Grewal *et al.* 2002). Recall that a canine model of this disease also was effectively treated by BMT (Shull *et al.* 1987, 1988). BMT on Hunter disease (MPS II) patients has in some cases produced measurable improvements but is mostly ineffective particularly in more severe forms and with late transplant (Shapiro *et al.* 1995; Vellodi *et al.* 1999; Peters and Krivit 2000; Neufeld and Muenzer 2001; Seto *et al.* 2001; Takahashi *et al.* 2001). MPS III disease typically evokes severe retardation and behavioural abnormalities, and neurologic decline appears to continue following BMT (Vellodi *et al.* 1992; Hoogerbrugge *et al.* 1995; Shapiro *et al.* 1995; Neufeld and Muenzer 2001). BMT in globoid cell leukodystrophy, which was partially successful in mice, has resulted in gains in intellect, cognition, and some other criteria, particularly in late onset forms (Hoogerbrugge *et al.* 1995; Shapiro *et al* 1995; Krivit *et al.* 1995*a*, 1998, 1999; Wenger *et al.* 2001). Results with metachromatic leukodystrophy are mixed and most promising for late onset forms (Hoogerbrugge *et al.* 1995; Krivit *et al.* 1995*a*, 1998, 1999; Shapiro *et al.* 1995; Kapaun *et al.* 1999; Von Figura *et al.* 2001). While very few transplants of α-mannosidosis and α-fucosidosis patients have been reported, they are worth noting given that BMT on the respective animal models was particularly effective on the CNS. A 7-year-old boy with α-mannosidosis receiving BMT died 18 weeks later, and no significant decrease in neuronal storage was evident (Will *et al.* 1987). However, a report on a boy transplanted at 22 months of age (Wall *et al.* 1998) indicated increases in IQ, language and social skills, and stabilization in other neurologic parameters. Overall, the rate of development was less than normal. A boy with α-fucosidosis transplanted at 8 months showed mild neurodevelopmental delay 18 months later and improvement by MRI (Vellodi *et al.* 1995). Another patient, transplanted at the onset of neurologic symptoms, has shown improved psychomotor development

(Miano *et al.* 2001). Two patients with GM2 gangliosidosis underwent BMT after their first year of life already showing neurologic signs (Hoogerbrugge *et al.* 1995). One with Tay–Sachs briefly showed some improvement followed by further deterioration and death 6 months later. One with Sandhoff disease only survived 1 month following transplant.

Findings from the above and transplants in other diseases have led to the opinion that BMT should not be performed in patients already fallen below a set developmental quotient, and clearly intervention at pre-symptomatic stages is most desirable. Furthermore, it generally appears that the procedure is most likely to alter the course of the neurologic decline in diseases that have milder CNS involvement. The simple conclusion is that BMT in humans has a limited impact on the CNS, sufficient only to address relatively minor deficiencies and largely unable to reverse pre-existing storage and cytopathology. However, the fact that it does have some positive effect, and consideration of findings in animal studies and on microglia, provides hope. It is reasonable to expect that further work on isolation and stable manipulation of human haematopoietic cells to over-secrete and research on ways to maximize CNS colonization will lead to significant improvements in human therapy. Also, more basic studies on secretion and uptake in cell culture with *human*, rather than animal, microglia and target neural cells, and on human microglial dynamics *in vivo* might prove insightful.

Studies on animal models have raised some important options for human therapy involving haematopoietic cell transplantation. BMT has been combined with other therapeutic modalities. MPS VII mice received weekly injections of β-glucuronidase beginning at birth and ending at 7 weeks (Sands *et al.* 1997). This was immediately followed by syngeneic BMT. The protocol produced CNS results similar to or better than mice receiving enzyme injections throughout their lifespan. In both cases, there was some long-term albeit limited reduction in neuronal storage, possibly due to enzyme entry through an incomplete BBB in the immature mice and greater neuronal requirement for enzyme during the developmental period. The combined therapy was more effective than ERT alone in reducing storage in meninges and retinal pigment epithelium, and produced higher total enzyme levels in brain, all presumably related to invaded bone marrow-derived cells. Detailed comparison to results from previous studies with BMT alone was not made, but the combined therapy was quite similar to BMT performed neonatally (Sands *et al.* 1993). The practical points are the following. The combined approach delays the use of the preparative regimens for BMT, which have significant deleterious effects on, for example, cerebellar development if applied perinatally (Sands *et al.* 1993). Furthermore, potentially productive early intervention with ERT in humans would allow more time for identification of suitable BMT donor or preparation and integration of transduced autologous haematopoietic cells. Bone marrow transplantation in a mouse model of Sandhoff disease also receiving *N*-butyldeoxynojirimycin to inhibit ganglioside synthesis, reducing the storage burden, resulted in greater efficacy than either treatment alone (Jeyakumar *et al.* 2001). Deterioration of neurologic function assessed by three motor-based behaviours was delayed or slowed more in mice with the combination therapy. This clearly complementary approach appears amenable to human application (see Chapter 15), offers similar temporal advantages as the ERT/BMT combination and may have additive or even synergistic benefit (Jeyakumar *et al.* 2001). Finally, as noted earlier, implantation of normal neural cells into Twitcher mice to give rise to new oligodendrocytes significantly extended survival of recipients when combined with BMT (Huppes *et al.* 1992). This kind of strategy is being further pursued (Wenger *et al.* 2000) and may provide neurologic benefit for Krabbe or other human diseases, particularly if limited anatomic sites of pathology most critical to function can be identified.

Anticipated advances and aspirations

Despite the rarity of lysosomal storage diseases in the human population, the history of sustained efforts towards treatment has led to recognition of several factors that if maximized could lead to success. In the context of CMT, these include deposition of ample and well-dispersed cells, adequate secretion level, and efficient uptake of released enzyme. The effectiveness of focal cell injections and BMT could be bolstered with a better understanding of requirements for cell migration. Early fetal replacement of endogenous haematopoietic lineages could increase macrophage/microglial population of the CNS, potentially attaining a donor population that corresponds to 10% or more of the native CNS population. While such initial studies for storage disease have been disappointing, improvements in engraftment and proper identification of microglial precursors which may stem from progenitors to the haematopoietic system itself (Cuadros *et al.* 1992; Alliot *et al.* 1999) will be essential before final judgment can be passed. Early introduction of neural stem or progenitor cells is highly promising in regard to cell number, and ventricular or generative zone introduction coupled with permissive developmental pathways of migration appear to produce extensive dissemination (Snyder *et al.* 1995). A conclusive appreciation of the soundness of neural integration may be the greatest challenge here. In all cases, strides in tackling the immunologic challenge presented by CMT are expected to continue through autologous *ex vivo* approaches and improved understanding of immune tolerance.

Beyond cellular seeding, further steps to improve enzyme delivery are clear. In many cases, the amount of secretion and its sustained operation through stable gene integration has not been maximized. Ensuring that the gene product is adequately endowed with appropriate moieties for receptor-mediated uptake will secure significant enhancement. Indeed for the many, if not most, cells within the CNS that see low levels of extracellular enzyme, glycosyl receptor systems may well not be saturated. This suggests that even minor improvement in secretion levels coupled with high-uptake enzyme forms could yield disproportionately greater improvement. As classical enzyme receptors on neural cells may be limited, exploring more novel acceptor and receptor systems is also worthwhile (Dobrenis *et al.* 1992; Xia *et al.* 2001). In sum, there are several rational and feasible means to attain improved cross-correction. Given the notable examples of significant CNS correction already obtained, yet with methods not fully optimized, it is reasonable to expect considerable success in the near future. This may be even closer than we think if one considers cross-correction in light of the chronic progressive nature of the relevant diseases. In terms of storage, CMT outcome evaluated over the long term is after all the consequence of an ever-widening cumulative process determined by the daily balance between substrate load and enzyme activity. Therefore, minor improvements in enzyme delivery may yield profound improvements over time. The question then becomes whether this is rapid enough to halt the functional neurophysiological deficits that arise in storage diseases and underscores the importance of better understanding the pathogenetic cascades involved (see Chapter 12).

Hidden within failures and successes lay clues to additional mechanisms that we suspect but know little about. The interactions between donor and recipient cells, and the factors determining the fate of extracellular enzyme within the complex fabric of the CNS are probably complicated. It is only recent studies that begin to better dissect this, such as ones showing that delivery of enzyme to distal neuronal lysosomes might be realized more through intracellular transport along axonal pathways than through simple diffusion (Passini *et al.* 2002). Another case in point is the potential contribution of so-called 'direct enzyme' transfer found to be very efficient in cell culture and independent of M6P-mediated uptake which may be limited in the adult CNS. Further investigation of this using relevant cell types and with appropriate *in vivo* experiments (Bou-Gharios *et al.* 1993*b*) could be valuable. A concept rarely addressed (Desnick *et al.* 1979) is that of indirect storage depletion. In diseases where storage substrates can be detected in the cerebrospinal fluid as well as the blood, to what extent might donor cells reduce the substrate load on enzyme-deficient cells by simply reducing extracellular substrate? It is possible that this 'sink' effect can help explain those instances where storage depletion has been reported in neurones without detectable enzyme uptake. It is also tempting to speculate that this played some role in the particularly effective result obtained with BMT on feline α-mannosidosis (Walkley *et al.* 1994*a*). Extracellular substrate loads of mannose-terminal oligosaccharides found in fluids including CSF (Warren *et al.* 1988) might have been efficiently reduced by donor-derived macrophages and microglia, given that these cell types express the mannose receptor (Linehan *et al.* 1999; Marzolo *et al.* 1999). Selection of appropriate cell types and transgene expression or amplification of appropriate receptors aimed at sequestering substrate might be worth exploring as another strategy for CMT. A greater understanding of the contribution of soluble agents such as toxic metabolites or disease-induced deleterious cytokines to compromise and loss of CNS cells is important, particularly to neural cell replacement strategies that could be challenged by their non-replaced cellular neighbours. Indeed, arguably the greatest merit for using neural cell replacement lies in diseases like the neuronal ceroid lipofuscinoses where cell death is a prominent feature. The use of neural cell progenitors appears exciting, and initial transplantation of progenitors derived from human tissue are encouraging (e.g. Flax *et al.* 1998; Buchet *et al.* 2002). Given technical and ethical issues associated with derivation of human cells, studies revealing the unexpected fate and generation of neural cells from primitive cells present in adult bone marrow (e.g. Brazelton *et al.* 2000; Mezey *et al.* 2000) opens important new and practical avenues of pursuit for human therapy (Koc *et al.* 1999; Mezey *et al.* 2003).

One can be considerably confident that dramatic new results of therapeutic success in mouse models will mark the next few years. Nevertheless, there is still a long bridge to cross to equivalent success with human disease. While many of the principles we have and continue to discover through animal studies are likely to apply to humans, the details and specific needs can be expected to be different. The solidification of CMT strategies for human trial merit the need to progress beyond development in transgenic mice, and ironically return to the larger naturally existing domestic animal models that were once the predominant test subjects. These stepping-stone models will allow consideration of the extent that developmental differences or the simple reality of having to address a larger brain pose additional challenge to adequate cell and enzyme delivery. Furthermore, the models will provide opportunity to assess more complex behaviours allowing superior evaluation of treatment benefit. This may be particularly critical to validating the more heroic approaches such as neural cell replacement.

The nature of the CMT strategy requires the consideration of more variables than other therapeutic modalities posed at storage diseases, but it also offers the potential to address more obstacles to success. The cell is more than just a pool of enzyme. Through intrinsic or manipulative genetic programming, it can respond appropriately to environmental cues to reach sites difficult to otherwise access and to perform multiple functions that may include debris removal, cell replacement, substrate removal, supply of neurotrophic factors, abrogate toxic elements, and even mediate gene delivery (Lynch *et al.* 1999). Based on advances that have already been made, one can anticipate that CMT will play a central role in overcoming the devastating consequences of human storage diseases that affect the CNS.

Summary

There is now substantial evidence that CMT can effect significant improvement in CNS pathology in lysosomal storage diseases. Much of this can be attributed to cross-correction where cells release enzymes for uptake by deficient cells, and the impact of the mechanism can be enhanced through gene overexpression and use of receptor-mediated uptake systems. Studies with animal models of disease support these concepts. Direct implantation of cells and use of BMT to deliver microglial/brain macrophage precursors to the CNS have both resulted in cross-correction. The mechanism has also proved an important component of *in vivo* gene replacement in neural cells, by dramatically extending correction to distal cells through enzyme secretion from transduced cells. Other mechanisms in CMT may also be involved such as indirect storage depletion by donor cells or direct cell–cell contact. BMT has been extremely successful in some animal disease models. One of the benefits of the approach is that it results in extremely widespread delivery of cells to the CNS, important in treating the global nature of the diseases. Cell-mediated therapy is also a tool by which to directly replace enzyme-deficient populations. This may underlie some of the success of BMT which can replace deleterious brain macrophages. The integrative potential of neural progenitor cells appears exciting and can be coupled with enzyme overexpression, but much more basic research is needed on this approach. In all its manifestations, CMT offers the potential to effect a permanent cure through stable cellular population of the CNS. Bone marrow transplantation has also yielded a positive neurologic impact in some storage disease patients. Ongoing efforts to successfully employ autologous transplantation incorporating *ex vivo* gene overexpression and/or earlier intervention will in principle increase the effectiveness of haematopoietic cell therapy and could extend it to diseases as yet untreatable. Specific use of macrophage/microglial lineage cells and bone marrow stromal cells also merits further investigation, as well as various combination therapies that could incorporate substrate deprivation or direct implantation of neural progenitor cells in critical sites of pathology.

Acknowledgements

The author's research has been supported in part by funds from the March of Dimes and the Kirby Foundation.

This chapter is dedicated to the memory of my father-in-law, Joseph M. Horris, who recently lost his personal battle with disease.

References

Abraham, D., Muir, H., Olsen, I. and Winchester, B. (1985). Direct enzyme transfer from lymphocytes corrects a lysosomal storage disease. *Biochem Biophys Res Comm*, **129**, 417–25.

Abraham, D., Muir, H., Winchester, B. and Olsen, I. (1988). Lymphocytes transfer only the lysosomal form of α-D-mannosidase during cell-to-cell contact. *Exp Cell Res*, **175**, 158–68.

Alliot, F., Godin, I. and Pessac, B. (1999). Microglia derive from progenitors, originating from the yolk sac, and which proliferate in the brain. *Dev Brain Res*, **117**, 145–52.

Andjelkovic, A. V., Nikolic, B., Pachter, J. S. and Zecevic, N. (1998). Macrophages/microglial cells in human central nervous system during development: an immunohistochemical study. *Brain Res*, **814**, 13–25.

Bach, G., Friedman, R., Weissmann, B. and Neufeld, E. F. (1972). The defect in the Hurler and Scheie syndromes: deficiency of alpha-L-iduronidase. *Proc Natl Acad Sci USA*, **69**, 2048–51.

Banati, R. B., Rothe, G., Valet, G. and Kreutzberg, G. W. (1993). Detection of lysosomal cysteine proteinases in microglia: flow cytometric measurement and histochemical localization of cathepsin B and L. *Glia*, **7**, 183–91.

Barker, J. E., Deveau, S., Lessard, M., Hamblen, N., Vogler, C., Levy, B. (2001) *In utero* fetal liver cell transplantation without toxic irradiation alleviates lysosomal storage in mice with mucopolysaccharidosis type VII. *Blood Cells Mol Dis*, **27**, 861–73.

Beccari, T., Orlacchio, A., Costanzi, E., Appolloni, M. G., Laurenzi, A. and Bocchini, V. (1997). Constitutive expression of β-N-acetylhexosaminidase in a microglia cell line: transcriptional modulation by lipopolysaccharide and serum factors. *J Neurosci Res*, **50**, 44–9.

Billinghurst, L. L., Taylor, R. M. and Snyder, E. Y. (1998). Remyelination: cellular and gene therapy. *Semin Pediatr Neurol*, **5**, 211–28.

Birkenmeier, E. H., Barker, J. E., Vogler, C. A. *et al.* (1991). Increased life span and correction of metabolic defects in murine mucopolysaccharidosis type VII after syngeneic bone marrow transplantation. *Blood*, **78**, 3081–92.

Biswas, S., Pinson, D. M., Bronshteyn, I. G. and LeVine, S. M. (2001). IL-6 deficiency allows for enhanced therapeutic value after bone marrow transplantation across a minor histocompatibility barrier in the Twitcher (globoid cell leukodystrophy) mouse. *J Neurosci Res*, **65**, 298–307.

Bosch, A., Perret, E., Desmaris, N., Trono, D. and Heard, J. M. (2000). Reversal of pathology in the entire brain of mucopolysaccharidosis type VII mice after lentivirus-mediated gene transfer. *Hum Gene Ther*, **11**, 1139–50.

Bou-Gharios, G., Abraham, D. and Olsen, I. (1993*a*). Lysosomal storage diseases: mechanism of enzyme replacement therapy. *Histochem J*, **25**, 593–605.

Bou-Gharios, G., Adams, G., Pace, P., Warden, P. and Olsen, I. (1993*b*). Correction of a lysosomal deficiency by contact-mediated enzyme transfer after bone-marrow transplantation. *Transplantation*, **56**, 991–6.

Bradbury, M. W. (1993). The blood–brain barrier. *Exp Physiol*, **78**, 453–72.

Bradel, E. J. and Sloan, H. R. (1988). Cultured neonatal rat oligodendrocytes are enriched in acid hydrolase activities. *Neurochem Res*, **13**, 929–36.

Brazelton, T. R., Rossi, F. M. V., Keshet, G. I. and Blau, H. M. (2000). From marrow to brain; expression of neuronal phenotypes in adult mice. *Science*, **290**, 1775–9.

Breider, M. A., Shull, R. M. and Constantopoulos, G. (1989). Long-term effects of bone marrow transplantation in dogs with mucopolysaccharidosis I. *Am J Pathol*, **134**, 677–92.

Brightman, M. W. (1965). The distribution within the brain of ferritin injected into the cerebrospinal fluid compartments. *Am J Anat*, **117**, 193–220.

Broadwell, R. D., Oliver, C. and Brightman, M. W. (1980). Neuronal transport of acid hydrolases and peroxidase within the lysosomal system of organelles: Involvement of agranular reticulum-like cisterns. *J Comp Neurol*, **190**, 519–32.

Brooks, A. I., Stein, C. S., Hughes, S. M. *et al.* (2002). Functional correction of established central nervous system deficits in an animal model of lysosomal storage disease with feline immunodeficiency virus-based vectors. *Proc Natl Acad Sci USA*, **99**, 6216–21.

Brustle, O., Jones, K. N., Learish, R. D. *et al.* (1999). Embryonic stem cell-derived glial precursors: a source of myelinating transplants. *Science*, **285**, 754–6.

Buchet, D., Serguera, C., Zennou, V., Charneau, P. and Mallet, J. (2002). Long-term expression of β-glucuronidase by genetically modified human neural progenitor cells grafted into the mouse central nervous system. *Mol Cell Neurosci*, **19**, 389–401.

Buckley, K. M., Melikan, H. E., Provoda, C. J. and Waring, M. T. (2000). Regulation of neuronal function by protein trafficking: a role for the endosomal pathway. *J Physiol*, **525**, 11–19.

Burudi, E. M. E., Riese, S., Stahl, P. D. and Regnier-Vigouroux, A. (1999). Identification and functional characterization of the mannose receptor in astrocytes. *Glia*, **25**, 44–55.

Casal, M. L. and Wolfe, J. H. (2001). In utero transplantation of fetal liver cells in the mucopolysaccharidosis type VII mouse results in low-level chimerism, but overexpression of β-glucuronidase can delay onset of clinical symptoms. *Gene Ther*, **97**, 1625–34.

Claus, V., Jahraus, A., Tjelle, T. *et al.* (1998). Lysosomal enzyme trafficking between phagosomes, endosomes, and lysosomes in J774 macrophages. *J Biol Chem*, **273**, 9842–51.

Consiglio, A., Quattrini, A., Martino, S. *et al.* (2001). In vivo gene therapy of metachromatic leukodystrophy by lentiviral vectors: correction of neuropathology and protection against learning impairments in affected mice. *Nat Med*, **7**, 310–6.

Couce, M. E., Weatherington, A. J. and McGinty, J. F. (1992). Expression of insulin-like growth factor-II (IGF-II) and IGF-II/mannose-6-phosphate receptor in the rat hippocampus: an *in situ* hybridization and immunocytochemical study. *Endocrinology*, **131**, 1636–42.

Cserr, H. F. (1988). Role of secretion and bulk flow of brain interstitial fluid in brain volume regulation. *Ann N Y Acad Sci*, **529**, 9–20.

Cuadros, M. A. and Navascues, J. (1998). The origin and differentiation of microglial cells during development. *Prog Neurobiol*, **56**, 173–89.

Cuadros, M. A., Coltey, P., Nieto, M. C. and Martin, C. (1992). Demonstration of a phagocytic cell system belonging to the hemopoietic lineage and originating from the yolk sac in the early avian embryo. *Development*, **115**, 157–68.

Cuadros, M. A., Martin, C., Coltey, P., Almendros, A. and Navascués, J. (1993). First appearance, distribution, and origin of macrophages in the early development of the avian central nervous system. *J Comp Neurol*, **330**, 113–29.

Davidoff, M. and Galabov, P. (1976). On the histochemistry of *N*-acetyl-β-D-glucosaminidase in the rat central nervous system. *Histochemistry*, **46**, 317–32.

Davies, P., Page, R. C. and Allison, A. C. (1974). Changes in cellular enzyme levels and extracellular release of lysosomal acid hydrolases in macrophages exposed to group A streptococcal cell wall substance. *J Exp Med*, **139**, 1262–82.

Dean, R. T., Hylton, W. and Allison, A. C. (1979). Lysosomal enzyme secretion by macrophages during intracellular storage of particles. *Biochim Biophys Acta*, **584**, 57–68.

DeGroot, C. J. A., Huppes, W., Sminia, T., Kraal, G. and Dijkstra, C. (1992). Determination of the origin and nature of brain macrophages and microglial cells in mouse central nervous system, using non-radioactive in situ hybridization and immunoperoxidase techniques. *Glia*, **6**, 301–9.

Desnick, R. J., Dean, K. J., Grabowski, G. A., Bishop, D. F. and Sweeley, C. C. (1979). Enzyme therapy in Fabry's disease: differential in vivo plasma clearance and metabolic effectiveness of plasma and splenic α-galactosidase-A isozymes. *Proc Natl Acad Sci USA*, **76**, 5326–30.

DiCioccio, R. A. and Miller, A. L. (1991). Biosynthesis, processing, and secretion of α-L-fucosidase in lymphoid cells from patients with I-cell disease and pseudo-Hurler polydystrophy. *Glycobiology*, **1**, 595–604.

Dittmer, F., Ulbrich, E. J., Hafner, A. *et al.* (1999). Alternative mechanisms for trafficking of lysosomal enzymes in mannose 6-phosphate receptor-deficient mice are cell type-specific. *J Cell Sci*, **112**, 1591–7.

Dobrenis, K. (1998). Microglia in cell culture and in transplantation therapy for central nervous system disease. *Methods*, **16**, 320–44.

Dobrenis, K., Joseph, A. and Rattazzi, M. C. (1992). Neuronal lysosomal enzyme replacement using fragment C of tetanus toxin. *Proc Natl Acad Sci USA*, **89**, 2297–301.

Dobrenis, K., Wenger, D. A. and Walkley, S. W. (1994). Extracellular release of lysosomal glycosidases in cultures of cat microglia. *Mol Biol Cell Suppl*, **5**, 113a.

Dobrenis, K., Finamore, P. S., Masui, R. and Walkley, S. U. (1996). Secretion of lysosomal glycosidases by microglia in culture. *Mol Biol Cell Suppl.*, **7**, 325a.

Dobrenis, K., Finamore, P. S., Walkley *et al.* (1998). Cell preparations for therapeutic transplantation studies from brain of hybrid transgenic animals expressing E. coli β-Gal, neo-resistance and immortalizing SV40 large T antigen. *Soc for Neurosci Abstr*, **24**, 1056.

Dobrenis, K., Pinto, L. A., German, R. *et al.* (2000). Widespread delivery of microglia to mouse CNS following intravenous injection. *Soc for Neurosci Abstr*, **26**, 1101.

Dore, S., Kar, S. and Quirion, R. (1997). Presence and differential internalization of two distinct insulin-like growth factor receptors in rat hippocampal neurons. *Neuroscience*, **78**, 373–83.

Earley, R. L., Pinto, L., Finamore, P., Walkley, S. U. and Dobrenis, K. (1999). Cytokine modulation of extracellular release of acid glycohydrolases by murine microglia. *Mol Biol Cell*, **10**, 112a.

Enomaa, N., Danos, O., Peltonen, L. and Jalanko, A. (1995). Correction of deficient enzyme activity in a lysosomal storage disease, aspartylglucosaminuria, by enzyme replacement and retroviral gene transfer. *Hum Gene Ther*, **6**, 723–31.

Fairbairn, L. J., Lashford, L. S., Spooncer, E. *et al.* (1996). Long-term in vitro correction of α-L-iduronidase deficiency (Hurler syndrome) in human bone marrow. *Proc Natl Acad Sci USA*, **93**, 2025–30.

Flax, J. D., Aurora, S., Yang, C. *et al.* (1998). Engraftable human neural stem cells respond to developmental cues, replace neurons, and express foreign genes. *Nat Biotechnol*, **16**, 1033–9.

Flugel, A., Bradl, M., Kreutzberg, G. W. and Graeber, M. B. (2001). Transformation of donor-derived bone marrow precursors into host microglia during autoimmune CNS inflammation and during the retrograde response to axotomy. *J Neurosci Res*, **66**, 74–82.

Francesco, C. D., Cracco, C., Tomanin, R. *et al.* (1997). In vitro correction of iduronate-2-sulfatase deficiency by adenovirus-mediated gene transfer. *Gene Ther*, **4**, 442–8.

Franklin, R. J. M. and Blakemore, W. F. (1998). Transplanting myelin-forming cells into the central nervous system: principles and practice. *Methods*, **16**, 311–9.

Fratantoni, J. C., Hall, C. W. and Neufeld, E. F. (1968). Hurler and Hunter syndromes: mutual correction of the deficits in cultured fibroblasts. *Science*, **162**, 570–2.

Freeman, B. J., Roberts, M. S., Vogler, C. A., Nicholes, A., Hofling, A. A. and Sands, M. S. (1999). Behavior and therapeutic efficacy of β-glucuronidase-positive mononuclear phagocytes in a murine model of mucopolysaccharidosis type VII. *Blood*, **94**, 2142–50.

Frisella, W. A., O'Connor, L. H., Vogler, C. A. *et al.* (2001). Intracranial injection of recombinant adeno-associated virus improves cognitive function in a murine model of mucopolysaccharidosis type VII. *Mol Ther*, **3**, 351–8.

Fu, H., Samulski, R. J., McCown, T. J., Picornell, Y. J., Fletcher, D. and Muenzer, J. (2002). Neurological correction of lysosomal storage in a mucopolysaccharidosis IIIB mouse model by adeno-associated virus-mediated gene delivery. *Mol Ther*, **5**, 42–9.

Gehrmann, J., Matsumoto, Y. and Kreutzberg, G. W. (1995). Microglia: intrinsic immuneffector cell of the brain. *Brain Res Rev*, **20**, 269–87.

Ghodsi, A., Stein, C., Derksen, T., Yang, G., Anderson, R. D. and Davidson, B. L. (1998). Extensive β-glucuronidase activity in murine central nervous system after adenovirus-mediated gene transfer to brain. *Hum Gene Ther*, **9**, 2331–40.

Ghodsi, A., Stein, C., Derksen, T., Martins, I., Anderson, R. D. and Davidson, B. L. (1999). Systemic hyperosmolality improves β-glucuronidase distribution in murine MPS VII brain following intraventricular gene transfer. *Exp Neurol*, **160**, 109–16.

Glickman, J. N. and Kornfeld, S. (1993). Mannose 6-phosphate-independent targeting of lysosomal enzymes in I-cell disease B lymphoblasts. *J Cell Biol*, **123**, 99–108.

Grewal, S. S., Krivit, W., Defor, T. E. *et al.* (2002). Outcome of second hematopoietic cell transplantation in Hurler syndrome. *Bone Marrow Transplant*, **29**, 491–6.

Griffiths, G. M. (1996). Secretory lysosomes – a special mechanism of regulated secretion in haemopoietic cells. *Trends Cell Biol*, **6**, 329–32.

Guidotti, J. E., Mignon, A., Haase, G. *et al.* (1999). Adenoviral gene therapy of the Tay–Sachs disease in hexosaminidase A-deficient knock-out mice. *Hum Mol Genet*, **8**, 831–8.

Hahn, C. N., del Pilar Martin, M., Zhou, X. Y., Mann, L. W. and d'Azzo, A. (1998). Correction of murine galactosialidosis by bone marrow-derived macrophages overexpressing human protective protein/cathepsin A under control of the colony-stimulating factor-1 receptor promoter. *Proc Natl Acad Sci USA*, **95**, 14880–85.

Haskins, M., Baker, H. J., Birkenmeier, E. *et al.* (1991). Transplantation in animal model systems. In *Treatment of genetic diseases* (Desnick, R.J., ed.), pp. 183–201. New York: Churchill Livingstone Inc.

Heinonen, O., Kyttala, A., Lehmus, E., Paunio, T., Peltonen, L. and Jalanko, A. (2000). Expression of palmitoyl protein thioesterase in neurons. *Mol Genet Metab*, **69**, 123–9.

Heuer, G. G., Skorupa, A. F., Alur, R. K. P., Jiang, K. and Wolfe, J. H. (2001). Accumulation of abnormal amounts of glycosaminoglycans in murine mucopolysaccharidosis type VII neural progenitor cells does not alter the growth rate or efficiency of differentiation into neurons. *Mol Cell Neurosci*, **17**, 167–78.

Hickey, W. F. and Kimura, H. (1988). Perivascular microglial cells of the CNS are bone marrow-derived and present antigen in vivo. *Science*, **239**, 290–2.

Hickey, W. F., Hsu, B. L. and Kimura, H. (1991). T-lymphocyte entry into the central nervous system. *J Neurosci*, **28**, 254–60.

Hickey, W. F., Vass, K. and Lassmann, H. (1992). Bone marrow-derived elements in the central nervous system: An immunohistochemical and ultrastructural survey of rat chimeras. *J Neuropathol Exp Neurol*, **51**, 246–56.

Hickman, S. and Neufeld, E. F. (1972). A hypothesis for I-cell disease: defective hydrolases that do not enter lysosomes. *Biochem Biophys Res Comm*, **49**, 992–9.

Hill, D. F., Bullock, P. N., Chiapelli, F. and Rome, L. H. (1985). Binding and internalization of lysosomal enzyme by primary cultures of rat glia. *J Neurosci Res*, **14**, 35–47.

Hirayama, M., Mutoh, T. and Tokudo, A. (2001). Acid hydrolase activity of cultured Bovine oligodendrocytes. *Neurochem Res*, **26**, 121–4.

Ho, J. L. and Klempner, M. S. (1985). Tetanus toxin inhibits secretion of lysosomal contents from human macrophages. *J Infect Dis*, **152**, 922–9.

Holtzman, E. (1989). *Lysosomes*, pp. 319–39. New York: Plenum Press.

Hoogerbrugge, P. M., Suzuki, K., Suzuki, K. *et al.* (1988). Donor-derived cells in the central nervous system of twitcher mice after bone marrow transplantation. *Science*, **239**, 1035–8.

Hoogerbrugge, P. M., Brouwer, O. F., Bordigoni, P. *et al.* (1995). Allogeneic bone marrow transplantation for lysosomal storage diseases. *Lancet*, **345**, 1398–402.

Huang, M. M., Wong, A. YuX., Kakkis, E. and Kohn, D. B. (1997). Retrovirus-mediated transfer of the human α-L-iduronidase cDNA into human hematopoietic progenitor cells leads to correction in trans of Hurler fibroblasts. *Gene Ther*, **4**, 1150–9.

Huppes, W., De Groot, C. J. A., Ostendorf, R. H. *et al.* (1992). Detection of migrated oligodendrocytes throughout the central nervous system of the galactocerebrosidase-deficient twitcher mouse. *J Neurocytol*, **21**, 129–36.

Imai, F., Sawada, M., Suzuki, H. *et al.* (1997). Migration activity of microglia and macrophages into rat brain. *Neurosci Lett*, **237**, 49–52.

Ioannou, Y. A., Bishop, D. F. and Desnick, R. J. (1992). Overexpression of human alpha-galactosidase A results in its intracellular aggregation, crystallization in lysosomes, and selective secretion. *J Cell Biol*, **119**, 1137–50.

Janzer, R. C. (1993). The blood–brain barrier: cellular basis. *J Inherit Metab Dis*, **16**, 639–47.

Jenkins, H. G., Martin, J. and Dean, M. F. (1988). Receptor-mediated uptake of beta-glucuronidase into primary astrocytes and C6 glioma cells from rat brain. *Brain Res*, **462**, 265–74.

Jessup, W. and Dean, R. T. (1980). Spontaneous lysosomal enzyme secretion by a murine macrophage-like cell line. *Biochem J*, **190**, 847–50.

Jessup, W. and Dean, R. T. (1982). Secretion by mononuclear phagocytes of lysosomal hydrolases bearing ligands for the mannose-6-phosphate receptor system of fibroblasts: evidence for a second mechanism of spontaneous secretion *Biochem Biophys Res Comm*, **105**, 922–7.

Jeyakumar, M., Norflus, F., Tifft, C. J. *et al.* (2001). Enhanced survival in Sandhoff disease mice receiving a combination of substrate deprivation therapy and bone marrow transplantation. *Blood*, **97**, 327–9.

Jin, H. K. Canrter, J. E., Huntley, G. W. and Schuchman, E. H. (2002). Intracerebral transplantation of mesenchymal stem cells into acid sphingomyelinase-deficient mice delays the onset of neurologic abnormalities and extend their life span. *J Clin Invest*, **109**, 1183–91.

Kapaun, P., Dittmann, R. W., Granitzny, B. *et al.* (1999). Slow progression of juvenile metachromatic leukodystrophy 6 years after bone marrow transplantation. *J Child Neurol*, **14**, 222–8.

Kaplan, A., Achord, D. T. and Sly, W. S. (1977). Phosphohexosyl components of a lysosomal enzyme are recognized by pinocytosis receptors on human fibroblasts. *Proc Natl Acad Sci USA*, **74**, 2026–30.

Kelly, R. B. (1993). Storage and release of neurotransmitters. *Cell*, **72**/*Neuron*, **10**, 43–53.

Kennedy, D. W. and Abkowitz, J. L. (1997). Rapid communication – kinetics of central nervous system microglial and macrophage engraftment: analysis using a transgenic bone marrow transplantation model. *Blood*, **90**, 986–93.

Kennedy, D. W. and Abkowitz, J. L. (1998). Mature monocytic cells enter tissues and engraft. *Proc Natl Acad Sci USA*, **95**, 14944–9.

Kessler, U., Aumeier, S., Funk, B. and Kiess, W. (1992). Biosynthetic labeling of β-hexosaminidase B: inhibition of the cellular uptake of lysosomal secretions containing [^{3}H]hexosaminidase B by insulin-like growth factor-II in rat C6 glial cells. *Mol Cell Endocrinol*, **90**, 147–53.

Kida, S., Steart, P. V., Zhang, E. and Weller, R. O. (1993). Perivascular cells act as scavengers in the cerebral perivascular spaces and remain distinct from pericytes, microglia and macrophages. *Acta Neuropathol*, **85**, 646–52.

Kiess, W., Thomas, C. L., Greenstein, L. A. *et al.* (1989). Insulin-like growth factor-II (IGF-II) inhibits both the cellular uptake of β-galactosidase and the binding of β-galactosidase to purified IGF-II/mannose 6-phosphate receptor. *J Biol Chem*, **264**, 4710–4.

Klatzo, I. and Miquel, J. (1960). Observations of pinocytosis in nervous tissue. *J Neuropathol Exp Neurol*, **19**, 475–87.

Koc, O. N., Peters, C., Aubourg, P. *et al.* (1999). Bone marrow-derived mesenchymal stem cells remain host-derived despite successful hematopoietic engraftment after allogeneic transplantation in patients with lysosomal and peroxisomal storage diseases. *Exp Hematol*, **27**, 1675–81.

Koenig, H., Goldstone, A. and Hughes, C. (1978). Lysosomal enzymuria in the testosterone-treated mouse. *Lab Invest*, **39**, 329–41.

Kosuga, M., Sasaki, K., Tanabe, A. *et al.* (2001). Engraftment of genetically engineered amniotic epithelial cells corrects lysosomal storage in multiple areas of the brain in mucopolysaccharidosis type VII mice. *Mol Ther*, **3**, 139–48.

Krall, W. J., Challita, P. M., Perimutter, L. S., Skelton, D. C. and Kohn, D. B. (1994). Cells expressing human glucocerebrosidase from a retroviral vector repopulate macrophages and central nervous system microglia after murine bone marrow transplantation. *Blood*, **9**, 2737–48.

Kramer, R., Zhang, Y., Gehrmann, J., Gold, R., Thoenen, H. and Wekerle, H. (1995). Gene transfer through the blood–nerve barrier: NGF-engineered neuritogenic T lymphocytes attenuate experimental autoimmune neuritis. *Nat Med*, **1**, 1162–6.

Kresse, H. and Neufeld, E. F. (1972). The Sanfilippo A corrective factor. Purification and mode of action. *J Biol Chem*, **247**, 2164–70.

Krivit, W. (2002). Stem cell bone marrow transplantation in patients with metabolic storage diseases. *Adv Pediatr*, **49**, 359–78.

Krivit, W., Lockman, L. A., Watkins, P. A., Hirsch, J. and Shapiro, E. G. (1995*a*). The future for treatment by bone marrow transplantation for adrenoleukodystophy, metachromatic leukodystrophy, globoid cell leukodystrophy and Hurler syndrome. *J Inherit Metab Dis*, **18**, 398–412.

Krivit, W., Sung, J. H., Shapiro, E. G. and Lockman, L. A. (1995*b*). Microglia: the effector cell for reconstitution of the central nervous system following bone marrow transplantation for lysosomal and peroxisomal storage diseases. *Cell Transplant*, **4**, 385–92.

Krivit, W., Shapiro, E. G., Peters, C. *et al.* (1998). Hematopoietic stem-cell transplantation in globoid-cell leukodystrophy. *N Engl J Med*, **338**, 1119–26.

Krivit, W., Peters, C. and Shapiro, E. G. (1999). Bone marrow transplantation as effective treatment of central nervous system disease in globoid cell leukodystrophy, metachromatic leukodystrophy, adrenoleukodystophy, mannosidosis, fucosidosis, aspartylglucosaminuria, Hurler, Maroteaux–Lamy, and Sly syndromes, and Gaucher disease type III. *Curr Opin Neurol*, **12**, 167–76.

Kurz, H. and Christ, B. (1998). Embryonic CNS macrophages and microglia do not stem from circulating, but from extravascular precursors. *Glia*, **22**, 98–102.

Kyttala, A., Heinonen, O., Peltonen, L. and Jalanko, A. (1998). Expression and endocytosis of lysosomal aspartylglucosaminidase in mouse primary neurons. *J Neurosci*, **18**, 7750–6.

Lacorazza, H. D., Flax, J. D., Snyder, E. Y., and Jendoubi, M. (1996). Expression of human β-hexosaminidase α-subunit gene (the gene defect of Tay Sachs disease) in mouse brains upon engraftment of transduced progenitor cells. *Nature Med*, **2**, 424–9.

Lassmann, H., Zimprich, F., Vass, K. and Hickey, W. F. (1991). Microglial cells are a component of the perivascular glia limitans. *J Neurosci Res*, **28**, 236–43.

Lassmann, H., Schmied, M., Vass, K. and Hickey, W. F. (1993). Bone marrow derived elements and resident microglia in brain inflammation. *Glia*, **7**, 19–24.

Lawson, L. J., Perry, V. H., Dri, P. and Gordon, S. (1990). Heterogeneity in the distribution and morphology of microglia in the normal adult mouse brain. *Neuroscience*, **39**, 151–70.

Lawson, L. J., Perry, V. H. and Gordon, S. (1992). Turnover of resident microglia in the normal adult mouse brain. *Neuroscience*, **48**, 405–15.

Learish, R., Ohashi, T., Robbins, P. A. *et al.* (1996). Retroviral gene transfer and sustained expression of human arylsulfatase A. *Gene Ther*, **3**, 343–9.

Leimig, T., Mann, L., Martin, M. D. P. *et al.* (2002). Functional amelioration of murine galactosialidosis by genetically modified bone marrow hematopoietic cells. *Gene Ther*, **99**, 3169–78.

Lesniak, M. A., Hill, J. M., Kiess, W., Rojecki, M., Pert, C. B. and Roth, J. (1988). Receptors for insulin-like growth factors I and II: autoradiographic localization in the rat brain and comparison to receptors for insulin. *Endocrinology*, **123**, 2089–99.

Linehan, S. A., Martinez-Pomares, L., Stahl, P. D. and Gordon, S. (1999). Mannose receptor and its putative ligands in normal murine lymphoid and nonlymphoid organs: in situ expression of mannose receptor by selected macrophages, endothelial cells, perivascular microglia, and mesenial cells, but not dendritic cells. *J Exp Med*, **189**, 1961–72.

Ling, E. A. (1976). Electron-microscopic identification of amoeboid microglia in the spinal cord of newborn rats. *Acta Anat*, **96**, 600–9.

Ling, E. A. (1977). Light and electron microscopic demonstration of some lysosomal enzymes in the amoeboid microglia in neonatal rat brain. *J Anat*, **123**, 637–48.

Ling, E. A., Penney, D. and Leblond, C. P. (1980). Use of carbon labeling to demonstrate the role of blood monocytes as precursors of the 'amoeboid cells' present in the corpus callosum of postnatal rats. *J Comp Neurol*, **193**, 631–57.

Liuzzo, J. P., Petanceska, S. S. and Devi, L. A. (1999*a*). Neurotrophic factors regulate cathepsin S in macrophages and microglia: a role in the degradation of myelin basic protein and amyloid β peptide. *Mol Med*, **5**, 334–43.

Liuzzo, J. P., Petanceska, S. S., Moscatelli, D. and Devi, L. A. (1999*b*). Inflammatory mediators regulate cathepsin S in macrophages and microglia: a role in attenuating heparan sulfate interactions. *Mol Med*, **5**, 320–33.

Lorinez, M. C., Parente, M. K., Roederer, M. *et al.* (1999). Single cell analysis and selection of living retrovirus vector-corrected mucopolysaccharidosis VII cells using a fluorescence-activated cell sorting-based assay for mammalian β-glucuronidase enzymatic activity. *J Biol Chem*, **274**, 657–65.

Luddi, A., Volterrani, M., Strazza, M. *et al.* (2001). Retrovirus-mediated gene transfer and galactocerebrosidase uptake into Twitcher glial cells results in appropriate localization and phenotype correction. *Neurobiol Dis*, **8**, 600–10.

Ludwig, T., Munier-Lehmann, H., Bauer, U. *et al.* (1994). Differential sorting of lysosomal enzymes in mannose 6-phosphate receptor-deficient fibroblasts. *EMBO J*, **13**, 3430–7.

Lynch, W. P., Sharpe, A. H. and Snyder, E. Y. (1999). Neural stem cells as engraftable packaging lines can mediate gene delivery to microglia: Evidence from studying retroviral *env*-related neurodegeneration. *J Virol*, **73**, 6841–51.

McKanna, J. A. (1993). Lipocortin I immunoreactivity identifies microglia in adult rat brain (1993). *J Neurosci Res*, **36**, 491–500.

McNamara, A., Jenne, B. M. and Dean, M. F. (1985). Fibroblasts acquire β-glucuronidase by direct and indirect transfer during co-culture with macrophages. *Exp Cell Res*, **160**, 150–7.

Marks, D. L. and Pagano, R. E. (2002). Endocytosis and sorting of glycosphingolipids in sphingolipid storage disease. *Trends Cell Biol*, **12**, 605–13.

Martino, S., Emiliani, C., Tancini, B. *et al.* (2002). Absence of metabolic cross-correction in Tay–Sachs cells. *J Biol Chem*, **277**, 20177–84.

Marzolo, M. P., von Bernhardi, R. and Inestrosa, N. C. (1999). Mannose receptor is present in a functional state in rat microglial cells. *J Neurosci Res*, **58**, 387–95.

Matsushima, G. K., Taniike, M., Glimcher, L. H. *et al.* (1994). Absence of MHC class II molecules reduces CNS demyelination, microglial/macrophage infiltration, and twitching in murine globoid cell leukodystrophy. *Cell*, **78**, 645–56.

Matsuura, F., Ohta, M., Ioannou, Y. A. and Desnick, R. J. (1998). Human alpha-galactosidase A; characterization of the N-linked oligosaccharides on the intracellular and secreted glycoforms overexpressed by Chinese hamster ovary cells. *Glycobiology*, **8**, 329–39.

Matteoli, M., Verderio, C., Rossetto, O. *et al.* (1996). Synaptic vesicle endocytosis mediates the entry of tetanus toxin into hippocampal neurons. *Proc Natl Acad Sci USA*, **93**, 13310–5.

Matzner, U., Habetha, M. and Gieselmann, V. (2000*a*). Retrovirally expressed human arylsulfatase A corrects the metabolic defect of arylsulfatase A-deficient mouse cells. *Gene Ther*, **7**, 805–12.

Matzner, U., Harzer, K., Learish, R. D., Barranger, J. A. and Gieselmann, V. (2000*b*). Long-term expression and transfer of arylsulfatase A into brain of arylsulfatase A-deficient mice transplanted with bone marrow expressing the arylsulfatase A cDNA from a retroviral vector. *Gene Ther*, **7**, 1250–7.

Matzner, U., Schestag, F., Hartmann, D. *et al.* (2001). Bone marrow stem cell gene therapy of arylsulfatase A-deficient mice, using an arylsulfatase A mutant that is hypersecreted from retrovirally transduced donor-type cells. *Hum Gene Ther*, **12**, 1021–33.

Matzner, U., Hartmann, D., Lullmann-Rauch, R. *et al.* (2002). Bone marrow stem cell-based gene transfer in a mouse model for metachromatic leukodystrpohy: effects on visceral and nervous system disease manifestations. *Gene Ther*, **9**, 53–63.

Mezey, E., Chandross, K. J., Harta, G., Maki, R. A. and McKercher, S. R. (2000). Turning blood into brain: cells bearing neuronal antigens generated in vivo from bone marrow. *Science*, **290**, 1779–82.

Mezey, E., Key, S., Vogelsang, G., Szalayova, I., Lange, G. D. and Crain, B. (2003). Transplanted bone marrow generates new neurons in human brains. *Proc Natl Acad Sci USA*, **100**, 1364–9.

Miano, M., Lanino, E., Gatti, R. *et al.* (2001). Four year follow-up of a case of fucosidosis treated with unrelated donor bone marrow transplantation. *Bone Marrow Transplant*, **27**, 747–51.

Miranda, S. R. P., Erlich, S., Visser, J. W. M. *et al.* (1997). Bone marrow transplantation in acid sphingomyelinase-deficient mice: engraftment and cell migration into the brain as a function of radiation, age, and phenotype. *Blood*, **90**, 444–52.

Moore, S. and Thanos, S. (1996). The concept of microglia in relation to central nervous system disease and regeneration. *Prog Neurobiol*, **48**, 441–60.

Muschol, N., Matzner, U., Tiede, S., Gieselmann, V., Ullrich, K. and Braulke, T. (2002). Secretion of phosphomannosyl-deficient arylsulfatase A and cathepsin D from isolated human macrophages. *Biochem J*, **368**, 845–53.

Nakajima, K. and Kohsaka, S. (1993). Characterization of brain microglia and the biological significance in the central nervous system. *Adv Neurol*, **60**, 7347–743.

Nakajima, K., Kikuchi, Y., Ikoma, E. *et al.* (1998). Neurotrophins regulate the function of cultured microglia. *Glia*, **24**, 272–89.

Nakata, T., Teraa, S. and Hirokawa, N. (1998). Visualization of the dynamics of synaptic vesicle and plasma membrane proteins in living axons. *J Cell Biol*, **140**, 659–74.

Naoi, M., Iwashita, T. and Nagatsu, T. (1987). Binding of specific glycoconjugates to human brain synaptosomes: studies using glycosylated β-galactosidase. *Neurosci Lett*, **79**, 331–6.

Neufeld, E. F. (1991). Lysosomal storage diseases. *Annu Rev Biochem*, **60**, 257–80.

Neufeld, E. F. and Fratantoni, J. C. (1970). Inborn errors of mucopolysaccharide metabolism. *Science*, **168**, 141–6.

Neufeld, E. F. and Muenzer, J. (2001). The mucopolysaccharidoses. In *The metabolic and molecular bases of inherited disease* (Scriver, C. R., Beaudet, A. L., Sly, W. S. and Valle, D, ed.), pp. 3421–52. New York: McGraw-Hill.

Neufeld, E. F., Sando, G. N., Garvin, A. J. and Rome, L. H. (1977). The transport of lysosomal enzymes. *J Supramol Struct*, **6**, 95–101.

Nielsen, F. C. and Gammeltoft, S. (1990). Mannose-6-phosphate stimulates proliferation of neuronal precursor cells. *FEBS Lett*, **262**, 142–4.

Nielsen, F. C., Wang, E., and Gammeltoft, S. (1991). Receptor binding, endocytosis, and mitogenesis of insulin-like growth factors I and II in fetal rat brain neurons. *J Neurochem*, **56**, 12–21.

Nixon, R. A. and Cataldo, A. M. (1995). The endosomal–lysosomal system of neurons: new roles. *Trends Neurosci*, **18**, 489–96.

Norflus, F., Tifft, C. J., McDonald, M. P. *et al.* (1998). Bone marrow transplantation prolongs life span and ameliorates neurologic manifestations in Sandhoff disease mice. *J Clin Invest*, **101**, 1881–8.

O'Brien, J. S., Storb, R., Raff, R. F. *et al.* (1990). Bone marrow transplantation in canine GM1 gangliosidosis. *Clin Genet*, **38**, 274–80.

Ocrant, I., Valentino, K. L., Eng, L. F., Hintz, R. L., Wilson, D. M. and Rosenfeld, R. G. (1988). Structural and immunohistochemical characterization of insulin-like growth factor I and II receptors in the murine central nervous system. *Endocrinology*, **123**, 1023–34.

Ohata, K., Marmarou, A. and Povlishock, J. T. (1990). An immunocytochemical study of protein clearance in brain infusion edema. *Acta Neuropathol*, **81**, 162–77.

Olsen, I., Dean, M. F., Harris, G. and Muir, H. (1981). Direct transfer of a lysosomal enzyme from lymphoid cells to deficient fibroblasts. *Nature*, **291**, 244–7.

Olsen, I., Dean, M. F., Muir, H. and Harris, G. (1982). Acquisition of β-glucuronidase activity by deficient fibroblasts during direct contact with lymphoid cells. *J Cell Sci*, **55**, 211–31.

Olsen, I., Muir, H., Smith, R., Fensom, A. and Watt, D. J. (1983). Direct enzyme transfer from lymphocytes is specific. *Nature*, **306**, 75–7.

Olsen, I., Abraham, D., Shelton, I., Bou-Gharios, G., Muir, H. and Winchester, B. (1988). Cell contact induces the synthesis of a lysosomal enzyme precursor in lymphocytes and its direct transfer to fibroblasts. *Biochim Biophys Acta*, **968**, 312–22.

Olsen, I., Oliver, T., Muir, H., Smith, R. and Partridge, T. (1986). Role of cell adhesion in contact-dependant transfer of a lysosomal enzyme from lymphocytes to fibroblasts. *J Cell Sci*, **85**, 231–44.

Olsen, I., Bou-Gharios, G., Abraham, D. and Chain, B. (1993). Lysosomal enzyme transfer from different types of lymphoid cell. *Exp Cell Res*, **209**, 133–9.

Ono, K., Takii, T., Onozaki, K., Ikawa, M., Okabe, M. and Sawada, M. (1999). Migration of exogenous immature hematopoietic cells into adult mouse brain parenchyma under GFP-expressing bone marrow chimera. *Biochem Biophys Res Comm*, **262**, 610–4.

Overly, C. C. and Hollenbeck, P. J. (1996). Dynamic organization of endocytic pathways in axons of cultured sympathetic neurons. *J Neurosci*, **16**, 6056–64.

Oya, Y., Proia, R., Norflus, F., Tifft, C. J., Langaman, C. and Suzuki, K. (2000). Distribution of enzyme-bearing cells in GM2 gangliosidosis mice: regionally specific pattern of cellular infiltration following bone marrow transplantation. *Acta Neuropathol*, **99**, 161–8.

Pagano, R. E., Puri, V., Dominguez, M. and Marks, D. L. (2000). Membrane traffic in sphingolipid storage diseases. *Traffic*, **1**, 807–15.

Parton, R. G., Simons, K. and Dotti, C. G. (1992). Axonal and dendritic pathways in cultured neurons. *J Cell Biol*, **119**, 123–37.

Passini, M. A., Lee, E. B., Heuer, G. G. and Wolfe, J. H. (2002). Distribution of a lysosomal enzyme in the adult brain by axonal transport and by cells of the rostral migratory stream. *J Neurosci*, **22**, 6437–46.

Petanceska, S., Canoll, P. and Devi, L. A. (1996). Expression of rat cathepsin S in phagocytic cells. *J Biol Chem*, **271**, 4403–9.

Peters, C. and Krivit, W. (2000). Hematopoietic cell transplantation for mucopolysaccharidosis IIB (Hunter syndrome). *Bone Marrow Transplant*, **25**, 1097–9.

Peters, A., de Palay, S. L. and Webster, H. (1991). *The fine structure of the nervous system*, pp. 273–311. New York: Oxford University Press.

Phaneuf, D., Wakamatsu, N., Huang, J.-Q. *et al.* (1996). Dramatically different phenotypes in mouse models of human Tay–Sachs and Sandhoff diseases. *Hum Mol Genet*, **5**, 1–14.

Priller, J., Flugel, A., Wehner, T. *et al.* (2001). Targeting gene-modified hematopoeitic cells to the central nervous system: use of green fluorescent protein uncovers microglial engraftment. *Nat Med*, **7**, 1356–61.

Rattazzi, M. C. and Dobrenis, K. (1991*a*). Enzyme replacement: overview and prospects. In *Treatment of genetic diseases* (Desnick, R. J., ed.), pp. 131–52. New York: Churchill Livingstone.

Rattazzi, M. C. and Dobrenis, K. (1991*b*). Behind the blood–brain barrier: transport of protein from the subarachnoid spaces to brain parenchyma induced by plasma hyperosmolality. *Pediatr Res*, **29**, 363A.

Rattazzi, M. C. and Dobrenis, K. (2001). Treatment of GM2 gangliosidosis: Past experiences and future prospects. In *Advances in genetics vol. 44; Tay-Sachs disease* (Desnick, R. J. and Kaback, M. M., ed.), pp. 317–39. San Diego: Academic Press.

Rattazzi, M. C., Dobrenis, K., Joseph, A. and Schwartz, P. (1987). Modified b-D-N-acetylhexosaminidase isozymes for enzyme replacement in GM2 gangliosidosis. *Isozymes: Curr Top Biol Med Research*, **16**, 49–65.

Rennels, M. L., Gregory, T. F., Blaumarnis, T. F. *et al.* (1985). Evidence for a paravascular fluid circulation in the mammalian central nervous system, provided by the rapid distribution of tracer protein throughout the brain from the subarachnoid space. *Brain Res*, **326**, 47.

Rezaie, P., Patel, K. and Male, D. K. (1999). Microglia in the human fetal spinal cord—patterns of distribution, morphology and phenotype. *Dev Brain Res*, **115**, 71–81.

Rhagavan, S. S., Rhoads, D. B. and Kanfer, J. N. (1972). Acid hydrolases in neuronal and glial enriched fractions of rat brain. *Biochim Biophys Acta*, **268**, 755–60.

Rio-Hortega, P. D. (1932). Microglia. In *Cytology and cellular pathology of the nervous system* (Penfield, W., ed.), pp. 483–534. New York: Hafner Publishing Co.

Rodriguez, A., Webster, P., Ortego, J. and Andrews, N. W. (1997). Lysosomes behave as Ca^{2+}-regulated exocytic vesicles in fibroblasts and epithelial cells. *J Cell Biol*, **137**, 93–104.

Rome, L. H., Weissmann, B. and Neufeld, E. F. (1979). Direct demonstration of binding of a lysosomal enzyme, alpha-L-iduronidase, to receptors on cultured fibroblasts. *Proc Natl Acad Sci USA*, **76**, 2331–4.

Sands, M. S., Barker, J. E., Vogler, C. *et al.* (1993). Treatment of murine mucopolysaccharidosis type VII by syngeneic bone marrow transplantation in neonates. *Lab Invest*, **68**, 676–86.

Sands, M. S., Vogler, C., Torrey, A. *et al.* (1997). Murine mucopolysaccharidosis type VII: long term therapeutic effects of enzyme replacement followed by bone marrow transplantation. *J Clin Invest*, **99**, 1596–605.

Sangalli, A., Taveggia, C., Salviata, A., Wrabetz, L., Bordignon, C. and Severini, G. M. (1998). Transduced fibroblasts and metachromatic leukodystrophy lymphocytes transfer arylsulfatase A to myelinating glia and deficient cells *in vitro*. *Hum Gene Ther*, **9**, 2111–9.

Sango, K., Yamanaka, S., Hoffman, A. *et al.* (1995). Mouse models of Tay–Sachs and Sandhoff diseases differ in neurologic phenotype and ganglioside metabolism. *Nat Genet*, **11**, 170–6.

Sawada, M., Suzumura, A., Yamamato, H. and Marunouchi, T. (1990). Activation and proliferation of the isolated microglia by colony stimulating factor-1 and possible involvement of protein kinase C. *Brain Res*, **509**, 119–24.

Schmid, J. A., Mach, L., Paschke, E. and Glossl, J. (1999). Accumulation of sialic acid in endocytic compartments interferes with the formation of mature lysosomes. *J Biol Chem*, **274**, 19063–71.

Schneider, C., Gennaro, R., de Nicola, G. and Romeo, D. (1978). Secretion of granule enzymes from alveolar macrophages. *Exp Cell Res*, **112**, 249–56.

Schnyder, J. and Bagglioni, M. (1978). Secretion of lysosomal hydrolases by stimulated and non-stimulated macrophages. *J Exp Med*, **148**, 435–50.

Sena-Esteves, M., Camp, S. M., Alroy, J., Breakefield, X. O. and Kaye, E. M. (2000). Correction of acid β-galactosidase deficiency in GM1 gangliosidosis human fibroblasts by retrovirus vector-mediated gene transfer: higher efficiency of release and crosscorrection by the murine enzyme. *Hum Gene Ther*, **11**, 715–27.

Seto, T., Kono, K., Morimoto, K. *et al.* (2001). Brain magnetic resonance imaging in 23 patients with mucopolysaccharidoses and the effect of bone marrow transplantation. *Ann Neurol*, **50**, 79–92.

Sferra, T. J., Qu, G., McNeely, D. *et al.* (2000). Recombinant adeno-associated virus-mediated correction of lysosomal storage within the central nervous system of the adult mucopolysaccharidosis type VII mouse. *Hum Gene Ther*, **11**, 507–19.

Shapiro, E. G., Lockman, L. A., Balthazor, M. and Krivit, W. (1995). Neuropsychological outcomes of several storage diseases with and without bone marrow transplantation. *J Inherit Metab Dis*, **18**, 413–29.

Shull, R. M., Hastings, N. E., Selcer, R. R. *et al.* (1987). Bone marrow transplantation in canine mucopolysaccharidosis I. *J Clin Invest*, **79**, 435–43.

Shull, R. M., Breider, M. A. and Constantopoulos, G. (1988). Long-term neurological effects of bone marrow transplantation in a canine lysosomal storage disease. *Pediatr Res*, **24**, 347–52.

Skorupa, A. F., Fisher, K. J., Wilson, J. M., Parente, M. K. and Wolfe, J. H. (1999). Sustained production of β-glucuronidase from localized sites after AAV vector gene transfer results in widespread distribution of enzyme and reversal of lysosomal storage lesions in a large volume of brain in mucopolysaccharidosis VII mice. *Exp Neurol*, **160**, 17–27.

Snyder, E. Y., Taylor, R. M. and Wolfe, J. H. (1995). Neural progenitor cell engraftment corrects lysosomal storage throughout the MPS VII mouse brain. *Nature*, **374**, 367–70.

Soper, B. W., Duggy, T. M., Vogler, C. A. and Barker, J. E. (1999). A genetically myeloablated MPS VII model detects the expansion and curative properties of as few as 100 enriched murine stem cells. *Exp Hematol*, **27**, 1691–704.

Soper, B. W., Lessard, M. D., Vogler, C. A. *et al.* (2001). Nonablative neonatal marrow transplantation attenuates functional and physical defects of β-glucuronidase. *Blood*, **97**, 1498–504.

Staddon, J. M. and Rubin, L. L. (1996). Cell adhesion, cell junctions and the blood–brain barrier. *Curr Opin Neurobiol*, **6**, 622–7.

Stewart, K., Brown, O. A., Morelli, A. E. *et al.* (1997). Uptake of α-(L)-iduronidase produced by retrovirally transduced fibroblasts into neuronal and glial cells in vitro. *Gene Ther*, **4**, 63–75.

Streit, W. J., Walter, S. A. and Pennel, N. A. (1999). Reactive microgliosis. *Prog Neurobiol*, **57**, 563–81.

Sudhof, T. C. and Jahn, R. (1991). Proteins of synaptic vesicles involved in exocytosis and membrane recycling. *Neuron*, **6**, 665–77.

Sun, H., Yang, M., Haskins, M. E., Patterson, D. F. and Wolfe, J. H. (1999). Retrovirus vector-mediated correction and cross-correction of lysosomal α-mannosidase deficiency in human and feline fibroblasts. *Hum Gene Ther*, **10**, 1311–9.

Suzuki, K., Hoogerbrugge, P. M., Poorthuis, B. J. H. M., Van Bekkum, D. W. and Suzuki, K. (1988). The twitcher mouse – central nervous system pathology after bone marrow transplantation. *Lab Invest*, **58**, 302–8.

Suzuki, H., Iai, F., Kanno, T. and Sawada, M. (2001). Preservation of neurotrophin expression in microglia that migrate into the gerbil's brain across the blood–brain barrier. *Neurosci Lett*, **312**, 95–8.

Takahashi, Y., Sukegawa, K., Aoki, M. *et al.* (2001). Evaluation of accumulated mucopolysaccharides in the brain of patients with mucopolysaccharidoses by (1) H-magnetic resonance spectroscopy before and after bone marrow transplantation. *Pediatr Res*, **49**, 349–55.

Takenaka, T., Murray, G. J., Qin, G., Quirk, J. M., Ohshima, T. *et al.* (2000). Long-term enzyme correction and lipid reduction in multiple organs of primary and secondary transplanted Fabry mice receiving transduced bone marrow cells. *Proc Natl Acad Sci USA*, **97**, 7515–20.

Taylor, R. M. and Wolfe, J. H. (1994). Cross-correction of β-glucuronidase deficiency by retroviral vector-mediated gene transfer. *Exp Cell Res*, **214**, 606–13.

Taylor, R. M. and Wolfe, J. H. (1997*a*). Glycosaminoglycan storage in cultured neonatal murine mucopolysaccharidosis type VII neuroglial cells and correction by β-glucuronidase gene transfer. *J Neurochem*, **68**, 2079–85.

Taylor, R. M. and Wolfe, J. H. (1997*b*). Decreased lysosomal storage in the adult MPS VII mouse brain in the vicinity of grafts of retroviral vector-corrected fibroblasts secreting high levels of β-glucuronidase. *Nat Med*, **3**, 771–4.

Taylor, R. M., Farrow, B. R. H., Stewart, G. J. and Healy, P. J. (1986). Enzyme replacement in nervous tissue after allogeneic bone-marrow transplantation for fucosidosis in dogs. *Lancet*, **2**, 772–4.

Taylor, R. M., Farrow, B. R. H., Stewart, G. J., Healy, P. J. and Tiver, K. (1988). The clinical effects of lysosomal enzyme replacement by bone marrow transplantation after total lymphoid irradiation on neurologic disease in fucosidase deficient dogs. *Transplantation Proc*, **XX**, 89–93.

Taylor, R. M., Farrow, B. R. H. and Stewart, G. J. (1992). Amelioration of clinical disease following bone marrow transplantation in fucosidase-deficient dogs. *Am J Med Genet*, **42**, 628–32.

Teixeira, C. A., Sena-Esteves, M., Lopes, L., Miranda, M. C. S. and Ribeiro, M. G. (2001). Retrovirus-mediated transfer and expression of β-hexosaminidase α-chain cDNA in human fibroblasts from GM2 gangliosidosis B1 variant. *Hum Gene Ther*, **12**, 1771–83.

Torchiana, E., Lulli, L., Cattaneo, E. *et al.* (1998). Retroviral-mediated transfer of the galactocerebrosidase gene in neural progenitor cells. *Neuroreport*, **9**, 3823–7.

Unger, E. R., Sung, J. H., Manivel, J. C., Chenggis, M. L., Blazar, B. R. and Krivit, W. (1993). Male donor-derived cells in the brains of female sex-mismatched bone marrow transplant recipients: a Y-chromosome specific in situ hybridization study. *J Neuropathol Exp Neurol*, **52**, 460–70.

Vellodi, A., Young, E., New, M., Pot-Mees, C. and Hugh-Jones, K. (1992). Bone marrow transplantation for Sanfilippo disease type B. *J Inherit Metab Dis*, **15**, 911–8.

Vellodi, A., Cragg, H., Winchester, B. *et al.* (1995). Allogeneic transplantation for fucosidosis. *Bone Marrow Transplant*, **15**, 153–8.

Vellodi, A., Young, E. P., Cooper, A. *et al.* (1997). Bone marrow transplantation for mucopolysaccharidosis type I: experience of two British centres. *Arch Dis Child*, **76**, 92–9.

Vellodi, A., Young, E., Cooper, A., Lidchi, V., Winchester, B., and Wraith, J. E. (1999). Long-term follow-up following bone marrow transplantation for Hunter disease. *J Inherit Metab Dis*, **22**, 638–48.

Vladutiu, G. D. and Rattazzi, M. C. (1979). Excretion-reuptake route of β-hexosaminidase in normal and I-Cell disease cultured fibroblasts. *J Clin Invest*, **63**, 595–601.

Von Figura, K. and Kresse, H. (1972). The Sanfilippo B corrective factor: a *N*-acetyl-alpha-D-glucosamindiase. *Biochem Biophys Res Comm*, **48**, 262–9.

Von Figura, K. and Kresse, H. (1974). Inhibition of pinocytosis by cytochalasin B. Decrease in intracellular lysosomal-enzyme activities and increased storage of glycosaminoglycans. *Eur J Biochem*, **48**, 357–63.

Von Figura, K., Gieselmann and Jaeken, J. (2001). Metachromatic leukodystrophy. In *The metabolic and molecular bases of inherited disease* (Scriver, C. R., Beaudet, A. L., Sly, W. S. and Valle, D., ed.), pp. 3695–724. New York: McGraw-Hill.

Wada, R., Tifft, C. J. and Proia, R. L. (2000). Microglial activation precedes acute neurodegeneration in Sandhoff disease and is suppressed by bone marrow transplantation. *Proc Natl Acad Sci USA*, **97**, 10954–9.

Walkley, S. U. and Dobrenis, K. (1995). Bone marrow transplantation for lysosomal diseases. *Lancet*, **345**, 1382–3.

Walkley, S. U., Thrall, M. A., Dobrenis, K. *et al.* (1994*a*). Correction of enzyme defect in CNS neurons in a lysosomal storage disease following bone marrow transplant. *Proc Natl Acad Sci USA*, **91**, 2970–4.

Walkley, S. U., Thrall, M. A., Dobrenis, K., March, P. and Wurzelmann, S. (1994*b*). Bone marrow transplantation in neuronal storage diseases. *Brain Pathol*, **4**, 376.

Walkley, S. U., Dobrenis, K., Siegel, D. and Thrall, M. A. (1995). Bone marrow transplantation for cell mediated delivery of lysosomal enzymes to neurons. *Acta Hematol*, **93**, 164.

Walkley, S. U., Thrall, M. A. and Dobrenis, K. (1996). Targeting gene products to the brain and neurons using bone marrow transplantation: A cell-mediated delivery system for therapy of inherited metabolic human disease. In *Protocols for gene transfer in neuroscience: towards gene therapy of neurological disorders* (Lowenstein, P. R. and Enquist, L. W., ed.), pp. 275–302. England: John Wiley and Sons.

Wall, D. A., Grange, D. K., Goulding, P., Daines, M., Luisiri, A. and Kotagal, S. (1998). Bone marrow transplantation for the treatment of α-mannosidosis. *J Pediatr*, **133**, 282–5.

Walter, H. J., Berry, M., Hill, D. J., Cwyfan-Hughes, S., Holly, J. M. P. and Logan, A. (1999). Distinct sites of insulin-like growth factor (IGF)-II expression and localization in lesioned rat brain: possible roles of IGF binding proteins (IGFBPs) in the mediation of IGF-II activity. *Endocrinology*, **40**, 520–32.

Warren, C. D., Azaroff, L. S., Bugge, B. and Jeanloz, R. W. (1988). The accumulation of oligosaccharides in tissues and fluids of cats with α-mannosidosis. *Carbohydrate Res*, **180**, 325–38.

Wenger, D. A., Rafi, M. A., Luzi, P., Datto, J. and Costantino-Ceccarini, E. (2000). Krabbe disease: genetic aspects and progress toward therapy. *Mol Genet Metab*, **70**, 1–9.

Wenger, D. A., Suzuki, K., Suzuki, Y. and Suzuki, K. (2001). Galactosylceramide lipidodis: globoid cell leukodystrophy (Krabbe disease). In *The metabolic and molecular bases of inherited disease* (Scriver, C. R., Beaudet, A. L., Sly, W. S. and Valle, D., ed.), pp. 3669–94. New York: McGraw-Hill.

Whitley, C. B., Belani, K. G., Chang, P.-N. *et al.* (1993). Long-term outcome of Hurler syndrome following bone marrow transplantation. *Am J Med Genet*, **46**, 209–18.

Will, A., Cooper, A., Hatton, C., Sardharwalla, I. B., Evans, D. I. K. and Stevens, R. F. (1987). Bone marrow transplantation in the treatment of α-mannosidosis. *Arch Dis Childhood*, **62**, 1044–9.

Wolburg, H. and Risau, W. (1995). Formation of the blood–brain barrier. In *Neuroglia* (Kettenmann, H. and Ransom, B. R., ed.), pp. 763–76. New York: Oxford University Press.

Wolfe, J. H., Kyle, J. W., Sands, M. S., Sly, W. S., Markowitz, D. G. and Parente, M. K. (1995). High level expression and export of beta-glucuronidase from murine mucopolysaccharidosis VII cells corrected by a double-copy retrovirus vector. *Gene Ther*, **2**, 70–8.

Wood, J. M. (1980). Physiology, pharmacology and dynamics of cerebrospinal fluid. In *Neurobiology of cerebrospinal fluid* (Wood, J. M., ed.), pp. 1–15. New York: Plenum Press.

Wu, Y.-P., McMahon, E., Kraine, M. R. *et al.* (2000). Distribution and characterization of GFP^{+} donor hematogenous cells in twitcher mice after bone marrow transplantation. *Am J Pathol*, **156**, 1849–54.

Xia, H., Mao, Q. and Davidson, B. L. (2001). The HIV Tat protein transduction domain improves the biodistribution of β-glucuronidase expressed from recombinant viral vectors. *Nat Biotechnol*, **19**, 640–4.

Yin, H. S. and Yang, M. F. (1992). Effect of monensin on the neuronal ultrastructure and endocytic pathway of macromolecules in cultured brain neurons. *Cell Mol Neurobiol*, **12**, 297–307.

Chapter 15

Inhibition of substrate synthesis: a pharmacological approach for glycosphingolipid storage disease therapy

Frances M. Platt and Terry D. Butters

Introduction

The neuronopathic lysosomal storage diseases are not currently amenable to therapy due to the difficulties of delivering functional enzyme/protein to the brain. Recently, progress has been made in delivery techniques, but there have been no clinical studies to date demonstrating efficacy in these diseases. Over two decades ago, an alternative strategy was suggested by Radin based on small-molecule enzyme inhibitors for treating a subset of these disorders, the glycosphingolipidoses. Recently, the efficacy of this approach has been demonstrated in animal disease models and in the clinic. Before discussing these studies, a brief background on glycosphingolipids (GSLs) and GSL storage diseases is warranted, as it provides insights into the potentials and the limitations of drug-based strategies for treating this family of predominantly neurodegenerative disorders.

Glycosphingolipids

Glycosphingolipids are glycoconjugates that consist of the lipid ceramide to which one or more monosaccharide is linked. There are two classes of GSLs that have either glucosyl ceramide (glucosphingolipids, GlcSLs) or galactosyl ceramide (galactosphingolipids, GalSLs) as the core structure. In higher organisms, including mammals, GlcSLs can be modified to carry sialic acid and are termed gangliosides. Gangliosides are expressed by many different cell types but are particularly abundant in the nervous system. Despite the fact that GSLs are ubiquitous components of eukaryotic cells, we have a relatively poor understanding of their biological roles. *In vitro* studies have implicated GlcSLs to contribute to cell growth, differentiation, cell–cell and cell–matrix interactions, and to membrane organization and signalling. The GalSLs are important components of myelin. With the advent of targeted gene disruption technology, their roles are currently being explored *in vivo* in mice engineered to lack key enzymes in the GSL biosynthetic pathways.

Biosynthesis of glycosphingolipids

The biosynthesis of GlcSLs has been elucidated in considerable detail with the enzymes, their co-factors, and their topology having been determined (van Echten and Sandhoff 1993; Sandhoff and van Echten 1994). Synthesis is initiated in the endoplasmic reticulum (ER) with the formation of ceramide. The first monosaccharide to be transferred to ceramide is glucose, and this occurs on the cytosolic face of an early Golgi compartment (Trinchera *et al.* 1991). The formation of glucosylceramide (GlcCer) is catalysed by the ceramide-specific glucosyltransferase (EC 2.4.1.80), using UDP-glucose as the nucleotide sugar donor (Ichikawa and Hirabayashi 1998). The GlcCer formed is the precursor for the GlcSLs that are found in peripheral tissues and the central nervous system (CNS). Glucosylceramide is converted to more complex GlcSL species through the action of sequentially acting transferases located in the lumen of the Golgi. In the CNS and kidney, a galactosyltransferase (EC 2.4.1.47) catalyses the transfer of galactose to ceramide to form galactosylceramide (GalCer), a prominent component of myelin (Burger *et al.* 1996; Coetzee *et al.* 1998). This GSL is further modified by sulphation to form sulfatide, can be galactosylated to form digalactosylceramide, although this is not an abundant GalSL in mammals (Coetzee *et al.* 1998), and sialylated to form GM4. The diversity of GSLs arises through the modification of GlcCer. The cell-specific expression of GlcSLs reflects the differential expression of the transferases involved in GlcSL biosynthesis, which can vary with cell differentiation (Taga *et al.* 1995). The synthesis of gangliosides in non-Golgi compartments may also occur. A ganglioside-specific sialyltransferase has been localized to axons and non-Golgi structures in neurones (Stern and Tiemeyer 2001). How general a phenomenon this is remains unclear at the present time. Glucosphingolipids are indispensable during mammalian development. When the ceramide glucosyltransferase gene is knocked out in mice, the phenotype is embryonic lethality (Yamashita *et al.* 1999). This could be a consequence of the absence of GlcSLs or an increase in free ceramide, or a combination of both biochemical changes. Circumstantial evidence that GlcSLs are also essential for early development in humans comes from the observation that no human disease states have been identified that result from defects in the genes involved in the biosynthesis of GlcCer. There are, however, rare examples of human diseases with defects in ganglioside biosynthesis (Max *et al.* 1974; Tanaka *et al.* 1975). Whether this implied embryonic lethality reflects the importance of GlcSLs or overabundance of the precursor ceramide is unclear. However, it should be noted that although severe diseases result from deficiencies in N-glycosylation, they have only recently been recognized as a group of related diseases and their biochemical bases elucidated (Schachter 2001). This raises the theoretical possibility that defects in GSL biosynthesis do occur but have not been clinically and biochemically characterized to date.

Following synthesis, GSLs are transported to the plasma membrane where they are thought to mediate the majority of their functions. They typically recycle via the Golgi compartment (Hakomori 2000; Galbiati *et al.* 2001). They are routed to lysosomes as part of general membrane turnover where they undergo sequential degradation of the oligosaccharide to yield ceramide, which can be further degraded or recycled (Sandhoff and Kolter 1997).

The catabolism of GSLs is understood in considerable detail and this is due in no small part to the study of human metabolic diseases which result from a failure to degrade GSLs in the lysosome (Sandhoff and Kolter 1996, 1997; Bierfreund *et al.* 2000). The lysosome contains numerous acid exoglycohydrolases that along with their protein co-factors (saposins and activator proteins) remove terminal sugars from GSLs (van Echten and Sandhoff 1993; Sandhoff and van Echten 1994; Sandhoff *et al.* 1998) (Chapter 8). The catabolic pathway is sequential, with the product of one reaction being the substrate for the next. Under normal circumstances, the lysosomal degradative capacity can fully degrade all GSLs entering the lysosome. The enzymes present in the lysosome are not limiting and are present at higher levels than are required to mediate complete GSL catabolism. This is known from the GSL storage diseases in which defects in the genes which encode these hydrolases result in a complete lack of enzyme, impaired catalysis, or enzyme instability (Schuette *et al.* 1999) (Chapter 4). Their inheritance is primarily autosomal recessive, with carriers typically being unaffected; 50% enzyme levels are therefore adequate to escape disease (Neufeld 1991).

Glycosphingolipid storage diseases

There is a disease associated with the majority of steps in GSL catabolism (Chapters 2 and 4). Steps in catabolism lacking a disease state indicate enzyme redundancy in the pathway, i.e. additional enzymes involved in the breakdown of other glycoconjugates can catabolize the GSL substrate. The frequency of individual diseases is not high, but collectively they are a significant and severe group of disorders. Approximately half of all lysosomal storage diseases involve the storage of GSLs and have a collective frequency of 1 : 18 000 live births (Meikle *et al.* 1999). Because GSLs, and in particular gangliosides, are abundantly expressed in the nervous system, the brain is frequently an organ affected by storage and these disorders are the commonest cause of paediatric neurodegenerative disease (Meikle *et al.* 1999) (Chapters 2–4). The individual disease states, the specific enzyme deficiencies, and the resulting storage lipids are listed in Table 15.1 (and reviewed in Chapter 2). The only disorder lacking CNS involvement is type 1 Gaucher disease, which involves storage of GlcCer in peripheral tissue macrophages.

The level of residual enzyme an affected individual has is a prognostic indicator of the age of disease onset, disease severity, and life expectancy (Conzelmann and Sandhoff 1983) (Chapter 4). Assaying lysosomal enzymes *in vitro* using artificial substrates is always problematic as it may not fully reflect the events that occur within the intact lysosome. However, even in the artificial environment in which enzyme is measured, the residual enzyme level determined is a reasonably accurate predictor of clinical outcome. Infantile-onset disease occurs when the mutation in the gene is very severe resulting in either no or very low levels of residual enzyme

Table 15.1 Enzyme Defects, Affected Genes, and Glycolipids Stored in Human Glycosphingolipid Lysosomal Storage Diseases

Disease	Enzyme defect	Glycosphingolipid stored
Gaucher types 1, 2,* and 3*	β-Glucocerebrosidase	Glucosylceramide
Fabry	α-Galactosidase	Globotriaosylceramide (Gb3)
Tay–Sachs*	Hexosaminidase A	GM2 Ganglioside
Sandhoff*	Hexosaminidases A and B	GM2 Ganglioside
GM1 Gangliosidosis*	β-Galactosidase	GM1 Ganglioside
Krabbe*	β-Galactocerebrosidase	Galactosylceramide
Metachromatic leukodystrophy*	ArylsulfataseA	Galactosylceramide sulfate

*Neurological involvement.

activity. Juvenile-onset variants have mutations that result in more residual enzyme activity, leading to a slower rate of storage, delayed symptom onset, and progression. Adult-onset (chronic) variants can develop symptoms at any stage of late childhood/adulthood and have appreciable levels of residual enzyme activity (Rapola 1994) (Chapter 4). The rate of storage is therefore slow, clinical presentation delayed, and disease progression protracted. It is difficult to obtain accurate frequencies of the occurrence of the late-onset variants as the majority of affected individuals are misdiagnosed, due to superficial similarity in clinical presentation with more common neuromuscular disorders. It is still the case that the neurological glycosphingolipidoses are erroneously perceived to be exclusively paediatric disorders, and a diagnosis of one of these diseases in the adult is rarely considered.

Therapeutic options

The GSL storage disorders are monogenic diseases. Mutations in the gene encoding the glycohydrolase can result in varying degrees of enzyme deficiency, depending on the specific nature of the mutation in question (Chapter 4). As the enzyme deficiency leads to disease, a logical approach to therapy is either to replace the gene (Chapter 16) or to replace the enzyme (enzyme replacement therapy (ERT) and bone marrow transplantation (BMT)) (Chapters 13 and 14). The former strategy is still experimental, whereas the latter is limited by lack of penetrance of the enzyme into the CNS. Direct intravenous infusion of enzyme as a therapy is restricted to type 1 Gaucher disease and more recently Fabry disease (Eng *et al.* 2001; Schiffmann *et al.* 2001) (Chapter 13). Bone marrow transplantation is limited by scarcity of matched donors, procedure-associated morbidity and mortality, and limited efficacy (Erikson *et al.* 1990; Ringden *et al.* 1995). However, exceptions do occur and the feline model of α-mannosidosis does respond very well to BMT (Walkley *et al.* 1994) (see Chapter 14). Many of the enzymes in question are not efficiently secreted and recaptured by neighbouring cells, limiting the efficacy of BMT (Walkley and Dobrenis 1995). Stem cell therapy has the potential to deliver enzyme to the brain and mediate cell replacement but is still at an experimental stage (Chapter 14). All these approaches require invasive delivery systems, and many are disease specific in nature (gene therapy, ERT, and engineered stem cell therapy). This chapter addresses an alternative therapeutic strategy based on the use of small molecules.

The pharmacological approach

Drug-based strategies for treating GSL storage disease have only recently been evaluated (Platt and Butters 1998; Butters *et al.* 2000a). Before discussing the specifics of this approach, it is worth making some general comments on the potential advantages of taking a pharmacological approach to therapy. Firstly, drug screening, pre-clinical development, toxicology, and clinical evaluation are the typical approaches taken to treat the majority of human diseases and do not involve the unknown elements associated with the biological therapies based on stem cells or gene therapy. This is not to belittle these approaches as they undoubtedly hold considerable future promise, it is simply that drug-based strategies can be evaluated immediately and they are not dependent on the practical and ethical considerations associated with novel biotherapies (Chapters 14 and 16). When specifically considering storage diseases of the brain, some small molecules can cross the blood–brain barrier, and therefore the possibility of effectively managing storage in the CNS is realistic, providing that a suitable agent is identified. There is also the potential of using one drug to treat multiple diseases, making commercial development more attractive, negating the requirement for disease-specific therapies. As many of these disorders are individually rare, this is an important factor. Drug therapies are cheaper than protein therapies, which again should facilitate the treatment of the majority of patients, not just those fortunate enough to reside in affluent countries. What is therefore needed is a biochemical target upon which to base the pharmacological approach. Such a target was suggested by the pioneer of this field, Norman Radin, who advocated inhibiting the synthesis of GlcSLs as a way of managing these disorders (Vunnam and Radin 1980; Radin, 1996). This approach was termed substrate-deprivation therapy (Beutler 1993) and over the years has been variously termed substrate inhibition, substrate reduction (Lachmann and Platt 2001), and substrate balance therapy. For the purpose of this chapter, we will refer to this approach as substrate reduction therapy (SRT) as it captures the essential element of this approach, reduction in substrate burden.

Substrate reduction therapy

Storage of GSLs in the endosomal–lysosomal system arises due to insufficient residual enzyme activity. The rate of synthesis proceeds as normal (no feedback inhibition), leading to a constant influx of GSLs into the endosomal–lysosomal system, of which only a proportion can be degraded, resulting in GSL storage. By reducing the rate of synthesis storage should be prevented. If full balance could not be achieved, it would be anticipated that severe forms could be converted into milder forms, i.e. the rate of GSL accumulation could be significantly slowed. As the synthesis of GlcSLs follows a single biosynthetic pathway with GlcCer as the common precursor (Fig. 15.1), inhibitors that block the transfer of glucose to ceramide (mediated by ceramide glucosyltransferase) would have the potential to be used in all storage diseases which involve the storage of GlcCer-based GSLs (Gaucher types 1, 2, and 3, Fabry, Tay–Sachs, Sandhoff, and GM1 gangliosidosis). Ideally, such an inhibitor would not block the transfer of galactose to ceramide (mediated by ceramide galactosyltransferase) and hence would not affect myelin. This would render such drugs ineffective for the treatment of Krabbe disease and metachromatic leukodystrophy (Table 15.1), which involve the storage of GalSLs (Neufeld 1991) (Chapter 2). If drugs could be identified which cross the blood–brain barrier, then storage diseases with neurological phenotypes (the majority and most challenging group for development of therapies) could also be treated. There is the additional prospect of combining substrate-lowering drugs with enzyme augmentation, to tackle the disease from both sides of the synthesis : catabolism equation. There is the potential that synergy could result, leading to more effective therapy, and reduce the level of drug and enzyme augmentation needed to effectively manage the disease.

Glycosyltransferase Inhibitors

Before considering the inhibitors specific for the first step in GSL biosynthesis, a brief overview of glycosyltransferase inhibitors is warranted. Glycosyltransferases are membrane-bound proteins involved in glycoconjugate biosynthesis and require the participation of an activated nucleotide sugar donor and an acceptor. Although many of the activities and genes for these enzymes have been identified, they are particularly difficult to study mechanistically because of the lack of sufficient purified protein in a native form. The transfer of sugar to acceptor presents technical difficulties for automating enzyme assays, and simple, high-throughput screening of chemical libraries for potential inhibitors has rarely been achieved. The search for inhibitors therefore has been restricted to rational design of nucleotide sugar

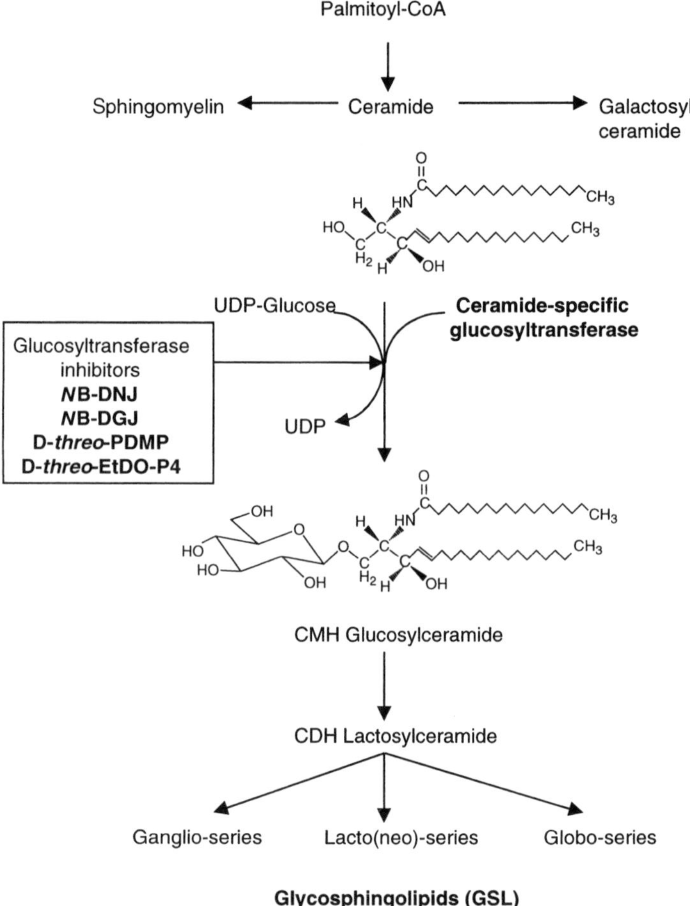

Fig. 15.1 Synthesis of glycosphingolipids indicating the step in biosynthesis inhibited by PDMP series and imino sugar compounds.

donor analogues that may mimic some part of a possible transition state during the reaction (Compain and Martin 2001). Good examples can be found among the sialyltransferases (Schaub *et al.* 1998; Schroder and Giannis 1999; Sun *et al.* 2001) where inhibitory constants in the 10–20 μM range have been reported.

The mechanism of catalytic transfer has been assumed to take place in a similar fashion to the well-characterized nucleophilic substitution of the anomeric carbon of the donor monosaccharide, which is characteristic of glycosidase-mediated cleavage of the glycosidic bond (Withers 2001). The use of imino sugars, which contain a protonatable cyclic nitrogen, as part of a complex that mimics the positive charge character of any reaction intermediate also provides some novel compounds for synergistic inhibition of fucosyltransferases with the GDP-fucose donor (Qiao *et al.* 1996; Jefferies and Bowen 1997; Schuster and Blechert 2001). Compounds with similar designs have proved efficient and selective inhibitors for α-and β-galactosyltransferases (Takayama *et al.* 1999). Recent progress in defining a general mechanism for catalytic transfer using crystallographic data to identify the molecular organization of the active site for glycosyltransferases offers new opportunities to develop further inhibitors (Unligil and Rini 2000; Persson *et al.* 2001).

For SRT, two approaches could be envisaged, either a generic approach to inhibit GSL biosynthesis at an early step or identify selective inhibitors of each transferase in the pathway responsible for generating the disease-specific storage GSL. Currently, we are restricted to the former approach as disease-specific transferase inhibitors have not as yet been identified.

Ceramide-specific glucosyltransferase inhibitors

Two classes of compound have been described that have inhibitory activity towards the first glycosyltransferase in the GlcSL biosynthetic pathway (ceramide glucosyltransferase)—the PDMP series and imino sugars (Fig. 15.2).

PDMP Series

Morpholino and pyrrolidino derivatives (PDMP series) that structurally resemble ceramide are low (10^{-8} M) inhibitors of transferase activity (Vunnam and Radin 1980; Inokuchi and Radin 1987; Lee et al. 1999). Some assumptions are made regarding the mode of action of this compound, but the competitive and reversible nature of the inhibition, despite the unnatural configuration, suggests transition state mimicry. The prototypic enantiomer, D-threo-PDMP, has shown limited application due to high toxicity and non-selectivity for ceramide-specific glucosyltransferase, eliciting elevated levels of potentially toxic ceramide

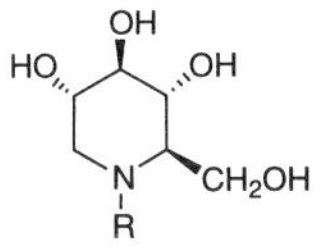

Deoxynojirimycin
R = $-(CH_2)_3CH_3$, *N*-butyl-DNJ (NB-DNJ)
R = $-(CH_2)_8CH_3$, *N*-nonyl-DNJ (NN-DNJ)

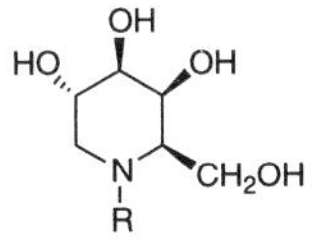

Deoxygalactonojirimycin
R = H, DGJ
R = $-(CH_2)_3CH_3$, *N*-butyl-DGJ (NB-DGJ)

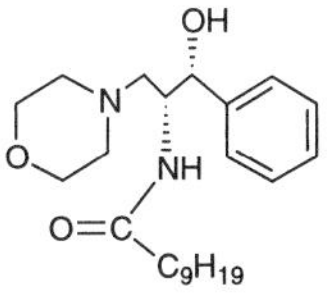

D-*threo*-1-phenyl-2-decanoylamino-3-morpholino-1-propanol (D-*threo*-PDMP)

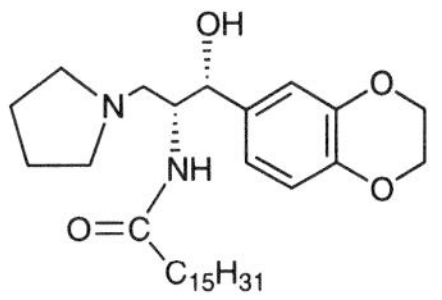

D-*threo*-1-(3',4'-ethylenedioxy)phenyl-2-palmitoylamino-3-pyrrolidino-1-propanol (D-*threo*-EtDO-P4)

Fig. 15.2 Structures of pharmacological compounds evaluated for the treatment of the glycosphingolipidoses.

in cells (see Table 15.2). Elevated ceramide levels could occur as the consequence of inhibition of the ceramide-specific glucosyltransferase through a failure to metabolize ceramide through other pathways. Experiments with PDMP suggest that the combined inhibition of enzymes that also convert ceramide, such as sphingomyelin synthase (ceramide cholinephosphotransferase, EC 2.7.8.3) and 1-O-acylceramide synthase (EC 2.3.1.-), directly leads to ceramide accumulation. Improvements in design, e.g. the D-threo-ethylenedioxy-P4 compound (D-threo-EtDO-P4), has reduced these unwanted activities to allow dose discrimination between inhibition of the glucosyltransferase and other ceramide-metabolizing enzymes (Lee et al. 1999)(Table 15.2). The cellular toxicity observed with the PDMP series is unrelated to the inhibition of GlcSL biosynthesis, based on dose, and depends more on the hydrophobic nature of these compounds perturbing membrane structure/integrity.

Imino sugar inhibitors

The imino sugar family of compounds are monosaccharide mimetics, many of which occur naturally in certain plants and micro-organisms. They have been used as glycohydrolase inhibitors for many years. They are characterized by having a nitrogen atom in place of the ring oxygen (Fig. 15.2). The nitrogen atom provides an additional point for modification, and simple alkylation of glucose or galactose analogues confers unexpected activities for additional enzyme targets, such as the ceramide-specific glucosyltransferase-mediated pathway, which is critical for GSL biosynthesis (Butters *et al.* 2000*b*). Imino sugars with either glucose or galactose stereochemistry is one requirement for inhibitory activity of the ceramide-specific glucosyltransferase (Platt *et al.* 1994*b*). Modifications to the hydroxyl groups demonstrate some selectivity since C2-OH inversion (mannose isomer), and C6-Me (fucose isomer) are non-inhibitory (Platt *et al.* 1994*b*), whereas C4-OH inversion (galactose isomer) does not affect inhibition. Substitution of the C3, C6 hydroxyl groups of deoxynojirimycin (DNJ) causes a loss in potency (Butters *et al.* 2000*b*). However, stereo-inversion of the C6 hydroxyl to provide either the altro or the ido-series does not reduce potency significantly (Butters, unpublished data). Substitution of the C1 position often leads to a dramatic reduction in inhibitory potency, a significant point of difference in the ability of similar analogues to inhibit α-glucosidases (Butters *et al.* 2000*b*). This is not the case for the pyrrolidine-based inhibitors which are also potent inhibitors of both glucosidases and glucosyltransferase (Butters *et al.* 2000*b*).

A second requirement for inhibitory activity of glucose and galactose analogues is alkylation of the ring nitrogen. A carbon chain of greater than three atoms is required for activity since methyl- and ethyl-derivatives are inactive and *N*-propyl analogues show only partial activity (Platt *et al.* 1994*b*). The major factor in promoting inhibitory activity appears to be hydrophobicity since *N*-benzyl-DNJ is as potent as *N*-butyl-DNJ (Butters *et al.* 1998). Further increases in alkyl chain length leads to a 10-fold improvement in potency in an *in vitro* assay; however, a greater increase in potency (1000-fold) has been obtained using a more lipophilic adamantane moiety (Overkleeft *et al.* 1998). The ability of large hydrophobic groups to insert into lipid bilayers is thought to promote the inhibition of the membrane-bound glucosyltransferase by inducing a high local concentration of compound in membrane protein complexes (Platt and Butters 1995). Although an increase in potency can be obtained by increasing hydrophobicity, the cytotoxicity of these compounds reduces their potential for therapeutic use (Table 15.2). With extended alkyl chain compounds the cytotoxicity property can be offset, with only marginal reduction in inhibitory potency by the use of an ether chain at C7 (van den Broek *et al.* 1994; Butters *et al.* 1998).

Table 15.2 Properties of Compounds used for *in vitro* Studies of Glycolipid Storage Disorders

Substrate reduction therapy: *in vitro* pre-clinical studies					
	CerGlcT IC_{50}				
Compound	***In vitro***	**In cells***	**Cytotoxicity(CC_{50})**	**Therapeutic index (CC_{50}/IC_{50})**	**Ceramide elevation in cells**
*N*B-DNJ	20 μM[1]	20 μM[1]	>10 mM[2]	>500	Not observed at 0.5 mM[3]
*N*B-DGJ	40 μM[1]	20 μM[1]	>10 mM[2]	>500	Not observed at 0.5 mM[3]
D-*threo*-PDMP	20 μM[4]	20 μM[5]	10–25 μM[6,7]	0.5–1.25	Threefold elevation at 12.5 μM[7]
D-*threo*-EtDO-P4	100 nM[8]	10 nM[8]	<1 μM[8]	<100	Elevated above 1 μM[8]

'Chaperone-mediated' enzyme folding: *in vitro* pre-clinical studies		
Compound	**Increase in mutant α-galactosidase activity[9]**	**Increase in mutant β-galactosidase activity[10]**
DGJ	Seven- to eightfold increase at 20 μM	1.7–6.0 increase at 0.5 mM
*N*B-DGJ	Slight increase at 100 μM[11]	1.1–6.1 increase at 0.5 mM
Compound	**Increase in mutant (N370S) β-glucosidase activity[12]**	
*N*N-DNJ	1.65 fold increase at 5 μM after 5 days	
*N*B-DNJ	No increase in activity at 100 μM	

Source: Platt *et al.* (1994*b*);[1] Durantel *et al.* (2001);[2] Mellor *et al.* (2003);[3] Miura *et al.* (1998);[4] Chatterjee *et al.* (1996);[5] Abe *et al* (1992);[6] Bieberich *et al.* (1999);[7] Lee *et al* (1999);[8] Fan *et al.* (1999);[9] Tominaga *et al.* (2001);[10] Asano *et al.* (2000);[11] Sawkar *et al.* (2002).[12]

*Reduction of ceramide glucosyltransferase in cells was obtained from literature data where the depletion of radiolabelled precursor incorporation into GlcCer was measured after 4 days of treatment with inhibitor.

The mechanism of action of imino sugars supports a substrate analogue mode of direct active-site inhibition. Using *in vitro* assays, both *N*B-DNJ and *N*B-DGJ are competitive for ceramide and non-competitive for UDP-glucose (Butters *et al.* 1998). Molecular modelling experiments based on the crystal structure of ceramide and the NMR solution structure of *N*B-DNJ reveals an unexpected homology between three chiral centres at C2, C3, and C6 and the *N*-alkyl chain of *N*B-DNJ with the *trans*-alkenyl and N-acyl chain of ceramide. The 3-hydroxyl group is a key component of this overlay, since the alignment with the C3–OH of ceramide is critical for enzymatic activity (Vunnam and Radin 1980). In support of these data, methylation of the C3 chiral centre in *N*B-DNJ completely ablates glucosyltransferase inhibitory activity (Butters *et al.* 1998).

Imino sugars as enzyme activity modulators—chemical chaperone therapy

Imino sugars have also been suggested as potential therapeutic agents for treating GSL storage disease by virtue of their ability to stabilize hydrolases deficient or unstable in these diseases. A disease-specific approach has been proposed using galactose analogue imino sugars, aiming to improve the catalytic activity of mutant α- and β-galactosidases (Table 15.2). At high concentrations, deoxygalactonojirimycin (DGJ) is a potent (10^{-9} M) inhibitor of α-galactosidase and deficiency in this enzyme leads to Fabry disease. However, if used at sub-inhibitory concentrations in fibroblasts containing a misfolded mutant form of α-galactosidase, DGJ accelerated transport and maturation of the enzyme (Fan *et al.* 1999). By analysing a number of galactose compounds including DGJ and *N*B-DGJ, some restoration of β-galactosidase activity was observed in enzyme-deficient knockout mouse fibroblasts and human β-galactosidosis fibroblasts (Tominaga *et al.* 2001). The authors concluded that the DGJ compounds work as intracellular activators, resulting in molecularly stable forms of the enzyme targeted normally to the lysosome. Further *in vivo* experiments are needed to validate this approach of 'chemical chaperone therapy'. Importantly, small molecules gain access to the brain, and their use would offer a novel pharmacological option for treating the neuronopathic forms of the glycosphingolipidoses, such as GM1 gangliosidosis or the galactosidase deficiency associated with Morquio B disease. The DGJs analysed to date for chaperone therapy are not selective for α- and β-galactosidases. Doses would have to be carefully managed to improve the activity of one enzyme form without inhibition of the other, thereby generating a lysosomal storage phenotype. *N*B-DGJ has been evaluated in normal mice and mouse models for lysosomal storage disease where it was well tolerated (Andersson *et al.* 2000). In intracellular GlcSL metabolism, the inhibitory activity of this compound favours reduction of synthase activity and not α- and β-galactosidase inhibition, therefore removing any doubts that an unwanted GlcSL storage phenotype could be generated.

A similar rationale has been proposed as a novel therapeutic strategy for treating Gaucher disease with an *N*-alkylated DNJ (*N*-nonyl-DNJ, *N*N-DNJ) (Sawkar *et al.* 2002). Using primary skin fibroblasts carrying the most common mutation in the glucocerebrosidase gene in Gaucher disease, N370S, the authors demonstrated that inclusion of 5 μM *N*N-DNJ in the medium for 5 days increased the activity of enzyme in intact cells 1.65 fold (Table 15.2). These data suggest that the N370S mutation has protein folding deficiencies that can be corrected by addition of an active-site inhibitor and could be used to therapeutically enhance lysosomal glycolipid degradation by mutant glucocerebrosidase in type 1 Gaucher disease. Glucocerebrosidase has greater affinity for hydrophobic compounds, and it is notable that although *N*B-DNJ does not appear to increase mutant enzyme activity at 100 μM, it does promote an increase in serum half-life (Priestman *et al.* 2000). Thus, both *N*B-DNJ and *N*N-DNJ protect the enzyme from thermal inactivation (Sawkar *et al.* 2002).

Given that modest increases in enzyme activity may be sufficient to alter lysosomal storage of GSLs by significant amounts, orally available small molecular chaperones may have an important clinical application in mild forms of disease.

Recently, improvement in cardiac function was reported in a patient with the cardiac variant of Fabry disease given intra-venous infusions of galactose to increase residual enzyme activity. The clinical improvement measured in this patient will provide the impetus for further studies with either galactose or a non-toxic analogue of galactose (Frustaci *et al.* 2001).

Potency, specificity, and cytotoxicity of imino sugars and PDMP series compounds

Both the imino sugars and PDMP series of compounds have been evaluated in tissue culture to determine the relative potency, specificity, and cytotoxicity (Table 15.2). Despite the high affinity of the improved pyrrolidino derivatives (e.g. D-*threo*-EtDO-P4) for the ceramide-specific glucosyltransferase, the hydrophobic nature of this compound induces cytotoxicity. If the therapeutic index for the two compounds is compared (half maximal cytotoxic concentration/half maximal inhibitory concentration, CC_{50}/IC_{50}), D-*threo*-EtDO-P4 has a value of <100, whereas *N*B-DNJ has a value greater than 500 (Table 15.2). The difference in compound concentrations needed to obtain inhibition of the transferase in cells between imino sugars and PDMP analogues argues for different modes of entry. Imino sugars rapidly cross the plasma membrane to the cytosol, the location of the transferase active site. To inhibit the cellular enzyme, an equivalent concentration to isolated enzyme inhibition of 20 μM is required extracellularly, suggesting a freely diffusable mode of access (Table 15.2). By contrast, 10-fold lower concentrations of D-*threo*-EtDO-P4 are required to inhibit the cellular enzyme, indicating a cytosolic concentration effect across the diffusion gradient. These data also indicate that a potential accumulation of hydrophobic compound could occur within the cell that could lead to toxicity after long-term administration.

How essential are glycosphingolipids *in vivo*?

Having defined classes of inhibitory drugs with which to evaluate SRT, an important question is can partial GSL depletion be tolerated? This is a controversial topic and merits some detailed discussion as our understanding of *in vivo* GSL functions is currently limited.

It is clear from a mutant melanoma cell line lacking ceramide glucosyltransferase that the total absence of GlcSLs is compatible with viability at the single-cell level (Ichikawa *et al.* 1994). In keeping with this, no toxicity has been observed in a range of *in vitro* cell lines extensively depleted of GlcSLs using *N*B-DNJ to inhibit GlcSL biosynthesis (Platt *et al.* 1994*a*). However, these studies provide no clues as to the functional roles of GlcSL in an intact organism where GlcSL depletion would have the potential to cause toxicity. There is an extensive literature which suggests that GSLs are critical for several functions, particularly in the CNS (Zeller and Marchase 1992; Rahmann 1995; Hadjiconstantinou and Neff 1998; Walkley *et al.* 1998).

Homologous recombination was used to generate a knockout mouse null for the ceramide glucosyltranferase responsible for initiating the GlcSL biosynthetic pathway (Yamashita *et al.* 1999). The knockout mouse had a lethal phenotype early in embryogenesis. However, later in development during post-implantation organogenesis, pharmacological (*N*B-DGJ treatment of normal mouse embryos in tissue culture) GlcSL depletion (not total ablation) did not result in overt morphological changes (Brigande *et al.* 1998; Brigande and Seyfried 1998). Similarly, development of a teleost, the Japanese Medaca fish (*Oryzias latipes*), also proceeded normally in the presence of a GSL-depleting agent (PDMP treatment) during late organogenesis (Fenderson *et al.* 1992). The embryos exhibited extensive GSL depletion in organs including brain but were viable and had no overt morphological or behavioural changes or deficits (Fenderson *et al.* 1992). There may therefore be developmental windows sensitive to GSL depletion and other stages, which can proceed as normal in their absence or when severely depleted.

Most research has focused on vertebrate and in particular mammalian systems. It is worth noting that although GSL species are conserved in all eukaryotes, their complexity has increased over evolutionary time (Gagneux and Varki 1999). For instance, invertebrates do not synthesize gangliosides yet clearly develop, metamorphose and have complex behavioural repertoires in their absence. It is not perhaps surprising therefore that when higher ganglioside synthesis was knocked out (GM2/GD2 synthase, β1,4-*N*-acetylgalactosaminyl transferase, EC 2.4.1.165-deficient mouse) brain development proceeded as normal and the mice were viable (Takamiya *et al.* 1996). Complex gangliosides may therefore not be required for neural development, dendritigenesis, or synaptogenesis in the murine brain which are processes which have evolved in their absence. Alternatively, functional substitution by the simpler gangliosides present in these mice may account for their lack of phenotype. It was only later in life that more subtle neurological abnormalities emerged in these mice, including myelination defects and Wallerian degeneration, suggesting that higher gangliosides function in central myelination and maintenance of integrity in axons and myelin (Sheikh *et al.* 1999).

It is worth considering the details of the knockout mouse models which provide the insights we currently have into GSL functions *in vivo*. For instance, embryonic lethality of animals null for GSLs may reflect the effects of increasing basal ceramide levels in the absence of the ceramide glucosylation pathway (Yamashita *et al.* 1999). In the case of the higher ganglioside knockout mouse, the adult phenotype could reflect a lack of higher gangliosides or the overexpression of simple gangliosides which could substitute for them.

A hypothesis has been proposed by Gagneux and Varki that oligosaccharide diversity (lipid and protein-linked glycans, including blood group antigens) has evolved primarily to evade pathogen recognition (Gagneux and Varki 1999). This would serve in part to explain the enormous diversity of glycan structures which exist in higher organisms and the singular lack of exclusive function ascribed to the majority of them. For example, they speculate that differential patterns of ganglioside expression in the brain may serve as a protective strategy to avoid death from neurotoxins. The inter-species variability (even amongst closely related species) in ganglioside expression in the brain may reflect the differential exposure of different species to different pathogens and toxins (and hence different selective pressures) due to differences in the ecology of each species (Gagneux and Varki 1999). As pathogens adapt to a new carbohydrate receptor through mutation, the host species diversifies its carbohydrates further in a perpetual co-evolutionary battle.

It is clear that we have much to learn about the natural history and evolution of GSLs, and it is pertinent to stress that our current level of understanding makes it impossible to predict what impact if any partial GSL depletion will have in an adult mammal. When considering potential adverse effects of depletion mediated by SRT, it is important to stress that a knockout scenario is not the desired objective. Partial depletion is the aim of this therapeutic strategy.

Two issues are relevant to SRT, one is how important are absolute expression levels of GSLs for maintenance of normal homoeostasis in adult mammals. One recent theme to emerge in GlcSL research is that GlcSLs may be important in membrane organization and endosomal trafficking of molecules within the cell (Kobayashi and Hirabayashi 2000). They are constituents of lipid rafts/microdomains, which may be important in mediating cell-signalling events. However, what is not known is the minimum complement of rafts required to maintain function and whether GSLs are essential components of rafts. Secondly, to what extent can ceramide accumulation be avoided if ceramide is not glucosylated due to transferase inhibition? Does the excess ceramide get converted into sphingomyelin, avoiding changes in basal ceramide levels? As free ceramide can lead to apoptosis, these issues have important implications for tolerability and cytotoxicity of these drugs *in vivo*. Data from experimental systems were therefore needed to begin to address these issues.

Glycosphingolipid depletion is tolerated in adult mice

Healthy C57Bl/6 mice were treated orally with *N*B-DNJ (Table 15.3). It was found that GSL depletion was dose dependent, and that 70% peripheral GSL depletion was well tolerated over a 4-month period (Platt *et al.* 1997*b*). This raises interesting questions concerning the biology of GlcSLs in adult mice, as they appear to be expressed at levels that are in excess of those required to maintain homoeostasis, under normal physiological conditions. It should however be emphasized that due to the very long *in vivo* half-lives of GlcSL in the CNS, minimal depletion was observed in brain tissue in *N*B-DNJ-treated mice after 4 months of drug treatment (Platt *et al.* 1997*b*). The long-term consequences of GSL depletion on brain function were therefore not revealed by this study. Some effects of drug treatment were, however, observed, including weight loss and partial lymphoid organ atrophy. However, when similar *in vivo* studies were carried out with the galactose analogue, *N*B-DGJ, no weight loss or lymphoid organ changes occurred (Andersson *et al.* 2000). As both drugs are equivalent GlcSL biosynthesis inhibitors *in vivo*, these effects of *N*B-DNJ are clearly not related to GlcSL depletion. Levels of GlcSLs can therefore be reduced without inducing pathology, paving the way for evaluation of GlcSL-lowering drugs in animal disease models. It is interesting to note that increases in sphingomyelin were observed in the drug-treated mice. This suggests that the increase in free ceramide which could result from inhibition of ceramide glucosyltransferase is instead shunted into the sphingomyelin biosynthetic pathway, avoiding ceramide-mediated cytotoxicity.

Evaluation of imino sugar inhibitors in models of glucosphingolipid storage diseases

To date, the majority of studies evaluating SRT as a therapeutic strategy has involved the use of the prototypic imino sugar *N*B-DNJ (Tables 2 and 3). Three phases of its evaluation have taken place: *in vitro* proof of concept in a tissue culture disease model, evaluation in two murine disease models which involve storage in the brain (either as monotherapy or in combination with the enzyme augmenting modality BMT), and finally clinical evaluation in type 1 Gaucher disease.

In vitro model of Gaucher disease

The cell type affected in Gaucher disease is the macrophage that acquires its storage burden as a result of the phagocytic ingestion of apoptotic cells (Cox and Schofield 1997). A macrophage cell line was therefore induced to resemble a Gaucher macrophage by treating it with an irreversible inhibitor of glucocerebrosidase (EC 3.2.1.45), conduritol β-epoxide (CBE) (Platt *et al.* 1994*a*). Cells were co-administered *N*B-DNJ and CBE and prevention of storage was achieved (as determined by biochemical and EM analysis) at doses between 5 and 50 μM (Platt *et al.* 1994*a*). This validated the approach at the cellular level.

Substrate reduction therapy in a mouse model of Tay–Sachs disease

Engineered (knockout) mouse models of the GSL storage diseases have provided *in vivo* systems in which to evaluate therapeutic strategies and study pathogenesis (Chapter 11). One criterion for the efficacy of SRT is that there be some residual enzyme activity present. A gene knockout model null for the disease-specific enzyme would therefore appear inappropriate. Fortuitously, there are some mouse models, such as the Tay–Sachs (*hexa* $^{-/-}$) mouse, where residual enzyme activity is present due to the activities of other enzymes (Sango *et al.* 1995; Suzuki and Mansson 1998; Suzuki and Proia 1998). Tay–Sachs disease results from mutations in the *HEXA* gene that encodes the α-subunit of β-hexosaminidase (EC 3.2.1.52) (Gravel *et al.* 2001) (Chapter 4, Fig 4.2). This results in a deficiency of the A isoenzyme which is required for the catabolism of GM2 ganglioside in lysosomes. The human disease is characterized by progressive neurodegeneration (Gravel *et al.* 2001). The Tay–Sachs mouse exhibits progressive storage of GM2, but the level of the stored ganglioside never crosses the threshold required to induce neurodegeneration (Cohen-Tannoudji *et al.* 1995; Sango *et al.* 1995; Phaneuf *et al.* 1996). This is because the mouse, in contrast to human, has significant sialidase activity that converts GM2 to GA2 that can then be catabolized by the hexosaminidase B isoenzyme (Sango *et al.* 1995). This feature of the murine catabolic pathway has led to the proposal by Gravel and colleagues of exploiting the sialidase as an alternative target for human Tay–Sachs disease gene therapy or to utilize a pharmacological approach to attempt to stimulate sialidase expression/activity (Igdoura *et al.* 1999).

When the Tay–Sachs mouse model was orally treated with *N*B-DNJ (Table 15.3) two observations were made. Firstly, *N*B-DNJ gained access to the brain and prevented GM2 accumulation, and secondly, the number of storage neurones and their storage burden were greatly reduced in *N*B-DNJ-treated Tay–Sachs mice, when compared with untreated controls (Platt *et al.* 1997*a*). Limiting the biosynthesis of the substrate (GM2) for the defective enzyme (β-hexosaminidase A) therefore prevents GSL accumulation and the neuropathology associated with its lysosomal storage (Platt *et al.* 1997*a*). This study provided proof of concept of SRT at the level of an animal disease model.

Table 15.3 Status of Compounds used for *In vivo* Studies of Glycolipid Storage Disorders

Compound	Pre-clinical Study	Evaluation period	Pre-clinical Study	Evaluation Period	Clinical Trials	Evaluation period	Regulatory status
	Substrate Reduction Therapy: *In vivo* Pre-clinical and Clinical Studies						
	Normal animals		**Disease models**		**Human Storage Disorders**		
*N*B-DNJ	Normal mouse[1] 600 mg/Kg/day 1200 mg/Kg/day 1800 mg/Kg/day 2400 mg/Kg/day Normal rat[2] 180 mg/Kg/day Normal cat[3] 50 mg/Kg/day	 50 days 50 days 20 days 14 days 8–13 weeks 19, 23, 54 & 144 days	Tay–Sachs mouse[4] 4800 mg/Kg/day Sandhoff mouse[5] 2400 mg/Kg/day NPC mouse[3] 1200 mg/Kg/day NPC cat[3] 50–150 mg/Kg/day MPS IIIA mouse[6] 2000 mg/Kg/day	 8 weeks 18 weeks 10 weeks 54 days 10 months	Type I Gaucher[7] 100 mg 3 times daily (TID) Type I Gaucher[8] 100–200 mg TID 100 mg 1–3 times daily Type 1 Gaucher[9] 50 mg TID Type 3 Gaucher[10] Late Onset Tay–Sachs[10] Niemann–Pick Type C[10]	12 months 24 months 6 months In progress In progress In progress	European Union (2002), Israel (2003), and USA (2003) approval for mild to moderate type 1 Gaucher disease – – –
*N*B-DGJ	Normal mouse[11] 2400 mg/Kg/day 300–4800 mg/Kg/day	 5 weeks 10 days	Sandhoff mouse[12] 1200–4800 mg/Kg/day NPC mouse[13]	 23 weeks 11 weeks	–	–	
D-*threo*-EtDO-P4	Normal mouse[14] 2 mg/Kg twice daily	 3 days	Fabry mouse[14] 10 mg/Kg twice daily	 8 weeks	– –	–	
D-*threo*-PDMP	Normal mouse[15] 100 mg/Kg/day	 10 days	–	–	– –	–	

'Chaperone-mediated' Enzyme Folding: *In vivo* Pre-clinical Studies

Compound	Increase in mutant α-galactosidase activity[16]
DGJ (3 or 30 mg/Kg/day)	4.8 or 18-fold in heart, 2 or 2.8 fold in kidney, 3.1 or 7.1 in spleen, 1.7 or 1.8 fold in liver

References: [1]Platt *et al.* 1997b. [2]Narita & Butters (unpublished). [3]Zervas *et al.* 2001. [4]Platt *et al.* 1997a. [5]Jeyakumar *et al.* 1999. [6]Walkley *et al.* unpublished. [7]Cox *et al.* 2000. [8]Zimran & Elstein, 2003. [9]Heitner *et al.* 2002. [10]Oxford GlycoSciences, (unpublished). [11]Andersson *et al.* 2000. [12]Andersson & Platt (unpublished). [13]Gondre-Lewis and Walkley (unpublished). [14]Abe *et al.* 2000. [15]Inokuchi *et al.* 1987. [16]Tominaga *et al.* 2001.

Substrate reduction therapy in a symptomatic model of Sandhoff disease

The mouse model of Sandhoff disease was generated through the targeted disruption of the *Hexb* gene and lacks hexosaminidase A and B isoenzymes, resulting in the storage of GM2 and GA2 gangliosides in the CNS and periphery (Sango *et al.* 1995) (Chapter 11). The Sandhoff disease mouse has very low levels of residual enzyme activity, conferred by the minor hexosaminidase S (α,α) isoenzyme. The mice undergo rapid, progressive neurodegeneration and die at 4–5 months of age (Sango *et al.* 1995). Substrate reduction therapy would be predicted to delay the onset of symptoms and partially extend life expectancy, but lack of residual enzyme will limit the efficacy of SRT. This is analogous to treating the human infantile-onset disease variants.

When Sandhoff disease mice were orally treated with *N*B-DNJ (Table 15.3), their life expectancy was increased by 40% and GSL storage was reduced in peripheral tissues and in the CNS (Jeyakumar *et al.* 1999). Following the onset of clinical signs, the rate of decline was significantly slower in the *N*B-DNJ-treated mice compared with untreated controls. The age at which deterioration could first be detected was approximately 100 days for untreated mice and approximately 135 days for *N*B-DNJ-treated mice. However, the terminal stage of the disease (when the mice are moribund) was prolonged in *N*B-DNJ treated mice. When GSL storage levels were measured in the untreated and *N*B-DNJ-treated Sandhoff mice at their end points (at 125 and 170 days, respectively), the levels of GM2 and GA2 were comparable, indicating that death correlated with the same levels of GSL storage in the brains of the two groups of mice. Histological examination of the mice at day 120 showed reduced storage in the brain of *N*B-DNJ-treated mice. At the ultrastructural level, the neurones showed greatly reduced storage burdens. The reduction in GSL storage was even more pronounced in the liver. In common with other peripheral organs, the liver is exposed to higher concentrations of *N*B-DNJ, whereas only approximately 5–10% of the concentration in the serum is detected in the cerebrospinal fluid (Platt *et al.* 1997*a*).

Substrate reduction therapy in a genetic model

The efficacy of SRT was further demonstrated in the Sandhoff mouse model by Proia and colleagues, who crossed the Sandhoff mouse with a mouse engineered to block the synthesis of the storage GSL (GalNAcT$^{-/-}$ mice) (Liu *et al.* 1999) (Table 15.3). GalNAcT transfers *N*-acetylgalactosamine onto GSL acceptors to synthesize complex GSLs including GM2 and GA2, the major storage GSLs in the Sandhoff mouse. The resulting mice (deficient in GalNAcT and the β-subunit of β-hexosaminidase), therefore, have defects in both GM2 ganglioside synthesis and GM2 ganglioside catabolism. They did not store GlcSL, lived longer, and had greatly improved neurological function.

It is interesting to note that these mice eventually developed storage of oligosaccharides derived from the catabolism of N-linked glycans. These are additional substrates for β-hexosaminidases and are known to accumulate in Sandhoff patients (Chapter 4, Fig. 4.2). This was the first clear indication that stored N-glycans also contribute to neuropathology in this disease. This study elegantly highlighted the potential of SRT and also the limitation of SRT in diseases where the defective enzyme has additional non-GlcSL substrates (Liu *et al.* 1999).

Combination therapy in the Sandhoff mouse

Both *N*B-DNJ-mediated SRT (Jeyakumar *et al.* 1999) and BMT (Norflus *et al.* 1998) have been independently shown to increase life expectancy in the Sandhoff mouse. The main factor that limits the efficacy of SRT in this mouse model is the lack of significant residual enzyme activity. Bone marrow transplantation is limited by the fact that few donor origin cells re-populate the brain and hence the enzyme reconstitution in brain is very low (2–5% of normal levels). It is unclear to what degree the disease process influences the rate of donor cell entry into the brain, and this may vary at different stages in disease progression.

Combining SRT and BMT could be complementary and potentially synergistic. The efficacy of combining these two therapies was therefore assessed. Sandhoff disease mice treated with BMT and *N*B-DNJ survived significantly longer than those treated with BMT or *N*B-DNJ alone. When the mice were subdivided into two groups on the basis of their donor bone marrow-derived CNS enzyme levels, the high-enzyme group exhibited a greater degree of synergy (25%) than the group as a whole (13%). It is interesting to note that the average brain reconstitution achieved in the low-enzyme group was only 1%, less than that in the high-enzyme group. This demonstrates that very modest increases in enzyme when combined with substrate-lowering drugs can have a profound impact on survival. These findings have important implications for future attempts at gene therapy in these diseases as even modest enzyme reconstitution may be adequate if combined with SRT. Combination therapy may therefore be the strategy of choice for treating the infantile-onset disease variants (Jeyakumar *et al.* 2001).

Substrate reduction therapy in a mouse model of Fabry disease

Fabry disease is an X-linked GSL storage disorder characterized by α-galactosidase A (EC 3.2.1.22) deficiency resulting in ceramide trihexoside storage. The primary clinical manifestations in humans include renal and cardiovascular disease, neuropathy, and angiokeratoma (Chapter 3). A mouse model of this disease (α-galactosidase A gene knockout) was generated by Kulkarni and colleagues (Ohshima *et al.* 1997) but lacks a clinical phenotype, presumably due to a salvage pathway in the mouse. Biochemical storage can, however, be demonstrated in this model and hence it is suitable for SRT evaluation. Shayman and colleagues treated the Fabry disease mouse model with the GSL biosynthesis inhibitor D-*threo*-EtDO-P4 (Abe *et al.* 2000). This compound is hydrophobic and was given in the form of liposomes by intraperitoneal injection for 4 or 8 weeks duration. They demonstrated a reduction in ceramide trihexoside levels in multiple organs including kidney and liver. No toxic effects were observed at doses up to 15 mg/kg/day, but weight loss occurred at 30 mg/kg/day, presumably due to this approaching the maximum tolerated dose.

Substrate reduction therapy in a mouse model of Niemann–Pick type C disease

Glycosphingolipid accumulation is not restricted to the "classical" GSL storage diseases in which the inherited defect is in a lysosomal hydrolase (Chapters 2–4). Other lysosomal disorders including Niemann–Pick disease type C (NPC) accumulate GSL in the brain, secondary to the primary defect (Chapter 5, 9 and 12) in the *NPC1* gene (and less commonly the *NPC2* gene). NPC1 is a protein that is localized to vesicles thought to recycle unesterified cholesterol from late endosomes/lysosomes to the ER and Golgi (Chapter 9). Niemann–Pick disease type C has therefore primarily been considered to be a disorder of cholesterol transport. However, certain GlcSLs are stored in the brain in NPC, suggesting that NPC1 may also play a role in both GSL and cholesterol homoeostasis. A critical question in NPC is what causes the neurodegeneration? As GlcSL accumulation in the classical GlcSL storage diseases is known to lead to neuronal dysfunction and death (although precisely how still remains to be determined), Walkley hypothesized that the stored GlcSLs may be contributors to the neuropathology associated with this disease (Zervas *et al.* 2001).

Two classes of GlcSls accumulate in the brain in NPC—neutral GlcSLs and gangliosides with the dominant species being GM2. GM2 is known to cause progressive neurodegeneration when it is stored in patients with Tay–Sachs and Sandhoff disease. Proia and colleagues investigated the contribution of the gangliosides to NPC pathology by crossing the NPC1 mouse (spontaneous model with a lesion in the *NPC1* gene, Chapter 11) with a mouse genetically engineered to prevent it synthesizing GM2 and some other higher GSL species (GalNAcT$^{-/-}$ mice). Neuronal GM2 storage was prevented, but it did not alter the disease course (Liu *et al.* 2000). If GSLs play a role in pathogenesis, it must therefore be the lipids which remain in the double-mutant mice, namely GM3, lactosylceramide, glucosylceramide and free sphingosine.

In an independent study, Walkley and colleagues generated NPC1$^{-/-}$ mice crossed with GalNAcT$^{-/-}$ mice (Gondre-Lewis *et al.* 2003). In this study life expectancy was highly variable in the double mutant mice with some surviving as long as 15 weeks while others died prematurely consistent with the earlier report (Liu, et al, 2000). Most significantly, cholesterol accumulation in neurones of the double mutants was found to be dramatically reduced. Furthermore, neurones storing cholesterol always exhibited GM3 storage but some GM3 positive neurones exhibited no cholesterol increase, findings consistent with cholesterol accumulation secondary to NPC1 deficiency being ganglioside dependent.

Walkley and colleagues used *N*B-DNJ treatment in the NPC1 mouse model (Table 15.3) to determine whether or not any GlcSLs were contributing to the pathology (Zervas *et al.* 2001). They found that life expectancy of the NPC1 mouse was significantly extended and the neuropathology significantly delayed. They obtained similar data in the NPC cat model (Table 15.3) (Zervas *et al.* 2001). These observations in two disparate mammalian species suggest that GlcSLs are involved in the neuropathology of NPC1. However, we currently do not know precisely which of the storage GSL species is contributing to the pathology. The other possibility is that *N*B-DNJ mediates the clinical improvement via a currently unidentified activity of this drug, independent of GSL depletion. However, the imino sugar *N*B-DGJ (galactose analogue) which also inhibits GSL biosynthesis, but does not cause any side effects attributable to *N*B-DNJ (Andersson *et al.* 2000), has the same effect in the NPC1 mouse (Gondré-Lewis and Walkley, unpublished). Life expectancy was extended to the same extent, making a GSL depletion-based mechanisms probable (Zervas *et al.* 2001) although still does not rule out a different biochemical property/activity shared by these compounds.

Clinical evaluation of *N*B-DNJ-mediated substrate reduction therapy in Type 1 Gaucher disease

Following the proof of principle studies *in vitro* and in animal disease models, *N*B-DNJ had the potential for clinical use. Normally, at this stage in drug development, a lengthy process of pre-clinical toxicology and scale up of drug would be required. However, in the case of *N*B-DNJ, this had already taken place due to the drug's previous development as an anti-viral compound. *N*B-DNJ was developed by Monsanto in the 1980s as an anti-human immunodeficiency virus (anti-HIV) compound and has been through phase II clinical testing (Fischl *et al.* 1994). This is based on the α-glucosidase I and II (EC 3.2.1.106 and EC 3.2.1.84, respectively) inhibitory properties of this drug. When N-glycan processing is arrested at the level of α-glucosidases I and II, immature glucosylated N-glycans are present on the HIV envelope glycoproteins gp120 and gp41 (Karlsson *et al.* 1993). Changes occur in the structure of the V1 and V2 loops of gp120 when it folds in the presence of these glucosylated N-glycans (Fischer *et al.* 1996*a*). As a consequence, the virus cannot undergo the post-CD4 binding conformational change required to expose the fusogenic peptide of gp41 (Fischer *et al.*, 1995, 1996*a*,*b*). Human immunodeficiency virus cannot therefore enter the host cell and cause infection. However, because the enzyme target is in the lumen of the ER, very high extracellular concentrations of the drug are needed to achieve α-glucosidase inhibition *in vitro*. For example, *N*B-DNJ has a *Ki* of 0.2 μM against isolated α-glucosidase I *in vitro*, but extracellular concentrations of 0.5 mM are required to achieve inhibition of α-glucosidase I in intact cells in tissue culture (Karlsson *et al.* 1993).

When evaluated in HIV patients, it was not possible to achieve high enough plasma concentrations of this drug, and hence no major impact on viraemia was observed (Fischl *et al.* 1994). However, despite its lack of anti-viral efficacy, several important pieces of information resulted from the HIV clinical trials. *N*B-DNJ was well tolerated, with the major side effect being gastrointestinal (GI) tract distress due to GI tract disaccharidase inhibition, resulting in osmotic diarrhoea. Serum levels in the range of 10–50 μM were achieved through oral dosing (Fischl *et al.* 1994). These levels of compound are known to inhibit GSL biosynthesis *in vitro* in human cells (Platt *et al.* 1994*a*,*b*) and *in vivo* in mice (Platt *et al.* 1997*b*). The glucosyltransferase inhibited by *N*B-DNJ is known to have its catalytic site on the cytosolic face of an early Golgi compartment (Platt and Butters 1995). This is why even though *N*B-DNJ is a weaker inhibitor of the transferase relative to α-glucosidases I and II (*Ki* of 20 and 0.2 μM respectively), high levels of GSL biosynthesis inhibition is achieved *in vivo*, as the enzyme target is more accessible to the drug (Platt *et al.* 1997*b*).

In 1998–1999, patients with non-neuronopathic Gaucher disease were recruited at four centres (Cambridge, Amsterdam, Prague, and Jerusalem) into a 1-year open-label clinical trial of *N*B-DNJ (Cox *et al.* 2000) (Table 15.3). Type 1 Gaucher disease was selected because it has clearly defined clinical end points, no involvement of the CNS, and an effective therapy with which to compare efficacy. Type 1 Gaucher disease is a macrophage disorder characterized by hepatosplenomegaly, anaemia, and bone disease (Chapter 3). The trial was co-ordinated by Oxford GlycoSciences and *N*B-DNJ was referred to as OGT-918. Twenty-eight adult patients (14 females and 14 males) were enrolled, seven of whom had had previous splenectomies. All patients were unable or unwilling to take ERT. Liver and spleen volumes were measured by magnetic resonance imaging (MRI) or computed tomography, and haematological parameters were monitored. In addition, several biochemical markers were measured including chitotriosidase (Aerts and Hollak 1997), cell-surface leucocyte GM1 as an indicator of whether GSL levels were depleted in response to OGT-918 treatment, and the plasma levels of GlcCer, the storage lipid. Most patients were treated with oral doses of 100 mg of OGT-918 three times per day. Three patients received 200 mg three times a day and four patients had their doses lowered to 100 mg once or twice a day. Individualized dosing was based on variation in the pharmacokinetics of the compound, tolerability, and organ volume response after 6 months of treatment.

Pharmacokinetics

On the basis of the *in vitro* studies (Platt *et al.* 1994*a,b*) in normal mice (Platt *et al.* 1997*b*) and animal disease models (Platt *et al.* 1997*a*), it was predicted that a serum level in humans of 5–10 μM should be sufficient to partially inhibit GSL synthesis and impact the disease (Platt and Butters 1998). Pharmacokinetic profiling in a subgroup of patients showed that the drug reached maximum plasma concentrations by 2.5 h with a plasma half-life of 6.3 h. Steady-state concentrations of OGT-918 were achieved by day 15 of dosing, and the mean peak level of OGT-918 over the 12-month study was 6.8 μM with trough values of 3.9 μM (Cox *et al.* 2000).

Side effects

A known side effect of OGT-918 is diarrhoea. This was noted in the previous trial with this compound when it was tested as an anti-viral agent (Fischl *et al.* 1994). The compound is a disaccharidase inhibitor and therefore prevents the breakdown of complex dietary carbohydrates at the intestinal brush border. Unabsorbed sugar molecules remain in the GI tract, leading to the osmotic influx of water into the intestinal lumen, resulting in diarrhoea and flatulence due to enhanced bacterial fermentation.

In the Gaucher clinical study, the dose given was 10-fold lower than in the HIV trial. In the Gaucher trial, it was found that although most patients reported GI tract symptoms as soon as they started taking OGT-918, the diarrhoea spontaneously resolved in most patients within several weeks and did not generally pose a significant problem (Cox *et al.* 2000).

Of the 28 patients enrolled in the trial six withdrew. Two were unable to tolerate the GI tract side effects (one suffered from Parkinson's disease and the other did a lot of business travel). Two patients withdrew due to pre-existing medical conditions (hepatocellular carcinoma and pulmonary hypertension), one additional patient left to start a family, and another was advised by her rabbi to withdraw after 1 day on study. The remaining 22 patients were monitored at 6 and 12 months for signs of clinical improvement. Two further patients withdrew from an extension study because of symptoms of peripheral neuropathy. At the time of writing, some patients in this study had received treatment for 36 months.

Biochemical efficacy

One of the critical issues concerning the use of OGT-918 in humans was whether GlcSL depletion can be achieved. The activity of *N*B-DNJ to inhibit GlcSL biosynthesis was unknown when the HIV clinical trial was conducted, so this property of the drug had never been investigated in humans prior to the Gaucher clinical trial. GlcSL depletion was assessed in three different ways. Firstly, a GlcSL unrelated to the disease was monitored on the cell surface of leucocytes [flow cytometric analysis of GM1, (Platt *et al.* 1994*a*)] to give a sensitive measure of general GSL depletion. A 38.5% reduction after 12 months of therapy (Cox *et al.* 2000) was observed. On a small number of samples, leucocyte LacCer levels (a GlcSL which contributes to the GlcCer storage burden in macrophages due to its abundance in the cells they phagocytose) were measured by TLC and also showed a time-dependent reduction (F. M. Platt and T.D. Butters, unpublished data). Finally, preliminary analysis of GlcCer itself was carried out in the plasma of several patients, and the initial analysis demonstrated reduced levels following treatment (Elstein *et al.* Submitted for publication). Taken together, these data show that at the plasma levels achieved in the study: (a) GlcSL expression is reduced in accordance with the mechanisms of action of this drug: (b) LacCer in leucocytes is reduced, thereby reducing the burden of this lipid ingested by macrophages; and (c) the disease storage product (GlcCer) present in the plasma was reduced from baseline. This therefore provides the biochemical foundation for the proposed SRT mechanism central to this treatment strategy. Furthermore, when the plasma was investigated for the presence of glucosylated N-glycans that arise due to ER α-glucosidase inhibition (the activity of *N*B-DNJ responsible for its anti-viral properties) only trace levels could be detected. Therefore, as predicted from previous studies (reviewed in Platt and Butters 2000), the low dose of compound used in the Gaucher trial has little impact on the other pathway inhibited by this drug, due to the inaccessibility of the α-glucosidase 1 enzyme target (located in the ER lumen).

Clinical efficacy: 1-year Study

Spleen and liver volumes showed a statistically significant reduction (15%, 11.8–18.4, $P < 0.001$and 7%, 3.4–10.5, $P < 0.001$ respectively) after 6 months of therapy. At 12 months, the decrease from baseline was 19% (14.3–23.7, $P < 0.001$) and 12% (7.8–16.4, $P < 0.001$), respectively (Cox *et al.* 2000). This was comparable to the response observed in patients of similar baseline disease severity receiving ERT (Lachmann and Platt 2001). When chitotriosidase, a marker of the disease activity, was measured, the macrophage-derived enzyme showed a time-dependent reduction, indicating a reduction in the total pool of Gaucher cells within the patients treated with OGT-918 (Cox *et al.* 2000). Haematological parameters of haemoglobin and platelet counts showed trends towards improvement, with a greater improvement in haemoglobin noted in patients who were anaemic at baseline. A statistically significant improvement in platelet counts was achieved following 12 months of treatment.

Extension study: 12–24 Months

Longer term efficacy and safety were evaluated in patients who had completed 12 months of therapy (Elstein *et al.* submitted for publication). Eighteen patients were followed up for a further year, and at 24 months a statistically significant improvement in all efficacy end points was observed (organ volumes and haematological parameters). No serious adverse events were reported and no further cases of peripheral neuropathy emerged in this study. Gastrointestinal tract side effects persisted in these patients but to a lesser extent than in the first 12 months. For example, 80% of patients reported diarrhoea as an adverse event in the first 12 months on therapy, but this declined to 14% by 20 months. Bone marrow fat fraction measurements were made in two patients, and the results showed an improvement in fat fraction from baseline by 12 months and an even greater improvement was noted in both individuals at 24 months. This indicates a reduction in the number of Gaucher cells in the bone marrow in response to therapy. In keeping with this observation, chitotriosidase levels continued to decline in the extension phase. The improvement in the key clinical features of the disease achieved after 1 year of therapy was therefore maintained during the extension phase of the study. In 2002, the European regulatory authority (EMEA) approved *N*B-DNJ for use in type 1 Gaucher patients (mild-to-moderate disease, unwilling or unable to receive ERT). In 2003 *N*B-DNJ was also approved in Israel and the USA.

Prospects for combination therapy in Gaucher disease

In principle, it would be predicted that in just the same way that BMT and SRT are synergistic in their action in the Sandhoff mouse model (Jeyakumar *et al.* 2001), combining intravenous ERT and SRT in Gaucher patients would be a potential treatment option. Multiple permutations could be envisaged including monotherapy, sequential therapy (enzyme followed by SRT maintenance), or co-administration (continuous *N*B-DNJ with periodic enzyme administration). One issue, which would restrict direct co-administration, would be inhibition of glucocerebrosidase by *N*B-DNJ, as this compound is a known inhibitor of this enzyme. The IC_{50} for β-glucocerebrosidase inhibition is 520 μM which is 25 times higher than that required to inhibit the ceramide-specific glucosyltransferease (IC_{50} 20 μM) (Platt *et al.* 1994b). Therefore, in the presence of serum concentration of *N*B-DNJ of 5–50 μM *N*B-DNJ will inhibit GSL biosynthesis but not cause inhibition of glucocerebrosidase (Platt *et al.* 1994*b*). This has been confirmed *in vivo* in healthy mice. When mice were treated with *N*B-DNJ 4800 mg/kg/day (50 μM serum level) and co-administered glucocerebrosidase (5–10 U/kg Ceredase™), no inhibition of enzyme was detected (even at inhibitor concentrations above those being achieved in the clinical studies) (Priestman *et al.* 2000). Therefore, co-administration is a viable option as no enzyme inhibition occurs and may increase considerably the therapeutic options for the management of this particular disease.

Future compounds for substrate reduction therapy

The compound *N*B-DGJ is a galactose analogue that is also a potent inhibitor of the ceramide glucosyltransferase (but not the galactosyltransferase important in GalCer synthesis for myelin function). *N*B-DGJ is a more selective enzyme inhibitor with fewer complicating inhibitory properties and will undergo pre-clinical toxicological testing in the near future (Andersson *et al.* 2000). It was found that none of the effects of *N*B-DNJ induced at high doses (10 times greater serum level than the clinical study), such as weight loss and lymphoid organ shrinkage (Platt *et al.* 1997*b*) is attributable to GSL depletion. They must be due to other properties of *N*B-DNJ, since *N*B-DGJ lacks these effects but is an equivalent inhibitor of GSL biosynthesis *in vivo* (Andersson *et al.* 2000) (Table 15.3). This compound does not inhibit sucrase isomaltase and therefore would be predicted to be even better tolerated than *N*B-DNJ due to lack of side effects in the GI tract (Andersson *et al.* 2000).

Current status of studies evaluating substrate reduction therapy for glucosphingolipid storage diseases

The studies to date which explore the use of SRT in mouse and humans are summarized in Table 15.3. More information is available for *N*B-DNJ by virtue of extensive pre-clinical and clinical evaluation. The PDMP series of compounds have yet to be evaluated for efficacy in mouse models with neuronopathic forms of these diseases, and it remains to be determined whether the improved pyrrolidino derivative, (D-*threo*-EtDO-P4) crosses the blood–brain barrier.

Summary

Over the past decade, considerable progress has been made in evaluating SRT using small-molecule inhibitors of the ceramide glucosyltransferase which catalyses the first step in GlcSL biosynthesis. Two classes of inhibitors have been characterized *in vitro* (PDMP series and N-alkylated imino sugars), and more recently the imino sugars have been evaluated in mouse models that have storage in the brain. Efficacy was demonstrated in mouse models of Tay–Sachs and Sandhoff disease. In addition, the D-*threo*-EtDO-P4 compound (PDMP series) has shown efficacy in Fabry mice where it reduced the biochemical storage burden in peripheral tissues. The 2-year clinical study of the imino sugar *N*B-DNJ in type 1 Gaucher disease has provided evidence for improvement in the signs and laboratory features of the disease. The recent approval of this drug for use in type 1 Gaucher patients in Europe, Israel and the USA paves the way for the evaluation of SRT for other sphingolipidoses.

An increase in therapeutic options for type 1 Gaucher disease will provide alternative regimes for treating patients. The fact that two therapeutic measures (ERT and SRT) approach disease therapy from different mechanistic sides of the synthesis : catabolism equation should permit a range of treatment and management protocols to be devised and evaluated clinically.

However, the principle additional contribution that SRT could make would be in the currently refractory and severe variants of Gaucher disease (types 2 and 3) and in the gangliosidoses which all involve storage in the brain. The pre-clinical studies in mouse models of Tay–Sachs and Sandhoff disease (Platt *et al.* 1997*a*; Jeyakumar *et al.* 1999) offer the prospect that these drugs may be of benefit to patients with these conditions, at least those with the juvenile-and adult-onset variants of these disorders. The intractable infantile-onset variants will undoubtedly need an additional enzyme augmenting modality if the pathology is to be improved (Jeyakumar *et al.* 2001). With the advent of more effective means for delivering enzymes to the CNS (Chapters 14 and 16), there is the prospect that over the next decade there may be a number of strategies available for improving the lives of patients suffering from these devastating neurological diseases. It is anticipated that SRT may play a role either as a monotherapy or in combination with other therapeutic modalities.

Acknowledgements

FNP is a Lister Institute Research Fellow. The authors thank Raymond Dwek for a critical reading of the manuscript.

References

Abe, A., Inokuchi, J., Jimbo, M., Shimeno, H., Nagamatsu, A., Shayman, J. A. *et al.* (1992). Improved inhibitors of glucosylceramide synthase. *J Biochem Tokyo*, **111**, 191–6.

Abe, A., Gregory, S., Lee, L., Killen, P. D., Brady, R. O., Kulkarni, A. *et al.* (2000). Reduction of globotriaosylceramide in Fabry disease mice by substrate deprivation. *J Clin Invest*, **105**, 1563–71.

Aerts, J. M. and Hollak, C. E. (1997). Plasma and metabolic abnormalities in Gaucher's disease. *Baillieres Clin Haematol*, **10**, 691–709.

Andersson, U., Butters, T. D., Dwek, R. A. and Platt, F. M. (2000). *N*-butyldeoxygalactonojirimycin: a more selective inhibitor of glycosphingolipid biosynthesis than *N*-butyldeoxynojirimycin, *in vitro* and *in vivo*. *Biochem Pharmacol*, **59**, 821–9.

Asano, N., Ishii, S., Kizu, H., Ikeda, K., Yasuda, K., Kato, A. *et al.* (2000). In vitro inhibition and intracellular enhancement of lysosomal alpha-galactosidase A activity in Fabry lymphoblasts by 1-deoxygalactonojirimycin and its derivatives. *Eur J Biochem*, **267**, 4179–86.

Beutler, E. (1993). Gaucher disease as a paradigm of current issues regarding single gene mutations of humans. *Proc Natl Acad Sci USA*, **90**, 5384–90.

Bieberich, E., Freischutz, B., Suzuki, M. and Yu, R. K. (1999). Differential effects of glycolipid biosynthesis inhibitors on ceramide-induced cell death in neuroblastoma cells. *J Neurochem*, **72**, 1040–9.

Bierfreund, U., Kolter, T. and Sandhoff, K. (2000). Sphingolipid hydrolases and activator proteins. *Methods Enzymol*, **311**, 255–76.

Brigande, J. V. and Seyfried, T. N. (1998). Glycosphingolipid biosynthesis may not be necessary for vertebrate brain development. *Ann N Y Acad Sci*, **845**, 215–8.

Brigande, J. V., Platt, F. M. and Seyfried, T. N. (1998). Inhibition of glycosphingolipid biosynthesis does not impair growth or morphogenesis of the postimplantation mouse embryo. *J Neurochem*, **70**, 871–82.

van den Broek, L. A. G. M., Vermaas, D. J., van Kemenade, F. J., Tan, M. C. C. A., Rotteveel, F. T. M., Zandberg, P. *et al.* (1994). Synthesis of oxygen-substituted N-alkyl 1-deoxynojirimycin derivatives: aza sugar α-glucosidase inhibitors showing antiviral (HIV-1) and immunosuppressive activity. *Recueil des Travaux Chimiques des Pays-Bas*, **113**, 507–16.

Burger, K. N., van der Bijl, P. and van Meer, G. (1996). Topology of sphingolipid galactosyltransferases in ER and Golgi: transbilayer movement of monohexosyl sphingolipids is required for higher glycosphingolipid biosynthesis. *J Cell Biol*, **133**, 15–28.

Butters, T. D., van den Broek, L. A. G. M., Fleet, G. W. J. T. M., Krulle, T. K., Wormald, M. R., Dwek, R. A. *et al.* (1998). Molecular requirements of imino sugars for the selective control of N-linked glycosylation and glycosphingolipid biosynthesis. *Revue Roumaine de Biochimie*, **35**, 75.

Butters, T., Dwek, R. and Platt, F. (2000*a*). Inhibition of glycosphingolipid biosynthesis: application to lysosomal storage disorders. *Chem Rev*, **100**, 4683–96.

Butters, T. D., van den Broek, L. A. G. M., Fleet, G. W. J., Krulle, T. M., Wormald, M. R., Dwek, R. A. *et al.* (2000*b*). Molecular requirements of imino sugars for the selective control of N-linked glycosylation and glycospingolipid biosynthesis. *Tetrahedron Assymetry*, **11**, 113–24.

Chatterjee, S., Cleveland, T., Shi, W. Y., Inokuchi, J. I. and Radin, N. S. (1996). Studies of the action of ceramide-like substances (D- and L-PDMP) on sphingolipid glycosyltransferases and purified lactosylceramide synthase. *Glycoconj J*, **13**, 481–6.

Coetzee, T., Suzuki, K. and Popko, B. (1998). New perspectives on the function of myelin galactolipids. *Trends Neurosci*, **21**, 126–30.

Cohen-Tannoudji, M., Marchand, P., Akli, S., Sheardown, S. A., Puech, J. P., Kress, C. *et al.* (1995). Disruption of murine Hexa gene leads to enzymatic deficiency and to neuronal lysosomal storage, similar to that observed in Tay-Sachs disease. *Mamm Genome*, **6**, 844–9.

Compain, P. and Martin, O. R. (2001). Carbohydrate mimetics-based glycosyltransferase inhibitors. *Bioorg Med Chem*, **9**, 3077–92.

Conzelmann, E. and Sandhoff, K. (1983). Partial enzyme deficiencies: residual activities and the development of neurological disorders. *Dev Neurosci*, **6**, 58–71.

Cox, T. M. and Schofield, J. P. (1997). Gaucher's disease: clinical features and natural history. *Baillieres Clin Haematol*, **10**, 657–89.

Cox, T., Lachmann, R., Hollak, C., Aerts, J., van Weely, S., Hrebicek, M. *et al.* (2000). Novel oral treatment of Gaucher's disease with *N*-butyldeoxynojirimycin (OGT 918) to decrease substrate biosynthesis. *Lancet*, **355**, 1481–5.

Durantel, D., Branza-Nichita, N., Carrouee-Durantel, S., Butters, T. D., Dwek, R. A. and Zitzmann, N. (2001). Study of the mechanism of antiviral action of iminosugar derivatives against bovine viral diarrhea virus. *J Virol*, **75**, 8987–98.

van Echten, G. and Sandhoff, K. (1993). Ganglioside metabolism. Enzymology, Topology, and regulation. *J Biol Chem*, **268**, 5341–4.

Eng, C. M., Guffon, N., Wilcox, W. R., Germain, D. P., Lee, P., Waldek, S. *et al.* (2001). Safety and efficacy of recombinant human alpha-galactosidase A – replacement therapy in Fabry's disease. *N Engl J Med*, **345**, 9–16.

Erikson, A., Groth, C. G., Mansson, J. E., Percy, A., Ringden, O. and Svennerholm, L. (1990). Clinical and biochemical outcome of marrow transplantation for Gaucher disease of the Norrbottnian type. *Acta Paediatr Scand*, **79**, 680–5.

Fan, J. Q., Ishii, S., Asano, N. and Suzuki, Y. (1999). Accelerated transport and maturation of lysosomal alpha-galactosidase A in Fabry lymphoblasts by an enzyme inhibitor. *Nat Med*, **5**, 112–5.

Fenderson, B. A., Ostrander, G. K., Hausken, Z., Radin, N. S. and Hakomori, S. (1992). A ceramide analogue (PDMP) inhibits glycolipid synthesis in fish embryos. *Exp Cell Res*, **198**, 362–6.

Fischer, P. B., Collin, M., Karlsson, G. B., James, W., Butters, T. D., Davis, S. J. *et al.* (1995). The alpha-glucosidase inhibitor *N*-butyldeoxynojirimycin inhibits human immunodeficiency virus entry at the level of post-CD4 binding. *J Virol*, **69**, 5791–7.

Fischer, P. B., Karlsson, G. B., Butters, T. D., Dwek, R. A. and Platt, F. M. (1996*a*). *N*-butyldeoxynojirimycin-mediated inhibition of human immunodeficiency virus entry correlates with changes in antibody recognition of the V1/V2 region of gp120. *J Virol*, **70**, 7143–52.

Fischer, P. B., Karlsson, G. B., Dwek, R. A. and Platt, F. M. (1996*b*). *N*-butyldeoxynojirimycin-mediated inhibition of human immunodeficiency virus entry correlates with impaired gp120 shedding and gp41 exposure. *J Virol*, **70**, 7153–60.

Fischl, M. A., Resnick, L., Coombs, R., Kremer, A. B., Pottage, J. C. Jr, Fass, R. J. *et al.* (1994). The safety and efficacy of combination N-butyl-deoxynojirimycin (SC-48334) and zidovudine in patients with HIV-1 infection and 200–500 CD4 cells/mm^3. *J Acquir Immune Defic Syndr*, **7**, 139–47.

Frustaci, A., Chimenti, C., Ricci, R., Natale, L., Russo, M. A., Pieroni, M. *et al.* (2001). Improvement in cardiac function in the cardiac variant of Fabry's disease with galactose-infusion therapy. *N Engl J Med*, **345**, 25–32.

Gagneux, P. and Varki, A. (1999). Evolutionary considerations in relating oligosaccharide diversity to biological function. *Glycobiology*, **9**, 747–55.

Galbiati, F., Razani, B. and Lisanti, M. P. (2001). Emerging themes in lipid rafts and caveolae. *Cell*, **106**, 403–11.

Gondre-Lewis, McGlynn, R. and Walkley, S.U. (2003). Cholesterol accumulation in NPC1-deficient neurons is ganglioside dependent. *Curr Biol*, **13**, 1324–9.

Gravel, R. A., Kaback, M. M., Proia, R. L., Sandhoff, K., Suzuki, K. and Suzuki, K. (2001). The GM2 gangaliosidoses. In *The metabolic and molecular bases of inherited disease* (Scriver, C. R., Beadet, A. L., Valle, D. and Sly, W. S., ed.), Vol. 3, pp. 3827–76. New York: McGraw-Hill.

Hadjiconstantinou, M. and Neff, N. H. (1998). GM1 ganglioside: in vivo and in vitro trophic actions on central neurotransmitter systems. *J Neurochem*, **70**, 1335–45.

Hakomori, S. I. (2000). Cell adhesion/recognition and signal transduction through glycosphingolipid microdomain. *Glycoconj J*, **17**, 143–51.

Heitner, R., Elstein, D., Aerts, J., van Weely, S. and Zimran, A. (2002). Low dose *N*-butyldeoxynojirimycin (OGT 918) for type 1 Gaucher disease. Blood Cells, *Molecules and Diseases*, **28**, 127–33.

Ichikawa, S. and Hirabayashi, Y. (1998). Glucosylceramide synthase and glycosphingolipid synthesis. *Trends Cell Biol*, **8**, 198–202.

Ichikawa, S., Nakajo, N., Sakiyama, H. and Hirabayashi, Y. (1994). A mouse B16 melanoma mutant deficient in glycolipids. *Proc Natl Acad Sci USA*, **91**, 2703–7.

Igdoura, S. A., Mertineit, C., Trasler, J. M. and Gravel, R. A. (1999). Sialidase-mediated depletion of GM2 ganglioside in Tay–Sachs neuroglia cells. *Hum Mol Genet*, **8**, 1111–6.

Inokuchi, J. and Radin, N. S. (1987). Preparation of the active isomer of 1-phenyl-2-decanoylamino-3-morpholino-1-propanol, inhibitor of murine glucocerebroside synthetase. *J Lipid Res*, **28**, 565–71.

Inokuchi, J., Mason, I. and Radin, N. S. (1987). Antitumor activity via inhibition of glycosphingolipid biosynthesis. *Cancer Lett*, **38**, 23–30.

Jefferies, I. and Bowen, B. R. (1997). Synthesis of inhibitors of [alpha]-1,3-fucosyltransferase. *Bioorg Med Chem Lett*, **7**, 1171–4.

Jeyakumar, M., Butters, T. D., Cortina-Borja, M., Proia, R. L., Perry, V. H., Dwek, R. A. *et al.* (1999). Delayed symptom onset and increased life expectancy in Sandhoff disease mice treated with *N*-butyldeoxynojirimycin. *Proc Natl Acad Sci USA*, **96**, 6388–93.

Jeyakumar, M., Norflus, F., Tifft, C. J., Cortina-Borja, M., Butters, T. D., Proia, R. L. *et al.* (2001). Enhanced survival in Sandhoff disease mice receiving a combination of substrate deprivation therapy and bone marrow transplantation. *Blood*, **97**, 327–29.

Karlsson, G. B., Butters, T. D., Dwek, R. A. and Platt, F. M. (1993). Effects of the imino sugar *N*-butyldeoxynojirimycin on the N-glycosylation of recombinant gp120. *J Biol Chem*, **268**, 570–6.

Kobayashi, T. and Hirabayashi, Y. (2000). Lipid membrane domains in cell surface and vacuolar systems. *Glycoconj J*, **17**, 163–71.

Lachmann, R. H. and Platt, F. M. (2001). Substrate reduction therapy for glycosphingolipid storage disorders. *Exp Opin Investig Drugs*, **10**, 455–66.

Lee, L., Abe, A. and Shayman, J. A. (1999). Improved inhibitors of glucosylceramide synthase. *J Biol Chem*, **274**, 14662–9.

Liu, Y., Wada, R., Kawai, H., Sango, K., Deng, C., Tai, T. *et al.* (1999). A genetic model of substrate deprivation therapy for a glycosphingolipid storage disorder. *J Clin Invest*, **103**, 497–505.

Liu, Y., Wu, Y. P., Wada, R., Neufeld, E. B., Mullin, K. A., Howard, A. C. *et al.* (2000). Alleviation of neuronal ganglioside storage does not improve the clinical course of the Niemann–Pick C disease mouse. *Hum Mol Genet*, **9**, 1087–92.

Max, S. R., Maclaren, N. K., Brady, R. O., Bradley, R. M., Rennels, M. B., Tanaka, J. *et al.* (1974). GM3 (hematoside) sphingolipodystrophy. *N Engl J Med*, **291**, 929–31.

Meikle, P. J., Hopwood, J. J., Clague, A. E. and Carey, W. F. (1999). Prevalence of lysosomal storage disorders. *JAMA*, **281**, 249–54.

Mellor, H.R., Platt, F.M., Dwek, R.A and Butters, T.D. (2003). Membrane disruption and cytotoxicity of hydrophobic N-alkylated imino sugars is independent of the inhibition of protein and lipid glycosylation. *Biochem J*, **374**, 307–14.

Miura, T., Kajimoto, T., Jimbo, M., Yamagishi, K., Inokuchi, J. C. and Wong, C. H. (1998). Synthesis and evaluation of morpholino- and pyrrolidinosphingolipids as inhibitors of glucosylceramide synthase. *Bioorg Med Chem*, **6**, 1481–9.

Neufeld, E. F. (1991). Lysosomal storage diseases. *Annu Rev Biochem*, **60**, 257–80.

Norflus, F., Tifft, C. J., McDonald, M. P., Goldstein, G., Crawley, J. N., Hoffmann, A. *et al.* (1998). Bone marrow transplantation prolongs life span and ameliorates neurologic manifestations in Sandhoff disease mice. *J Clin Invest*, **101**, 1881–8.

Ohshima, T., Murray, G. J., Swaim, W. D., Longenecker, G., Quirk, J. M., Cardarelli, C. O. *et al.* (1997). alpha-Galactosidase A deficient mice: a model of Fabry disease. *Proc Natl Acad Sci USA*, **94**, 2540–4.

Overkleeft, H. S., Renkema, G. H., Neele, J., Vianello, P., Hung, I. O., Strijland, A. *et al.* (1998). Generation of specific deoxynojirimycin-type inhibitors of the non-lysosomal glucosylceramidase. *J Biol Chem*, **273**, 26522–7.

Persson, K., Ly, H. D., Dieckelmann, M., Wakarchuk, W. W., Withers, S. G. and Strynadka, N. C. J. (2001). Crystal structure of the retaining galactosyltransferase LgtC from *Neisseria meningitidis* in complex with donor and acceptor sugar analogs. *Nat Struct Biol*, **8**, 166–75.

Phaneuf, D., Wakamatsu, N., Huang, J. Q., Borowski, A., Peterson, A. C., Fortunato, S. R. *et al.* (1996). Dramatically different phenotypes in mouse models of human Tay–Sachs and Sandhoff diseases. *Hum Mol Genet*, **5**, 1–14.

Platt, F. M. and Butters, T. D. (1995). Inhibitors of glycosphingolipid biosynthesis. *Trends in Glycosci Glycotechnol*, **7**, 495–511.

Platt, F. M. and Butters, T. D. (1998). New therapeutic prospects for the glycosphingolipid lysosomal storage diseases. *Biochem Pharmacol*, **56**, 421–30.

Platt, F. M. and Butters, T. D. (2000). Substrate deprivation: A new therapeutic approach for the glycosphingolpid lysosomal storage diseases. *Expert Reviews in Molecular Medicine.* http://www-ermm.cbcu.cam.ac.uk

Platt, F. M., Neises, G. R., Dwek, R. A. and Butters, T. D. (1994*a*). *N*-butyldeoxynojirimycin is a novel inhibitor of glycolipid biosynthesis. *J Biol Chem*, **269**, 8362–5.

Platt, F. M., Neises, G. R., Karlsson, G. B., Dwek, R. A. and Butters, T. D. (1994*b*). *N*-butyldeoxygalactonojirimycin inhibits glycolipid biosynthesis but does not affect N-linked oligosaccharide processing. *J Biol Chem*, **269**, 27108–14.

Platt, F. M., Neises, G. R., Reinkensmeier, G., Townsend, M. J., Perry, V. H., Proia, R. L. *et al.* (1997*a*). Prevention of lysosomal storage in Tay–Sachs mice treated with *N*-butyldeoxynojirimycin. *Science*, **276**, 428–31.

Platt, F. M., Reinkensmeier, G., Dwek, R. A. and Butters, T. D. (1997*b*). Extensive glycosphingolipid depletion in the liver and lymphoid organs of mice treated with *N*-butyldeoxynojirimycin. *J Biol Chem*, **272**, 19365–72.

Priestman, D. A., Platt, F. M., Dwek, R. A. and Butters, T. D. (2000). Imino sugar therapy for type 1 Gaucher disease. *Glycobiology*, **10**, iv–vi.

Qiao, L., Murray, B. W., Shimazaki, M., Schultz, J. and Wong, C.-H. (1996). Synergistic inhibition of human alpha-1,3-fucosyltransferase V. *J Am Chem Soc*, **118**, 7653–62.

Radin, N. S. (1996). Treatment of Gaucher disease with an enzyme inhibitor. *Glycoconj J*, **13**, 153–7.

Rahmann, H. (1995). Brain gangliosides and memory formation. *Behav Brain Res*, **66**, 105–16.

Rapola, J. (1994). Lysosomal storage diseases in adults. *Pathol Res Pract*, **190**, 759–66.

Ringden, O., Groth, C. G., Erikson, A., Granqvist, S., Mansson, J. E. and Sparrelid, E. (1995). Ten years' experience of bone marrow transplantation for Gaucher disease. *Transplantation*, **59**, 864–70.

Sandhoff, K. and van Echten, G. (1994). Ganglioside metabolism: enzymology, topology and regulation. *Prog Brain Res*, **101**, 17–29.

Sandhoff, K. and Kolter, T. (1996). Topology of glycosphingolipid degradation. *Trends Cell Biol*, **6**, 98–103.

Sandhoff, K. and Kolter, T. (1997). Biochemistry of glycosphingolipid degradation. *Clin Chim Acta*, **266**, 51–61.

Sandhoff, K., Kolter, T. and Van Echten Deckert, G. (1998). Sphingolipid metabolism. Sphingoid analogs, sphingolipid activator proteins, and the pathology of the cell. *Ann N Y Acad Sci*, **845**, 139–51.

Sango, K., Yamanaka, S., Hoffmann, A., Okuda, Y., Grinberg, A., Westphal, H. *et al.* (1995). Mouse models of Tay–Sachs and Sandhoff diseases differ in neurologic phenotype and ganglioside metabolism. *Nat Genet*, **11**, 170–6.

Sawkar, A. R., Cheng, W.-C., Beutler, E., Wong, C.-H., Balch, W. E. and Kelly, J. W. (2002). Chemical chaperones increase the cellular activity of N370S -glucosidase: a therapeutic strategy for Gaucher disease. *Proc Natl Acad Sci USA*, **99**, 15428–33.

Schachter, H. (2001). Congenital disorders involving defective N-glycosylation of proteins. *Cell Mol Life Sci*, **58**, 1085–104.

Schaub, C., Muller, B. and Schmidt, R. R. (1998). New sialyltransferase inhibitors based on CMP-quinic acid: development of a new sialyltransferase assay. *Glycoconj J*, **15**, 345–54.

Schiffmann, R., Kopp, J. B., Austin, H. A. III, Sabnis, S., Moore, D. F., Weibel, T. *et al.* (2001). Enzyme replacement therapy in Fabry disease: a randomized controlled trial. *JAMA*, **285**, 2743–9.

Schroder, P. N. and Giannis, A. (1999). From substrate to transition state analogues: The first potent inhibitor of sialyltransferases. *Angew Chem Int Ed*, **38**, 1379–80.

Schuette, C. G., Doering, T., Kolter, T. and Sandhoff, K. (1999). The glycosphingolipidoses-from disease to basic principles of metabolism. *Biol Chem*, **380**, 759–66.

Schuster, M. and Blechert, S. (2001). Inhibition of fucosyltransferase V by a GDP-azasugar. *Bioorg Med Chem Lett*, **11**, 1809–11.

Sheikh, K. A., Sun, J., Liu, Y., Kawai, H., Crawford, T. O., Proia, R. L. *et al.* (1999). Mice lacking complex gangliosides develop Wallerian degeneration and myelination defects. *Proc Natl Acad Sci USA*, **96**, 7532–7.

Stern, C. A. and Tiemeyer, M. (2001). A ganglioside-specific sialyltransferase localizes to axons and non-Golgi structures in neurons. *J Neurosci*, **21**, 1434–43.

Sun, H. B., Yang, J. S., Amaral, K. E. and Horenstein, B. A. (2001). Synthesis of a new transition-state analog of the sialyl donor. Inhibition of sialyltransferases. *Tetrahedron Lett*, **42**, 2451–3.

Suzuki, K. and Mansson, J.-E. (1998). Animal models of lysosomal disease: an overview. *J Inher Metab Dis*, **21**, 540–7.

Suzuki, K. and Proia, R. L. (1998). Mouse models of human lysosomal diseases. *Brain Pathol*, **8**, 195–215.

Taga, S., Tetaud, C., Mangeney, M., Tursz, T. and Wiels, J. (1995). Sequential changes in glycolipid expression during human B cell differentiation: enzymatic bases. *Biochim Biophys Acta*, **1254**, 56–65.

Takamiya, K., Yamamoto, A., Furukawa, K., Yamashiro, S., Shin, M., Okada, M. *et al.* (1996). Mice with disrupted GM2/GD2 synthase gene lack complex gangliosides but exhibit only subtle defects in their nervous system. *Proc Natl Acad Sci USA*, **93**, 10662–7.

Takayama, S., Chung, S. J., Igarashi, Y., Ichikawa, Y., Sepp, A., Lechler, R. I. *et al.* (1999). Selective inhibition of [beta]-1,4- and [alpha]-1,3-galactosyltransferases: donor sugar-nucleotide based approach. *Bioorg Med Chem*, **7**, 401–9.

Tanaka, J., Garcia, J. H., Max, S. R., Viloria, J. E., Kamijyo, Y., McLaren, N. K. *et al.* (1975). Cerebral sponginess and GM3 gangliosidosis; ultrastructure and probable pathogenesis. *J Neuropathol Exp Neurol*, **34**, 249–62.

Tominaga, L., Ogawa, Y., Taniguchi, M., Ohno, K., Matsuda, J., Oshima, A. *et al.* (2001). Galactonojirimycin derivatives restore mutant human beta-galactosidase activities expressed in fibroblasts from enzyme-deficient knockout mouse. *Brain Dev*, **23**, 284–7.

Trinchera, M., Fabbri, M. and Ghidoni, R. (1991). Topography of glycosyltransferases involved in the initial glycosylations of gangliosides. *J Biol Chem*, **266**, 20907–12 (ISSN: 0021–9258).

Unligil, U. M. and Rini, J. M. (2000). Glycosyltransferase structure and mechanism. *Curr Opin Struct Biol*, **10**, 510–7.

Vunnam, R. R. and Radin, N. S. (1980). Analogs of ceramide that inhibit glucocerebroside synthetase in mouse brain. *Chem Phys Lipids*, **26**, 265–78.

Walkley, S. U. and Dobrenis, K. (1995). Bone marrow transplantation for lysosomal diseases [comment]. *Lancet*, **345**, 1382–3.

Walkley, S. U., Thrall, M. A., Dobrenis, K., Huang, M., March, P. A., Siegel, D. A. *et al.* (1994). Bone marrow transplantation corrects the enzyme defect in neurons of the central nervous system in a lysosomal storage disease. *Proc Natl Acad Sci USA*, **91**, 2970–4.

Walkley, S. U., Siegel, D. A., Dobrenis, K. and Zervas, M. (1998). GM2 ganglioside as a regulator of pyramidal neuron dendritogenesis. *Ann N Y Acad Sci*, **845**, 188–99.

Withers, S. G. (2001). Mechanisms of glycosyl transferases and hydrolases. *Carbohyd Polym*, **44**, 325–37.

Yamashita, T., Wada, R., Sasaki, T., Deng, C., Bierfreund, U., Sandhoff, K. *et al.* (1999). A vital role for glycosphingolipid synthesis during development and differentiation. *Proc Natl Acad Sci USA*, **96**, 9142–7.

Zeller, C. B. and Marchase, R. B. (1992). Gangliosides as modulators of cell function. *Am J Physiol*, **262**, C1341–55.

Zervas, M., Somers, K. L., Thrall, M. A. and Walkley, S. U. (2001). Critical role for glycosphingolipids in Niemann–Pick disease type C. *Curr Biol*, **11**, 1283–7.

Zimran, A. and Elstein, D. (2003). Gaucher disease and the clinical experience with substrate reduction therapy. *Phil Trans R Soc Lond B*, **358**, 961–6.

Chapter 16

Gene therapy

Mark S. Sands

Introduction

Gene replacement represents a therapeutic approach that is conceptually very simple (Friedmann 1999). This approach entails delivering a functional copy of the mutant gene to cells so that they now produce the deficient protein. Gene therapy for lysosomal storage diseases may offer several advantages over enzyme replacement therapy (ERT)(Chapter 13) or bone marrow transplantation (BMT)(Chapter 14) strategies. Although ERT is effective at reducing lysosomal storage, it is extremely expensive and transient in nature requiring repeated injections for the life of the patient (Eng *et al.* 2001; Kakkis *et al.* 2001). In addition, in most cases, soluble enzyme is incapable of crossing the blood–brain barrier when administered systemically, thereby, making ERT ineffective for central nervous system (CNS) disease (Shull *et al.* 1994; Vogler *et al.* 1999) (Chapter 13). In theory, gene therapy may provide a means to permanently alter the genetic makeup of a subset of cells so that they produce the therapeutic enzyme for the life of the patient. While allogeneic BMT can also achieve this goal, graft rejection and graft-versus-host disease are often associated with this procedure and can severely limit its efficacy (Chapter 14). A gene therapy approach directed to the patient's own haematopoietic system would eliminate these adverse consequences. Finally, depending on the type of gene transfer vector used and the route of administration, gene therapy may be able to be performed without any severe conditioning regimens.

Lysosomal storage diseases are considered excellent candidates for gene therapy (Daly and Sands 1998). Most lysosomal storage diseases are caused by single gene defects and are inherited in an autosomal recessive fashion (Neufeld 1991; Neufeld and Muenzer 1995). A child must inherit one defective gene from each parent to have the enzyme deficiency and present with the clinical signs of disease. The fact that the parents are asymptomatic heterozygotes, usually with 50% normal enzyme levels, suggests that the normal amount of enzyme is not required for a therapeutic response. In fact, the results from several studies suggest that enzyme levels as low as 1–10% normal may be efficacious (Wolfe *et al.* 1992*a*; Marechal *et al.* 1993; Moullier *et al.* 1993). This is an important point since it is often difficult to fully reconstitute normal levels of expression using a gene therapy approach. Furthermore, since these genetic diseases are not dominant in nature, the mutant genes in the affected children do not interfere with the function of the normal gene product. Rather, the defective genes simply are not producing any protein or are producing a protein that is enzymatically inactive. Therefore, it is not necessary to actually correct the defective genes. Simply adding a functional copy of the gene to a cell should correct the biochemical defect. Although several lysosomal enzyme deficiencies are inherited as X-linked traits (Chapter 3), it is likely that a gene replacement strategy would also provide a therapeutic response for those disorders. Finally, due to the phenomenon of cross correction, successful gene transfer to a relatively small subset of cells may be sufficient to reduce lysosomal storage throughout an organ or tissue (Neufeld and Fratantoni 1970) (Chapter 13).

Although conceptually simple, the delivery of genetic material and subsequent expression of a therapeutic protein in a whole animal or patient has proven technically difficult. The transfer of genetic material into cultured cells has been accomplished by microinjection-, chemical- (dextran, calcium phosphate, and cationic lipids), receptor ligand-, and viral-mediated approaches. Most of these approaches are either impractical or far too inefficient for *in vivo* applications. However, viral-mediated approaches take advantage of the mechanisms that viruses have evolved to efficiently transfer their genetic material into cells. Thus, viral vectors represent one of the most promising methods of gene transfer. Most of the progress with gene therapy approaches in whole animal models of human disease has been made using viral gene transfer vectors. Therefore, the discussion of gene therapy for CNS manifestations of lysosomal storage diseases will be limited to studies utilizing viral-mediated approaches.

Therapeutic principle

The same basic principle underlying other therapeutic strategies for lysosomal storage diseases, such as BMT and ERT, also applies for gene therapy approaches. Most therapeutic strategies rely on the fact that a small percentage of lysosomal enzymes are secreted from a cell and are then recaptured by either the same cell or an adjacent cell by a receptor-mediated mechanism. The enzymes that are endocytosed from the extracellular milieu are trafficked to the lysosomal compartment where they function normally. This biological process, originally referred to as 'cross correction' was first described by Dr E. Neufeld (Neufeld and Fratantoni 1970). A number of groups have since dissected the molecular mechanisms underlying this biological process (Kornfeld 1992; Kornfeld and Sly 1995). The original discovery of cross correction and the subsequent understanding of the mechanisms involved have led to a more systematic approach to the development of effective therapies (Chapter 13).

In a gene therapy approach, it would be ideal to permanently modify all of the affected cells in a patient so that they could produce normal levels of the deficient enzyme for the remainder of the patient's life. This would preclude the need for repeated administration of exogenous enzyme. Unfortunately, the technology required to faithfully regulate gene expression or to stably modify the genetic makeup of virtually every cell in a tissue or in the entire body does not currently exist. Therefore, a gene therapy approach for most lysosomal storage diseases will take advantage of the process of cross correction. In theory, it may be possible to genetically modify a few cells, which can stably overexpress the deficient enzyme. The genetically modified cells could then secrete higher levels of enzyme and correct adjacent cells. If the expression level is high enough, the modified cells would secrete sufficient levels of enzyme into the circulation to provide a systemic response.

The basic gene therapy approach outlined above would likely be effective for many of the lysosomal storage diseases since most lysosomal enzymes are modified and trafficked through the cell similarly. However, it is unlikely that all lysosomal disorders would respond to this approach. For example, diseases affecting lysosome function such as Niemann–Pick C (Carstea *et al.* 1997) and the juvenile form of neuronal ceroid lipofuscinosis (The International Batten Disease Consortium 1995) are both caused by defects in membrane-bound proteins (Chapter 9). Cross correction would not occur since these proteins are not soluble and cannot be secreted and recaptured by adjacent cells. In this situation, all or most of the affected cells would have to be corrected by gene therapy or replaced (for example by stem cell transplantation). The techniques required to accomplish these goals do not currently exist.

Barriers to effective therapy for central nervous system diseases

The progressive accumulation of undegraded material in the brain and the accompanying cognitive deficits associated with many of the lysosomal storage diseases represent some of the most severe clinical features of these diseases (Chapter 3). In addition, there are anatomical features of the brain that create significant obstacles to the development of effective CNS-directed therapies. Numerous studies have demonstrated that BMT or ERT can prevent or reduce the accumulation of undegraded substrates in many tissues outside of the CNS (Chapters 13 and 14). However, with a few notable exceptions (Taylor *et al.* 1986, 1992; Walkley *et al.* 1994*a*), these approaches are only minimally effective at reducing the lysosomal storage that accumulates in the CNS. The decreased efficacy is probably due to the presence of the blood–brain barrier, which effectively blocks most soluble molecules from entering the brain (Lattera *et al.* 1992; Kennedy and Abkowitz 1997; Vogler *et al.* 1999). Safe and effective methods to open (hyperosmotic agents such as mannitol), bypass (intracranial or intrathecal injections), or transport (TAT-mediated protein transduction) enzyme, virus particles, or cells across the blood–brain barrier will have to be developed in order to deliver therapeutic amounts of the deficient enzyme to the brain.

Another characteristic of the CNS that has limited the effectiveness of gene therapy approaches is the fact that most neurons in the brain are post-mitotic. This precludes the use of murine-based retroviral vectors for CNS-directed therapy since cell division is required for the recombinant retroviral genome to enter the cell nucleus. This obstacle has been at least partially overcome by the recent development of adeno-associated virus (AAV) and lentiviral gene transfer vectors, both of which can infect neurons of the brain (Muzyczka 1994; Naldini *et al.* 1996). However, viral gene transfer vectors that have a greater tropism for neurons, such as replication-defective herpes or rabies viruses, would probably increase the efficacy of CNS-directed gene therapy. Similarly, the efficacy of CNS-directed gene therapy may be limited if it is initiated in the advanced stages of the disease when there has been significant neuronal loss or irreversible damage (Chapter 12). In this case, the dead or permanently damaged cells may not be readily replaced as might occur in other tissues that have a greater regenerative capacity. Therefore, the therapeutic intervention may have to be initiated prior to the onset of CNS-associated symptoms. Alternatively, in cases where the onset of CNS disease is delayed, therapeutic intervention after the initial signs of cognitive dysfunction are detected could greatly slow disease progression and improve the quality of life.

Gene therapy for lysosomal storage diseases affecting the brain

Ex vivo gene therapy

Ex vivo gene therapy refers to the genetic modification of autologous, allogeneic, or xenogeneic cells outside the body, then transplantation of those modified cells into an affected individual. Most of the *ex vivo* gene therapy approaches attempted so far involve the manipulation of cells derived from the haematopoietic system. Therapies involving the haematopoietic system are covered in detail in Chapter 14 and will be discussed here only as they relate to gene therapy and the CNS. Haematopoietic-directed therapy for lysosomal storage diseases is based on the principle that if an affected patient's haematopoietic system could be replaced by one that expresses the deficient enzyme, then those cells should have access to most tissues of the body and be able to correct surrounding cells through the process of cross correction (Hobbs *et al.*1981).

Haematopoietic-directed gene therapy has the potential to treat lysosomal storage diseases that affect the brain, since haematopoietic-derived cells (microglia) are found throughout the CNS. There are examples in animal models where BMT or haematopoietic-directed gene therapy provided enzyme activity to the brain or demonstrated efficacy for certain lysosomal storage diseases (Yeager *et al.* 1984; Taylor *et al* 1986, 1992; Shull *et al.* 1987; Hoogerbrugge *et al.* 1988; Walkley *et al.* 1994*a*; Miranda *et al.* 1997, 1998; Norflus *et al.* 1998). However, studies in other animal models of lysosomal storage disease suggest that a haematopoietic-directed approach will not be effective for the disease in the brain (Birkenmeier *et al.* 1991, Poorthuis *et al.* 1994, Walkley *et al.* 1994b). In fact, even if the therapy was initiated in mice with mucopolysaccharidosis type VII at a time when there was little or no evidence of storage (newborns), there was still little or no reduction of disease in the brain (Sands *et al.* 1993). The exact reasons for the different CNS responses to BMT in various lysosomal storage diseases are not clear. However, a number of factors such as differences in enzyme secretion, differences in cell migration and the effects of different storage products on brain development or toxicity could affect efficacy (Walkley and Dobrenis 1995).

Results from haematopoietic-directed gene therapy experiments generally mimic the experience with BMT. The reduction of storage, reduced Purkinje cell loss, and delayed onset of ataxia observed in the arylsulfatase A-deficient mouse following BMT were also observed following haematopoietic stem cell-directed gene therapy (Miranda *et al.* 2000). The results of BMT and hematopoietic stem cell-directed gene therapy in mucopolysaccharidosis type VII (MPS VII) mice were also similar. Both BMT and haematopoietic-directed gene therapy resulted in a dramatic reduction of lysosomal storage in some visceral organs in a murine model of β-glucuronidase deficiency but neither form of therapy reduced storage in the brain (Wolfe *et al.* 1992*a*; Marechal 1993). However, it may be possible to increase the efficacy of haematopoietic-directed gene therapy by simply increasing the level of expression in the transplanted cells. This has been demonstrated in principle in the murine model of galactosialidosis [protective protein/cathepsin A (PPCA) deficiency]. Bone marrow cells overexpressing lysosomal PPCA from either an erythroid- or myeloid-specific promoter provided more complete correction than bone marrow-derived cells expressing normal levels of protein (Zhou *et al.* 1995; Hahn *et al.* 1998). Most notably, there was less Purkinje cell loss and improved motor coordination following transplantation with bone marrow overexpressing PPCA in the monocyte/macrophage lineages.

Although most *ex vivo* gene therapy experiments for lysosomal storage diseases have been directed to the haematopoietic system, it may be possible to obtain similar or perhaps more complete levels of correction by targeting other cell types. Syngeneic or autologous fibroblasts have been engineered to overexpress β-glucuronidase activity, incorporated into an inert matrix, and then implanted into the peritoneum of MPS VII mice or dogs, respectively (Moullier *et al.* 1993; Wolfe *et al.* 2000). In a similar approach, cells overexpressing β-glucuronidase were encapsulated in alginate microspheres and then implanted into the peritoneum of MPS VII mice (Ross *et al.* 2000*a*). In each case, lysosomal storage was reduced in several tissues. Although there was no reduction of lysosomal storage in the CNS, these approaches may be effective if the artificial organoids or engineered cells themselves were implanted into the brain. For example, microencapsulated cells over expressing β-glucuronidase were implanted into the lateral ventricles of MPS VII mice (Ross *et al.* 2000*b*). These cells produced high levels of enzyme, reduced lysosomal storage in the brain and partially corrected the circadian rhythm abnormalities observed in the MPS VII mouse. In another experiment, both low level expression and reduction of lysosomal storage near the graft were observed in the brains of MPS VII mice following implantation of syngeneic fibroblasts expressing β-glucuronidase from a retroviral vector (Taylor and Wolfe 1997). Similar results were obtained following transplantation of amniotic epithelial cells transduced with a recombinant adenoviral vector into the brains of MPS VII mice (Kosuga *et al.* 2000). In both cases, although the implanted cells appeared to persist, the expression from retroviral and adenoviral vectors decreased with time. It is well known that in most cases, *in vivo* expression from murine-based retroviruses and adenoviruses is transient (Palmer *et al.* 1991; Yang *et al.* 1994). However, these studies represent proof-of-principle experiments demonstrating the potential of this strategy. Perhaps more promising is the use of multipotent neuronal progenitor cells that have the capacity to migrate throughout the brain and differentiate into many different types of neuronal cells. Widespread reduction of lysosomal storage was observed in the brains of MPS VII mice after implantation of neuronal progenitor cells expressing normal levels of β-glucuronidase activity (Snyder *et al.* 1995). When the biology of neuronal progenitors is better understood and the technology advances so that autologous neuronal progenitor cells could be isolated and genetically engineered to express the deficient enzyme, this may represent a viable therapeutic approach.

Ex vivo gene therapy is a promising approach for the treatment of certain lysosomal storage diseases that affect the CNS. However, before this can be widely and effectively used in patients, additional research is required to better understand the underlying pathophysiology of lysosomal storage diseases, to determine the appropriate target cells, gene transfer vectors and transplantation protocols, and finally to define the ages at which therapy will be most efficacious.

In vivo gene therapy

In vivo gene therapy refers to the direct genetic manipulation of cells in the body. Although this approach may appear straightforward and perhaps technically easier than an *ex vivo* approach, it will be more difficult to precisely direct the gene therapy to specific cell types. To date, direct *in vivo* gene therapy approaches for lysosomal storage diseases affecting the CNS have been performed exclusively in small animal models (Table 16.1). In fact, most of the gene therapy experiments have been performed in the β-glucuronidase (GUSB) deficient mouse, an authentic model of the lysosomal storage disease MPS VII. Although MPS VII is extremely rare in humans, the MPS VII mouse is a powerful experimental model and has been used extensively for a number of reasons: (1) It is an established model caused by a spontaneous mutation and was first described prior to the generation of other mouse models by the use of 'knockout' technology (Birkenmeier *et al.* 1989; Sands and Birkenmeier 1993). (2) It is a small animal model on a uniform genetic background and relatively large numbers of animals can be generated. (3) It is a very well-characterized model that closely mimics the human disease and affects many organ systems (Sly *et al.* 1973; Vogler *et al.* 1990; Sands *et al.* 1995; Ohlemiller *et al.* 2000). (4) It has lysosomal storage throughout the brain, measurable cognitive deficits and has been used previously as a model for CNS-directed therapies (Chang *et al.* 1993; Levy *et al.* 1996; Wolfe and Sands 1996; O'Connor *et al.* 1998). (5) A very sensitive histochemical stain for GUSB activity is available that permits the

Table 16.1 Summary of *in vivo* central nervous system (CNS)-directed gene therapy studies performed in murine models of lysosomal storage disease

Disease	Vector	Approach	Results	Reference
MPS VII	HV	Ocular	(+) Enz	Wolfe *et al.* (1992*b*)
MPS VII	Ad	Intracranial	(+) Enz, ↓ Stor	Ohashi *et al.* (1997)
MPS VII	Ad	Intracranial	(+) Enz, ↓ Stor	Ghodsi *et al.* (1998)
MPS VII	Ad	Intracranial	(+) Enz, ↓ Stor	Stein *et al.* (1999)
MPS VII	Ad	Intraventricular + mannitol	(+) Enz, ↓ Stor	Ghodsi *et al.* (1999)
MPS VII	AAV	Intracranial	(+) Enz, ↓ Stor	Skorupa *et al.* (1999)
MPS VII	HIV	Intracranial	(+) Enz, ↓ Stor	Bosch *et al.* (2000*b*)
MPS VII	AAV	Newborn, intrathecal	(+) Enz, ↓ Stor	Elliger *et al.* (1999)
GS	AAV	Intracranial	(+) Enz, ↓ Stor	Leimig *et al.* (1999)
MPS VII	AAV	Intracranial	(+) Enz, ↓ Stor	Bosch *et al.* (2000*a*)
MPS VII	AAV	Intracranial	(+) Enz, ↓ Stor	Sferra *et al.* (2000)
MPS VII	HV	Intracranial	(+) Enz, ↓ Stor	Zhu *et al.* (2000)
MPS VII	AAV	Newborn, intracranial	(+) Enz, ↓ Stor, ↑ Funct	Frisella *et al.* (2001)
MPS VII	AAV	Intracranial	(+) Enz, ↓ Stor, ↑ Funct	Heth *et al.* (2001)

MLD	HIV	Intracranial	(+) Enz, ↓ Stor, ↑ Funct	Consiglio *et al.* (2001)
MPS IIIB	AAV	Intracranial	(+) Enz, ↓ Stor	Fu *et al.* (2001)
GLD	AAV	Intracranial	(+) Enz, Min/No Improvement	Fantz *et al.* (2001)
GLD	Ad	Intracranial	(+) Enz, Min/No Improvement	Shen *et al.* (2001)
MPS VII	AAV	Newborn, intraventricular	(+) Enz	Passini and Wolfe (2001)
MPS VII	FIV	Intracranial	(+) Enz, ↓ Stor, ↑ Funct	Brooks *et al.* (2002)
MPS VII	AAV	Intracranial	(+) Enz	Passini *et al.* (2002)
MPS VII	AAV	Intravitreal	(+) Enz, ↓ Stor	Hennig *et al.* (2003)

These studies were performed in adult animals unless otherwise noted. q Funct, improved electrophysiologic or cognitive function; p Stor, decreased storage material; (1) Enz, detectable enzyme activity; AAV, adeno-associated virus; Ad, adenovirus; FIV, feline immunodeficiency virus; GLD, globoid-cell leukodystrophy; GS, galactosialidosis; HIV, human immunodeficiency virus; HV, herpes virus; Min/No Improvement, extensive brain disease persists with only a marginal increase (5–10 days) in lifespan; MLD, metachromatic leukodystrophy; MPS IIIB, mucopolysaccharidosis type IIIB; MPS VII, mucopolysaccharidosis type VII.

detection of single enzyme-positive cells *in situ* (Birkenmeier *et al.* 1991; Wolfe and Sands 1996). These characteristics make the MPS VII mouse model a very powerful tool to develop and carefully evaluate various gene therapy approaches.

Since most lysosomal storage diseases are progressive in nature, it would be preferable to initiate therapy as early as possible, either at birth or *in utero*. However, since widespread newborn screening for these diseases does not currently exist, most affected children are not identified until after they present with clinical signs of disease (Chapter 3). Therefore, in most cases the goal of the therapy will be to stop the progression of, or perhaps even reverse, the disease process. The majority of gene therapy experiments performed in the MPS VII mouse model have been performed in adult animals with established disease. One of the first CNS-directed gene therapy experiments was performed with a recombinant herpesvirus vector encoding the GUSB cDNA. Herpes-based vectors are promising gene therapy tools for the brain since the virus has a natural tropism for the CNS (Breakefield and Geller 1988). Successful gene transfer to the brain of MPS VII mice was accomplished following ocular administration of the virus (Wolfe *et al.* 1992*b*). However, the number of transduced cells in the brain was very low and the level of GUSB expression from the vector was not sufficient to reduce lysosomal storage. A recent study showed that modifications to the Herpes vector greatly increased the transduction efficiency and level of GUSB expression (Zhu *et al.* 2000). However, in that study, the virus was delivered by direct intracranial injection rather than by ocular administration, thereby increasing the invasiveness of the approach. Although the data are promising, the herpesvirus genome is relatively large (150 kb) and poorly understood when compared to other viral gene transfer vectors. A more complete understanding of the biology of these recombinant vectors will be required to ensure their safety and efficacy.

Several studies describe a more direct and invasive approach using adenoviral vectors for CNS gene therapy in young adult MPS VII mice with established disease. Adenoviral gene transfer vectors efficiently transduce cells *in vivo* and can mediate very high levels of expression (Rosenfeld *et al.* 1992). Following a single intracranial injection of a GUSB-expressing adenovirus vector, relatively high levels of GUSB activity were measured in the injected hemisphere and GUSB activity was observed histochemically in a relatively large area of the brain around the injection site (Ohashi *et al.* 1997; Ghodsi *et al.* 1998; Stein *et al.* 1999). Although the enzyme activity was detected histochemically at quite a distance from the injection site, a relatively small number of cells were actually transduced as determined by *in situ* hybridization for GUSB mRNA (Ghodsi *et al.* 1998). Of particular significance is the fact that a single injection of virus in one hemisphere resulted in measurable GUSB activity in the contralateral hemisphere and was able to reduce lysosomal storage in both cerebral hemispheres. Following an intraventricular injection of an adenovirus vector, intense GUSB staining was localized primarily in the ependymal cells lining the ventricles (Ghodsi *et al.* 1999). Injection of the adenoviral vector alone resulted in a reduction of storage that was limited to the periventricular space. Interestingly, mannitol-induced systemic hyperosmolality caused the GUSB activity in the ventricle to penetrate into the brain parenchyma (Ghodsi *et al.* 1999). This mannitol-induced diffusion of GUSB resulted in a reduction of storage that extended well beyond the periventricular region.

The adenovirus-mediated gene therapy experiments represent proof-of-principle experiments showing that overexpression of GUSB in a few cells can have a more global effect on lysosomal storage. These data suggest that a direct intracranial gene transfer approach may be appropriate for the treatment of lysosomal storage diseases affecting the brain. However, adenovirus-based gene transfer vectors have a number of severe limitations. Although the level of expression from adenovirus vectors can be very high, it is usually transient in nature. For lysosomal storage diseases, in fact for most inherited metabolic disorders, the expression of the deficient protein product will have to be maintained for the life of the patient. It has been demonstrated previously that lysosomal storage reaccumulates in virtually every tissue including the brain of MPS VII mice once the therapy is discontinued (Vogler *et al.* 1996). It seems likely that storage material will also reaccumulate in other lysosomal storage diseases if expression from a gene transfer vector decreases. Another major limitation of recombinant adenoviral vectors is that they elicit a strong cellular and humoral immune reaction in injected animals. The severe immune response rapidly eliminates the transduced cells and precludes the possibility of readministering the gene therapy vector (Yang *et al.* 1994). Although the brain is an immune privileged site and the reactions against adenoviral vectors appear to be less severe when compared with systemic injections, the expression is still transient and immune reactions do occur. Therefore, at the current level of recombinant adenovirus development, it seems unlikely that these vectors will provide long-term therapeutic benefits. However, recent reports of lower toxicity and long-term expression from 'gutless' adenoviral vectors suggest that they may have promise as an efficacious gene therapy tool (Schiedner *et al.* 1998).

Immune reactions that are independent of the gene transfer vector may also impact on the efficacy of CNS-directed gene therapy. Chronic inflammation of the brain has been reported in certain lysosomal storage diseases (Wada *et al.* 2000). Pre-existing inflammation may interfere with the delivery of any viral gene transfer vector. Therefore, immune modulation may be required for effective CNS-directed gene therapy in some lysosomal storage diseases. However, this may be disease-specific and will probably have to be determined experimentally.

Until recently, virtually all of the commonly used gene therapy vectors were limited by the inability to transduce non-dividing cells (murine-based oncoretroviruses), the lack of persistent *in vivo* expression (oncoretroviruses and adenoviruses), or toxicity (herpes and adenoviruses). Several newly developed viral gene transfer vectors may overcome some of these limitations. Adeno-associated virus is a replication-defective human parvovirus that infects dividing and non-dividing cells and integrates site-specifically in human chromosome 19 (Muzyczka 1994). Adeno-associated virus was first used as a gene transfer vector in 1984 (Hermonat and Muzyczka 1984) but was not widely utilized due to the fact that only a relatively small (<5 kb) expression cassette could be packaged and the vectors were difficult to produce in large quantities. However, as the methods for AAV production improved (Grimm *et al.* 1998; Zolotukhin *et al.* 1999), more groups experimented with the vectors. It soon became apparent that AAV could transduce post-mitotic cells, including neurones, *in vivo*, and expression of the transgene persisted for extended periods of time (Mccown *et al.* 1996; Klein *et al.* 1998). In addition, recombinant AAV vectors do not appear to elicit as robust an immune response as that observed with adenoviral vectors (Chirmule *et al.* 1999). These attributes represent a major advance in the field of gene therapy. Unfortunately, the ability of wild-type AAV to integrate site-specifically appears to be lost in the recombinant forms (McLaughlin *et al.* 1988). However, if the positive *in vivo* results obtained in small and large animal models can be translated to humans, then AAV vectors may represent very effective gene therapy tools.

The first experiments using AAV in a model of lysosomal storage disease were performed in the MPS VII mouse and involved intramuscular and intravenous injections.

Intramuscular injections of AAV in newborn and adult, or intravenous injections in adult MPS VII mice resulted in relatively high levels of GUSB expression and reductions in lysosomal storage in some visceral organs (Watson *et al.* 1998; Daly *et al.* 1999*a*). Not surprisingly, there was no reduction of storage in the brain probably due to the inability of GUSB to cross the blood–brain barrier (Vogler *et al.* 1999). Nonetheless, it was encouraging that AAV could mediate relatively high-level expression and reduce lysosomal storage in a broad range of tissues in an animal model of lysosomal storage disease.

Several groups have since reported that a single intracranial injection of AAV in adult MPS VII mice resulted in persistent (≅20 weeks) high-level expression (Skorupa *et al.* 1999; Bosch *et al.* 2000*a*; Sferra *et al.* 2000). Similar to the adenovirus-mediated gene therapy experiments, a relatively small number of transduced cells resulted in a rather large area of detectable GUSB activity. Likewise, the area of lysosomal storage reduction exceeded the area of histochemically demonstrable GUSB activity. It is important to note that the animals treated in these studies were young adult MPS VII mice with established lysosomal storage in the brain. Therefore, these data indicate that the accumulation of storage material in the brains of MPS VII mice is reversible. This is encouraging and consistent with other studies showing that the accumulation of glycosaminoglycans in other tissues is reversible. It is also important to note that unlike adenovirus-mediated gene therapy, there was little or no evidence of acute toxicity associated with the administration of AAV. Although these data are both impressive and encouraging, it is unclear from these studies whether cognitive functions are improved by the treatment. However, a recent study showed that the electrophysiologic response (long-term potentiation) of the hippocampus in young adult MPS VII mice was normalized after an intracranial injection of an AAV5 vector (Heth *et al.* 2001). Although this does not directly address cognitive function, it suggests that improvements in CNS function may be possible after lysosomal storage is established and then reduced following therapy.

Recently, lentiviruses, which include human (HIV) and feline (FIV) immunodeficiency viruses, have been developed as gene therapy vectors (Naldini *et al.* 1996; Poeschla *et al.* 1998). Like AAV, these viruses are capable of infecting non-dividing cells, and recombinant forms have been shown to transduce neurones in the brain. In addition, the lentiviral vectors mediate long-term *in vivo* expression with little or no acute toxicity. Therefore, these vectors share several positive gene transfer characteristics with AAV vectors. The lentiviral vectors also have several advantages over AAV. First, lentiviral vectors can accommodate a larger insert size ranging from 7–9 kb. Second, peak expression from lentiviral vectors occurs within several days after administration, whereas it may take from 4–8 weeks to achieve maximum expression from an AAV vector. This delay in AAV expression is believed to be due, at least in part, to the relatively slow rate of second strand synthesis (Ferrari *et al.* 1996; Fisher *et al.* 1996).

Although the lentiviral vectors have characteristics that are desirable for a gene therapy vector, there are obvious concerns about their safety, especially the HIV-based vectors. As with other viral gene transfer vectors, many of the lentivirus genes have been removed from the recombinant vectors. In the case of the HIV vectors, most of the HIV genes have been deleted, and those functions essential for vector production are supplied in trans (Naldini *et al.* 1996). Therefore, several precise recombination events would be required to reconstitute a viral genome that resembles wild-type, and even then not all of the wild-type open reading frames would be present. Murine-based recombinant retroviral gene transfer vectors are often produced in stable packaging cell lines that supply the viral helper functions. It is possible that recombination events capable of generating a wild-type viral genome can occur over time in those stable lines (Markowitz *et al.* 1988). To minimize the possibility of producing wild-type HIV or FIV, most recombinant lentiviral vectors are produced in 293T cells using transient transfection of several independent plasmids encoding the helper functions (Naldini *et al.* 1996; Dull *et al.* 1998). Transient transfection minimizes the time that the various plasmids are in the same cell together and reduces the chance of recombination. In addition, there is little or no sequence homology shared between the different helper plasmids, further minimizing the possibility of homologous recombination. Because of these safeguards, the chance of generating a wild-type lentivirus is extremely remote. Therefore, the recombinant lentiviruses represent gene therapy vectors that are probably as safe as any currently available vector.

A recent study showed that a single intracranial injection of an HIV-based lentiviral vector in adult (10-week-old) MPS VII mice resulted in high-level GUSB activity that persisted for at least 16 weeks (Bosch *et al.* 2000*b*). Like previous studies with different gene transfer vectors, the area of lysosomal storage reduction exceeded the area of histochemically demonstrable GUSB activity. Similar results were observed in a separate study in the MPS VII mouse using an FIV-based vector (Brooks *et al.* 2002). The FIV study has particular significance since cognitive studies were performed on the same animals before and after the CNS-directed gene therapy. The MPS VII mice had measurable deficits in a repeated acquisition and performance chamber assay (RAPC) when compared to age-matched normal littermates prior to the initiation of the gene therapy studies. Following direct intracranial injection of the lentiviral vector, treated MPS VII mice performed significantly better than untreated MPS VII mice and were not significantly different from the normal controls in this behavioral test. These data suggest that some of the cognitive deficits may be reversible following localized delivery of a gene therapy vector. This is an important finding since it was unclear whether the cognitive deficits could be reversed once established. It is now critical to determine the time beyond which there is no cognitive improvement following this therapeutic approach.

As mentioned above, lysosomal storage diseases are progressive in nature and it would be preferable to initiate therapy during the newborn period or perhaps even *in utero*. Although widespread newborn screening for lysosomal storage diseases does not currently exist, prenatal or early postnatal diagnoses can be made if there is a history of disease in the family (Chapter 3). In that case, it may be possible to initiate therapy early in life before the onset of clinical signs. This situation has been extensively modelled in the MPS VII mouse (Sands *et al.* 1993, 1994, 1995, 1997). Intravenous administration of a recombinant AAV vector to newborn (1–2 days old) MPS VII mice resulted in widespread GUSB expression and a reduction of storage in many tissues including the brain (Daly *et al.* 1999*b*). It was confirmed that the enzyme activity in the brain was due, at least in part, to virus entering the brain and stably transducing cells that appeared to be neurones. Although this finding is encouraging, similar results may not be obtained in newborn children. It is known that the blood–brain barrier in newborn rodents is not completely formed (Lattera *et al.* 1992; Vogler *et al.* 1999). This could explain the presence of viral genome and enzyme activity in the brains of MPS VII mice treated at birth with AAV. It is believed that the blood–brain barrier is fully formed in newborn infants and this would probably prevent viral particles from entering the brain. Therefore, to more closely model the human situation, newborn MPS VII mice were injected intracranially with a similar AAV vector (Frisella *et al.* 2001). As with AAV injections in young adult mice, high levels of GUSB activity were localized near the injection sites (Fig. 16.1). The distribution and level of AAV genome correlated

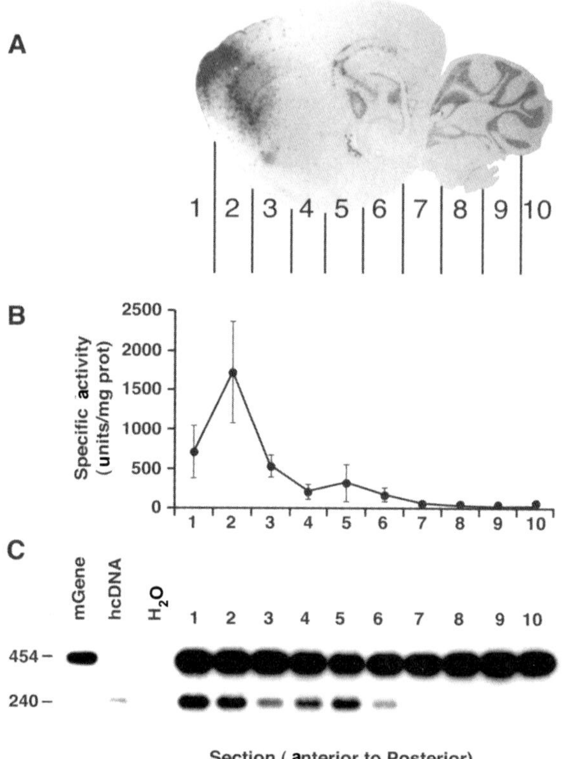

Fig. 16.1 β-Glucuronidase (GUSB) activity and the recombinant adeno-associated virus (AAV) genome are concentrated near the injection sites in mucopolysaccharidosis VII (MPS VII) mice that received intracranial injections of AAV at birth. Histochemical staining demonstrates a concentration of GUSB activity (red) near the injection sites in the anterior cortex and hippocampus (A). Quantitative biochemical assays performed on homogenates from 1 mm coronal sections show that increased GUSB-specific activities are observed in the cortex and hippocampus (B). The data represent the mean and one standard deviation from assays performed on sections from three AAV-injected mice. Relatively more polymerase chain reaction (PCR) product from the AAV-encoded human GUSB cDNA (240, hcDNA) is observed in sections from the anterior cortex and hippocampus when compared to other regions of the brain (C). The PCR product (454, mGene) from the murine GUSB gene served as an internal control. The numbers (1–10) in each panel correspond to the specific 1 mm section from the injected brains. **See Plate 10.**

with the high levels of GUSB activity. Lysosomal storage was greatly reduced or eliminated in neuronal and non-neuronal cells throughout the brain with the notable exception of the cerebellum (Fig. 16.2). Importantly, localized expression of GUSB and widespread reduction of lysosomal storage disease prevented the development of cognitive deficits in the MPS VII mice. AAV-treated MPS VII mice performed significantly better in most phases of the Morris water maze behavioral test when compared to untreated MPS VII mice, and there was no significant difference between the treated MPS VII and normal animals (Fig. 16.3).

Another study showed that an intrathecal injection of AAV in newborn MPS VII mice resulted in detectable GUSB activity in the brain and a reduction of lysosomal storage in

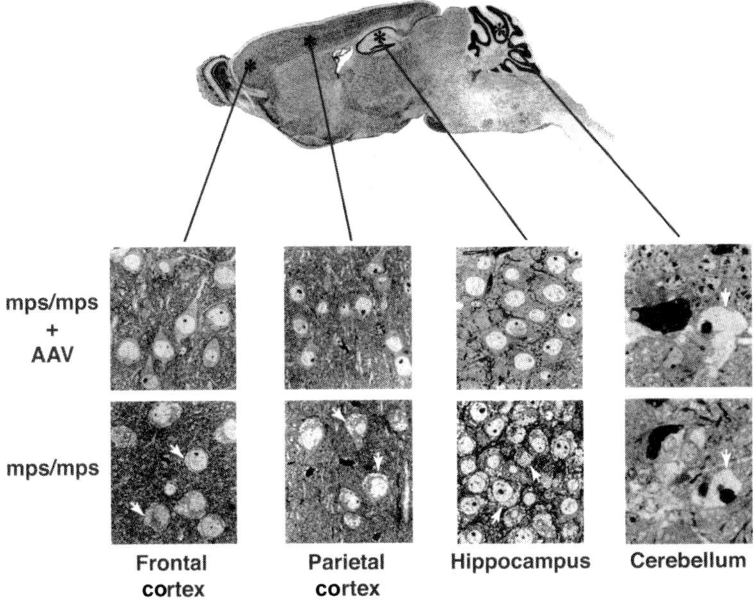

Fig. 16.2 Lysosomal storage is reduced in many regions of the brain at 8 weeks following adeno-associated virus (AAV)-mediated gene transfer performed in newborn mucopolysaccharidosis VII (MPS VII) mice. Distended lysosomes (white arrows) can be seen in the frontal cortex, parietal cortex, hippocampus, and cerebellum of untreated age-matched MPS VII (mps/mps) mice. Histopathologic evidence of lysosomal storage (distended lysosomes) is prevented in the frontal cortex, parietal cortex, and the hippocampus of AAV-treated MPS VII (mps/mps + AAV) mice. There were comparable amounts of lysosomal storage (white arrows) in cells of the cerebellum from both treated and untreated MPS VII mice.

some neurones (Elliger *et al.* 1999). This represents a less invasive approach; however, it is not clear how extensive the correction was throughout the brain or whether cognitive functions were spared. Intraventricular injections of an AAV vector into newborn MPS VII mice also resulted in a relatively widespread distribution of GUSB expression at levels that were probably therapeutic (Passini and Wolfe 2001).

Although considerable work has been performed in the MPS VII model, it remains to be demonstrated that similar approaches will be effective in other models of lysosomal storage disease. Recently, several groups have shown that CNS-directed *in vivo* gene therapy appears to be effective in other animal models of lysosomal storage disease. An elegant study demonstrating the efficacy of CNS-directed gene therapy was performed in the mouse model of metachromatic leukodystrophy (MLD, arylsulfatase A deficiency) (Consiglio *et al.* 2001). Five-month-old MLD mice received a single injection in each cerebral hemisphere of a lentiviral vector encoding arylsulfatase A. The lentiviral-treated mice had dramatically reduced storage, and more importantly, performed significantly better in several behavioral tests than MLD mice injected with a similar vector encoding a marker gene. In another study, injection of an AAV vector encoding lysosomal PPCA directly into the cerebellum of mice with galactosialidosis resulted in expression of the deficient protein and decreased Purkinje cell loss (Leimig *et al.* 1999). Similarly, when an AAV vector

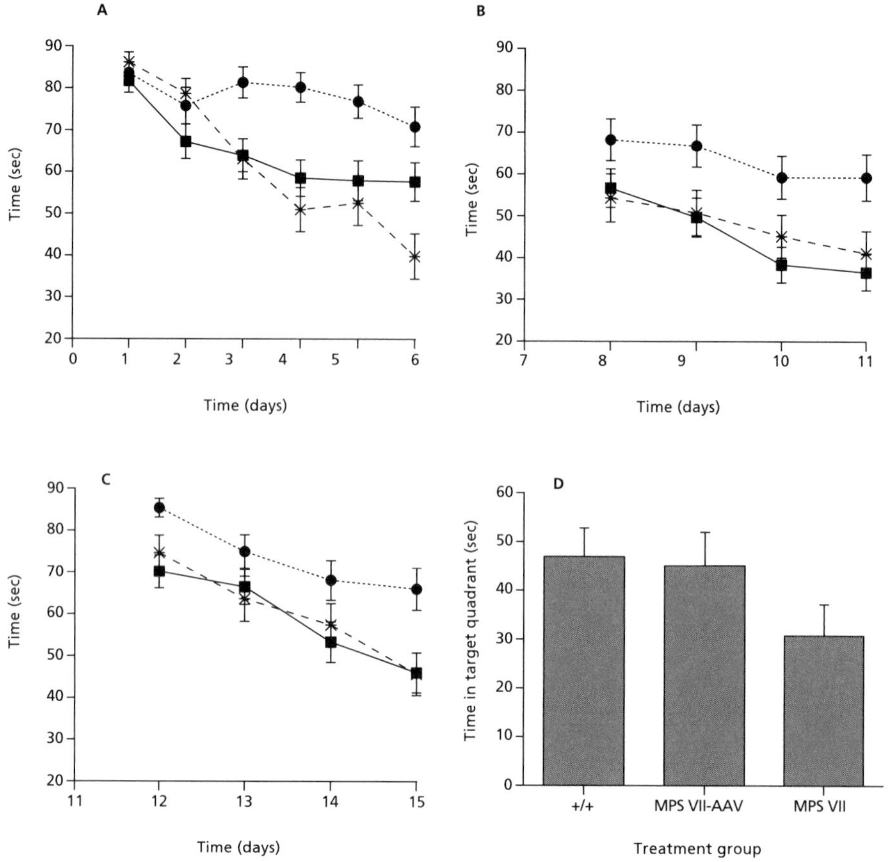

Fig. 16.3 Adeno-associated virus (AAV)-treated mucopolysaccharidosis VII (MPS VII) mice perform significantly better than untreated mutant animals in some phases of the Morris water maze test. AAV-treated MPS VII mice (asterisk) perform similarly to normal (filled square) and significantly ($P = 0.0151$) better than untreated mutants (filled circle) in the Acquisition (A), Relearning (B) and Relocation (C) phases of the test. The average performance of AAV-treated MPS VII mice was better than untreated MPS VII mice in the Probe (D) phase of the test. However, the difference was not statistically significant ($P < 0.16$).

encoding α-*N*-acetylglucosaminidase was injected into the brains of mice with MPS IIIB (Sanfilippo syndrome B), both persistent expression and a reduction of storage were observed (Fu *et al.* 2001).

The results from CNS-directed *in vivo* gene therapy are encouraging and suggest that if a viral gene transfer vector can be safely delivered to the brain of an affected patient then lysosomal storage may be reduced and improvements in cognitive functions might be possible.

Challenges and future directions

Although both *ex vivo* and *in vivo* gene therapy for the CNS component of lysosomal storage diseases are promising and will probably represent viable therapeutic modalities in the future, considerable research is required before these approaches can be translated into humans. One of the biggest challenges is the effective delivery and widespread distribution of the gene therapy vector or genetically engineered cells to the brain. Most of the gene therapy experiments have been performed in murine models of lysosomal storage disease where the volume of the brain is several thousand fold smaller than a human brain. It is unlikely that a single or a few injections will be sufficient to deliver the therapeutic agent throughout the entire human brain. This goal may require transient disruption of the blood-brain barrier to allow cells or viral vectors administered systemically to enter the brain. Alternatively, newly developed viral vectors with different tropisms may naturally distribute more extensively throughout the CNS. For example, many of the CNS-directed *in vivo* gene therapy experiments have been performed with AAV type 2, which does not diffuse far from the site of injection. It has recently been shown that AAV type 5 diffuses much more extensively throughout the brain when compared to AAV2 (Davidson *et al.* 2000). A related issue is the distribution of enzyme within the brain. Due to the blood-brain barrier and high cell density within the brain, lysosomal enzymes do not readily enter the CNS from the circulation or diffuse freely once inside. Therefore, it would be of great benefit to be able to modify the proteins such that they could enter the brain and more freely diffuse. A recent study showed that there was a 1.5-fold increase in the distribution of β-glucuronidase activity in the brains of MPS VII mice when the enzyme was fused to the TAT sequence derived from HIV (Xia *et al.* 2001). This small stretch of amino acids is referred to as a protein transduction domain and can mediate the transport of various proteins across the blood-brain barrier and increase the distribution of enzyme in a tissue (Scwarze *et al.* 1999). Alternatively, it may be possible to disseminate the gene product throughout the brain by axonal transport. A recent study showed that GUSB activity could be detected in the contralateral hippocampus of MPS VII mice following a single injection of AAV in the opposite hippocampus. The enzyme activity in the uninjected side was observed in the absence of any detectable expression and was likely transported axonally through the hippocampal commissure (Passini *et al.* 2002). The level of activity transported to the contralateral side was sufficient to reduce lysosomal storage in the hippocampus. It has also been demonstrated that both a marker gene (green fluorescent protein) (Dudas *et al.* 1999) and a lysosomal enzyme (β-glucuronidase) (Hennig *et al.* 2003) can be transported throughout the visual pathways of the brain following an intraocular injection of a gene transfer vector. As a result of this approach, the reduction of lysosomal storage in the CNS of the MPS VII mouse extended beyond the eye and visual pathways into the hippocampus and cortex (Hennig *et al.* 2003).

Once methods are developed to increase the distribution of both gene transfer vector and enzyme, then experiments must be performed in larger animal models to establish that widespread expression and reduction of lysosomal storage can be achieved in a brain that more closely resembles a human brain in size. Historically, it has been difficult to translate gene therapy approaches developed in rodent models to larger animals and humans. Therefore, successful gene therapy experiments performed in other animal models of lysosomal storage disease will raise the confidence level that a similar approach may be efficacious in humans.

Another aspect of gene transfer approaches that must be carefully scrutinized is the potential for long-term toxicity. Since the ideal gene therapy approach for an inherited metabolic disease would involve a permanent genetic change to a cell or organism, acute toxicology studies may not be sufficient to reveal any long-term adverse effects. This was recently illustrated when hepatic tumours were discovered in a large proportion of aged (1–1.5 years old) MPS VII mice treated with a recombinant AAV vector at birth (Daly *et al.* 2001;

Donsante *et al.* 2001). In contrast, there were no tumours discovered in a nearly identical experiment performed by the same group in the same strain of mouse but for a shorter period of time (4 months) (Daly *et al.* 1999*b*). Although it remains unclear what the underlying cause of the tumour formation was, this observation highlights the need for long-term toxicology studies. Furthermore, the immunologic consequences of vector administration as well as transgene expression must be carefully studied. It has been shown in experimental models of lysosomal storage disease that immunologic reactions to either the gene transfer vector or transgene product can severely limit the effectiveness of a gene therapy approach (Shull *et al.* 1996; Ohashi *et al.* 1997).

It is tempting to extrapolate the positive results observed in one form of lysosomal storage disease to other forms due to the similarities in the processing and trafficking of many of the lysosomal enzymes. However, two recent studies showed that the direct injection of either adenoviral or AAV vectors into the CNS of galactocerebrosidase-deficient mice (Twitcher mice) resulted in little or no efficacy (Fantz *et al.* 2001; Shen *et al.* 2001). This is in sharp contrast to the positive results obtained in several mouse models of other lysosomal storage diseases and highlights the need to perform similar experiments in authentic animal models of different diseases. Finally, widespread newborn screening may provide one of the biggest benefits for effective treatment of these progressive disorders since it would facilitate treatment initiation prior to the onset of clinical symptoms. It has been shown that it is more efficacious to initiate BMT or ERT early in life prior to the onset of severe clinical symptoms (Sands *et al.* 1993, 1997). Once these issues have been thoroughly researched and the appropriate technologies have been developed, gene therapy may hold enormous potential as an effective long-term treatment for these disorders.

Summary

Gene therapy may be an effective approach for the CNS disease associated with many lysosomal storage diseases. Lysosomal storage diseases represent good candidates for gene therapy since they are single gene defects, expression of lysosomal enzymes need not be precisely regulated, genetic modification of a relatively small percentage of cells can result in widespread correction, and in many cases the accumulated storage material can be reversed. One of the challenges of treating the CNS disease is that it has proven difficult to efficiently deliver a gene therapy vector to the brain through a systemic route. However, results obtained in small animal models of lysosomal storage disease suggest that direct administration of a gene therapy vector to the brain can reduce storage material and in some cases improve cognitive functions. Based on previous studies showing a positive correlation between the results obtained in animal models of lysosomal storage disease and children with these disorders following BMT or ERT, it seems likely that a gene therapy approach for the CNS disease will be successful. However, the studies performed in small animal models represent proof-of-principle experiments and should be viewed with caution. As mentioned above, there are many obstacles that remain to be overcome before these approaches can be successfully translated to affected humans. However, as our understanding of the disease processes, brain biology and gene transfer technology advances, many of these obstacles will be overcome and gene therapy will likely represent an effective therapeutic approach for the CNS disease associated with lysosomal storage disorders.

Acknowledgements

The author thanks Anne Hennig and Marie Roberts for critically reading the manuscript and providing helpful comments. This work was partially supported by a grant (DK 57586) from the National Institutes of Health

References

Birkenmeier, E. H., Davisson, M. T., Beamer, W. G. *et al.* (1989). Murine mucopolysaccharidosis VII – characterization of a mouse with β-glucuronidase deficiency. *J Clin Invest*, **83**, 1258–66.

Birkenmeier, E. H., Barker, J. E., Vogler, C. A. *et al.* (1991). Increased life span and correction of the metabolic defects in murine mucopolysaccharidosis type VII after syngeneic bone marrow transplantation. *Blood*, **78**, 3081–92.

Bosch, A., Perret, E., Desmaris, N. and Heard, J. M. (2000*a*). Long-term and significant correction of brain lesions in adult mucopolysaccharidosis type VII mice using recombinant AAV vectors. *Mol Ther*, **1**, 63–70.

Bosch, A., Perret, E., Desmaris, N., Trono, D. and Heard, J. M. (2000*b*). Reversal of pathology in the entire brain of mucopolysaccharidosis type VII mice after lentivirus-mediated gene transfer. *Hum Gene Ther*, **11**, 1139–50.

Breakefield, X. O. and Geller, A. I. (1988). A defective HSV-1 vector expresses *Eschericia coli* β-galactosidase in cultured peripheral neurons. *Science*, **241**, 1667–9.

Brooks, A. I., Stein, C. S., Hughes, S. M. *et al.* (2002). Functional correction of established central nervous system deficits in an animal model of lysosomal storage disease with feline immunodeficiency virus-based vectors. *Proc Natl Acad Sci*, **99**, 6216–21.

Carstea, E. D., Morris, J. A., Coleman, K. G. *et al.* (1997). Niemann–Pick C1 disease gene: homology to mediators of cholesteraol homeostasis. *Science*, **277**, 228–31.

Chang, P. L., Lambert, D. T. and Pisa, M. A. (1993). Behavioral abnormalities in a murine model of a human lysosomal storage disease. *Neuroreport*, **4**, 507–10.

Chirmule, N., Propert, K. J., Magosin, S. A., Qian, Y., Qian, R. and Wilson, J. M. (1999). Immune responses to adenovirus and adeno-associated virus in humans. *Gene Ther*, **6**, 1574–83.

Consiglio, A., Quattrini, A., Martino, S. *et al.* (2001). *In vivo* gene therapy of metachromatic leukodystrophy by lentiviral vectors: correction of neuropathology and protection against learning impairments in affected mice. *Nat Med*, **7**, 310–6.

Daly, T. M. and Sands, M. S. (1998). Gene therapy for lysosomal storage diseases. *Expert Opin Investig Drugs*, **7**, 1673–82.

Daly, T. M., Okuyama, T., Vogler, C., Haskins, M. E., Muzyczka, N. and Sands, M. S. (1999*a*). Neonatal intramuscular injection with recombinant adeno-associated virus results in prolonged α-glucuronidase expression *in situ* and correction of liver pathology in mucopolysaccharidosis type VII mice. *Hum Gene Ther*, **10**, 85–94.

Daly, T. M., Vogler, C., Levy, B., Haskins, M. E. and Sands, M. S. (1999*b*). Neonatal gene transfer leads to widespread correction of pathology in a murine model of lysosomal storage disease. *Proc Natl Acad Sci*, **96**, 2296–300.

Daly, T. M., Ohlemiller, K. K., Roberts, M. S., Vogler, C. A. and Sands, M. S. (2001). Prevention of clinical disease in MPS VII mice following AAV-mediated neonatal gene transfer. *Gene Ther* (in press).

Davidson, B. L., Stein, C. S., Heth, J. A. *et al.* (2000). Recombinant adeno-associated virus type 2, 4, and 5 vectors: transduction of variant cell types and regions in the mammalian central nervous system. *Proc Natl Acad of Sci*, **97**, 3428–32.

Donsante, A., Vogler, C. A., Muzyczka, N. *et al.* (2001). Observed incidence of tumorigenesis in long-term rodent studies of rAAV vectors. *Gene Ther* (in press).

Dudas, L., Anand, V., Acland, G. M. *et al.* (1999). Persistent transgene product in retina, optic nerve and brain after intraocular injection of rAAV. *Vision Res*, **39**, 2545–53.

Dull, T., Zuffery, R., Kelly, M. *et al.* (1998). A third generation lentivirus vector with a conditional packaging system. *J Virol*, **72**, 8463–71.

Elliger, S. S., Elliger, C. A., Aguilar, C. P., Raju, N. R. and Watson, G. L. (1999). Elimination of lysosomal storage in brains of MPS VII mice treated by intrathecal administration of an adeno-associated virus vector. *Gene Ther*, **6**, 1175–78.

Eng, C. M., Guffon, N., Wilcox, W. R. *et al.* (2001). Safety and efficacy of recombinant human α-galactosidase: A replacement therapy in Fabry's disease. *N Engl J Med*, **345**, 9–16.

Fantz, C., Wenger, D. and Sands, M. S. (2001). Neonatal and *in utero* gene transfer utilizing adeno-associated virus and lentiviral vectors for the treatment of Krabbe's disease. *Mol Ther*, **3**, S228 (Abstract).

Ferrari, F. K., Samulski, T., Shenk, T. and Samulski, R. J. (1996). Second-strand synthesis is a rate limiting step for efficient transduction by recombinant adeno-associated virus vectors. *J Virol*, **70**, 3227–34.

Fisher, K. J., Gao, G. P., Weitzman, M. D., DeMatteo, R., Burda, J. F. and Wilson, J. M. (1996). Transduction with recombinant adeno-associated virus for gene therapy is limited by leading-strand synthesis. *J Virol*, **70**, 520–32.

Friedmann, T. (1999). The origins, evolution and directions of human gene therapy. In *The development of human gene therapy* (Friedmann, T., ed.) pp. 1–20. New York: Cold Spring Harbor Laboratory Press.

Frisella, W. A., O'Connor, L. H., Vogler, C. A. *et al.* (2001). Intracranial injection of recombinant adeno-associated virus improves cognitive function in a murine model of mucopolysaccharidosis type VII. *Mol Ther*, **3**, 351–8.

Fu, H., Picornell, Y., Fletcher, D. and Muenzer, J. (2001). *In vivo* correction of lysosomal storage in the brain of a MPS IIIB mouse model by AAV-mediated gene therapy. *Mol Ther*, **3**, S227 (Abstract).

Ghodsi, A., Stein, C., Derksen, T., Yang, G., Anderson, R. D. and Davidson, B. L. (1998). Extensive α-glucuronidase activity in murine central nervous system after adenovirus-mediated gene transfer to brain. *Hum Gene Ther*, **9**, 2331–40.

Ghodsi, A., Stein, C., Derksen, T., Martins, I., Anderson, R. D. and Davidson, B. L. (1999). Systemic hyperosmolality improves α-glucuronidase distribution and pathology in murine MPS VII brain following intraventricular gene transfer. *Exp Neurol*, **160**, 109–16.

Grimm, D., Kern, A., Rittner, K. and Klienschmidt, J. A. (1998). Novel tools for purification of recombinant adenoassociated virus vectors. *Hum Gene Ther*, **9**, 2745–60.

Hahn, C. A., Martin, M. D. P., Zhou, X. Y., Mann, L. W. and D'Azzo, A. (1998). Correction of murine galactosialidosis by bone marrow-derived macrophages overexpressing human protective protein/cathepsin A under control of the colony-stimulating factor-1 receptor promoter. *Proc Natl Acad Sci*, **95**, 14880–5.

Hennig, A. K., Levy, B., Ogilvie, J. M. *et al.* (2003). Intravitreal gene therapy reduces lysosomal storage in specific areas of the CNS in Mucopolysaccharidosis VII mice. *J Neurosci*, **23**, 3302–7.

Hermonat, P. L. and Muzyczka, N. (1984). Use of adeno-associated virus as a mammalian DNA cloning vector: transduction of neomycin resistance into mammalian tissue culture cells. *Proc Natl Acad Sci*, **81**, 6466–70.

Heth, J. A., Martins, I. H., Chen, J. *et al.* (2001). AAV5-mediated gene transfer corrects hippocampal learning defects in murine MPS VII. *Mol Ther*, **3**, S318 (Abstract).

Hobbs, J. R., Barrett, A. J., Chambers, D. *et al.* (1981). Reversal of clinical features of Hurler's disease and biochemical improvement after treatment by bone marrow transplantation. *Lancet*, **2**, 709–16.

Hoogerbrugge, P. M., Suzuki, K., Suzuki, K. *et al.* (1988). Donor-derived cells in the central nervous system of twitcher mice after bone marrow transplantation. *Science*, **239**, 1035–8.

Kakkis, E. D., Muenzer, J., Tiller, G. E. *et al.* (2001). Enzyme replacement therapy in mucopolysaccharidosis I. *N Engl J Med*, **344**, 182–8.

Kennedy, D. W. and Abkowitz, J. L. (1997). Kinetics of central nervous system microglial and macrophage engraftment: analysis using a transgenic bone marrow transplantation model. *Blood*, **90**, 986–93.

Klein, R. L., Lewis, M. H., Muzyczka, N. and Meyer, E. M. (1998). Neuron-specific transduction in the rat septohippocampal or nigrostriatal pathway by recombinant adeno-associated virus vectors. *Exp Neurol*, **150**, 183–94.

Kornfeld, S. (1992). Structure and function of the mannose-6-phosphate/insulin like growth factor receptors. *Annu Rev Biochem*, **61**, 307–30.

Kornfeld, S. and Sly, W. S. (1995). I-Cell disease and pseudo-Hurler polydystrophy: disorders of lysosomal enzyme phosphorylation and localization. In *The metabolic basis of inherited disease* (Scriver, C. R., Beaudet, A. L., Sly, W. S. and Valle, D. ed.) pp. 2495–508. New York: McGraw-Hill.

Kosuga, M., Sasaki, K., Tanabe *et al.* (2000). Engraftment of genetically engineered amniotic epithelial cells corrects lysosomal storage in multiple areas of the brain in mucopolysaccharidosis type VII mice. *Mol Ther*, **3**, 139–48.

Lattera, J. J., Stewart, P. A. and Goldstein, G. W. (1992). Development of the blood brain barrier. In *Fetal and neonatal physiology* (Polin, A. and Fox, W. W., ed.) pp. 1525–31. Philadelphia: W.B. Saunders Co.

Leimig, T., Hargrove, P., Mann, L. *et al.* (1999). AAV vectors for the *in vivo* correction of brain pathology in galactosialidosis and GM1 gangliosidosis mice. *Am Soc Gene Ther Annu Meeting* (Abstract).

Levy, B., Galvin, N., Vogler, C., Birkenmeier, E. H. and Sly, W. S. (1996). Neuropathology of murine mucopolysaccharidosis type VII. *Acta Neuropathol*, **92**, 562–8.

Marechal, V., Naffakh, N., Danos, O. and Heard, J. M. (1993). Disappearance of lysosomal storage in spleen and liver of mucopolysaccharidosis VII mice after transplantation of genetically modified bone marrow stem cells. *Blood*, **82**, 1358.

Markowitz, D., Goff, S. and Bank, A. (1988). A safe packaging line for gene transfer: separating viral genes on two different plasmids. *J Virol*, **62**, 1120–4.

McCown, T. J., Xiao, X., Li, J., Breese, G. R. and Samulski, R. J. (1996). Differential and persistent expression patterns of CNS gene transfer by an adeno-associated virus (AAV) vector. *Brain Res*, **713**, 99–107.

McLaughlin, S. K., Collis, P., Hermonat, P. I. and Muzyczka, N. (1988). Adeno-associated virus general transduction vectors: analysis of proviral structures. *J Virol*, **62**, 1963–73.

Miranda, S. R. P., Erlich, S., Visser, J. W. M. *et al.* (1997). Bone marrow transplantation in acid sphingomyelinase-deficient mice: engraftment and cell migration as a function of radiation, age, and phenotype. *Blood*, **90**, 444–52.

Miranda, S. R. P., Erlich, S., Friedrich, V. L., Haskins, M. E., Gatt, S. and Schuchman, E. H. (1998). Biochemical, pathological, and clinical response to transplantation of normal bone marrow cells into acid sphingomyelinase-deficient mice. *Transplantation*, **65**, 884–92.

Miranda, S. R. P., Erlich, S., Friedrich, V. L., Gatt, S. and Schuchman, E. H. (2000). Hematopoietic stem cell gene therapy leads to marked visceral organ improvements and a delayed onset of neurological abnormalities in the acid sphingomyelinase deficient mouse model of Niemann–Pick disease. *Gene Ther*, **7**, 1768–76.

Moullier, P., Bohl, D., Heard, J. M. and Danos, O. (1993). Correction of lysosomal storage in the liver and spleen of MPS VII mice by implantation of genetically modified bone marrow stem cells. *Nat Genet*, **4**, 154–9.

Muzyczka, N. (1994). Adeno-associated virus (AAV) vectors: will they work. *J Clin Invest*, **94**, 1351.

Naldini, L., Blomer, U., Gallay, P. *et al.* (1996). *In vivo* gene delivery and stable transduction of nondividing cells by a lentiviral vector. *Science*, **272**, 263–7.

Neufeld, E. F. (1991). Lysosomal storage diseases. *Annu Rev Biochem*, **60**, 257–80.

Neufeld, E. F. and Fratantoni, J. C. (1970). Inborn errors of mucopolysaccharide metabolism. *Science*, **169**, 141–6.

Neufeld, E. F. and Muenzer, J. (1995). The mucopolysaccharidoses. In *The metabolic basis of inherited disease* (Scriver, C. R., Beaudet, A. L., Sly, W. S. and Valle, D. ed.) pp. 2465–94. New York: McGraw-Hill.

Norflus, F., Tiffts, C. J., McDonald, M. P., Goldstein, G., Crawley, J. N., Hoffmann, A., Sandhoff, K., Suzuki, K. and Proia, R. L. (1998). Bone marrow transplantation prolongs life span and ameliorates neurologic manifestations in Sandhoff mice. *J Clin Invest*, **101**, 1881–8.

O'Connor, L. H., Erway, L. C., Vogler, C. A. *et al.* (1998). Enzyme replacement therapy for murine mucopolysaccharidosis type VII leads to improvements in behavior and auditory function. *J Clin Invest*, **101**, 1394–400.

Ohashi, T., Watabe, K., Uehara, K., Sly, W. S., Vogler, C. and Eto, Y. (1997). Adenovirus-mediated gene transfer and expression of human α-glucuronidase in the liver, spleen and central nervous system in mucopolysaccharidosis type VII. *Proc Natl Acad Sci*, **94**, 1287–92.

Ohlemiller, K. K., Vogler, C. A., Roberts, M. *et al.* (2000). Retinal function is improved in a murine model of a lysosomal storage disease following bone marrow transplantation. *Exp Eye Res*, **71**, 469–81.

Palmer, T. D., Rosman, G. J., Osborne, W. R. A. and Miller, A. D. (1991). Genetically modified skin fibroblasts persist long after transplantation but gradually inactivate introduced genes. *Proc Natl Acad Sci*, **88**, 1330–4.

Passini, M. A. and Wolfe, J. H. (2001). Widespread gene delivery and structure-specific patterns of expression in the brain after intraventricular injections of neonatal mice with an adeno-associated virus vector. *J Virol*, **75**, 12382–92.

Passini, M. A., Lee, E. B. and Heuer, G. G. (2002). Distribution of a lysosomal enzyme in the adult brain by axonal transport and by cells of the rostral migratory stream. *J Neurosci*, **22**, 6437–46.

Poeschla, E. M., Wong-Staal, F. and Looney, D. (1998). Efficient transduction of nondividing human cells by feline immunodeficiency virus lentiviral vectors. *Nat Med*, **4**, 354–7.

Poorthuis, B. J. H. M., Romme, A. E., Willemsen, R. and Wagemaker, G. (1994). Bone marrow transplantation has a significant effect on enzyme levels and storage of glycosaminoglycans in tissues and in isolated hepatocytes of mucopolysaccharidosis type VII mice. *Pediatr Res*, **36**, 187–93.

Rosenfeld, M. A., Yoshimura, K., Trapnell, B. C. *et al.* (1992). *In vivo* gene transfer of the human cystic fibrosis transmembrane conductance regulator gene to the airway epithelium. *Cell*, **68**, 143–55.

Ross, C. J. D., Bastedo, L., Maier, S. A., Sands, M. S. and Chang, P. L. (2000*a*). Treatment of a lysosomal storage disease, mucopolysaccharidosis VII, with microencapsulated recombinant cells. *Hum Gene Ther*, **11**, 2117–27.

Ross, C. J. D., Ralph, M., Chang, P. L. (2000*b*). Somatic gene therapy for a neurodegenerative disease using micro encapsulated recombinant cells. *Exp Neurol*, **166**, 276–86.

Sands, M. S. and Birkenmeier, E. H. (1993). A single-base-pair deletion in the β-glucuronidase gene accounts for the phenotype of murine mucopolysaccharidosis type VII. *Proc Natl Acad Sci*, **90**, 6567–71.

Sands, M. S., Barker, J. E., Vogler, C. A. *et al.* (1993). Treatment of murine mucopolysaccharidosis type VII by syngeneic bone marrow transplantation in neonates. *Lab Invest*, **68**, 676–86.

Sands, M. S., Vogler, C. A., Kyle, J. W. *et al.* (1994). Enzyme replacement therapy for murine mucopolysaccharidosis type VII. *J Clin Invest*, **93**, 2324–31.

Sands, M. S., Erway, L. C., Vogler, C. A., Sly, W. S. and Birkenmeier, E. H. (1995). Syngeneic bone marrow transplantation reduces the hearing loss associated with murine mucopolysaccharidosis type VII. *Blood*, **86**, 2033–40.

Sands, M. S., Vogler, T., Torrey, A. *et al.* (1997). Murine mucopolysaccharidosis type VII. Long-term therapeutic effects of enzyme replacement and enzyme replacement followed by bone marrow transplantation. *J Clin Invest*, **99**, 1596–605.

Schiedner, G., Morral, N., Parks, R. J. *et al.* (1998). Genomic DNA transfer with a high-capacity adenovirus vector results in improved *in vivo* gene expression and decreased toxicity. *Nat Genet*, **18**, 180–3.

Scwarze, S. R., Ho, A., Vocero-Akbani, A. and Dowdy, S. F. (1999). In vivo protein transduction: delivery of a biologically active protein into the mouse. *Science*, **285**, 1569–72.

Sferra, T. J., Qu, G., McNeely, D. *et al.* (2000). Recombinant adeno-associated virus-mediated correction of lysosomal storage within the central nervous system of the adult mucopolysaccharidosis type VII mouse. *Hum Gene Ther*, **11**, 507–19.

Shen, J., Ohashi, T. and Eto, Y. (2001). Adenovirus-mediated gene therapy of neonatal twitcher mice. *Mol Ther*, **3**, S234 (Abstract).

Shull, R. M., Hastings, N. E., Selcer, R. R. *et al.* (1987). Bone marrow transplantation in canine mucopolysaccharidosis. I. Effects within the central nervous system. *J Clin Invest*, **79**, 435–43.

Shull, R. M., Kakkis, E. D., McEntee, M. F., Kania, S. A., Jonas, A. J. and Neufeld, E. F. (1994). Enzyme replacement in a canine model of Hurler syndrome. *Proc Natl Acad Sci*, **91**, 12937–41.

Shull, R. M., Lu, X., Dube, I. *et al.* (1996). Humoral immune response limits gene therapy in canine MPS I. *Blood*, **88**, 377–9.

Skorupa, A. F., Fisher, K. J., Wilson, J. M., Parente, M. K. and Wolfe, J. H. (1999). Sustained production of α-glucuronidase from localized sites after AAV vector gene transfer results in widespread distribution of enzyme and reversal of lysosomal storage lesions in a large volume of brain in mucopolysaccharidosis VII mice. *Exp Neurol*, **160**, 17–27.

Sly, W. S., Quinton, B. A., McAllister, W. H. and Rimoin, D. L. (1973). Beta glucuronidase deficiency: report of clinical, radiologic, and biochemical features of a new mucopolysaccharidosis. *J Pediatr*, **82**, 249–57.

Snyder, E. Y., Taylor, R. M. and Wolfe, J. H. (1995). Neuronal progenitor cell engraftment corrects lysosomal storage throughout the MPS VII mouse brain. *Nature*, **374**, 367–70.

Stein, C. S., Ghodsi, A., Derksen, T. and Davidson, B. L. (1999). Systemic and central nervous system correction of lysosomal storage in mucopolysaccharidosis type VII mice. *J Virol*, **73**, 3424–9.

Taylor, R. M. and Wolfe, J. H. (1997). Decreased lysosomal storage in the adult MPS VII mouse brain in the vicinity of grafts of retroviral-corrected fibroblasts secreting high levels of α-glucuronidase. *Nat Med*, **3**, 771–4.

Taylor, R. M., Stewart, G. J., Farrow, B. R. H. and Healy, P. J. (1986). Enzyme replacement in nervous tissue after allogeneic bone marrow transplantation for fucosidosis in dogs. *Lancet*, **2**, 772–4.

Taylor, R. M., Farrow, B. R. H. and Stewart, G. J. (1992). Amelioration of clinical disease following bone marrow transplantation in fucosidase-deficient dogs. *Am J Med Genet*, **42**, 628–32.

The International Batten Disease Consortium (1995). Isolation of a novel gene underlying Batten disease (CLN3). *Cell*, **82**, 949–57.

Vogler, C., Birkenmeier, E. H., Sly, W. S. *et al.* (1990). A murine model of mucopolysaccharidosis VII–gross and microscopic findings in β-glucuronidase-deficient mice. *Am J Pathol*, **136**, 207–17.

Vogler, C., Sands, M. S., Levy, B., Galvin, N., Birkenmeier, E. H. and Sly, W. S. (1996). Enzyme replacement with recombinant β-glucuronidase in murine mucopolysaccharidosis type VII – Impact of therapy during the first six weeks of life on subsequent lysosomal storage, growth, and survival. *Pediatric Res*, **39**, 1050–4.

Vogler, C., Levy, B., Galvin, N. J. *et al.* (1999). Enzyme replacement in murine mucopolysaccharidosis type VII: neuronal and glial response to α-glucuronidase requires early initiation of enzyme replacement therapy. *Pediatric Res*, **45**, 838–44.

Wada, R., Tiffts, C. J. and Proia, R. L. (2000). Microglial activation precedes acute neurodegeneration in Sandhoff disease and is suppressed by bone marrow transplantation. *Proc Natl Acad Sci*, **97**, 10954–9.

Walkley, S. U. and Dobrenis, K. (1995). Bone marrow transplantation for lysosomal storage diseases. *Lancet*, **345**, 1382–3.

Walkley, S. U., Thrall, M., Dobrenis, K., March, P. and Wurzelmann, S. (1994*a*). Bone marrow transplantation in neuronal storage diseases. *Brain Path*, **4**, 376.

Walkley, S. U., Thrall, M. A., Dobrenis, K. *et al.* (1994*b*). Bone marrow transplantation corrects the defect in neurons of the central nervous system in a lysosomal storage disease. *Proc Natl Acad Sci*, **91**, 2970–4.

Watson, G. L., Sayles, J. N., Chen, C. *et al.* (1998). Treatment of lysosomal storage disease in MPS VII mice using a recombinant adeno-associated virus. *Gene Ther*, **5**, 1642–9.

Wolfe, J. H. and Sands, M. S. (1996). Murine mucopolysaccharidosis type VII: a model system for somatic gene therapy of the central nervous system. In *Gene transfer into neurones, towards gene therapy of neurological disorders* (Lowenstein, P., and Enquist, L. ed.) pp. 263–74. Essex: J. Wiley and Sons.

Wolfe, J. H., Sands, M. S., Barker, J. E. *et al.* (1992*a*). Reversal of pathology in murine mucopolysaccharidosis type VII by somatic cell gene transfer. *Nature*, **360**, 749–51.

Wolfe, J. H., Deshmane, S. L. and Fraser, N. W. (1992*b*). Herpesvirus vector gene transfer and expression of β-glucuronidase in the central nervous system of MPS VII mice. *Nat Genet*, **1**, 379–84.

Wolfe, J. H., Sands, M. S., Harel, N. *et al.* (2000). Gene transfer of low levels of β-glucuronidase corrects hepatic lysosomal storage in a large animal model of mucopolysaccharidosis VII. *Mol Ther*, **2**, 552–61.

Xia, H., Mao, Q. and Davidson, B. L. (2001). The HIV Tat protein transduction domain improves the biodistribution of b-glucuronidase expressed from recombinant viral vectors *Nature Biotech*, **19**, 640–4.

Yang, Y., Ertl, H. C. J. and Wilson, J. M. (1994). MHC class I-restricted cytotoxic T lymphocytes to viral antigens destroy hepatocytes in mice infected with E1-deleted recombinant adenoviruses. *Immunity*, **1**, 433–42.

Yeager, A. M., Brennan, S., Tiffany, C., Moser, H. W. and Santos, G. W. (1984). Prolonged survival and remyelination after hematopoietic cell transplantation in the twitcher mouse. *Science*, **225**, 1052–4.

Zhou, X. Y., Morreau, H., Rottier, R. *et al.* (1995). Mouse model for the lysosomal storage disorder galactosialidosis and correction of the phenotype with overexpressing erythroid precursor cells. *Genes Dev*, **9**, 2623–34.

Zhu, J., Kang, W., Wolfe, J. A. *et al.* (2000). Significantly increased expression of β-glucuronidase in the central nervous system of mucopolysaccharidosis type VII mice from the latency-associated transcript promoter in a nonpathogenic herpes simplex virus type 1 vector. *Mol Ther*, **2**, 82–94.

Zolotukhin, S., Byrne, B. J., Mason, E. *et al.* (1999). Recombinant adeno-associated virus purification using novel methods improves infectious titer and yield. *Gene Ther*, **6**, 973–85.

Index